Damage Control Management
in the Polytrauma Patient

Hans-Christoph Pape · Andrew B. Peitzman
C. William Schwab · Peter V. Giannoudis
Editors

Damage Control Management in the Polytrauma Patient

Forewords by

Roy Sanders, MD
Donald D. Trunkey, MD

Springer

Editors

Hans-Christoph Pape, MD, FACS
Professor of Surgery
University of Pittsburgh
Department of Orthopedic Surgery
Pittsburgh, PA
USA

C. William Schwab, MD, FACS
Professor of Surgery
University of Pennsylvania
  School of Medicine
University of Pennsylvania Medical Center
Department of Surgery
Philadelphia, PA
USA

Andrew B. Peitzman, MD
Mark M. Ravitch Professor
Executive Vice-Chairman
Department of Surgery
University of Pittsburgh
Pittsburgh, PA
USA

Peter V. Giannoudis, BSc, MB, MD,
EEC(ortho)
Professor
University of Leeds
Leeds General Infirmary University Hospital
Trauma and Orthopedic Surgery
Leeds, Yorkshire
United Kingdom

ISBN 978-0-387-89507-9   e-ISBN 978-0-387-89508-6
DOI 10.1007/978-0-387-89508-6
Springer New York Dordrecht Heidelberg London

Library of Congress Control Number: 2009933462

Printed on acid-free paper

Springer is part of Springer Science+Business Media (www.springer.com)

To those who put themselves in harm's way in their mission to provide care for the injured, to all the physicians and nurses who place the saving of life as the ultimate reason to be, and to all the patients who have taught us how to save lives.

Hans-Christoph Pape, MD, FACS
Andrew B. Peitzman, MD
C. William Schwab, MD, FACS
Peter V. Giannoudis, BSc, MB, MD, EEC(ortho)

To my parents, Klaus and Marie Luise, who enabled and inspired me to pursue a career in medicine, and to my wife, Claudia, and my children, Julia and Eva, who supported me throughout.

Hans-Christoph Pape, MD, FACS

To my partners and housestaff, who teach us; to our families, who provide our strength.

Andrew B. Peitzman, MD

To my fellows, faculty, and partners, who have selflessly labored to care for the injured, expand knowledge, and share experience as we advanced the concepts of Damage Control.

C. William Schwab, MD, FACS

To my wife, Rania, and my children, Marilena and Vasilis. Their love, understanding, and ongoing support throughout my career have been vital sources of energy, creativity, and commitment to education.

Peter V. Giannoudis, BSc, MB, MD, EEC(ortho)

Foreword

Orthopedic trauma is largely limited to the stabilization and subsequent surgical management of fractures and dislocations, with most patients presenting to their local emergency departments with isolated injuries. Modern techniques and implants have made outcomes for these injuries more predictable. Intramedullary nailing, for example, has become standard treatment for a displaced fracture of the femoral shaft. These conditions can be managed by the majority of general orthopedists being trained today. Interestingly, they most likely do not even understand or remember that this treatment evolved from the management of the polytraumatized patient with fractures.

The polytraumatized patient is, of course, a completely different matter. For many years, the only experience with these types of injuries was in casualties sustained by combatants during armed conflicts. Basic concepts such as anesthesia, blood transfusions, intravenous therapy, wound management, and even the development of nursing and the modern hospital were all learned and founded in armed conflicts such as the Crimean War, the Boer War, and World War I. The Second World War saw improvements in the management of both abdominal and extremity wounds, and this was further refined in the Korean and Vietnam Conflicts. These, however, were limited to saving lives and limbs that benefited from very basic care. Understanding even the most rudimentary physiological concepts now taken for granted eluded us, and this showed how limited knowledge was at that time.

Beginning in the 1960s, various technological advances occurred that would radically change the methods of management. The introduction of arterial blood gas machines, the Swan-Ganz catheter, PEEP, and volume-cycled ventilators all became commonplace, decreasing the risk of cardiopulmonary failure. Recovery rooms and intensive care units were developed at this time as well, finally allowing for the monitoring of patients in the peri-operative period. Amazingly, before that, postoperative cardiopulmonary failure was undiagnosed and left untreated. After successful resuscitation of the patient from the initial cardiopulmonary insult, the prolonged septic state ended in a cachectic and malnourished patient. The development of hyperalimentation was critical in reversing this, only to lead to the multiple organ system failure syndrome, which was then addressed in the 1970s and 1980s.

While all this cardiothoracic and thoraco-abdominal care was proceeding, fracture management was lagging behind. The recognition of the systemic consequences of leaving a patient in traction became evident in the 1970s, with the understanding of the fat embolus syndrome. Furthermore, it was shown that the length of time in traction, and not the Injury Severity Score, was the only variable that correlated to multiple organ system failure and pulmonary failure in these patients. It also became clear at this time that cardiopulmonary failure and the septic states of the post-severe trauma patient were due to treatment modalities employed and not to the original injury. Similarly, compartment syndromes and their complications were better understood and managed, both in the extremities and abdominal cavity.

At the same time, high speed motor vehicular trauma began a spectacular rise in the West. Although fatalities from these accidents were initially high, when basic safety precautions came into being such as the seat belt, patients who formerly would expire at the scene now became severely traumatized civilian casualties. The attempt to save these lives brought methods formerly reserved for the military into everyday use, namely Emergency Medical Service ambulances and the development of civilian trauma units. In the United States, one of the first such units was the Baltimore Shock-Trauma Center. This center managed polytrauma patients with a minimum of three organ system injuries from a five-state region, using three helicopters with resuscitative capabilities onboard for rapid transport to the facility. This was, in essence, a civilian M.A.S.H. unit.

Today, benefits of these advances are apparent. Emergency medical systems coupled to regional trauma centers allow for the timely response to injuries in almost any location. Across the world, lessons learned in resuscitation, anesthesia, and critical care allow for the management of patients with varying degrees of general and extremity injury. Specialists in each of the many disciplines address the specific problems of the patient in an orderly, algorithmic manner, maximizing outcomes based on firm scientific knowledge learned over the last half century. Truly, this is a better place.

Damage Control Management in the Polytrauma Patient attempts to carefully collate and combine current knowledge in this field, which in today's parlance is known as "Damage Control." This implies the ability to actually manage these patients rather than to chase their problems, as was done in the past.

This monumental task has been performed by editors and contributors who have a deep understanding of the management of severely injured patients who have also sustained skeletal trauma. The scientific basis for treatment, starting with the epidemiology and pathophysiology of the trauma state, is clearly and expertly covered. Similarly, phases of management as well as treatment of individual organ systems are explained so that each member of the team will have better insight into the decision-making process of the other. Finally, a frank discussion of the complications and limitations associated with these patients is included so that the reader is aware of where scientific endeavors need to continue in order to solve present-day problems.

This book is a testament to past limitations, the present concepts of management, and where the future lies. The editors are to be commended for putting together a superb volume on the current state of the art. The surgeon and patient alike will be better off for having their traumatologist read this text.

Roy Sanders, MD
Chief, Department of Orthopedics
Tampa General Hospital
Director, Orthopedic Trauma Services
Florida Orthopedic Institute
Tampa, Florida
USA

Foreword

The ravages of limb compartment syndrome were first reported by Volkmann in 1881. This led to treatment by releasing compartment pressure using fasciotomy. General surgeons soon encountered the same phenomenon in the abdomen, primarily related to management of severe liver injuries. The anatomy of the liver was not well understood, and resectional debridement or formal lobectomy was simply not done. Treatment consisted of packs, drains, and the electrocautery unit. Attempts to close the abdomen in such patients were fraught with difficulty, and it was soon recognized that it was better to stage and delay abdominal closure, an approach now recognized as damage control.

Compartment syndromes are now recognized to occur in any closed space in which blood, fluid, or air causes expansion of the space and meets resistance of the container. Compartment syndrome can occur in the cranial vault and is usually associated with blood in the epidural and subdural space or intraparenchymal tissue. Each hemithorax is subject to compartment syndrome that is caused by blood, air, or chyle. Compartment syndromes in the abdomen, including the retroperitoneum and pelvis, are frequently common following severe injury. The complexity and the anatomy of the extremities are such that there are multiple compartments in both the upper and lower extremity. Even the hand is subject to compartment syndromes.

Although compartment syndromes existed prior to the mid-twentieth century, they were exacerbated by advances in surgical care and resuscitation. During the late 1950s, pressure-regulated ventilators were introduced, followed shortly by surgical intensive care units, and patients were managed on ventilators following their initial surgery. It was not uncommon to attempt to close all abdominal incisions following major injury, only to have the anesthesiologist tell the surgeon that the patient was difficult to ventilate. It soon was recognized that this was associated with an increase in peak inspiratory pressures, and patients often went on to have multiple pneumothoraces and deterioration of pulmonary function. This did not improve when volume-regulated ventilators became more popular than the older pressure-regulated ventilators.

Another advance occurred in 1964 when the work of Shires and others changed our fluid resuscitation of the trauma patient. During World War II and the Korean Conflict, acute renal failure occurred in 80% of all patients who presented in shock, and, of those, a high percentage died until the introduction of renal dialysis.

In 1964, Shires showed in an animal model that, during resuscitation following severe shock, the interstitial space was constricted and intracellular water increased, which could only be addressed by increasing the amount of crystalloid solution during the resuscitation period. As a consequence, acute renal failure almost disappeared as a major problem during the Vietnam Conflict, but a new syndrome was recognized: Da Nang lung. There is no question that some of these patients were over-resuscitated with crystalloid since the prevailing concept at that time was that one had to "fill the pump" to get maximum cardiac output.

Since the Vietnam Conflict, another physiologic phenomenon has been on the scene: the lethal triad of hypothermia, coagulopathy, and acidosis. A fourth component to this lethal triad is reperfusion injury, which also occurs during prolonged shock when resuscitation is initiated. The combination of these four factors aggravates the pathophysiology of compartment syndromes wherever they occur in the multiply-injured patient.

In *Damage Control Management in the Polytrauma Patient*, the editors have focused on approaching damage control surgery in a logical and comprehensive fashion. They have appropriately introduced the subject with epidemiology and pathophysiology. This is comprehensive and primarily focuses on extremity trauma and the patient with polytrauma. Importantly, the editors have divided damage control into phases, emphasizing that the problem begins in the prehospital setting and that prevention is far better than most treatment. The timing of surgery is addressed. The importance of early second operation when the physiology has been corrected is also emphasized. Reconstruction during what the editors term phase four and adjunctive maneuvers are also presented to the reader.

Special aspects of damage control are important and also addressed. The editors approach this topic from an anatomic standpoint, but they also look at the very young patient and the older patient. It would have been inappropriate not to have also discussed the military situation, which is done nicely here. Finally, the editors address complications and outcomes, emphasizing again that this book is comprehensive and will be a reference book for orthopedic and general surgery residents and practicing surgeons, as well as a book that will be referred to often in academic centers.

Donald D. Trunkey, MD
Department of Surgery
Oregon Health and Sciences University
Portland, Oregon
USA

Preface

The sustained improvements in the observed survival rates of polytrauma patients within the last two decades are attributable to multiple factors. While advances in rescue and intensive care management have been widely recognized in the past, the dramatic management changes performed regarding surgical management have occurred more quietly.

Nevertheless, all surgical subspecialties involved in the care of these patients have been commonly affected, thus requiring closer cooperation than ever. The common goal is to control life-threatening conditions first, such as severe hemorrhage, impaired oxygenation, and cerebral herniation. Fixation of major pelvic and extremity fractures then follows, thus preventing secondary hemorrhage and secondary soft tissue damage. The overall goal is to achieve all these tasks in a timely fashion, where all surgical specialties must respect the effects of prolonged shock, coagulopathy, hypothermia, and untreated soft tissue necrosis.

The limitations in the duration of initial operations and the reduction in complication rates have been so striking that they justify the compromises associated with this management change. For general surgeons, the downsides may imply inability to close the abdominal incision initially and to deal with the complications induced by large abdominal wall defects. For orthopedic surgeons, temporary external fixation requires re-operations, and local infections can occur along the Schanz screws. Considerations of these issues are included in this book.

In view of these aspects, the editors have purposefully tried to compile a cooperative approach among all major subspecialties involved in the care of polytrauma patients. The major goal of this book is to improve the overall understanding of every reader towards a common, integrated approach to polytrauma care. The editors hope that this book will help combine the vision required to perform life-saving operations with the vision required to treat limb-threatening conditions, resulting in the best possible clinical outcome for every individual patient. The editors are grateful to outstanding clinician scientists who have achieved this difficult task.

Hans-Christoph Pape, MD, FACS
Andrew B. Peitzman, MD
C. William Schwab, MD, FACS
Peter V. Giannoudis, BSc, MB, MD, EEC(ortho)

Contents

Contributors

Michel B. Aboutanos, MD, MPH, FACS
Associate Professor of Surgery, Virginia Commonwealth University Health System, Division of Trauma and Critical Care, Department of Surgery, Richmond, VA, USA

Roxana Alexandrescu, MD, MPH
University of Manchester/Hope Hospital, TARN, Salford, Manchester, United Kingdom

Omar Bouamra, PhD
University of Manchester, Department of Medicine, TARN at Hope Hospital, Salford, Manchester, United Kingdom

Benjamin Braslow, MD
Assistant Professor of Surgery, Department of Surgery, University of Pennsylvania School of Medicine, Philadelphia, PA, USA

Robert V. Cantu, MD
Assistant Professor of Orthopedic Surgery, Dartmouth Hitchcock Medical Center, Department of Orthopedics, Lebanon, NH, USA

Bryan A. Cotton, MD
Assistant Professor of Surgery, Vanderbilt University School of Medicine, Department of Surgery, Nashville, TN, USA

Clinton James Devin, MD
Fondren Orthopedics at Texas Orthopedic Hospital, Houston, TX, USA

Thérèse M. Duane, MD
Associate Professor of Surgery, Virginia Commonwealth University Health System, Department of Surgery, Richmond, VA, USA

Timothy C. Fabian, MD, FACS
Harwell Wilson Alumni Professor and Chairman, University of Tennessee Health Science Center, Department of Surgery, Memphis, TN, USA

Henri R. Ford, MD, FACS, FAAP
Post-Doctoral Research Fellow, Vice-President and Surgeon-in-Chief,
Childrens Hospital Los Angeles, Vice Dean for Medical Education, Keck School
of Medicine, University of Southern California, Department of Pediatric Surgery,
Los Angeles, CA, USA

Peter V. Giannoudis, BSc, MB, MD, EEC(ortho)
Professor, University of Leeds, Leeds General Infirmary University Hospital,
Trauma and Orthopedic Surgery, Leeds, Yorkshire, United Kingdom

Claudia E. Goettler, MD, FACS
Assistant Professor, Department of Surgery, Brody School of Medicine,
East Carolina University, Greenville, NC, USA

Yigit S. Guner, MD
Post-Doctoral Research Fellow, Childrens Hospital Los Angeles/University
of Southern California, University of California Davis Medical Center,
Resident in General Surgery, Department of Pediatric Surgery, Los Angeles,
CA, USA

Rao R. Ivatury , MD, FACS
Professor of Surgery, Chief, Trauma, Critical Care, and Emergency Surgery,
Virigina Commonwealth University Health System, Department of Surgery,
Richmond, VA, USA

Donald H. Jenkins, Col, USAF, MC, MD
Trauma Medical Director, Chairman of General Surgery, Assistant Professor
of Surgery, Wildord Hall USAF Medical Center, Uniformed Services University
(Bethesda, Maryland), Lackland Air Force Base, TX, USA

Kenneth J. Koval, MD
Professor, Dartmouth Hitchcock Medical Center, Department of Orthopedics,
Lebanon, NH, USA

Fiona E. Lecky, CS(Ed), PhD, FCEM
University of Manchester, Trauma Audit and Research Network,
Salford Royal Hospital, Alford, Manchester, United Kingdom

Joon Y. Lee, MD
Assistant Professor, University of Pittsburgh Medical Center, Department
of Orthopedics and Neurological Surgery, Pittsburgh, PA, USA

Luke P.H. Leenen, MD, PhD, FACS
Professor of Trauma, University Medical Center Utrecht, Department
of Surgery, Utrecht, The Netherlands

Philipp M. Lenzlinger, MD
University Hospital Zürich, Department of Surgery, Zürich, Switzerland

Gary Lombardo, MD
Assistant Professor of Surgery, New York Medical College, Westchester Medical
Center, Department of Trauma, Surgical Critical Care, and Emergency Surgery,
Valhalla, NY, USA

Ajai K. Malhotra, MBBS(MD), MS, DNB, FRCS, FACS
Associate Professor and Vice Chair, Division of Trauma, Critical Care,
and Emergency General Surgery, Associate Medical Director, Level I Trauma
Center, Virginia Commonwealth University Health System,
Department of Surgery, Richmond, VA, USA

Patrick C. Malloy, MD
Interventional Radiologist, Hartford Hospital, Department of Radiology,
Hartford, CT, USA

Andrew Marcantonio, DO
Orthopedic Trauma Fellow, University of Pittsburgh School of Medicine,
Department of Orthopedic Surgery, Pittsburgh, PA, USA

Julie A. Mayglothling, MD
Assistant Professor, Virginia Commonwealth University Health System,
Department of Surgery, Division of Trauma/Critical Care,
Department of Emergency Surgery, Richmond, VA, USA

Frans L. Moll, MD, PhD
Professor of Vascular Surgery, Utrecht University Hospital, Department
of Vascular Surgery, Utrecht, The Netherlands

John A. Morris Jr., MD
Professor of Surgery, Director, Division of Trauma and Surgical Critical Care,
Vanderbilt University, Division of Trauma and Surgical Critical Care,
Department of Surgery, Nashville, TN, USA

Rami Mosheiff, MD
Associate Professor, Director, Orthopedic Trauma Center, Hadassah Hebrew
University Medical Center, Department of Orthopedic Surgery, Jerusalem, Israel

Nathan T. Mowery, MD
Assistant Professor of Surgery/Trauma Services, Wake Forest University,
Department of Surgery, Winston-Salem, NC, USA

Alan D. Murdock, Lt Col, USAF, MC, MD
Consultant to the Surgeon General for Surgical Services, Wilford Hall USAF
Medical Center, Trauma/Surgical Critical Care, Lackland Air Force Base,
TX, USA

Dieter Nast-Kolb, MD
Professor, University Hospital Essen, Department of Trauma Surgery,
Essen, Germany

Sarah Jane O'Brien, MB, BS, DTM&H, MFPHM
Professor, University of Manchester, School of Translational Medicine,
Hope Hospital, Salford, Manchester, United Kingdom

Gbolahan O. Okubadejo, MD
Orthopedic Surgeon, University of Pittsburgh Medical Center,
Department of Orthopedic Surgery, Pittsburgh, PA, USA

Hans-Christoph Pape, MD, FACS
Professor, University of Pittsburgh, Department of Orthopedic Surgery,
Pittsburgh, PA, USA

Andrew B. Peitzman, MD
Mark M. Ravitch Professor, Executive Vice-Chairman, Department of Surgery,
University of Pittsburgh, Pittsburgh, PA, USA

Brad A. Prather, MD
University of Louisville, Department of Orthopedic Surgery,
Louisville, KY, USA

John P. Pryor, MD
Assistant Professor of Surgery, Trauma Program Director, Division
of Traumatology and Surgical Critical Care, University of Pennsylvania
Medical Center, Philadelphia, PA, USA

Jörn Redeker, MD
Professor, Hannover Medical School, Department of Plastic, Hand,
and Reconstructive Surgery, Hannover, Germany

Craig S. Roberts, MD
Professor, University of Louisville, Department of Orthopedic Surgery,
Louisville, KY, USA

Michael F. Rotondo, , MD, FACS
Professor and Chairman, Chief, Trauma and Surgical Critical Care,
Department of Surgery, Brody School of Medicine, East Carolina University,
Greenville, NC, USA

Steffen Ruchholtz, MD
Professor of Surgery, University of Marburg, Department of Trauma,
Hand, and Reconstructive Surgery, Marburg, Germany

Babak Sarani, MD
Assistant Professor of Surgery, University of Pennsylvania, Department
of Surgery, Division of Traumatology and Surgical Critical Care,
Philadelphia, PA, USA

Thomas M. Scalea, MD
Physician-in-Chief, R. Adams Cowley Shock-Trauma Center, Baltimore,
MD, USA

James M. Schuster, MD, PhD
Assistant Professor of Neurosurgery, Trauma Coordinator, University
of Pennsylvania, Department of Neurosurgery, Philadelphia, PA, USA

C. William Schwab, MD, FACS
Professor of Surgery, University of Pennsylvania School of Medicine, University
of Pennsylvania Medical Center, Department of Surgery, Philadelphia, PA, USA

Malek Tabbara, MD
Research Fellow in Surgery, Harvard Medical School, Massachusetts General
Hospital, Department of Surgery, Boston, MA, USA

Georg Taeger, MD, PhD
Assistant Director, Department of Trauma Surgery, University Hospital Essen,
Essen, Germany

Ivan S. Tarkin, MD
Assistant Professor, University of Pittsburgh School of Medicine,
Department of Orthopedic Surgery, Pittsburgh, PA, USA

Otmar Trentz, MD
Professor, University Hospital Zürich, Department of Surgery, Zürich, Switzerland

Christopher C. Tzioupis, MBBS, MD, EEC (ortho)
Trauma Fellow, University of Leeds School of Medicine, Leeds General Infirmary,
Trauma and Orthopedic Surgery, Leeds, Yorkshire, United Kingdom

Jeffrey S. Upperman, MD
Director, Trauma Program, Associate Professor of Surgery, Childrens Hospital
Los Angeles, Keck School of Medicine, University of Southern California,
Department of Pediatric Surgery, Los Angeles, CA, USA

Martijn van Griensven, MD, PhD
Professor, Ludwig Boltzmann Institute for Experimental and Clinical
Traumatology, Vienna, Austria

George C. Velmahos, MD, PhD, MSEd
Professor of Surgery, Harvard Medical School, Department of Surgery,
Boston, MA, USA

Peter M. Vogt, MD, PhD
Professor and Chief, Hannover Medical School, Department of Plastic,
Hand, and Reconstructive Surgery, Hannover, Germany

Christian Waydhas, MD
Professor, Department of Trauma Surgery, University Hospital Essen,
Essen, Germany

Yoram A. Weil, MD
Attending, Hadassah Hebrew University Hospital, Orthopedic Trauma Service,
Jerusalem, Israel

Maralyn Woodford, BSc
University of Manchester, Trauma Audit and Research Network,
Salford Royal Hospital, Alford, Manchester, United Kingdom

Boris A. Zelle, MD
Orthopedic Resident, University of Pittsburgh School of Medicine,
Department of Orthopedic Surgery, Pittsburgh, PA, USA

Part I
Epidemiology and Pathophysiology

Chapter 1
The Damage Control Approach

Claudia E. Goettler, Michael F. Rotondo, and Peter V. Giannoudis

1.1 Historical Management of Injury

"Trauma surgery is just general surgery, but faster and under blood." – Anonymous

As the majority of trauma resuscitation and operation was historically performed by general surgeons, the practice of trauma and surgical critical care developed slowly as a general surgical subspecialty by those with special interest in this patient population. Surgical procedures for injury care, therefore, have been based entirely on elective general surgical procedures. Hence, injury to the stomach would receive an operative approach similar to that of a perforated ulcer. This was gradually modified by war experiences. Patients from the war zone generally had massive destructive wounds, and there was also delay to definitive care. This resulted in the development of novel operative techniques for trauma, such as pyloric exclusion, which are gradually finding their way back into general surgery for severe diseases.

1.2 Failure of a General Surgical Approach in Trauma

"The operation was a success but the patient died anyway." – Anonymous

Since general surgeons have long been trained to identify and repair operatively any diagnosed injury or disease, prolonged operative procedures for definitive repair were the norm. Patients who bleed during elective operative procedures either have control maneuvers instituted prior to the vascular incision as in vascular surgery, or

C.E. Goettler(✉)
Department of Surgery, Brody School of Medicine, East Carolina University,
 600 Moye Blvd, Greenville, NC, 27858, USA
e-mail: cgoettle@pcmh.com

H.-C. Pape et al. (eds.), *Damage Control Management in the Polytrauma Patient*,
DOI 10.1007/978-0-387-89508-6_1, © Springer Science+Business Media, LLC 2010

rapid pressure or clamp control of inadvertent vascular injury during a case. Additionally, hemorrhage nearly always occurs only moments before control is achieved when the patient is already in an operating suite, draped and in many cases already open.

This is radically different from the physiologic pattern in trauma patients who are injured minutes to hours prior to arriving in the operating room, and hence have been bleeding for an extended period of time prior to instituting surgical control. Additionally, this bleeding results in difficulty in obtaining rapid surgical control by obscuring the operative field and tissue planes. Similarly, intestinal contamination, ongoing prior to operative control, results in an increased degree of contamination by virtue of both the length of contamination time and the high energy of intestinal content distribution.

Finally, elective general surgeons usually have time and information, such as imaging and history, to allow planning for operative procedures, even if only during the brief initial work-up. In contrast, surgeons faced with a trauma patient do not know what disease process they will find on opening, even when guided by a CT scan, resulting in further delay in control while determining injuries. Moreover, these patients are more likely to be unstable and/or unresponsive, resulting in less information and time for operative planning.

Taken in their entirety, these factors – delay in operative presentation, unknown pathology at the start of operation, difficult and delayed control of hemorrhage and contamination – result in a major difference between general surgical and trauma patients. This is the concept of physiologic exhaustion that is found commonly in traumatized patients and occasionally in emergency general surgical patients. While elective general surgical patients should be fully evaluated and optimized before surgery, and emergency general surgical patients should be briefly "tuned-up" prior to surgery with fluid boluses, blood, and/or antibiotics, many trauma patients cannot wait even minutes for operative intervention due to extreme instability. These patients do not have any physiologic reserve and arrive in the OR in extremis. They may not tolerate the time under anesthesia needed to complete a full operative exploration and repair. Hence, using traditional approaches, these patients died either on the table during the course of their operation, or shortly thereafter, due to ongoing non-mechanical bleeding, usually from coagulopathy, or from subsequent multi-system organ failure.

1.3   The Development of the Abbreviated Laparotomy

"He who fights and runs away, may live to fight another day." – JA Aulls, 1876

Gradually, changes in the operative approach towards this group of extremely ill trauma patients began to be discussed and published in the literature. Stone and colleagues were the first to describe aborting a laparotomy by use of an abdominal packing when intraoperative coagulopathy developed [1]. This report was published in 1983. Several subsequent reports of this technique, specifically for hepatic injury, and then a large series showing survival advantage by Burch and colleagues followed [2]. Unfortunately, adoption of this technique was slow and in some cases was deemed a failure to finish operating or an attempt to shift work to another time.

The next iteration of this technique by Rotondo and colleagues resulted in renaming this care pattern "Damage Control" [3]. It should be noted that despite the name, derived from the navy ship damage management, this was a civilian trauma development rather than military. The "Damage Control" sequence was defined. Since then, and with a new name, the technique has become increasingly accepted and has resulted in undoubted decreases in mortality.

1.4 Basic Tenants of Damage Control

1.4.1 Damage Control Part 0: Rapid Transport to Definitive Care

Defined relatively lately, a crucial part of salvage in the selected extremely unstable trauma patients is the rapid transportation to a center capable of providing definitive care. The most direct method of transportation with fewest delays in transitional facilities is necessary to maximize survival [4]. During this period, judicious resuscitation should be under way. This period also refers to the management in the trauma center, where large-bore intravenous access and rapid recognition and transit to the operative suite are mandatory.

1.4.2 Damage Control Part 1: Rapid Control of Hemorrhage and Contamination

Operative intervention is focused on full exposure and rapid hemorrhage control. For major hepatic injury, packing is optimal, though multiple other more time-consuming methods may be necessary. Major vascular injury that cannot be safely treated by ligation can be considered for vascular shunting. Intestinal contamination should be controlled by whipstitch, intestinal ligation, or stapling. No attempts at formal resection are undertaken, and the intestine is left discontinuous. Details of management of specific organs are found in further chapters. The abdomen is closed by one of many quick temporary methods. The entire operative intervention should take about 1 h and certainly no longer than 90 min.

1.4.3 Damage Control Part 2: Resuscitation

Once out of the operating room, attention is turned to full resuscitation in the intensive care unit. Coagulapathy, anemia, acidosis, electrolyte abnormalities, and hypothermia should be aggressively corrected. Normalization of physiology is an indication to return for definitive operative care and is usually accomplished in 24–36 h.

Patients who fail to improve or have subsequent worsening of parameters must be considered as having either ongoing bleeding or a missed injury. These patients are returned to the operating room as an emergency for another look, which should be thought of as a return to Damage Control Part 1, with limited goals of hemorrhage control, identification of injury, and prevention of ongoing contamination. In some patients, several cycles through Damage Control Parts 1 and 2 may be necessary.

1.4.4 Damage Control Part 3: Return for Completion of Operative Repairs

When fully resuscitated and physiologically normalized, patients will tolerate a second surgical insult and longer operative times. They are then returned to the operating room for unpacking, second look, and definitive management of injuries. During this operation, all injuries should be clearly identified and repaired, including recreation of intestinal continuity. The luxury of the second look as well as potential difficulties with abdominal wall closure has led to an increase in primary anastomosis for colonic injuries, with good results. Feeding access should be considered in all of these patients. About half of this selected population will be able to tolerate primary fascial closure during this operation. The remainder is managed with sequential closure methods, primary allograft closure, or granulation and skin grafting (Figs. 1.1 and 1.2).

1.4.5 Damage Control Part 4: Definitive Abdominal Closure

A section of patients managed with Damage Control are not able to be safely closed at the completion of Damage Control Part 3, either due to high intraabdominal pressures or contamination requiring repeated washouts. Some can be closed subsequently during their hospital course. About 50–60% of Damage Control patients are discharged with definitive abdominal closure.

The remaining patients are treated with a temporizing method, such as vicryl mesh and skin grafting, until they have completely recovered from their metabolic insult. Typically, these patients will be at home for 6–9 months, recovering mobility

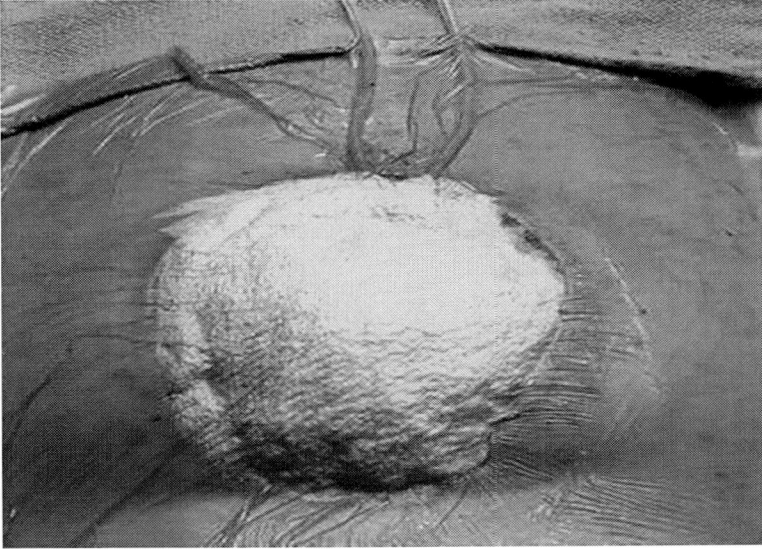

Fig. 1.1 As edema resolves, the defect becomes smaller and may be able to be closed primarily. The vacuum dressing is easily and inexpensively created with plastic sheeting against the bowels, gauze, drains, and an adhesive dressing

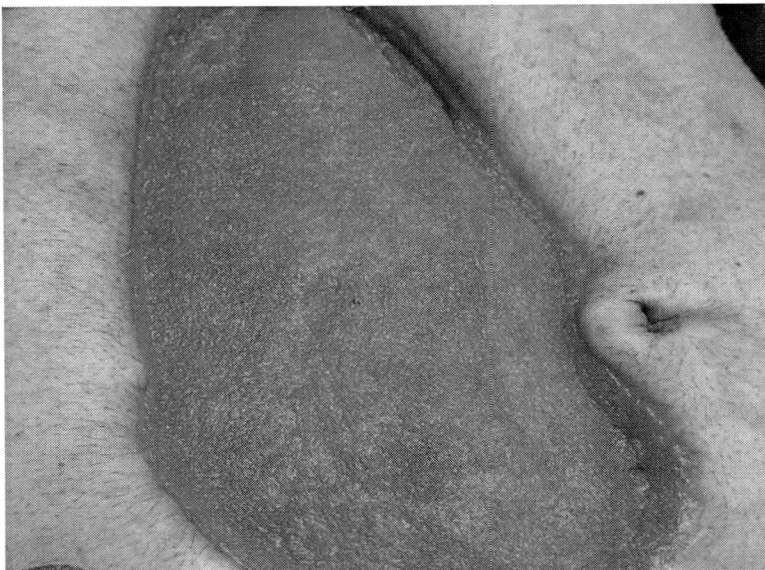

Fig. 1.2 Abdominal defects that cannot be closed primarily are allowed to granulate, usually via absorbable mesh, and then are skin-grafted

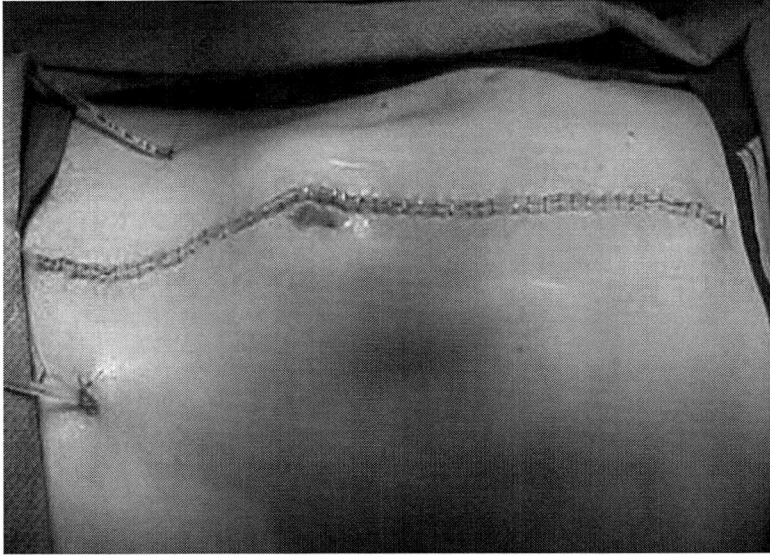

Fig. 1.3 Once the skin graft can be separated from the underlying intestines, the patient can undergo component separation and reconstruction of the abdominal wall

and optimal nutritional condition during which time the skin graft separates from the underlying intestines. At this time, an elective return to the operating room is undertaken for abdominal closure, with component separation and/or mesh or allograft, as well as stoma reversal if needed (Fig. 1.3). Long-term outcomes in these patients have been shown to be quite good.

1.5 Indications for Damage Control

1.5.1 Early Decision Making

In order for patients to benefit from a Damage Control sequence, the decision to abort operative intervention must be made early. It should be considered even prior to the arrival of the patient if there is hypotension in transport or in the trauma resuscitation area. While hypotension may well resolve with resuscitation, it is an early indicator that the patient is not prepared to tolerate a prolonged operation. Elevated lactate and/or base deficit are also early warning signs of physiologic derangement. While neither alone is an indicator for abbreviated laparotomy, they should induce the thought process. Absolute indicators will be discussed below; however, it cannot be stressed enough that a Damage Control operation should take only 60–90 min, and hence the decision to abort should be made early in the operation. Waiting to abort until the patient has reached physiologic exhaustion makes salvage extremely unlikely and results in almost certain death.

1.5.2 Triad of Death

There is extensive evidence that coagulopathy, acidosis, and hypothermia all interact to worsen each other in a vicious spiral that eventually results in ongoing hemorrhage and death. Early recognition of any of these findings is an indicator for abbreviated laparotomy. While many studies indicate varying absolute numbers, temperature less than 34 , pH less than 7.2 (or base excess greater than 8 in a patient with a corrected pH due to hyperventilation), and/or laboratory or clinical evidence of coagulopathy should result in abbreviation of the laparotomy and initiation of the Damage Control sequence [5]. Continued interaction with the anesthesia team is necessary to maintain awareness of these factors while operating.

1.5.3 Associated Injuries

Other injuries may contribute to the decision to interrupt laparotomy. Patients with multiple intraabdominal injuries should be considered for abbreviated laparotomy at each stage of repair, as the time necessary for complete repair becomes rapidly prohibitive. This is seen in patients with multiple widely spaced intestinal injuries or combined vascular and intestinal injuries. Other sources of blood loss also contribute, though they are of lesser immediate concern, such as extremity fractures and lacerations; but they cause concern as the loss of blood from these is often underestimated when hidden either by the skin or the drapes.

Multi-compartment injuries also call for Damage Control, such as management of hemorrhage of the abdomen and the chest. Clearly, full management of abdominal injuries and closure would compromise a patient who also requires thoracic exploration. Hence, rapid termination and temporization within one compartment followed rapid control and temporization within another compartment cuts the total operative time, blood loss, and heat and evaporative losses. This will rarely result in patients with Damage Control dressings on both abdominal and thoracic incisions or on combined abdominal and sternotomy incisions (Fig. 1.4).

Any other potentially life-threatening extra-abdominal injury that requires timely intervention is an indicator to stop operating after hemorrhage and contamination control and provide a temporary closure. This allows for more rapid evaluation of these associated injuries such as severe intracranial injury or aortic transection, as well as early and aggressive correction of coagulopathy, which could contribute to mortality in these injuries. This is also the most efficient way to get patients with liver or pelvic injuries to angiogram if indicated.

Lastly, the variability of the physiologic reserve should be assessed for the patient. Older patients and/or those with comorbidities are likely to be intolerant of long operative times and should have frequent reassessment of the need for abortion of the procedure.

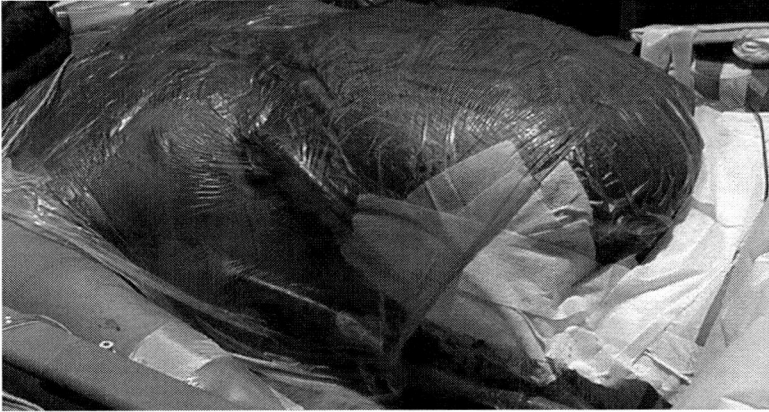

Fig. 1.4 Damage control of combined sternotomy and laparotomy. Note massive abdominal distention

1.5.4 Predicted or Present Abdominal Compartment Syndrome

One of the expansions of the Damage Control concept is the prediction of patients who are likely to develop abdominal compartment syndrome, and therefore selectively leaving these patients open with a temporary abdominal closure rather than closing fascia. This is done even in patients with definitive completion of their operation to prevent the cascade of physiologic injury occurring with abdominal compartment syndrome. Patients at risk are those who have received more than 10–15 units of blood products and/or more than 5 L of crystalloid [6]. Additionally, any patient with increasing peak ventilatory pressures of more than 10 points at fascial approximation is at extremely high risk.

1.5.5 Planned Reoperation

Finally, temporary abdominal closure can be done in any patient who requires further evaluation prior to completion of repair of injuries, such as planned second look or serial washouts or debridement.

1.6 Expansion of Damage Control Principles

With the success of the Damage Control sequence in visceral trauma and its general adoption by the trauma community, it is increasingly utilized in other traumatic injuries [7, 8]. Vascular, and now orthopedic injures, are treated by Damage Control techniques, which is the focus of this text. The utilization of this technique can be expected to improve the limb salvage, though data from large studies are not yet available. Additionally, the concept of damage control and the lethal triad has also spilled over into general surgery and is likely resulting in improved outcomes in this population as well.

1.7   Summary and Conclusion

The evolution of the abbreviated laparotomy or "Damage Control" for trauma has improved patient survival by decreasing the operative stress on patients in physiologic exhaustion. This technique requires rapid control of bleeding and contamination, temporary abdominal closure, and then intensive care resuscitation of physiology with return to the operating room for eventual definitive operative repair. This sequence should be utilized in patients with coagulopathy, acidosis, and hypothermia. While mortality in a subset of critically ill trauma patients has decreased with this modality, these patients have a very high incidence of morbidity and frequently require prolonged hospitalization and multiple operative procedures. The success of Damage Control in management of abdominal pathology has led to the expansion of the concept into orthopedic and vascular trauma, and into general surgical care.

References

1. Stone HH, Strom PR, Mullins RJ Management of the major coagulopathy with onset during laparotomy. Ann Surg 1983; 197: 532–535.
2. Burch JM, Ortiz VB, Richardson RJ, Martin RR, Mattox KL, Jordan GL Abbreviated laparotomy and planned reoperation for critically injured patients. Ann Surg 1992; 215: 476–484.
3. Rotondo MF, Schwab CW, McGonigal MD, Phillips, III, GR, Fruchterman TM, Kauder DR, Latenser BA, Angood PA "Damage control": An approach for improved survival in exsanguinating penetrating abdominal injury. J Trauma 1993; 3: 375–382.
4. Sagraves SG, Rotondo MF, Toschlog EA, Schenarts PJ, Bard MR, Goettler CE Brief interval transfer (BIT): The morbid consequence of delay to the trauma center in a rural patient demographic (abstract). J Trauma 2002; 53(6): 1209.
5. Morris JA, Eddy VA, Blirman TA, Rutheford EJ, Sharp EW The staged celiotomy for trauma: Issues in unpacking and reconstruction. Ann Surg 1993; 217: 576–586.
6. Cué JI, Cryer HG, Miller FB, Richardson JD, Polk HC Jr. Packing and planned reexploration for hepatic and retroperitoneal hemorrhage: Critical refinements of a useful technique. J Trauma 1990; 30: 1007–1013.
7. Reilly PM, Rotondo MF, Carpenter JP, Sherr SA, Schwab CW Temporary vascular continuity during damage control: Intraluminal shunting of proximal superior mesenteric artery injury. J Trauma 1995; 39(4): 757–760.
8. Porter JM, Ivatury RR, Nassoura ZE Extending the horizons of "damage control" in unstable trauma patients beyond the abdomen and gastrointestinal tract. J Trauma 1997; 42(3): 559–561.

Chapter 2
Epidemiology of Polytrauma

Fiona E. Lecky, Omar Bouamra, Maralyn Woodford, Roxana Alexandrescu, and Sarah Jane O'Brien

Epidemiology is the study of health and disease in populations, the scientific approach typifying public health medicine. The paradigms are somewhat different from the reductionist approach of much clinical science, which seeks to understand disease processes at an "omic" level. The rationale that underpins epidemiology suggests that effective disease control must begin and end by understanding the impact of a disease (and its prevention/management strategies) at a population level – globally, nationally, and locally – including the identification of vulnerable groups, etiological factors, and societal costs.

An epidemiological perspective on polytrauma – significant injuries affecting more than one body region – and its management must draw from the significant "injury control" literature. The latter often does not distinguish between polytrauma and major injury to a single body system. However, it sets an important context for more detailed descriptions of polytrauma found in trauma registries. This chapter will therefore first describe the global injury burden prior to a polytrauma focus.

2.1 Global Burden of Injury

Trauma fulfills the disease classification criteria for a global pandemic, this being a recurrent and significant cause of morbidity and mortality over time and across continents despite efforts to control its impact. Worldwide, about 16,000 people die every day as a result of an injury (5.8 million deaths per year), and the projections for 2020 show that 8.4 million deaths per year are expected [1, 2]. Consequently, injury will be the second most common cause of disability adjusted years of life lost

F.E. Lecky (✉)
Trauma Audit and Research Network, Salford Royal Hospital, University of Manchester, Alford, Manchester, M6 8HD, UK
e-mail: fiona.lecky@manchester.ac.uk

H.-C. Pape et al. (eds.), *Damage Control Management in the Polytrauma Patient*,
DOI 10.1007/978-0-387-89508-6_2, © Springer Science+Business Media, LLC 2010

within the next 13 years (second only to HIV/AIDS). Undoubtedly, the major burden of injury is increasingly occurring in the developing world as it industrializes, adopts motorized transportation, and remains the major center for armed conflict [2]. Despite a lower population incidence, injury remains the most common cause of death and disability in children and young adults in the developed world [2].

Incidence and trends vary across the developed world. National statistics are quoted as showing crude annual rates of approximately 1,095/100,000 injury deaths and hospitalizations in England and Wales [3, 4]. These data are obtained from national statistics that use International Classification of Disease codes, a taxonomy with limited descriptions of injury severity. The abbreviated injury scale (AIS) dictionary has a greater level of detail (over 2,000 injury codes) and allocates to every injury a severity score between 1 (mild) and 6 (maximal) [5]. These can be summated into the injury severity score (ISS) [6] as a global reflection of the anatomical severity of injury suffered by each individual patient. Severe injury is defined as ISS >15. Within Europe, most hospital admissions with injury have much lower ISS values (range 4–9), due to single isolated limb fractures in children or the elderly (falls), and isolated mild head injury (blunt assault) in young adults.

This latter AIS/ISS taxonomy has been utilized to describe injury incidence in continental Europe and the US; consequently, rates appear considerably lower than in England and Wales. Across continental Europe, the annual rates of death and severe injury (ISS >15) varies from 25 per 100,000 in Germany to 52.2 [7] in one region of Italy [8]. In Canada, the annual rate of death and severe injury (with ISS >12) is estimated at 71.5 per 100,000 [9]; a lower ISS is utilized here, but, in fact, the occurrence of ISS scores 13–15 is low, so this probably reflects a truly higher incidence of injury morbidity in Canada compared to continental Western Europe.

The incidence in most of continental Europe has declined in recent years (Figs. 2.1 and 2.2). There is limited literature available on the economics of injury, but they are an important source of direct medical costs as well as indirect costs resulting from economic production losses; in the Netherlands, for example, the direct costs of injury represents 5% of the health care budget, whereas in Spain, the total costs associated with traffic injuries alone account for 1.35% of the gross national product [10, 11]. In both countries, injury has been shown to be a more expensive disease than cancer or cardiovascular disease once societal costs are accounted for.

2.2 Etiology and Vulnerable Groups

Etiology and vulnerable groups are inextricably linked and reflect the nature of the disease. Injury results from a transfer of energy – most commonly kinetic, but, within armed conflict, thermal, chemical, blast, and radiation become important – to the patient. The nature/severity of the injuries sustained depends on the type and magnitude of impacting energy and vulnerability of the host.

Clearly, risk-taking behavior involving transportation ± alcohol, more prevalent in younger males, conveys a higher likelihood of injury. Indeed, statistics

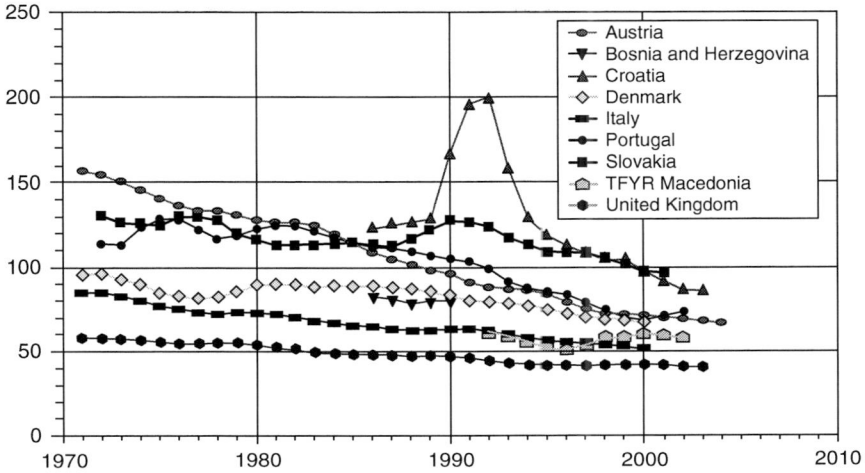

Fig. 2.1 SDR (standardized death rates), external cause injury and poison, all ages per 100,000 male. (Reprinted with permission by WHO from Appendix V. Health of All Database, June 2006, WHO. http://www.euro.who.int/eprise/main/WHO/InformationSources/Data/2005117 3;http://www.euro.who.int/eprise/main/WHO/InformationSources/Data/2005117%203.)

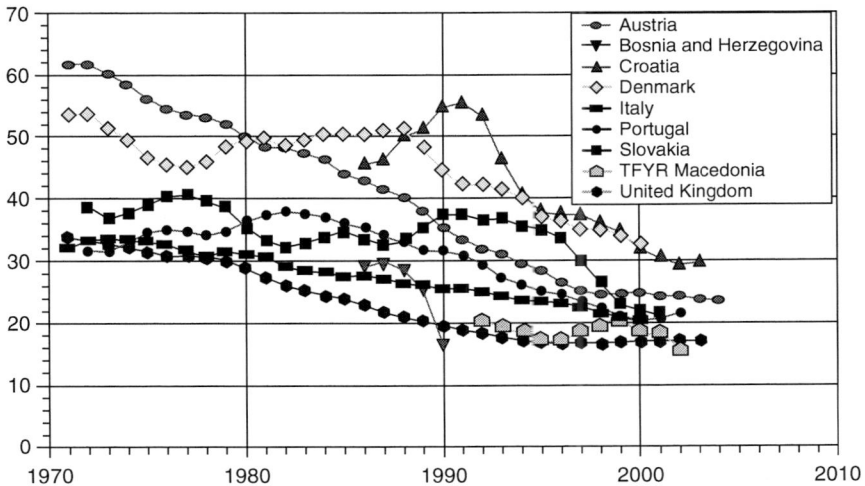

Fig. 2.2 SDR (standardized death rates), external cause injury and poison, all ages per 100,000 female. (Reprinted with permission by WHO from Appendix V. Health of All Database, June 2006, WHO. http://www.euro.who.int/eprise/main/WHO/InformationSources/Data/2005117 3;http://www.euro.who.int/eprise/main/WHO/InformationSources/Data/2005117%203.)

show that males predominate in injury hospitalizations up until the age of 65 [3, 4]. Among senior citizens, this type of risk-taking behavior is less common but falls secondary to medical diseases, sensory impairment, and musculoskeletal conditions, which occur increasingly with age. Osteoporosis in older women makes them more vulnerable to injury from falls at home – usually hip and upper limb fractures – but true polytrauma is relatively rare amongst this group.

As polytrauma usually results from high energy impact to more than one body system, it is not surprising that Road Traffic Crashes predominate as the causal mechanism for deaths and severe injuries in Europe [8]. In areas where interpersonal violence/firearms are more commonly used, intentional injury is sometimes the primary etiological factor in death and hospitalization for severe injury [12]. However, the latter may not truly reflect polytrauma, as single high velocity gunshot wounds (GSW) to vital organs carry a high morbidity. There is a well-described social class gradient, particularly among younger patients who are more vulnerable to intentional and non-intentional injury [13].

2.3   Data Sources for the Study of Polytrauma

A large European trauma registry has been employed to enable description of demography, mechanism/patterns of injury, and mortality from polytrauma. The advantage of using hospital-based trauma registries is that accurate injury descriptions are made using AIS codes, making it possible to identify true polytrauma – significant injury to more than one body region. AIS grades the severity of each single injury from 1 (mild) to 6 (maximal) on an ordinal scale: A serious injury to any body region is usually regarded as an AIS >2 [5, 6]. Therefore, polytrauma can be regarded as an AIS >2 in more than one of the following six body regions (ISS >17). It is often impossible to identify patients in this way from the ICD-based injury description in routine statistics.

Polytrauma can be defined as significant injury in at least two out of the following six body regions:

Head, neck, and cervical spine
Face
Chest and thoracic spine
Abdomen and lumbar spine
Limbs and bony pelvis
External (skin)

It is important to note that the limbs and bony pelvis constitute one body region; therefore multiple limb fractures, or a limb and pelvic fracture, will not constitute polytrauma without injuries to either head/abdomen/thorax.

The disadvantage of utilizing hospital trauma registries for descriptive epidemiology is that they are not easily linked to defined populations and often do not include pre-hospital deaths. Not an insignificant consideration, in urban environments more than 50% of deaths from injury occur in the pre-hospital environment [14]; in rural areas, this figure may be as high as 75% [15].

This potentially limits the epidemiological usefulness of trauma registries for primary and secondary prevention initiatives; however, many effective programs are already well proven:

primary = reducing the likelihood of an injury event occurrence: speed restrictions, gun control, drink driving legislation,

secondary = reducing the likelihood of injury in the event of an occurrence: helmets for motorcyclists, seatbelts for car occupants)

However, due to the interplay of human behavior and powerful vectors, injury remains a major health problem even where prevention programs have had an impact. It probably is reasonable to assume that a significant proportion of poly-trauma victims (reaching hospital alive) in a region covered by a trauma registry will be detailed therein in terms of injuries and clinical care. Therefore, for the purposes of injury control, large and well-established trauma registries can inform post-event injury care or tertiary prevention that reduces the effects of injury in patients who reach hospital alive.

Data on victims of polytrauma has been taken from the Trauma Audit and Research Network (TARN [16]). TARN records data from patients of all ages who sustain injury resulting in immediate admission to hospital for 3 days or longer and/or subsequent death/critical care or inter-hospital transfer. This is in line with the original "Major Trauma Outcome Study (MTOS)" trauma registry criteria [17]. Approximately 50% of the trauma-receiving hospitals in England and Wales and some European hospitals submit data to TARN. Glasgow Coma Scale, blood pressure, and respiratory rate are recorded when the patient enters the Emergency Department. Every injury is recorded and defined according to the AIS [5]. This is used by trained coders to enable calculation of the ISS [6]. Each hospital transfers leads to the generation of a separate record that is attached to the records from the initial presentation. The patient's age (but no patient identi-fier) is also recorded, and outcome in terms of survival or death is based on assessment at discharge or 30 days, whichever is first. Patients over 65 years with isolated fracture of the femoral neck or pubic ramus and those with single uncom-plicated or single closed limb injuries (excepting femoral fractures) are prospec-tively excluded.

Table 2.1 describes all cases in the TARN database by age group from 1989 to 2007. It can be seen that, for all age groups, most cases are not polytrauma as for there to be significant trauma to more than one body region the ISS should be >17; the median ISS for all age groups is 9 or 10 in the trauma reg-istry sample. The mortality rates increase significantly after age 65 when RTC causes a much lower proportion of injuries. Within this age group, there is also a reversal of male preponderance and an association of higher mortality with male gender, which is probably due to comorbidity and has been described elsewhere [18].

Table 2.1 Trauma audit and research network (TARN) data: all injured patients submitted from 1989 to 2007, by age group

Age groups		0–15 $N=22,281$	16–65 $N=108,881$	$65N=31,203$
Age (years)	Male	8.70	34.30	75.80
Median	Female	8.00	43.40	80.00
ISS (median)	Male	9	10	10
	Female	9	9	9
% male		67.4	74.3	36.4
% injured by RTC		45.7	45.1	23.7
Mortality	Male	4.2	6.5	20.7
%	Female	4.9	5.5	12.6

Data from Appendix V. Health of All Database, June 2006, WHO

Table 2.2 Trauma audit and research network (TARN): polytrauma cases by age group, 1989–2007

		0–15	16–65	>65	Total
Overall total		2811	20121	3582	26514
Proportion of all trauma cases %		12.6	18.5	11.5	16.3
Age (years)	Median age	11.0	32.5	76.0	33.3
ISS	median ISS	26	25	25	25
Cause of injuries	RTC	2305	14507	2359	19171
	%	82.0	72.1	65.9	72.3
Gender	Male	1820	15807	1771	19398
	%	64.7	78.6	49.4	73.2
Mortality at 30 days	Male	18.1	17.1	42.7	19.5
	Female	19.0	17.9	35.6	22.6

Data from Appendix V. Health of All Database, June 2006, WHO

2.4 Polytrauma Demography and Causes, Incidence within Trauma Registry, and Outcome

It can be seen from Table 2.2 that approximately 16% of trauma registry cases have polytrauma, that is, significant injuries in more than one body region (given that the limbs and pelvis constitute one body region). The proportion is lowest in the elderly. The median ages for polytrauma do not differ significantly from that from other trauma registry cases: children with polytrauma tending to be slightly older, 11 vs. 8.4 years, whereas the proportion of cases caused by road traffic collisions almost doubles across all age groups to 65–82%. Penetrating trauma is responsible for 2.4% (629) of all polytrauma cases over this timeframe. The degree of male preponderance does not change among the younger age groups. Among the elderly, there is almost a 50:50 gender split in terms of polytrauma cases, which differs from the female preponderance in all elderly trauma registry cases. ISS scores increase by a factor of 2.5, and mortality increases three- to fourfold in the younger age groups to approximately 20% in the young, and doubles to 39% in the over 65 years age group. However, 75% of deaths occur in children and adults of working age

2.4.1 Patterns of Injury as Markers for Polytrauma

Of the 26,541 polytrauma cases detailed here, 71.3% (18,904/26,514) have at least one limb± or pelvic fracture that is open, displaced, or comminuted. However, most limb/pelvic fractures on the registry have ((49,200/68,014)=72.3%) occurred in isolation. Half of all polytrauma cases have either a head and/or a thoracic injury, but, in contrast to thoracic injury, significant head injury occurs in isolation in two-thirds of head injury patients. Significant thoracic trauma is more likely to occur in the context of polytrauma (13,625/25,355=53.7% of patients with any thoracic injury) as is significant abdominal trauma (4,249/6,874=61.8% of patients with any abdominal injury). Significant abdominal trauma, however, is present in only 16.0% of polytrauma cases (4,249/26,514). Injuries to the face and external (skin) body regions are rare in the context of polytrauma.

2.4.2 Polytrauma Mortality: Impact of Age and Body Area

In terms of mortality, polytrauma with abdominal injury has the highest rate across all age groups (36.9%, 33.3%, 64.1%). In children, polytrauma with thoracic trauma confers the next highest risk of mortality (30.3%), whereas, in adults, it is polytrauma with head injury (29.3%, 56.2%). For isolated injuries and polytrauma, mortality does not appear significantly different between children and adults of working age, but there is a sharp rise in mortality for all patterns of injury after 65 years; interestingly, the relative increase in mortality with age is greater for cases of isolated injury where rates always more than double the mortality in younger age groups, perhaps suggesting that it is the younger, fitter elderly patients who fall victim to polytrauma. The relative impact of age in terms of mortality is greatest for limb/pelvic trauma, indicating the vulnerability of older patients to the complications of immobility.

In terms of overall mortality, it is first interesting to note that the impact of polytrauma is greater than the sum of its parts for children and young adults. For example, if the rates of mortality for isolated injuries of limb/pelvis, head, thorax, and abdomen are summed for children from Table 2.3, this comes to 14.3%, which is less than the polytrauma mortality rates for children with head/chest or abdominal injuries. Finally, although polytrauma accounted for only 16% of cases in this trauma registry sample, it accounted for almost half the deaths (5,393/12,611=43%), the remainder occurring mainly in the context of isolated significant head injury and

Table 2.3 Patterns of injury and mortality in polytrauma and isolated injury, by age group, 1989–2007

		0–15 years mortality %, No. of deaths	16–65 years mortality %, No. of deaths	>65 years mortality %, No. of deaths	Overall mortality %, No. of deaths
Limb/pelvis (n)Isolated	49,200	0.1%10	0.9%263	6.8%750	2.1%N=1023
Limb/pelvis (n)with polytrauma	18,904	12.2%236	13.1%1878	33.2%885	15.9%N=2999[a]
Head (n)isolated	25,776	6.9%371	12.9%2099	35.4 %1477	15.3%N=3947
Head (n)with polytrauma	12,340	25.5%477	29.3%2579	56.2%941	32.4%N=3997[a]
Thorax (n)isolated	11,730	5.2%24	4.9%442	16%356	7.0%N=822
Thorax (n)with polytrauma	13,625	30.3%358	25.3%2704	54.9%973	29.6%N=4035[a]
Abdomen (n)isolated	2,625	2.1%10	5.1%104	22%24	5.3%N=138
Abdomen (n)with polytrauma	4,249	36.9%152	33.3%1152	64.1%239	36.3%N=1543[a]

[a]Not mutually exclusive
Data from Appendix V. Health of All Database, June 2006, WHO

limb fractures in the elderly. This analysis has not dealt in detail with the disability consequences of polytrauma; inevitably, they are considerable, but large studies are rare due to the challenges of follow-up [19].

2.5 Summary and Conclusion

Injury is a global pandemic, and the second most costly disease worldwide, with the burden set to increase. Within civilian European MTOS-type trauma registries, true polytrauma using AIS criteria occurs in only 10% of cases, but causes up to half of all deaths in patients reaching hospital alive, mainly in male children and adults <65 years. Road traffic collisions are the predominant cause. The extremities and the pelvis are the most frequently injured body areas; however, thoracic trauma and abdominal trauma are specific markers for polytrauma and carry the greatest mortality risk in the young. Overall, most polytrauma deaths occur in the context of head and thoracic trauma. Polytrauma is rare in those over 65 years, and has double the mortality of younger adults. Within the younger age groups, the mortality associated with polytrauma is greater than the sum of its parts, suggesting a role for targeted improvements in care.

Acknowledgment The following hospitals have contributed data and funding to TARN allowing this work to take place: Addenbrooke's Hospital, Cambridge; Heatherwood & Wexham Park

Hospital, Slough; Rotherham District General Hospital, Rotherham; The Princess Royal Hospital, Shropshire; Airedale General Hospital, Yorkshire; Hillingdon Hospital, Middlesex; Royal Albert Edward Infirmary, Wigan; Torbay Hospital, Devon; Arrowe Park Hospital, Merseyside; Hinchingbrooke Hospital, Cambridgeshire; Royal Berkshire Hospital, Reading; Trafford General Hospital, Manchester; Ashford General Hospital, London; Homerton Hospital, London; Royal Bolton Hospital, Farnworth; University Hospital Lewisham, London; Atkinson Morley's Hospital, London; Hope Hospital, Salford; Royal Cornwall Hospital, Truro; University Hospital of Hartlepool, Hartlepool; Barnsley District General Hospital, Yorkshire; Huddersfield Royal Infirmary; Royal Devon & Exeter Hospital; University Hospital of North Staffordshire; Basildon Hospital, Essex; Hull Royal Infirmary, North Humberside; Royal Gwent Hospital, Newport; University Hospital of North Tees; Cleveland Bassetlaw Hospital, Nottinghamshire; Ipswich Hospital, Suffolk; Royal Hallamshire Hospital, Sheffield; University Hospital of Wales; Cardiff Bedford Hospital; James Cook University Hospital, Cleveland; Royal Hampshire County Hospital, Winchester; University Hospital, Aintree Liverpool; Birmingham Heartlands Hospital; James Paget Hospital, Norfolk; Royal Lancaster Infirmary; Walton Centre for Neurology, Liverpool; Blackburn Royal Infirmary, Lancashire; Jersey General Hospital; Royal Liverpool Childrens Hospital, Alder Hey; Wansbeck General Hospital, Northumberland; Blackpool Victoria Hospital; John Coupland Hospital; Royal Liverpool University Hospital; Warrington Hospital Cheshire; Booth Hall Children's Hospital, Manchester; John Radcliffe Hospital, Oxon; Royal London Hospital; Warwick Hospital, Warwick; Bradford Royal Infirmary, Yorkshire; Kent & Canterbury Hospital; Royal Manchester Children's Hospital, Pendlebury; Waterford Regional Hospital, Ireland; Bristol Royal Infirmary; Kent & Sussex Hospital; Royal Oldham Hospital; Watford General Hospital, Herts; Bromley Hospital, Kent; Kettering General Hospital, Northamptonshire; Royal Preston Hospital; West Cumberland Hospital Cumbria; Broomfield Hospital, Essex; Kings College Hospital; London Royal Shrewsbury Hospital, Shropshire; West Middlesex University Hospital; Burnley General Hospital; Kings Mill Hospital, Nottinghamshire; Royal Surrey County Hospital; West Wales General Hospital, Dyfed; Calderdale Royal Hospital, Halifax; Leeds General Infirmary; Royal Sussex County Hospital, Brighton; Weston General Hospital, Avon; Cheltenham General Hospital; Leicester Royal Infirmary; Royal United Hospital Bath Weymouth & District Hospital Dorset; Chesterfield & Nth Derbyshire Royal Hospital; Leigh Infirmary; Royal Victoria Hospital, Belfast N Ireland; Whipps Cross Hospital, London; Chorley District General Hospital; Leighton Hospital, Cheshire; Royal Victoria Infirmary, Newcastle Upon Tyne; Whiston Hospital, Liverpool; City Hospital, Birmingham; Lincoln County Hospital; Sandwell District General Hospital, West Midlands; William Harvey Hospital, Kent; Colchester General Hospital, Essex; Maidstone General Hospital, Kent; Scarborough Hospital North, Yorkshire; Withington Hospital, Manchester; Conquest Hospital East, Sussex; Manchester Royal Infirmary; Scunthorpe General Hospital, South Humberside; Withybush General Hospital, Dyfed; Countess of Chester Hospital; Medway Hospital, Kent; Selly Oak Hospital, Birmingham; Worcester Royal Infirmary; County Hospital, Hereford; Milton Keynes Hospital Sheffield Children's Hospital; Worthing Hospital, West Sussex; Coventry & Warwickshire Hospital; Morriston Hospital, Swansea; Skegness & District Hospital, Lincolnshire; Wrexham Maelor Hospital, Clwyd; Craigavon Area Hospital Co. Armagh; Nevill Hall Hospital, Wales; South Tyneside District Hospital Tyne & Wear Wycombe Hospital, High Bucks; Crawley Hospital, West Sussex; Newcastle General Hospital; Southampton General Hospital; Wythenshawe Hospital Manchester; Cumberland Infirmary, Cumbria; Norfolk & Norwich General Hospital; Southend Hospital, Essex; York District Hospital; Daisy Hill Hospital, County Down, Northern Ireland; North Manchester General Hospital; Southmead Hospital Bristol Ysbyty Gwynedd District General; Darrent Valley Hospital, Kent; North Tyneside General Hospital Tyne & Wear Southport & Formby District General Hospital; Derbyshire Royal Infirmary; Northampton General Hospital; St Bartholomews Hospital, London; Derriford Hospital, Plymouth; Northern General Hospital, Sheffield; St George's Hospital, London; Dewsbury District Hospital, Yorkshire; Northwick Park Hospital, Middlesex; St Helier Hospital, Surrey; Diana, Princess of Wales Children's Hospital, Birmingham; Nottingham University Hospital St James' University Hospital, Leeds; Diana, Princess of Wales Hospital, South Humberside; Ormskirk & District Hospital St Mary's Hospital,

London; Doncaster Royal Infirmary; Peterborough District Hospital; St Peters Hospital, Surrey; Ealing Hospital, Middlesex; Pilgrim Hospital, Lincs; St Thomas' Hospital, London; East Surrey Hospital, Redhill; Surrey Pinderfields General Hospital, Wakefield; Stepping Hill Hospital, Stockport; Eastbourne District General Hospital, East Sussex; Pontefract General Infirmary; Stoke Mandeville Hospital, Buckinghamshire; Epsom Hospital, Surrey; Queen Elizabeth Hospital; Kings Lynn; Sunderland Royal Hospital, Fairfield; General Hospital, Bury; Queen Elizabeth, Queen Mother Hospital, Kent; Tameside General Hospital Ashton Under Lyne Hammersmith Hospital, London; Regional Spinal Injuries Unit, Southport Merseyside; Taunton & Somerset Hospital; Harrogate District Hospital, Yorkshire; Rochdale Infirmary, Lancashire; The Horton Hospital, Oxfordshire.

References

1. Krug EG, Sharma GK, Lozano R. The Global Burden of Injuries. *Am J Public Health* 2000; 90: 523–526.
2. Murray CL, Lopez AD. Alternative projections of mortality and disability by cause 1990–2020. *Lancet* 1997; 349: 1498–1504.
3. Cryer PC, Davidson L, Styles CP, Langley JD. Descriptive epidemiology of injury in the South East: identifying priorities for action. *Publ Health* 1996; 110: 331–338.
4. Lyons RA, Jones SJ, Deacon T, Heaven M. Socioeconomic variation in injury in children and older people: a population based study. *Inj Prev* 2003; 9: 33–37.
5. Committee on injury scaling, Association for the Advancement of Automotive Medicine. *The Abbreviated Injury Scale. 1990 Revision. Update 98.* Des Plaines, Illinois: 1990.
6. Baker SP, O'Neill B, Haddon W, Long WB. The injury severity score: a method for describing patients with multiple injuries and evaluating emergency care. *J Trauma* 1974; 14: 187–196.
7. Liener UC, Rapp U, Lampl L, Helm M, Richter G, Gaus M, Wildner M , Kinzl L, Gebbhard F. Incidence of severe injuries. Results of a population – based analysis. *Unfallchirurg* 2004; 107: 483–490.
8. Di Bartolomeo S, Sanson G, Michelutto V, Nardi G, Burba I, Francescutti C, Lattuada L, Scian F. The regional study-group on major injury. Epidemiology of major injury in the population of Friuli Venezia Giulia – Italy. *Injury, Int J Care Injured* 2004; 35: 391–400.
9. Karmali S, Laupland K, Harrop AR, Findlay C, Kirkpatrick AW, Winston B, Kortbeek J, Crowshoe L, Hameed M. Epidemiology of severe trauma among status aboriginal Canadians: a population-based study. *CMAJ* 2005; 172: 1007–1011.
10. Van Beeck EF, Van Roijen L, Mackenbach JP. Medical costs and economic production losses due to injuries in the Netherlands. *J Trauma* 1997; 42: 1116–1123.
11. Bastida JL, Aguilar PS, González BD. The economic costs of traffic accidents in Spain. *J Trauma* 2004; 56: 883–889.
12. Demetriades D, Murray J, Sinz B, Myles D, Chan L, Sathyaragiswaran L, Noguchi T, Bongard FS, Cryer GH, Gaspard DJ. Epidemiology of major trauma and trauma deaths in Los Angeles County. *J Am Coll Surg* 1998; 187: 373–383.
13. Brookes M, MacMillan R, Cully S, Anderson E, Murray S, Mendelow AD, Jennett B. Head injuries in accident and emergency departments. How different are children from adults? *Journal of Epidemiology and Community Health* 1990;44(2):147–151.
14. Driscoll P, Lecky F. Primary prevention is better than cure. Emergency Medicine Australasia 2004;16:265–266.
15. Wyatt JP, Beard D, Gray A, Busuttil A, Robertson CE. Rate, causes and prevention of deaths from injuries in south-east Scotland. *Injury* 1996;27(5):337–340
16. www.tarn.ac.uk

17. Champion HC, Copes WS, Sacco WJ, Lawnick MM, Keast SC, Frey CF. The major trauma outcome study: establishing national norms for trauma care. *Journal of Trauma* 1990;30:1356–1365
18. Bouamra O, Wrotchford AS, Hollis S, Vail A, Woodford M, Lecky FE. A new approach to outcome prediction in trauma: a comparison with the TRISS model. *Journal of Trauma* 2006;61:701–710
19. Pape H-C, Zelle B, Lohse R, Hildebrand F, Krettek C, Panzica M, Duhme V, Sittaro NA. Evaluation and outcome of patients after polytrauma – Can patients be recruited for long-term follow up? *Injury* 2006;37(12):1197–1203

Chapter 3
Pathogenetic Changes: Isolated Extremity Trauma and Polytrauma

Martijn van Griensven

3.1 Outlining the Problem

Polytrauma is a term referring to the presence of multiple injuries and thus an array of different pathologies. Fractures of the skeleton are common findings in this setting, with femoral fractures displaying the highest incidence. Overall, isolated polytrauma represents a syndrome with a bandwidth of severities. The body reacts to such an accidental event by means of a "standard" program in order to restore the physiological state. A normal wound healing consists of:

1. vasoconstriction
2. coagulation
3. inflammation
4. tissue healing

The body will try to repair the encountered injury by this sequence of events independent of the extent of the injury. The first two stages were a major problem in the management of a multiple-injury victim decades ago. Technological advances and shorter rescue times shifted the problem from early and effective resuscitation to treatment of the victim's response to injury. This chapter will give an overview of the pathogenetic changes occurring during the posttraumatic course. These pathogenetic changes are strongly related to the posttraumatic disparity of the immune system [1, 2]. Furthermore, immune-monitoring can support clinical decision making, especially in borderline cases, with the choice of damage-control orthopedics.

M.V. Griensven (✉)
Ludwig Boltzmann Institute for Experimental and Clinical Traumatology,
Donaueschingenstrasse 13, Vienna, 1200, Austria
e-mail: Martijn.van.Griensven@lbitrauma.org

H.-C. Pape et al. (eds.), *Damage Control Management in the Polytrauma Patient*,
DOI 10.1007/978-0-387-89508-6_3, © Springer Science+Business Media, LLC 2010

3.2   From Systemic Inflammatory Response Syndrome to Multiple Organ Dysfunction Syndrome

As stated earlier, the clinical problems in the posttraumatic phase, besides the surgical ones, are mainly caused by the patient's inflammatory reaction. Multiple traumatized patients are at risk of progressive organ dysfunction from what appears to be a distorted immunologic process. In recent years, increasing understanding of the pathophysiology of the immunologic events occurring in both traumatic and surgical injuries has contributed enormously to the debate surrounding the etiology of septic complications and Multiple Organ Dysfunction Syndrome (MODS) after trauma [3–5]. The immunologic system displays dichotomous actions. In some instances, the immune system exerts an exaggerated response, with the potential to cause cell-mediated damage in remote organs. Conversely, an inhibition of the immune activity, called immunosuppression, can be observed. This contributes to the development of infection and sepsis after trauma [6, 7]. Multiple alterations in inflammatory and immunologic functions have been demonstrated in clinical and experimental situations within hours of trauma and hemorrhage, suggesting that a cascade of abnormalities that ultimately leads to ARDS and MODS is initiated in the immediate postinjury period [8, 9]. Damage-control orthopedics is indeed associated with a less severe Systemic Inflammatory Response Syndrome (SIRS) compared to early total care [10].

The initial immune response to a traumatic event is mainly the activation of the immune response. When this immune response is overwhelming, it is called SIRS. The development of SIRS can be divided in three stages:

1. local immune response
2. initial systemic immune response
3. exacerbating systemic inflammation [11, 12]

3.2.1   Local Immune Response

The local immune response is a reaction to the local trauma. Humoral and cellular immune mediators are locally activated in order to restore or minimize subsequent damages [13]. Damaged tissue is degraded and tissue repair is stimulated. Furthermore, mechanisms to clear pathogens, tissue debris, and antigens are activated [14]. Concomitantly, anti-inflammatory mediators are released to ensure that an overwhelming proinflammatory response does not cause any negative side effects [14, 15].

3.2.2   Initial Systemic Immune Response

When the local immune response is not able to control the initial damage, some of the mediators are released in the systemic circulation. These mediators attract and activate macrophages, thrombocytes, coagulation factors, etc., that oppose the damage more vigorously. This process continues until the wound or wounds have healed and homeostasis has been restored [16–18].

3.2.3   Exacerbating Systemic Inflammation

The systemic immune response becomes destructive when homeostasis cannot be restored; SIRS has developed [11, 16, 19]. The progressive endothelial dysfunction leads to an increased microvascular permeability with transudation into the organs [20–22]. In addition, microthrombi develop that obstruct microcirculation with subsequent local ischemia [23, 24]. Reperfusion of these local ischemic areas may cause reperfusion injury [7] and induce heat shock proteins [25]. Loss of regulation of vasodilatory and vasoconstrictory mechanisms results in a prominent vasodilatation with worsening of transudation and local ischemia [26, 27]. These circumstances may lead to a loss of organ function. If this occurs in several organs, an MODS would be developed. All signs of (systemic) inflammation can be clinically determined: Rubor, Calor, Tumor, Dolor, and Functio laesa (Redness, Heat, Swelling, Pain, and Loss or Disturbance of Function) [28].

This excessive inflammation with MODS results in death in 50–80% of the cases. The body, however, tries to counterregulate this inflammation via anti-inflammatory mediators. This anti-inflammation can also be exaggerated, leading to immune paralysis [29–32]. This is called Compensatory Anti-inflammatory Response Syndrome (CARS) [12, 16, 33, 34]. Microorganisms can easily invade the body during this period when it is with less or no immunosurveillance. Patients are prone to develop sepsis with subsequent septic shock [35, 36]. However, sometimes the anti-inflammation is initiated, but the inflammatory mediators sustain. This complex is called Mixed Antagonist Response Syndrome (MARS) [12, 16, 34]. Both CARS and MARS may develop in MODS. All these possible reactions (SIRS, CARS, MARS, and MODS) are called CHAOS (Cardiovascular shock, Homeostasis, Apoptosis, Organ dysfunction and immune Suppression) [12, 34].

3.3   Ischemia/Reperfusion

Not only trauma *per se* (with hypovolemic shock), but also operations to the extremities are accompanied by states of ischemia. Ischemia leads to necrosis, but this is not the main destroying mechanism. During reperfusion, systemic damage is induced [37]. In this phase, oxygen is delivered to the compromised ischemic area. In this area, normal physiologic metabolic processes are (partly) disabled, and anaerobic metabolism is performed. The oxygen is directly transformed in Radical Oxygen Species (ROS) [38]. These ROS are one of the most potent chemoattractants and activators for Polymorphonuclear Granulocytes (PMN) [37].

The eminent role for ROS was evidenced by a reduction in PMN accumulation, with concomitant pulmonary injury after Ischemia/Reperfusion (I/R) using several radical scavengers [38].

PMN, on the other hand, play a major role in the commencement phase after trauma. They seem to be crucial for both the healing and for the detrimental effects. Neutropenia reduced I/R injury in several animal models [39–41]. These facts make PMN the key players in I/R injury, SIRS, and MODS [38, 42–44]. These effects are augmented by interleukin-6 (IL-6) concerning recruitment, phagocytosis, and superoxidanion production [45, 46]. Similar disturbances are detected in the tissue counterpart of the PMN, the reticuloendothelial system [47].

3.4 Humoral Immune Response

Several humoral cascade systems are activated upon trauma including the complement system, cytokines, kinin-kallikrein system, coagulatory system, etc. Most of these systems are interconnected in their actions (Fig. 3.1). They are able to activate, inhibit, or modulate each other or even exert synergistic effects. The complement system, the cytokine system, and the coagulation system are the most well investigated systems in the context of trauma and sepsis.

3.4.1 Complement System

The complement system is the first humoral system activated in trauma. The cascade can be elicited by the classical, alternative, and lectin pathway. The important mediators concerning trauma and sepsis in this matter are the anaphylatoxins C3a and C5a. Several studies have shown a correlation between activated complement factors and mortality after trauma [39]. C5a regulates neutrophil adhesion associated processes and cytotoxic associated processes [40]. In recent experimental

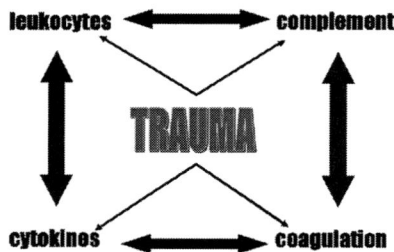

Fig. 3.1 The most investigated systems during trauma are the leukocytes, cytokine system, coagulation system, and complement system. Trauma by itself activates each system. The systems are also interconnected to each other

studies, blocking of complement leads to a reduction in pulmonary and intestinal permeability [41]. The accumulation of neutrophils in the lung was reduced by blocking the complement factor C5 [41]. Moreover, an antibody against C5a markedly restored the susceptibility of neutrophils to undergo apoptosis [42]. The PI3-Kinase seems to play an important role in this respect [43]. As the complement system is activated very early in trauma, intervention is hardly possible. Only in the context of posttraumatic sepsis might these therapies play a role.

3.4.2 Cytokine System

3.4.2.1 TNF-α and Its Receptors

TNF-α is one of the main players in inflammatory processes. Hemorrhagic shock *per se* causes secretion of TNF-α [44]. TNF-α exerts many effects on an array of cell types. TNF-α induces increased endothelial permeability in synergy with IL-1β [48]. Expression of adhesion molecules like Intercellular Adhesion Molecule-1 (ICAM-1) and E-selectin on endothelial cells is increased by TNF-α [49]. This leads to an activation and adhesion of PMN. Increased TNF-α serum levels are observed in patients with sepsis or septic shock. These are associated with bad prognosis [50]. Elevated concentrations in serum and bronchoalveolar lavages are associates with the occurrence of ARDS [45–47]. Interestingly, monocytes produce less TNF-α upon endotoxin stimulation in trauma patients with increased TNF-α serum levels. This coincided with a decreased mRNA expression of TNF-α [51]. This phenomenon indicates the possibility of CARS.

Two different membrane-bound receptors transduce TNF-α effects. TNF-RI (55 kDa) and TNF-RII (75 kDa) can be found in all cell types except on erythrocytes. Soluble forms of both receptors are present in plasma. There, they function antagonistically by binding bioactive TNF-α [52, 53]. Increased levels of sTNF-RI and sTNF-RII are found 3 h after trauma, with normalization at 12 h [54]. Most TNF-α mediated endotoxin effects are exerted by TNF-RI. TNF-RI knock-out mice are resistant to low-dose endotoxin, not to high doses. Interestingly, TNF-RI influences lymphocyte subpopulations and is needed for survival in polymicrobial sepsis [55]. Apoptosis induction in most cell types seems to be dependent on both TNF-receptors [56]. TNF-RI is also crucial for survival from sepsis in a traumatic setting [57]. This receptor is increased on PMN and monocytes in patients suffering from SIRS [58]. TNF-RII is responsible for proliferation of T-lymphocytes [59–61]. A downregulation on monocytes is noted during SIRS [58].

3.4.2.2 Interleukin-1

Mainly IL-1β is involved in inflammatory processes [62, 63]. IL-1β is produced from monocytes, macrophages, and endothelial cells upon stimulation with TNF-α or endotoxin [64]. Administration of endotoxin leads to maximal IL-1β levels after

3 h [65]. Effects of IL-1β resemble those of TNF-α. It induces production of pros-
taglandin E2, thromboxane, and IL-6. Stimulation of mononuclear cells derived
from septic trauma patients with endotoxin shows a reduced IL-1β secretion like
that observed for TNF-α. However, mRNA levels are not decreased, implying a
posttranscriptional inhibition [51, 66].

3.4.2.3 Interleukin-6

The most important secondary cytokine in trauma patients is IL-6 [4, 67]. In an
increasing number of hospitals, IL-6 is used as a prognostic marker for outcome in
trauma patients for SIRS, sepsis, and MODS. High IL-6 levels are associated with
poor outcome [50]. At the scene of an accident and in the emergency room, IL-6
serum levels are increased and correlate with the injury severity score, incidence of
complications, and mortality [68, 69]. IL-6 levels are even more increased in
patients suffering from sepsis. A correlation exists with the progression to septic
shock [70]. Significant higher IL-6 plasma levels are observed in nonsurvivors
compared to survivors [71]. A similar association is observed in trauma patients
developing ARDS [46, 47, 72]. A correlation also exists between the IL-6 concentrations after intramedullary osteosynthesis and the development of ARDS [73].
Nailing of femur fractures acts as a second hit and increases systemic IL-6 levels
[74]. These facts show that IL-6 is a marker for the intensity of trauma. It can therefore be helpful in stratifying trauma patients in risk groups. Especially for secondary
operations, IL-6 can assist in deciding the time point of operation [75] and the
procedures used [76, 77]. Interestingly, IL-6 is differentially secreted according to
age and gender [78].

3.4.2.4 Interleukin-10

Traumatized patients display significantly increased IL-10 plasma levels. In the early
phase after trauma, this can be related to PMN production [79], whereas in the later
phase Th-cells may be the source. IL-10 levels are correlated with ISS, ARDS,
MODS, and sepsis [80, 81], possibly due to the immunosuppressive features of IL-10.
Concomitantly, overproduction of IL-10 plays a role in the development of CARS
[34]. Neutralizing IL-10 reduces the susceptibility for secondary infections after
trauma [82]. This has to be timely adapted [83], as an early inhibition of IL-10 with
antibodies increased TNF-α levels and subsequent mortality [84].

3.4.2.5 Granulocyte-Monocyte Colony-Stimulating-Factor

Granulocyte-Monocyte Colony-Stimulating-Factor (GM-CSF) is a cytokine known
from a hematological perspective. It enhances myelopoiesis. However, it not only

increases the production of these cell types, but it also modulates their functions. Humans treated with recombinant GM-CSF exhibit increased MHC class II molecule expression on the surface of their PMN and monocytes [85–87]. The decreased HLA-DR expression in immunoparalysis after trauma may be due to diminished production of GM-CSF [88]. Administration of recombinant GM-CSF to whole blood of polytraumatized patients restored the monocyte HLA-DR expression *ex vivo* [89]. Thereby, it restored the responsiveness to endotoxin as measured by TNF-α production [89]. Administration of GM-CSF in an in vivo sepsis model was associated with improved survival [90, 91]. First treatments of sepsis patients show concordant positive effects [92].

3.5 Cellular Immune Response

The humoral immune system interacts with the cellular immune system and activates, inhibits, or modulates cellular immune responses (Fig. 3.1). Cell systems included are PMN, lymphocytes, and monocytes. These cells are responsible for different phases during the posttraumatic course. PMN play an eminent role in the early phase (prehospital until second or third day) [93, 94]. Lymphocytes and monocytes are important in the secondary phase of the posttraumatic course (after day 4).

3.5.1 Polymorphonuclear Granulocytes

PMN play a major role in the early phase after trauma. They seem to be crucial for both the positive ("healing") and for the detrimental effects. PMN are the key players of the innate immune response in SIRS and MODS [95–97]. Interestingly, in multiple traumatized patients suffering from SIRS, a reduced apoptosis rate of PMN was detected [98, 99]. This implies that PMN survive longer and are able to exert more detrimental effects [100]. These effects are regulated by IL-6 concerning recruitment, phagocytosis, and superoxidanion production [101, 102]. Similar disturbances are detected in the tissue counterpart of the PMN, the reticuloendothelial system [103].

3.5.2 PMN-Endothelial Interaction

PMN in the circulation are not detrimental. The deleterious effects of the PMN occur once they enter the organs [104]. In order to enter the tissue, PMN have to interact with the endothelium in the microcirculation. This process is multistaged and uses adhesion molecules expressed on both PMN and endothelial cells [105]. Landmarks of this interaction are: "rolling," "attachment," and "diapedesis" [106].

Selectins are important mediators for the process of PMN-"rolling" [107]. L-selectin is found on the surface of PMN, whereas P- and E-selectin are found in endothelial cells [108].

Secondly, PMN are attached to the endothelium via stable cell-cell-interaction induced by integrins. The β_2-subunit of the integrins (CD18) plays an important role for PMN.

The last group of adhesion molecules consists of the immunoglobulin-like ones. These are characterized by one or more homologous immunoglobulin-like domains. The most well-known member of this group is ICAM-1 [108]. This molecule is important in the pathogenesis of posttraumatic sepsis [109].

3.5.2.1 L-Selectin

The expression of L-selectin on PMN has been partly investigated in the case of trauma and has been shown to have important functions [110]. Kerner and colleagues described a correlation between L-selectin on monocytes and the incidence of MODS during the first 6 days after trauma [111]. On PMN, the maximum expression of L-selectin is detected from 3 to 12 h after trauma [112–116]. In contrast, some authors found a decreased membrane L-selectin expression correlating with SIRS [117, 118] or MODS having also a gender discrepancy [116]. Upon interaction with the endothelium, L-selectin is shed from the PMN surface. Therefore, this shedding is associated with the activity level of PMN. Maximum sL-selectin serum levels were observed 6 h after trauma [112, 114, 119]. This shedding correlated with reduced exudation of PMN in patients with SIRS [118].

Blocking L-selectin showed protective effects in trauma-associated animal models without increasing the risk of infection [120–124]. However, using an anti-L-selectin antibody in a clinical phase II study did not display decreased incidence of MODS [125].

3.5.2.2 ICAM-1

Nonactivated cells display a basal expression that is maximally increased 8 h after a traumatic insult [126–128]. Recently, the role of ICAM-1 in trauma and sepsis has been recognized [109]. Pulmonary microcirculatory endothelial cells reveal a huge increased expression of ICAM-1 in combination with an increased β2 integrin expression in PMN in patients deceased from sepsis [129]. A decreased ICAM-1 expression was detected in monocytes of these patients [130]. Trauma patients who did not die from septic complications had basal expressions of ICAM-1 on the pulmonary endothelial cells [129].

3.5.3 Lymphocytes

During the first 24 h after trauma, total lymphocyte numbers decrease [131, 132]. Patients with the most severe loss of lymphocytes were most prone to die, most likely from infections [131, 133]. This lymphocyte depletion may be related to increased levels of apoptosis that were also associated with subsequent MODS [134, 135]. Simultaneously, the lymphocytes were defective in their capacity to proliferate and in their function ("anergy"). This was due to a reduced expression of mRNA for IL-2 with subsequent diminished secretion [136].

Depending on the patient population, differences in the ratio T-helper to T-suppressor cells are described. In trauma patients developing sepsis and subsequent MODS, an inverse CD4+/CD8+ ratio was observed compared to healthy controls [131]. No change in this ratio was observed when MODS was due to trauma and SIRS but not due to sepsis [133]. The CD4+ T-helper cells can be differentiated into Th1 and Th2 cells. The pattern of circulating Th1/Th2 ratio is not altered in patients with multiple injuries [137]. The numbers of CD4+, CD8+, and NK-cells are increased in patients developing MODS [131]. Similar results were obtained in an experimental model with sepsis and MODS [138]. Elimination of NK-cells from mice abrogated the toxicity and the mortality from cytokine induced shock [139]. NK-cells interact with macrophages in order to clear bacteria during septic peritonitis [140].

3.5.4 Monocytes

The posttraumatic course is characterized by significant monocytosis, showing twice as much monocytes compared to normal control subjects [141]. Trauma leads to reduced responsiveness of blood monocytes to LPS and a decreased secretion of proinflammatory reacting cytokines [142]. This decreased responsiveness may be associated with a decreased CD14 expression. CD14 is the receptor for LPS. Trauma leads to a decrease in monocyte CD14 expression [143, 144]. Surprisingly, the percentage of monocytes expressing CD14 in trauma patients does not differentiate them from normal controls. However, monocyte CD14 receptor density demonstrates a significant reduction in septic trauma patients versus normal controls 3 days after trauma [144]. The decrease of membrane-bound CD14 is due to a shedding of the molecule. Therefore, soluble CD14 (sCD14) is increased after trauma [143, 144]. Those trauma patients with increased sCD14 during the first 24 h after trauma are prone to develop infectious complications [144]. In severely multiply traumatized patients, sCD14 serum levels remained elevated during the first 14 posttraumatic days. This phenomenon occurred for 6 days in less severely injured patients [143].

Furthermore, not only is the LPS responsiveness impaired, but the antigen-presenting function is as well. The antigen-presenting function depends on the expression of the MHC class II molecule HLA-DR. Trauma results in immediate and profound depression in monocyte HLA-DR class II antigen expression compared with controls [145]. Monocyte HLA-DR class III antigen expression returned to normal between days 7 and 14 in uninfected patients, despite subnormal production of interferon gamma. Failure to increase interferon gamma production and monocyte HLA-DR antigen expression was associated with an episode of major infection [145].

3.6   Coagulation System

3.6.1   Coagulopathy

Due to injury, with subsequent exposition of tissue factor, a large-scale activation of the coagulation cascade occurs. This leads to neutrophil homing to the tissues and activation on the site of injury. Coagulopathy following major trauma is conventionally attributed to activation and consumption of coagulation factors. It may be caused by hypothermia, acidosis, hyperfibrinolysis, low hemoglobin, and platelet function [146]. Coagulopathy is common, affecting as many as 25–36% of trauma victims, and may develop early after injury [147]. Very early after the traumatic event, patients present with a hypercoagulability [148]. The incidence of coagulopathy increases with severity of injury, but it is not related to the volume of intravenous fluid administered [146, 149]. Diffuse coagulopathy is one of the most challenging situations faced by physicians treating these patients and is associated with high morbidity and mortality. Because objective measurement of coagulopathy is often unattainable in the clinical setting, current guidelines recommend empirical replacement therapy for the coagulopathic patient with diffuse microvascular bleeding [150, 151]. Current management involves replacing coagulation factors (fresh frozen plasma, platelets, and cryoprecipitate) and correcting acidosis and hypothermia. A growing number of case series and reports have described the safe and effective hemostatic properties of rFVIIa in trauma patients with uncontrolled hemorrhage refractory to conventional therapy [152, 153].

3.6.2   Interaction Coagulation and Complement Systems

In trauma, both coagulation factors and tissue damage activate the complement cascade [154]. In the absence of bacterial or altered self products, the complement system can be activated by a connection with the coagulation system. The coagulation cascade and the complement cascade are connected through plasmin, a product of the thrombolytic route that regulates homeostasis in the coagulation. Human C5 incubated with thrombin generated C5a that was biologically active [155]. Thrombin may substitute for the C3-dependent C5 convertase.

3.7 Decision-Making Factors

From all the pathogenetic mediators described in this chapter, only a few have already entered the clinically arena (IL-6, HLA-DR). However, they are still not part of the routine protocol, except for IL-6 in a number of hospitals (like Lorenz Böhler Trauma Hospital). Immune monitoring is important to determine the "inflammatory state" of the patient. When the patient is immune-compromised (HLA-DR measurements), activating factors could be administered (like G-CSF). In case the immune system shows overt activation, surgeries should be postponed in order not to cross the threshold of the "patient's tolerance" (Fig. 3.2).

IL-6 serum values may be used to determine the surgical management of the multiply-injured patients, with special reference to the borderline patient. According to our data [73, 76, 156], no distinct clinical advantage to carrying out secondary definitive fracture fixation early could be determined. In contrast, in patients who demonstrated initial IL-6 values above 500 pg/ml, it may be advantageous to delay the interval between primary temporary fracture stabilization and secondary definitive fracture fixation for more than 4 days. In patients with blunt multiple injuries undergoing primary temporary fixation of major fractures, the timing of secondary definitive surgery should be carefully selected, because it may act as a second hit phenomenon and cause a deterioration of the clinical status.

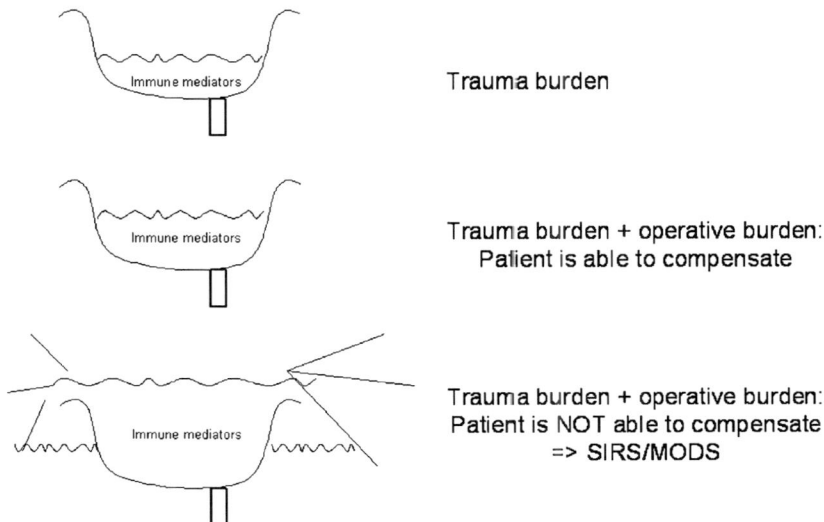

Fig. 3.2 Trauma leads to an inflammatory burden as represented by the immune mediators filling the bathtub. Patients who are able to compensate the operative burden mostly have moderately high IL-6 levels. The body is able to cope with the increased burden. When the patient, however, is borderline, the operative burden may be too much, and the immune system may be overactivated. This leads to SIRS and eventually may result in the development of MODS. Damage-control orthopedics is especially helpful in this last situation

Early, definitive fracture fixation is associated with increased perioperative liberation of proinflammatory cytokines and a higher incidence of MODS.

3.8   Summary and Conclusion

Trauma itself leads to an activation of cascade systems such as the complement system, cytokine system, leukocyte system, and the coagulation system. These systems are closely interconnected. The surgeon has to be aware that operating on a trauma patient can draw the delicate balance of these systems to the detrimental side. Biomarkers can assist the surgeon and the anesthesiologist in determining the physiological state of the patient. This is especially useful in borderline patients. IL-6 and HLA-DR are important markers in this respect. When IL-6 is high or increasing during the posttraumatic course in the intensive care, Damage Control Principles should be applied.

References

1. Lin E, Lowry SF, Calvano S. The systemic response to injury. In: Schwartz S, Shires GT, Spencer F, editors. *Principles of Surgery.* New York: McGraw-Hill, 1999: 3–51.
2. Guirao X, Lowry SF. Biologic control of injury and inflammation: much more than too little or too late. *World J Surg* 1996; 20:437–446.
3. Tompkins RG. The role of proinflammatory cytokines in inflammatory and metabolic responses. *Ann Surg* 1997; 225(3):243–245.
4. Nast-Kolb D, Waydhas C, Gippner-Steppert C, Schneider I, Trupka A, Ruchholtz S, Zettl R, Schweiberer L, Jochum M. Indicators of the posttraumatic inflammatory response correlate with organ failure in patients with multiple injuries. *J Trauma* 1997; 42(3):446–454.
5. Keel M, Trentz O. Pathophysiology of polytrauma. *Injury* 2005; 36:691–709.
6. Polk HC, Jr. Non-specific host defense stimulation in the reduction of surgical infection in man. *Br J Surg* 1987; 74(11):969–970.
7. Cipolle MD, Pasquale MD, Cerra FB. Secondary organ dysfunction. From clinical perspectives to molecular mediators. *Crit Care Med* 1993; 9:261–298.
8. Abraham E. Host defense abnormalities after hemorrhage, trauma, and burns. *Crit Care Med* 1989; 17(9):934–939.
9. Smith RM, Giannoudis PV. Trauma and the immune response. *J R Soc Med* 1998; 91(8):417–420.
10. Harwood PJ, Giannoudis PV, van Griensven M, Krettek C, Pape H-C. Alterations in the systemic inflammatory response after early total care and damage control procedures for femoral shaft fracture in severely injured patients. *J Trauma* 2005; 58:446–452.
11. Bone RC. Toward a theory regarding the pathogenesis of the systemic inflammatory response syndrome: what we do and do not know about cytokine regulation. *Crit Care Med* 1996; 24:163–172.
12. Davies MG, Hagen P-O. Systemic inflammatory response syndrome. *Br J Surg* 1997; 84:920–935.
13. Regel G, Dwenger A, Gratz KF, Nerlich ML, Sturm JA, Tscherne H. Humorale und zelluläre Veränderungen der unspezifischen Immunabwehr nach schwerem Trauma. *Unfallchirurg* 1989; 92:314–320.

14. Dinarello CA, Gelfland JA, Wolff SM. Anticytokine strategies in the treatment of the systemic inflammatory response syndrome. *JAMA* 1993; 269:1829–1835.
15. Platzer C, Meisel C, Vogt K, Platzer M, Volk HD. Up-regulation of monocytic IL-10 by tumor necrosis factor-α and cAMP elevating drugs. *Int Immunol* 1995; 7:517–523.
16. Bone RC. Immunologic dissonance: a continuing evolution in our understanding of the systemic inflammatory response syndrome (SIRS) and the multiple organ dysfunction syndrome (MODS). *Ann Intern Med* 1996; 125(8):680–687.
17. Bone RC. The pathogenesis of sepsis. Ann Intern Med 1991; 115:457–469.
18. Fukushima R, Alexander JW, Gianotti L, Ogle CK. Isolated pulmonary infection acts as a source of systemic tumor necrosis factor. *Crit Care Med* 1994; 22:114–120.
19. Regel G, Sturm JA, Pape H-C, Gratz KF, Tscherne H. Das Multiorganversagen (MOV) – Ausdruck eines generalisierten Zellschadens aller Organe nach schwerem Trauma. *Unfallchirurg* 1991; 94:487–497.
20. Kreuzfelder K, Joka T, Keinecke H-O. Adult respiratory distress syndrome as a specific manifestation of a general permeability defect in trauma patients. *Am Rev Respir Dis* 1988; 137:95–99.
21. Lucas CE, Ledgerwood AM, Rachwal WJ, Grabow D, Saxe J. Colloid oncotic pressure and body water dynamics in septic and injured patients. *J Trauma* 1991; 31:927–933.
22. Pape H-C, Regel G, Kleemann W, Goris JA, Regel G, Tscherne H. Posttraumatic multiple organ failure – A report on clinical and autopsy findings. *Shock* 1994; 2(3):228–234.
23. Sigurdsson GH, Christenson JT, el-Rakshy MB, Sadek S. Intestinal platelet trapping after traumatic and septic shock. An early sign of sepsis and multiorgan failure in critically ill patients? *JAMA* 1992; 20:458–467.
24. Gando S, Kameke T, Nanzaki S, Nakanishi Y. Disseminated intravascular coagulation is a frequent complication of systemic inflammatory response syndrome. *Thromb Haemost* 1996; 75:224–228.
25. Rinaldo JE, Gorry M, Strieter R, Cowan H, Abdolrasulnia R, Shepherd V. Effect of endotoxin-induced cell injury on 70-kD heat shock proteins in bovine lung endothelial cells. Am *J Respir Cell Mol Biol* 1990; 3:207–216.
26. Gomez-Jimenez J, Salgado A, Mourelle M, Martín MC, Segura RM, Peracaula R, Moncada S. L-arginine: nitric oxide pathway in endotoxemia and human septic shock. *Crit Care Med* 1995; 23:253–258.
27. Miyauchi T, Tomobe Y, Shiba R, Ishikawa T, Yanagisawa M, Kimura S, Sugishita Y, Ito I, Goto K, Masaki T. Involvement of endothelin in the regulation of human vascular tonus. Potent vasoconstrictor effect and existence in endothelial cells. *Circulation* 1990; 81:1874–1880.
28. Bone RC, Sibbald WJ, Sprung CL. The ACCP-SCCM consensus conference on sepsis and organ failure [editorial; comment]. *Chest* 1992; 101(6):1481–1483.
29. Randow F, Syrbe U, Meisel C, Krausch D, Zuckermann H, Platzer C, Volk HD. Mechanisms of endotoxin desensitization: involvement of interleukin-10 and transforming growth factor beta. *J Exp Med* 1995; 181:1887–1892.
30. Syrbe U, Meinecke A, Platzer C, Makki A, Asadullah K, Klug C. Improvement of monocyte function – A new therapeutic approach? In: Reinhart K, Eyrich K, Sprung CL, editors. *Sepsis: Current Perspectives in Pathophysiology and Therapy.* Berlin: Springer, 1994: 473–500.
31. Mills CD, Caldwell MD, Gann DS. Evidence of a plasma-mediated "window" of immundeficiency in rats following trauma. *J Clin Immunol* 1989; 9:139–150.
32. Kremer JP, Jarrar D, Steckholzer U, Ertel W.. Interleukin-1, -6 and tumor necrosis factor-alpha release is down-regulated in whole blood from septic patients. *Acta Haematol* 1996; 95(3–4):268–273.
33. Bone RC. Why the sepsis trials failed. *JAMA* 1996; 276(7):565–566.
34. Bone RC. Sir Isaac Newton, sepsis, SIRS, and CARS. *Crit Care Med* 1996; 24:1125–1128.
35. Moore FA. The role of the gastrointestinal tract in postinjury multiple organ failure. *Am J Surg* 1999; 178(6):449–453.

36. Volk HD, Lohmann T, Heym S, Golosubow A, Ruppe U, Reinke P, Thieme M, Nieter B, Tausch W, Döcke WD, von Baehr R. Decrease of the proportion of HLA-DR+ monocytes as prognostic parameter for the clinical outcome of septic disease. In: Masihi KN, Lange W, editors. *Immunotherapeutic prospects of infectious disease.* Berlin: Springer, 1990: 298-301.
37. Seekamp A, Ward PA. Ischemia-reperfusion injury. In: Oppenheim JJ, editor. *Inflammatory disease therapy.* Basel: Birkhauser Verlag, 1993: 137.
38. Bulger EM, Maier RV. An argument for vitamin E supplementation in the management of systemic inflammatory response syndrome. *Shock* 2003; 19(2):99-103.
39. Nuytinck JK, Goris RJ, Redl H, Schlag G, van Munster OJ. Posttraumatic complications and inflammatory mediators. *Arch Surg* 1986; 121:886-90.
40. Riedemann NC, Guo RF, Bernacki KD, Reuben JS, Laudes IJ, Neff TA, Gao H, Speyer C, Sarma VJ, Zetoune FS, Ward PA. Regulation by C5a of neutrophil activation during sepsis. *Immunity* 2003; 19:193-202.
41. Harkin DW, Marron CD, Rother RP, Romaschin A, Rubin BB, Lindsay TF. C5 complement inhibition attenuates shock and acute lung injury in an experimental model of ruptured abdominal aortic aneurysm. *Br J Surg* 2005; 92:1227-34.
42. Guo RF, Sun L, Gao H, Shi KX, Rittirsch D, Sarma VJ, Zetoune. FS, and Ward PA. In vivo regulation of neutrophil apoptosis by C5a during sepsis. *J Leukoc Biol* 2006; 80:1575-83.
43. Wrann CD, Tabriz NA, Barkhausen T, Klos A, van Griensven M, Pape HC, Kendoff DO, Guo R, Ward PA, Krettek C, Riedemann NC. The phosphatidylinositol 3-kinase signaling pathway exerts protective effects during sepsis by controlling C5a-mediated activation of innate immune functions. *J Immunol* 2007; 178:5940-48.
44. Ayala A, Perrin MM, Meldrum DR, Ertel W, Chaudry IH. Hemorrhage induces an increase in serum TNF which is not associated with elevated levels of endotoxin. *Cytokine* 1990; 2: 170-74.
45. Bogdan C, Vodovotz Y, Nathan C. Macrophage deactivation by interleukin 10. *J Exp Med* 1991; 174(6):1549-55.
46. Meduri GU, Headley S, Kohler G, Kohler G, Tolley E, Leeper KV, Umberger R. Persistent elevation of inflammatory cytokines predicts a poor outcome in ARDS. Plasma IL-1 beta and IL-6 levels are consistent and efficient predictors of outcome over time. *Chest* 1995; 107(4):1062-73.
47. Meduri GU, Kohler G, Headley S, Tolley E, Streutz F, Postlethwaite A. Inflammatory cytokines in the BAL of patients with ARDS. Persistent elevation over time predicts poor outcome. *Chest* 1995; 108(5):1303-14.
48. van Griensven M, Stalp M, Seekamp A. Ischemia-reperfusion directly increases pulmonary permeability in vitro. *Shock* 1999; 11(4):259-63.
49. Redl H, Schlag G, Kneidinger R, Dinges H, Davies J. Activation/adherence phenomena of leukocytes and endothelial cells in trauma and sepsis. In: Schlag G, Redl H, editors. *Pathophysiology of Shock, Sepsis and Organ Failure.* Springer-Verlag, pp 33-51,
50. Casey LC, Balk RA, Bone RC. Plasma cytokine and endotoxin levels correlate with survival in patients with the sepsis syndrome. *Ann Intern Med* 1993; 119:771-778.
51. Ertel W, Kremer JP, Kenney J, Steckholzer U, Jarrar D, Trentz O, Schildberg FW. Downregulation of proinflammatory cytokine release in whole blood from septic patients. *Blood* 1995; 85(5):1341–1347.
52. Moldawer LL. Interleukin-1, TNF alpha and their naturally occurring antagonists in sepsis. *Blood Purif* 1993; 11(2):128–133.
53. Peschon JJ, Torrance DS, Stocking KL, Glaccum MB, Otten C, Willis CR, Charrier K , Morrissey PJ, Ware CB, Mohler KM. TNF receptor-deficient mice reveal divergent roles for p55 and p75 in several models of inflammation. *J Immunol* 1998; 160(2):943–952.
54. Hensler T, Sauerland S, Bouillon B, Raum M, Rixen D, Helling HJ, Andermahr J, Neugebauer EAM. Association between injury pattern of patients with multiple injuries and circulating levels of soluble tumor necrosis factor receptors, interleukin-6 and interleukin-10, and polymorphonuclear neutrophil elastase. *J Trauma* 2002; 52(5):962–970.

55. Hildebrand F, Pape H-C, Harwood P, Wittwer T, Krettek C, van Griensven M. Are alterations of lymphocyte subpopulations in polymicrobial sepsis and DHEA treatment mediated by the tumour necrosis factor (TNF)-alpha receptor (TNF-RI)? A study in TNF-RI (TNF-RI(-/-)) knock-out rodents. *Clin Exp Immunol* 2004; 138:221–229.

56. Vandenabeele P, Declercq W, Vanhaesebroeck B, Grooten J, Fiers W. Both TNF receptors are required for TNF-mediated induction of apoptosis in PC60 cells. *J Immunol* 1995; 154(6):2904–2913.

57. van Griensven M, Wittwer T, Brauer N, Pape H-C. DHEA wirkt protektiv bei einer experimentellen polymikrobiellen Sepsis durch CLP – Besteht eine pathogenetische Bedeutung des TNF-α? *Chirurgisches Forum* 2001; 30:383–385.

58. Hubl W, Wolfbauer G, Streicher J, Andert S, Stanek G, Fitzal S, Bayer PM. Differential expression of tumor necrosis factor receptor subtypes on leukocytes in systemic inflammatory response syndrome. *Crit Care Med* 1999; 27(2):319–324.

59. Grell M, Becke FM, Wajant H, Männel DN, Scheurich P. TNF receptor type 2 mediates thymocyte proliferation independently of TNF receptor type 1. *Eur J Immunol* 1998; 28(1):257–263.

60. Stelzner TJ, Weil JV, O'Brien RF. Role of cyclic adenosine monophosphate in the induction of endothelial barrier properties. *J Cell Physiol* 1989; 139:157–166.

61. Tartaglia LA, Goeddel DV, Reynolds C, Figari LS, Weber RF, Fendly BM, Palladino MA. Stimulation of human T-cell proliferation by specific activation of the 75-kDa tumor necrosis factor receptor. *J Immunol* 1993; 151(9):4637–4641.

62. Dinarello CA. The biological properties of interleukin-1. *Eur Cytokine Netw* 1994; 5(6): 517–531.

63. Dinarello CA. The interleukin-1 family: 10 years of discovery. *FASEB J* 1994; 8(15): 1314–1325.

64. Angele MK, Xu YX, Ayala A, Schwacha MG, Catania RK, Cioffi WG, Bland KI, Chaudry IH. Gender dimorphism in trauma-hemorrhage-induced thymocyte apoptosis. *Shock* 1999; 12(4):316–322.

65. Cannon JG, Tompkins RG, Gelfand JA, Michie HR, Stanford GG, van der Meer JW, Endres S, Lonnemann G, Corsetti J Chernow B et al. Circulating interleukin-1 and tumor necrosis factor in septic shock and experimental endotoxin fever. *J Infect Dis* 1990; 161(1):79-84.

66. Schinkel C, Zimmer S, Kremer JP, Walz A, Rordorf-Adam C, Henckel von Donnersmarck G, Faist E. Comparative analysis of transcription and protein release of the inflammatory cytokines interleukin-1 beta (IL-1 beta) and interleukin-8 (IL-8) following major burn and mechanical trauma. *Shock* 1995; 4(4):241–246.

67. Martin C, Boisson C, Haccoun M, Thomachot L, Mege JL. Patterns of cytokine evolution (tumor necrosis factor-alpha and interleukin-6) after septic shock, hemorrhagic shock, and severe trauma. *Crit Care Med* 1997; 25(11):1813–1819.

68. Pape HC, Remmers D, Grotz M, Schedel I, von Glinski S, Oberbeck R, Dahlweit M, Tscherne H. Levels of antibodies to endotoxin and cytokine release in patients with severe trauma: does posttraumatic dysergy contribute to organ failure? *J Trauma* 1999; 46(5):907–913.

69. Gebhard F, Pfetsch H, Steinbach G, Strecker W, Kinzl L, Bruckner UB. Is interleukin 6 an early marker of injury severity following major trauma in humans? *Arch Surg* 2000; 135(3):291–295.

70. Terregino CA, Lopez BL, Karras DJ, Killian AJ, Arnold GK. Endogenous mediators in emergency department patients with presumed sepsis: are levels associated with progression to severe sepsis and death? *Ann Emerg Med* 2000; 35(1):26–34.

71. Presterl E, Staudinger T, Pettermenn M, Lassnigg A, Burgmann H, Winkler S, Frass M, Graninger W. Cytokine profile and correlation to the APACHE III and MPM II scores in patients with sepsis. *Am J Respir Crit Care Med* 1997; 156:825–832.

72. Clerici M, Shearer GM. A TH1-->TH2 switch is a critical step in the etiology of HIV infection [see comments]. *Immunol Today* 1993; 14(3):107–111.

73. Pape HC, Grimme K, van Griensven M, Sott AH, Giannoudis P, Morley J, Roise O, Ellingsen E, Hildebrand F, Wiese B, Krettek C. Impact of intramedullary instrumentation versus damage control for femoral fractures on immunoinflammatory parameters: prospective randomized analysis by the EPOFF Study Group. *J Trauma* 2003; 55(1):7–13.

74. Giannoudis PV, Smith RM, Bellamy MC, Morrison JF, Dickson RA, Guillou PJ. Stimulation of the inflammatory system by reamed and unreamed nailing of femoral fractures. An analysis of the second hit. *J Bone Joint Surg Br* 1999; 81(2):356–361.

75. Pape H-C, Stalp M, van Griensven M, Weinberg A, Dahlweit M, Tscherne H. Optimaler Zeitpunkt der Sekundäroperation bei Polytrauma. *Chirurg* 1999; 70:1287–1293.

76. Pape HC, van Griensven M, Rice J, Gansslen A, Hildebrand F, Zech S, Winny M, Lichtinghagen R, Krettek C. Major secondary surgery in blunt trauma patients and perioperative cytokine liberation: determination of the clinical relevance of biochemical markers. *J Trauma* 2001; 50(6):989–1000.

77. Pape H-C, Schmidt RE, Rice J, van Griensven M, das Gupta R, Krettek C, Tscherne H. Biochemical changes after trauma and skeletal surgery of the lower extremity: quantification of the operative burden. *Crit Care Med* 2000; 28(10):3441–3448

78. Frink M, Pape H-C, van Griensven M, Krettek C, Chaudry IH, Hildebrand F. Influence of sex and age on mods and cytokines after multiple injuries. *Shock* 2007; 27:151–156.

79. Wolk K, Docke W, von Baehr V, Volk H, Sabat R. Comparison of monocyte functions after LPS- or IL-10-induced reorientation: importance in clinical immunoparalysis. *Pathobiology* 1999; 67(5–6):253–256.

80. Neidhardt R, Keel M, Steckholzer U, Safret A, Ungethuem U, Trentz O, Ertel W. Relationship of interleukin-10 plasma levels to severity of injury and clinical outcome in injured patients. *J Trauma* 1997; 42(5):863–870.

81. Giannoudis PV, Smith RM, Perry SL, Windsor AJ, Dickson RA, Bellamy MC. Immediate IL-10 expression following major orthopaedic trauma: relationship to anti-inflammatory response and subsequent development of sepsis. *Intensive Care Med* 2000; 26(8): 1076–1081.

82. Steinhauser ML, Hogaboam CM, Kunkel SL, Lukacs NW, Stricter RM, Standiford TJ. IL-10 is a major mediator of sepsis-induced impairment in lung antibacterial host defense. *J Immunol* 1999; 162:392–399.

83. Song GY, Chung C-S, Chaudry IH, Ayala A. What is the role of interleukin 10 in polymicrobial sepsis: anti-inflammatory agent or immunosuppressant? *Surgery* 1999; 126:378–383.

84. van der Poll T, Marchant A, Buurman WA, Berman L, Keogh CV, Lazarus DD, Nguyen L, Goldman M, Moldawer LL, Lowry SF. Endogenous IL-10 protects mice from death during septic peritonitis. *J Immunol* 1995; 155(11):5397–5401.

85. Spagnoli GC, Juretic A, Rosso R, Van Bree J, Harder F, Heberer M. Expression of HLA-DR in granulocytes of polytraumatized patients treated with recombinant human granulocyte macrophage-colony-stimulating factor. *Hum Immunol* 1995; 43(1):45–50.

86. Drossou-Agakidou V, Kanakoudi-Tsakalidou F, Sarafidis K, Tzimouli V, Taparkou A, Kremenopoulos G, Germenis A. In vivo effect of rhGM-CSF and rhG-CSF on monocyte HLA-DR expression of septic neonates. *Cytokine* 2002; 18(5):260–265.

87. Caulfield JJ, Fernandez MH, Sousa AR, Lane SJ, Lee TH Hawrylowicz, CM. Regulation of major histocompatibility complex class II antigens on human alveolar macrophages by granulocyte-macrophage colony-stimulating factor in the presence of glucocorticoids. *Immunology* 1999; 98(1):104–110.

88. Wu JC, Livingston DH, Hauser CJ, Deitch EA, Rameshwar P. Trauma inhibits erythroid burst-forming unit and granulocyte-monocyte colony-forming unit growth through the production of TGF-beta1 by bone marrow stroma. *Ann Surg* 2001; 234(2):224–232.

89. Flohe S, Borgermann J, Dominguez FE, Majetschak M, Lim L, Kreuzfelder E, Obertacke U, Nast-Kolb D, Schade FU. Influence of granulocyte-macrophage colony-stimulating factor (GM-CSF) on whole blood endotoxin responsiveness following trauma, cardiopulmonary bypass, and severe sepsis. *Shock* 1999; 12(1):17–24.

90. Austin OM, Redmond HP, Watson WG, Cunney RJ, Grace PA, Bouchier-Hayes D. The beneficial effects of immunostimulation in posttraumatic sepsis. *J Surg Res* 1995; 59(4):446–449.
91. Gennari R, Alexander JW, Gianotti L, Eaves-Pyles T, Hartmann S. Granulocyte macrophage colony-stimulating factor improves survival in two models of gut-derived sepsis by improving gut barrier function and modulating bacterial clearance. *Ann Surg* 1994; 220(1):68–76.
92. Nierhaus A, Montag B, Timmler N, Frings DP, Gutensohn K, Jung R, Schneider CG, Pothmann W, Brassel AK, Schulte Am Esch J. Reversal of immunoparalysis by recombinant human granulocyte-macrophage colony-stimulating factor in patients with severe sepsis. *Intensive Care Med* 2003; 29(4):646–651.
93. Botha AJ, Moore FA, Moore EE, Sauaia A, Banerjee A, Peterson VM. Early neutrophil sequestration after injury: a pathogenic mechanism for multiple organ failure. *J Trauma* 1995; 39:411–417.
94. Botha AJ, Moore FA, Moore EE. Postinjury neutrophil priming and activation: an early vulnerable window. *Surgery* 1995; 118:358.
95. Korthuis RJ, Grisham MB, Granger DN. Leucocyte depletion attenuates vascular injury in postischemic skeletal muscle. *Am J Physiol* 1988; 254:H823–H827.
96. Vedder NB, Fouty BW, Winn RK, Harlan JM, Rice CL. Role of neutrophils in generalized reperfusion injury associated with resuscitation from shock. *Surgery* 1989; 106:509–516.
97. Fujishima S, Aikawa N. Neutrophil-mediated tissue injury and its modulation. *Intensive Care Med* 1995; 21(3):277–285.
98. Ertel W, Keel M, Ungethum U, Trentz O. Proinflammatorische Zytokine regulieren die Apoptose von Granulozyten während der systemischen Entzundung. *Langenbecks Arch Chir Suppl Kongressbd* 1997; 114:627–629.
99. Jimenez MF, Watson RW, Parodo J, Evans D, Foster D, Steinberg M, Rotstein OD, Marshall JC. Dysregulated expression of neutrophil apoptosis in the systemic inflammatory response syndrome. *Arch Surg* 1997; 132(12):1263–1269.
100. Zallen G, Moore EE, Johnson JL, Tamura DY, Aiboshi J, Biffl WL, Silliman CC. Circulating postinjury neutrophils are primed for the release of proinflammatory cytokines. *J Trauma* 1999; 46(1):42–48.
101. Mullen PG, Windsor AC, Walsh CJ, Cook DJ, Fisher BJ, Blocher CR, Leeper-Woodford SK, Sugerman HJ, Fowler AA III. Tumor necrosis factor-alpha and interleukin-6 selectively regulate neutrophil function in vitro. *J Surg Res* 1995; 58(2):124–130.
102. Call DR, Nemzek JA, Ebong SJ, Bolgos GL, Newcomb DE, Remick DG. Ratio of local to systemic chemokine concentrations regulates neutrophil recruitment. *Am J Pathol* 2001; 158:715–721.
103. Pape H-C, Remmers D, Grotz M, Kotzerke J, von Glinski S, van Griensven M, Dahlweid M, Sznidar S, Tscherne H. Reticuloendothelial system activity and organ failure in patients with multiple injuries. *Arch Surg* 1999; 134:421–427.
104. van Griensven M, Kuzu M, Breddin M, Bottcher F, Krettek C, Pape HC, Tschernig T. Polymicrobial sepsis induces organ changes due to granulocyte adhesion in a murine two hit model of trauma. *Exp Toxic Pathol* 2002; 54:203–209.
105. Kurose I, Anderson DC, Miyasaka M, Tamatani T, Paulson JC, Todd RF, Rusche JR, Granger DN. Molecular determinants of reperfusion-induced leukocyte adhesion and vascular protein leakage. *Circ Res* 1994; 74:336–343.
106. Butcher EC. Leukocyte-endothelial cell recognition: three (or more) steps to specificity and diversity. *Cell* 1991; 67:1033–1036.
107. Bargatze RF, Kurk S, Watts G, Kishimoto T K, Speer CA, Jutila MA. In vivo and in vitro functional examination of a conserved epitope of L- and E-Selectin crucial for leukocyte-endothelial cell interactions. *J Immunol* 1994; 152:5814–5825.
108. Springer TA. Adhesion receptors of the immune system. *Nature* 1990; 346:425–434.
109. van Griensven M, Probst C, Müller K, Hoevel P, Pape HC. Leukocyte-endothelial interactions via ICAM-1 are detrimental in polymicrobial sepsis. *Shock* 2006; 25:254–259.

110. Barkhausen T, Krettek C, van Griensven M. L-selectin: adhesion, signalling and its impor-
     tance in pathologic posttraumatic endotoxemia and non-septic inflammation. *Exp Toxic
     Pathol* 2005; 57:39–52.
111. Kerner T, Ahlers O, Spielmann S, Keh D, Buhrer C, Gerlach M, Hofler S, Gerlach H..
     L-selectin in trauma patients: a marker for organ dysfunction and outcome? *Eur J Clin Invest*
     1999; 29(12):1077–1086.
112. Seekamp A, van Griensven M, Hildebrandt F, Brauer N, Jochum M, Martin M. The effect of
     trauma on neutrophil L-selectin expression and sL-selectin serum levels. *Shock* 2001;
     15(4):254-60.
113. Muller JC, Buhrer C, Kiening KL, Kerner T, Gerlach H, Obladen M, Unterberg AW, Lanksch
     WR. Decreased soluble adhesion moleculeL-selectin plasma concentrations after major
     trauma. *J Trauma* 1998; 45(4):705–708.
114. Maekawa K, Futami S, Nishida M, Terada T, Inagawa H, Suzuki S, Ono K. Effects of trauma
     and sepsis on soluble L-Selectin and cell surface expression of L-selectin and CD11b.
     J Trauma 1998; 44(3):460–467.
115. Cocks RA, Chan TY, Rainer TH. Leucocyte L-selectin is up-regulated after mechanical
     trauma in adults. *J Trauma* 1998; 45(1):1–6.
116. van Griensven M, Barkhausen T, Hildebrand F et al. L-selectin shows time and gender
     dependency in association with MODS. *Injury* 2004; 35:1087–1095.
117. Ahmed NA, Christou NV. Decreased neutrophil L-selectin expression in patients with
     systemic inflammatory response syndrome. *Clin Invest Med* 1996; 19(6):427–434.
118. McGill SN, Ahmed NA, Hu F, Michel RP, Christou NV. Shedding of L-selectin as a mecha-
     nism for reduced polymorphonuclear neutrophil exudation in patients with the systemic
     inflammatory response syndrome. *Arch Surg* 1996; 131:1141–1147.
119. Stengel D, Orth M, Tauber R, Sehouli J, Hentsch S, Thielemann H, Laun R, Ekkernkamp A.
     Shed L-selectin (sCD62L) load in trauma patients. *J Surg Res* 2001; 99:321–327.
120. Schlag G, Redl H, Till GO, Davies J, Martin U, Dumont L. Anti-L-selectin antibody treat-
     ment of hemorrhagic-traumatic shock in baboons. *Crit Care Med* 1999; 27(9):1900–1907.
121. Ramamoorthy C, Sharar SR, Harlan JM, Tedder TF, Winn RK. Blocking L-selectin function
     attenuates reperfusion injury following hemorrhagic shock in rabbits. *Am J Physiol* 1996;
     271:H1871–H1877.
122. Seekamp A, Regel G, Rother K, Jutila M. The effect of anti-L-selectin (EL-246) on remote
     lung injury after infrarenal ischemia/reperfusion. *Shock* 1997; 7(6):447–454.
123. Redl H, Martin U, Khadem A, Pelinka LE, van Griensven M. Anti-L-selectin antibody
     therapy does not worsen the postseptic course in a baboon model. *Crit Care* 2005;
     9:R735–R744.
124. Seekamp A, van Griensven M, Breyhahn K, Pohlemann T. The effect of fucoidin on the
     remote pulmonary injury in a two-hit trauma model in mice. *Eur J Trauma* 2001;
     27(6):317–326.
125. Seekamp A, van Griensven M, Dhondt E, Diefenbeck M, Demeyer I, Vundelinckx G, Haas
     N, Schaechinger U, Wolowicka L, Rammelt S. The effect of anti-L-selectin (aselizumab) in
     multiply traumatized patients – Results of a phase II clinical trial. *Crit Care Med* 2004;
     32:2021–2028.
126. Rothlein R, Dustin ML, Marlin SD, Springer TA. A human intercellular adhesion molecule
     (ICAM-1) distinct from LFA-1. *J Immunol* 1986; 137:1270–1274.
127. Staunton DE, Dustin ML, Springer TA. Functional cloning of ICAM-2, a cell adhesion
     ligand for LFA-1 homologous to ICAM-1. *Nature* 1989; 339:61–64.
128. Staunton DE, Marlin SD, Stratowa C, Dustin ML, Springer TA. Primary structure of
     ICAM-1 demonstrates interaction between members of the immunoglobulin and integrin
     supergene families. *Cell* 1988; 52:925–933.
129. Tsokos M, Fehlauer F. Post-mortem markers of sepsis: an immunohistochemical study using
     VLA-4 (CD49d/CD29) and ICAM-1 (CD54) for the detection of sepsis-induced lung injury.
     Int J Legal Med 2001; 114(4–5):291–294.

130. Muller Kobold AC, Tulleken JE, Zijlstra JG, Sluiter W, Hermans J, Kallenberg CG. Leukocyte activation in sepsis; correlations with disease state and mortality. *Intensive Care Med* 2000; 26(7):883–892.
131. Menges T, Engel J, Welters I, Wagner RM, Little S, Ruwoldt R, Wollbrueck M, Hempelmann G. Changes in blood lymphocyte populations after multiple trauma: association with posttraumatic complications. *Crit Care Med* 1999; 27(4):733–740.
132. Fosse E, Trumpy JH, Skulberg A. Alterations in T-helper and T-suppressor lymphocyte populations after multiple injuries. *Injury* 1987; 18(3):199–202.
133. Cheadle WG, Pemberton RM, Robinson D, Livingston DH, Rodriguez JL, Polk HC Jr. Lymphocyte subset responses to trauma and sepsis. *J Trauma* 1993; 35(6):844–849.
134. Pellegrini JD, De AK, Kodys K, Puyana JC, Furse RK, Miller-Graziano C. Relationships between T lymphocyte apoptosis and anergy following trauma. *J Surg Res* 2000; 88(2):200–206.
135. Hotchkiss RS, Schmieg RE, Jr., Swanson PE, Freeman BD, Tinsley KW, Cobb JP, Karl IE, Buchman TG. Rapid onset of intestinal epithelial and lymphocyte apoptotic cell death in patients with trauma and shock. *Crit Care Med* 2000; 28(9):3207–3217.
136. Faist E, Schinkel C, Zimmer S, Kremer JP, Von Donnersmarck GH, Schildberg FW. Inadequate interleukin-2 synthesis and interleukin-2 messenger expression following thermal and mechanical trauma in humans is caused by defective transmembrane signalling. *J Trauma* 1993; 34(6):846–853.
137. Wick M, Kollig E, Muhr G, Koller M. The potential pattern of circulating lymphocytes TH1/TH2 is not altered after multiple injuries. *Arch Surg* 2000; 135(11):1309–1314.
138. van Griensven M, Dahlweid M, Giannoudis PV, Wittwer T, Bottcher F, Breddin M, Pape HC. Dehydroepiandrosterone (DHEA) modulates the activity and the expression of lymphocyte subpopulations induced by cecal ligation and puncture. *Shock* 2002; 18(5):445–449.
139. Carson WE, Yu H, Dierksheide J, Pfeffer K, Bouchard P, Clark R, Durbin J, Baldwin AS, Peschon J, Johnson PR, Ku G, Baumann H, Caligiuri MA. A fatal cytokine-induced systemic inflammatory response reveals a critical role for NK cells. *J Immunol* 1999; 162:4943–4951.
140. Godshall CJ, Scott MJ, Burch PT, Peyton JC, Cheadle WG. Natural killer cells participate in bacterial clearance during septic peritonitis through interactions with macrophages. *Shock* 2003; 19(2):144–149.
141. Faist E, Mewes A, Strasser T, Walz A, Alkan S, Baker C, Ertel W, Heberer G. Alteration of monocyte function following major injury. *Arch Surg* 1988; 123(3):287–292.
142. Keel M, Schregenberger N, Steckholzer U, Ungethüm U, Kenney J, Trentz O, Ertel W. Endotoxin tolerance after severe injury and its regulatory mechanisms. *J Trauma* 1996; 41(3):430–437.
143. Kruger C, Schutt C, Obertacke U, Joka T, Müller FE, Knöller J, Köller M, König W, Schönfeld W. Serum CD14 levels in polytraumatized and severely burned patients. *Clin Exp Immunol* 1991; 85(2):297–301.
144. Carrillo EH, Gordon L, Goode E, Davis E, Polk HC Jr. Early elevation of soluble CD14 may help identify trauma patients at high risk for infection. *J Trauma* 2001; 50(5):810–816.
145. Livingston DH, Appel SH, Wellhausen SR, Sonnenfeld G, Polk HC Jr. Depressed interferon gamma production and monocyte HLA-DR expression after severe injury. *Arch Surg* 1988; 123(11):1309–1312.
146. Cosgriff N, Moore EE, Sauaia A, Kenny-Moynihan M, Burch JM, Galloway B. Predicting life-threatening coagulopathy in the massively transfused trauma patient: hypothermia and acidoses revisited. *J Trauma* 1997; 42(5):857–861.
147. MacLeod JB, Lynn M, McKenney MG, Cohn SM, Murtha M. Early coagulopathy predicts mortality in trauma. *J Trauma* 2003; 55(1):39–44.
148. Kaufmann CR, Dwyer KM, Crews JD, Dols SJ, Trask AL. Usefulness of thrombelastography in assessment of trauma patient coagulation. *J Trauma* 1997; 42(4):716–720.

149. Brohi K, Singh J, Heron M, Coats T. Acute traumatic coagulopathy. *J Trauma* 2003; 54(6):1127–1130.
150. Practice Guidelines for blood component therapy: A report by the American Society of Anesthesiologists Task Force on Blood Component Therapy. *Anesthesiology* 1996; 84(3):732–747.
151. Hardy JF, De Moerloose P, Samama M. Massive transfusion and coagulopathy: pathophysiology and implications for clinical management. *Can J Anaesth* 2004; 51(4):293–310.
152. Dutton RP, McCunn M, Hyder M, D'Angelo M, O'Connor J, Hess J, Scalea TM. Factor VIIa for correction of traumatic coagulopathy. *J Trauma* 2004; 57(4):709–718.
153. Martinowitz U, Michaelson M. Guidelines for the use of recombinant activated factor VII (rFVIIa) in uncontrolled bleeding: a report by the Israeli Multidisciplinary rFVIIa Task Force. *J Thromb Haemost* 2005; 3(4):640–648.
154. Roumen RM, Redl H, Schlag G, Zilow G, Sandtner W, Koller W, Hendriks T, Goris RJA. Inflammatory mediators in relation to the development of multiple organ failure in patients after severe blunt trauma. *Crit Care Med* 1995; 23(3):474–480.
155. Huber-Lang M, Sarma JV, Zetoune FS, Rittirsch D, Neff TA, McGuire SR, Lambris JD, Warner RL, Flierl MA, Hoesel LM, Gebhard F, Younger JG, Drouin SM, Wetsel RA, Ward PA. Generation of C5a in the absence of C3: a new complement activation pathway. *Nat Med* 2006; 12:682–687.
156. Pape HC, Schmidt RE, Rice J, van Griensven M, Das Gupta R, Krettek C, Tscherne H. Biochemical changes after trauma and skeletal surgery of the lower extremity: quantification of the operative burden. *J Orthop Trauma* 2004; 18(8 Suppl):S24–S31.

Chapter 4
Pathogenetic Changes: Secondary Abdominal Compartment Syndrome

Rao R. Ivatury, Ajai K. Malhotra, Michel B. Aboutanos, Thérèse M. Duane, and Julie A. Mayglothling

4.1 Introduction

The World Society of Abdominal Compartment Syndrome (WSACS), formed by a group of investigators interested in the syndrome, has had three sessions as world congresses. The most recent one was in Antwerp, Belgium, in March 2007. The society reviewed the existing literature on the syndrome and proposed consensus definitions and recommendations [1, 2] for several key elements. State-of-the-art concepts have also been published as a monograph [3]. The consensus definition of Intra-Abdominal Hypertension (IAH) is a persistently elevated Intra-Abdominal Pressure (IAP) greater than 12 mmHg. Abdominal Compartment Syndrome (ACS) is defined by the WSACS as 'the presence of IAH accompanied by organ dysfunction(s) such as cardiac, respiratory, and renal [1] dysfunction.' ACS is referred to as "secondary" when there are no conditions originating from the abdomino-pelvic region.

4.2 Incidence

Based on a prospective shock trauma database, Balogh and colleagues [4] reported the incidence of postinjury secondary ACS to be 0.09% of all trauma admissions, 0.70% of all trauma ICU admissions, and 8.00% of shock/trauma patients requiring aggressive resuscitation (with ISS > 15, requiring more than 6 units of Packed Red Blood Cell (PRBC) transfusions during the first 12 h and having initial Base Deficit (BD) greater than 6 mEq/L) [5–7]. Burn patients,

R.R. Ivatury (✉)
Department of Surgery, Virginia Commonwealth University Health System,
1200 East Broad Street, W15E, Richmond, VA, 23298, USA
e-mail: rivatury@hsc.vcu.edu

H.-C. Pape et al. (eds.), *Damage Control Management in the Polytrauma Patient*,
DOI 10.1007/978-0-387-89508-6_4, © Springer Science+Business Media, LLC 2010

particularly with >70% BSA burns or inhalation injury, are also potentially susceptible for this syndrome [8, 9]. Postinjury secondary ACS occurs early in resuscitation, within 12–14 h after hospital admission [4–7]. Rodas and colleagues [10] described a "hyperacute ACS" among 0.13% of trauma patients from excessive resuscitation, identified within 4.8 h of admission, during initial resuscitation.

4.3 Pathogenesis and Rationale

Secondary ACS is typically seen in clinical situations in which massive, uncontrolled resuscitation is taking place. Classic examples are extensive burns, multisystem injuries with multiple extremity injuries, and severe penetrating chest injuries or extremity vascular injuries [4–10]. Trauma patients with multiple pelvic and long bone fractures may undergo resuscitation primarily in uncontrolled areas such as the interventional radiology suite, where there is a potential for massive fluid resuscitation. The syndrome can also be seen in patients with peritonitis, sepsis, and hypothermia [11]. Hemorrhagic or septic shock with or without tissue injury may lead to whole body ischemia/reperfusion injury due to the effects of inflammatory cells and mediators. The resulting increased permeability and hydrostatic pressure are the key early driving forces for interstitial fluid accumulation. Massive crystalloid resuscitation that is perhaps inevitable in the early phases of resuscitation will contribute to the problem of third space fluid losses into the peritoneal cavity, bowel lumen, bowel wall, as well as the retroperitoneal tissues – all contributing to intra-abdominal hypertension. The elevated intra-abdominal pressure impairs venous and lymphatic outflow from the gut and thus worsens gut edema by increasing capillary filtration pressure. Associated gastrointestinal ileus and reduced abdominal wall compliance may aggravate the IAP elevation [11]. Balogh and colleagues [4, 12], in a prospective trauma database, identified supranormal resuscitation as an important contributor for the development of IAH. Greater than 6 L of resuscitation and greater than 6 units of packed cell transfusions in a 6-h period have been mentioned as predictive of secondary ACS [7]. Ivy [8] observed, in burn patients, that greater than 0.25 L/Kg crystalloid resuscitation is a marker for development of ACS. Balogh and colleagues [12] showed from their data that independent risk factors for ACS may be identified very early, with 0.88 accuracy at the time of emergency department discharge and with 0.99 accuracy 1 h after ICU admission with adequate monitoring. These risk factors in the ED include: crystalloid infusion >3 L, no urgent surgery, and PRBC transfusion >3 units. In the ICU, gastric mucosal $paCO_2$ (by gastric tonometry) >16, crystalloid infusion >7.5 L, and urine output <150 ml (ICU) predicted secondary ACS. It is evident that all of these factors are surrogates for a patient in cellular anaerobiosis receiving massive, uncontrolled resuscitation.

The exact pathogenesis for the secondary ACS and subsequent onset of multiorgan failure is not established. In a series of experiments, one of the authors (Ivatury) has shown that the combined effects of sequential ischemia-reperfusion (shock and resuscitation) followed by intra-abdominal hypertension are additive, with the effects more than those of either insult alone. There is an amplified response with reduction of splanchnic flow as well as cytokine response and lung injury in pigs subjected to hemorrhagic shock, resuscitation, and subsequent intra-abdominal hypertension; this is a clinically pertinent model [13–15]. Moore and colleagues [16–18] have demonstrated that the postinjury neutrophil priming exhibits augmented elastase release for membrane degradation, increased CD11b/CD18 expression for adhesion, increased release of IL-8 to attract more neutrophils, and delayed apoptosis prolonging cytotoxicity. This augmented response pattern occurs maximally 3–16-h postinjury. Importantly, this corresponds to the time period when ACS most commonly occurs. ACS then acts as a second-hit to start the cascade of multiorgan failure. Mesenteric lymph may play an important role as the carrier of the primed neutrophils to distant circulation and cause distant organ failure. The role of bacterial translocation has not been uniformly defined [18–20]. The pathogenesis of the syndrome is summarized in Fig. 4.1.

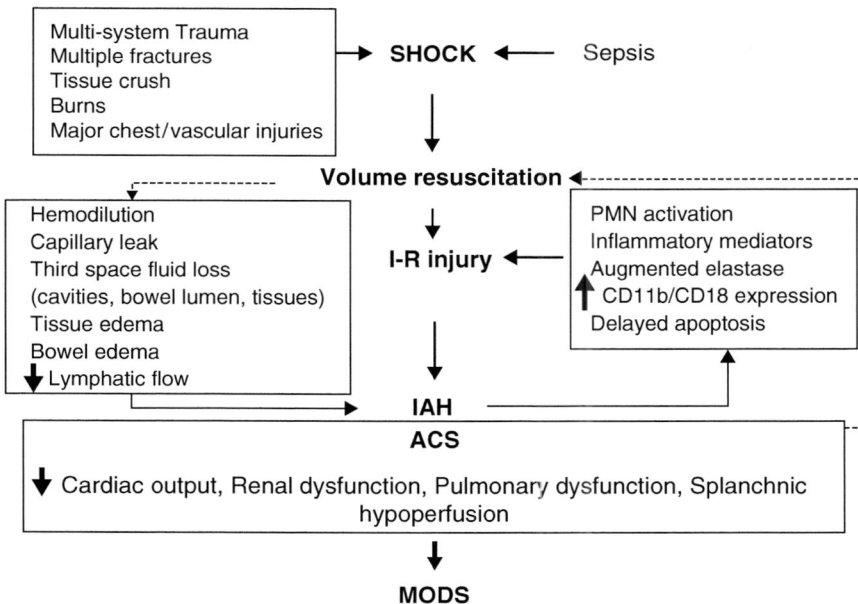

Fig. 4.1 Pathogenesis of secondary abdominal compartment syndrome. *I-R* ischemia-reperfusion; *IAH* intra-abdominal hypertension; *ACS* abdominal compartment syndrome; *MODS* multiorgan dysfunction syndrome

4.4 Decision Making Factors

The clinical indicators of secondary ACS are elevated IAP, elevated Peak Airway Pressure (PAP), poor cardiac index and low urine output, decreased tidal volume, and fictitiously elevated central venous pressure. Measurement of IAP by bladder pressure measurement, preferably by continuous measurement but at least intermittently, is the recommended method. Clinical examination, for example, palpation of the abdomen and measurement of abdominal girth, are inaccurate predictors of elevated IAP [21, 22]. In some clinical situations (e.g., massive extremity injuries with fractures and crush injury, exsanguinating vascular injuries in patients in profound shock), there may not be an opportunity to institute IAP monitoring. These are the patients who are transported urgently to the operating room for control of hemorrhage and resuscitation. The authors have described intra-operative diagnosis of secondary ACS in such patients by the observation that the patient's ventilation is becoming increasingly difficult [10]. (A special pitfall: This has been misdiagnosed as a tension pneumothorax, and a chest tube has been inserted into the lower chest, inadvertently into the abdomen under the diaphragm, which is elevated from the IAH.) As described earlier, the consequences of delayed diagnosis and treatment of secondary ACS are profound.

4.5 Strategies and Recommendations for Treatment

The standard treatment of secondary ACS is surgical decompression and the application of temporary abdominal closure. Since outcome depends upon the rapidity with which the diagnosis is made and decompression performed, the earlier the decompression, the better the outcome. In a series in which all secondary ACS patients were decompressed within 24 h, there was no difference between earlier and later decompression. Decompression may be performed nonoperatively by percutaneous drainage of the excessive peritoneal fluid. It does not affect bowel edema or tissue edema, yet the results of such an approach are effective, especially in the burn population. This may be combined with a judicious use of diuretics, once tissue acidosis and oxygen debt are corrected. If this does not reduce IAP or if the paracentesis is unsuccessful, surgical decompression is essential. This may be accomplished in the operating room or in the ICU, if the patient is critical and will not tolerate transport. After abdominal decompression, a temporary vacuum dressing is applied, and the "open abdomen" is managed by the many options that are available [23–27]. Unless the decompression is performed late after the onset of ACS, the immediate response is uniformly good. If decompression is delayed until there is tense abdomen and high IAP, there is the danger of "reperfusion syndrome," which may manifest as sudden hypotension and cardiac arrest. Perhaps because of this variability in the time for decompression, the ultimate results reported in the literature have been variable [4–7].

4.6 Strategies and Recommendations for Prevention and Surveillance

Postinjury secondary ACS can be prevented by exquisite treatment of hemorrhagic shock with attention to timely hemorrhage control and avoidance of supranormal oxygen delivery and "over-resuscitation." Multisystem injuries with extensive soft tissue trauma may be particularly prone for reperfusion injury and should prompt careful resuscitation based on end-points and the institution of IAP monitoring. *Controlled resuscitation* is the key, and the patient should spend less time in uncontrolled, unmonitored circumstances. Burn resuscitation may be initiated by standard resuscitation formulas, but it should be guided as soon as possible by the hourly urine output of 0.5 ml/kg/h. Recent studies suggest that colloid solutions may be preferable to crystalloids in burn patients, and hypertonic saline resuscitation may minimize secondary ACS as compared to conventional crystalloid resuscitation [28, 29]. Many anti-inflammatory approaches have been or are being investigated to ameliorate the primary insult, including hypertonic saline resuscitative strategies. Closed loop computer-driven resuscitation using fluid administration proportional to the measured value of a predefined end-point may achieve favorable outcomes with less over-all fluid administration and avoidance of over-resuscitation [16].

4.7 Summary and Conclusion

Secondary ACS is a preventable complication. Recognizing the patient population at risk, resuscitation must be fastidious and not uncontrolled. Tireless efforts at prevention of secondary ACS must be the goal, and "over-resuscitation" must be avoided. Resuscitation must be guided by measured end-points, and indiscriminate fluid infusion must be avoided. Both inadequate resuscitation and "over-resuscitation" are harmful to the patient. In this context, it is worth remembering the admonition by Pruitt [30]: 'Push the pendulum of resuscitation back from the realm of excess.' Early diagnosis of the impending abdominal compartment syndrome by a high index of suspicion is crucial in those circumstances in which the patients are taken to the operating room emergently. The operating team (including subspecialists in orthopedic surgery, neurosurgery, etc.) as well as the anesthesiologists must all be familiar with the syndrome, so that the "hyperacute" secondary ACS is recognized promptly and the abdomen decompressed immediately for the patient to survive the initial operation. In patients who are taken to the Intensive Care Unit, bladder pressure monitoring must be instituted early. Recognition and rapid and appropriate therapy are the cornerstones for a successful outcome.

References

1. Malbrain ML, Cheatham ML, Kirkpatrick A, Sugrue M, Parr M, De Waele J, Balogh Z, Leppäniemi A, Olvera C, Ivatury R, D'Amours S, Wilmer A, Wendon J, Hillman K. Results from the International Conference of experts on intra-abdominal hypertension and abdominal compartment syndrome. I. Definitions. Intensive Care Medicine 2006;32(11):1722–1732.
2. Cheatham ML, Malbrain ML, Kirkpatrick A, Sugrue M, Parr M, De Waele J, Balogh Z, Leppaniemi A, Olvera C, Ivatury R, D'Amours S, Wendon J, Hillman K, Johansson K, Kolkman K, Wilmer A. Results from the International Conference of experts on intra-abdominal hypertension and abdominal compartment syndrome II Recommendations. Intensive Care Med 2007;33(6):951–962.
3. Ivatury RR, Cheatham ML, Malbrain ML, Sugrue M (eds) *Abdominal Compartment Syndrome*. Georgetown: Landes Bioscience, 2006.
4. Balogh Z, McKinley BA, Cocanour CS, Kozar RA, Holcomb JB, Ware DN, Moore FA. Secondary abdominal compartment syndrome: an elusive complication of traumatic shock resuscitation. Am J Surg 2002;184:538–544.
5. Maxwell RA, Fabian TC, Croce MA, Davis KA. Secondary abdominal compartment syndrome: an underappreciated manifestation of severe hemorrhagic shock. J Trauma 1999;47:995–999.
6. Kopelman T, Harris C, Miller R, Arrillaga A. Abdominal compartment syndrome in patients with isolated extraperitoneal injuries. J Trauma 2000;49:744–749.
7. Biffl WL, Moore EE, Burch JM, Offner PJ, Franciose RJ, Johnson JL. Secondary abdominal compartment syndrome is a highly lethal event. Am J Surgery 2001;182:645–648.
8. Ivy ME. Secondary mabdominal compartment syndrome in burns. In: Ivatury RR, Cheatham ML, Malbrain ML, Sugrue M (eds), *Abdominal Compartment Syndrome*. Georgetown: Landes Bioscience, 2006
9. Tuggle D, Skinner S, Garza J, Vandijck D, Blot S. The abdominal compartment syndrome in patients with burn injury. Acta Clinica Belg 2007;62(Suppl 1):136–140.
10. Rodas EB, Malhotra AK, Chhitwal R, Aboutanos MB, Duane TM, Ivatury RR. Hyperacute abdominal compartment syndrome: an unrecognized complication of massive intraoperative resuscitation for extra-abdominal injuries. Am Surg 2005;75(11):977–981.
11. Kirkpatrick AW, De Waele JJ, Ball CG, Ranson K, Widder S, Laupland KB. The secondary and recurrent abdominal compartment syndrome. Acta Clin Belg 2007;62(Suppl 1):60–65.
12. Balogh Z, McKinley BA, Holcomb JB, Miller CC, Cocanour CS, Kozar RA, Moore FA. Both primary and secondary abdominal compartment syndrome (ACS) can be predicted early and are harbingers of multiple organ failure. J Trauma 2003;54:848–861.
13. Simon RJ, Friedlander MH, Ivatury RR, DiRaimo R, Machiedo GW. Hemorrhage lowers the threshold for intra-abdominal hypertension (IAH) induced pulmonary dysfunction. J Trauma 1997;42:398–405.
14. Friedlander M, Simon RJ, Ivatury RR, DiRaimo R. The effect of hemorrhage on SMA flow during increased intra-abdominal pressure. J Trauma 1998;45:433–439.
15. Oda J, Ivatury RR, Blocher CR, Malhotra AJ, Sugerman HJ. Amplified cytokine response and lung injury by sequential hemorrhagic shock and abdominal compartment syndrome in a laboratory model of ischemia-reperfusion. J Trauma 2002;52:625–631.
16. Rezende-Neto JB, Moore EE, Masuno T, Moore PK, Johnson JL, Sheppard FR, Cunha-Melo JR, Silliman CC. The abdominal compartment syndrome as a second insult during systemic neutrophil priming provokes multiple organ injury. Shock 2003;20:303–308.
17. Rezende-Neto J, Moore EE, Melo de Andrade MV, Teixeira MM, Lisboa FA, Arantes RM , De Souza DG, Da Cunha-Melo JR. Systemic inflammatory response secondary to abdominal compartment syndrome: stage for multiple organ failure. J Trauma 2002;53:1121–1128.
18. Raeburn C, Moore EE. Abdominal compartment syndrome provokes multiple organ failure: Animal and human supporting evidence. In: Ivatury RR, Cheatham ML, Malbrain ML, Sugrue M (eds.) *Abdominal Compartment Syndrome*. Georgetown: Landes Bioscience, 2006

19. Balogh Z, McKinley BA, Cox Jr CS, Allen SJ, Cocanour CS, Kozar RA, Moore EE, Miller IC, Weisbrodt NW, Moore FA. Abdominal compartment syndrome: The cause or effect of postinjury multiple organ failure. Shock 2003;20:483–492.
20. Doty JM, Oda J, Ivatury RR, Blocher CR, Christie GE, Yelon JA, Sugerman HJ. The effects of hemodynamic shock and increased intra-abdominal pressure on bacterial translocation. J Trauma 2002;52:13–17.
21. Kirkpatrick AW, Brenneman FD, McLean RF, Rapanos T, Boulanger BR. Is clinical examination an accurate indicator of raised intra-abdominal pressure in critically injured patients? Can J Surg 2000;43:207–211.
22. Sugrue M, Bauman A, Jones F, Bishop G, Flabouris A, Parr M, Stewart A, Hillman K, Deane SA. Clinical examination is an inaccurate predictor of intra-abdominal pressure. World J Surg 2002;26:1428–1431.
23. Ivatury RR, Kolkman KA, Johansson K. Management of open abdomen. Acta Clin Belg Suppl 2007;62(1):206–209.
24. Schechter W, Ivatury RR, Rotondo MF, Hirshberg A. Open abdomen after trauma and abdominal sepsis: A strategy for management. J Am Coll Surg 2006;203(3):390–396.
25. Ivatury RR, Latifi R, Malhotra AK. Abdominal compartment syndrome, recognition and management. In: Cameron J (ed.), *Current Surgical Therapy* 8th edition, Philadelphia, PA: Elsevier Mosby, 2004.
26. Ivatury RR, Malhotra AK, Aboutanis MB et al. The abdomen that won't close. In: Cameron J (ed), *Current Surgical Therapy*, 9th edition. Philadelphia: Mosby 2009, pp. 1019–1027.
27. Cothren CC, Moore EE, Johnson JL, Moore JB, Burch JM. One hundred percent fascial approximation with sequential abdominal closure of the open abdomen. Am J Surg 2006;192(2):238–242.
28. O'Mara MS, Slater H, Goldfarb IW, Caushaj PF. A prospective, randomized evaluation of intra-abdominal pressures with crystalloid and colloid resuscitation in burn patients. J Trauma 2005;58:1011–1018.
29. Oda J, Ueyama M, Yamashita K, Inoue T, Noborio M, Ode Y, Aoki Y, Sugimoto H. Hypertonic lactated saline resuscitation reduces the risk of abdominal compartment syndrome in severely burned patients. J Trauma 2006;60:64–71.
30. Pruitt BA. Protection from excessive resuscitation: "Pushing the pendulum back." J Trauma 2000;49:567–568.

Chapter 5
Impact of Head and Chest Trauma on General Condition

Otmar Trentz and Philipp M. Lenzlinger

5.1 Epidemiology

The clinical course and outcome of the polytraumatized patient is largely determined by the severity and the pattern of injuries sustained. Blunt chest trauma and Traumatic Brain Injury (TBI) represent the two major single injury entities with the highest risk of causing complications during treatment and recovery from severe multiple injuries.

A study based on the registry of the German Society of Trauma Surgery (DGU) reported relevant (Abbreviated Injury Scale AIS score >3) chest injury to be present in up to 52% of polytraumatized patients, depending on the cause of accident, while severe TBI was reported in 38% of motor Vehicle Accident (MVA) victims and 47% of pedestrians [1]. Similarly, in a prospective cohort of over 1,000 multiply-injured patients with orthopedic injuries, 81% also suffered from TBI and 52% from blunt chest trauma [2]. Moreover, about half of the polytraumatized patients who suffer from severe TBI, also sustain a blunt chest injury [3].

The presence of significant (AIS >3) chest or head injuries, respectively, increase both Length of Stay (LOS) in the Intensive Care Unit (ICU) as well as the number of days on respirator [1]. Furthermore, at around 27% ,severe TBI is the most common cause of death in injured patients and has a significantly elevated lethality (3.4%) as compared to overall mortality from trauma (2.2%) [4]. Similarly, chest injury may account for 20–25% of polytrauma deaths [5].

O. Trentz (✉)
Department of Surgery, University Hospital Zürich, Raemistrasse 100,
Zürich, 8091, Switzerland
e-mail: otmar.trentz@usa.ch

H.-C. Pape et al. (eds.), *Damage Control Management in the Polytrauma Patient*,
DOI 10.1007/978-0-387-89508-6_5, © Springer Science+Business Media, LLC 2010

5.2   Pathophysiology

Death due to trauma follows a trimodal time distribution:

During the first phase of seconds to minutes following trauma, patients succumb to immediate organ failure due to direct primary injury to the central nervous system (CNS) or exsanguination from rupture of the heart or the thoracic aorta.

A large number of patients die within the first few hours after trauma due to intracranial compression (epidural and subdural hematomas, generalized brain edema) or uncontrollable bleeding from lacerated intra-abdominal or intrathroacic organs as well as from retroperitoneal bleeding following pelvic ring disruption.

During the third phase, which lasts a few days to several weeks, patients suffer from secondary injuries due to hypoxia and infection, leading too often to fatal organ dysfunction.

Understanding the pathophysiology of this tertiary phase is essential for the treatment of multiply-injured patients in order to avoid the so-called "second hit" phenomena due to operative interventions.

Both the injured brain and lungs are important targets as well as effector organs in the systemic response to trauma. Therefore, TBI and blunt chest injury – or worse, the combination of both – put the patient at a high risk of complications during this phase of recovery from severe trauma.

5.3   The Host Defense Response

The reaction of the body to trauma is the result of a multitude of complex defense mechanisms aimed at isolating the damaged zone, reducing necrotic tissue, and inducing regeneration of the ensuing tissue defect. These mechanisms comprise a centrally regulated neuroendocrine activation, metabolic changes, and a pronounced systemic inflammatory response including an activation of the innate immune system. The sum of these processes is termed as the "host defense response," which is reversible and may be regarded as a physiologic reaction to trauma.

However, if these defense mechanisms become overwhelmed by the trauma and antigenic load and are additionally challenged through surgical interventions, it may lead to a pathologic, irreversible state commonly referred to as "host defense failure disease." This, in turn, may affect primarily uninjured organ systems and may lead to their impairment or failure (Multiple Organ Failure Syndrome, MODS), with potentially lethal outcome.

5.3.1   Neuroendocrine Reaction

The primary mechanical trauma as well as its secondary consequences stimulate a complex neuroendocrine response. Pain, stress, and fear as well as hypovolemia, hyperkapnia, acidosis, and endogenous and exogenous mediators from the injured region comprise the substantial afferent input of this axis. The efferent branch in turn leads to a massive release of stress hormones and inflammatory mediators, which influence the vegetative nervous system as well as the immune system (Fig. 5.1). The activation of the hypothalamic-pituitary-adrenal axis aims at

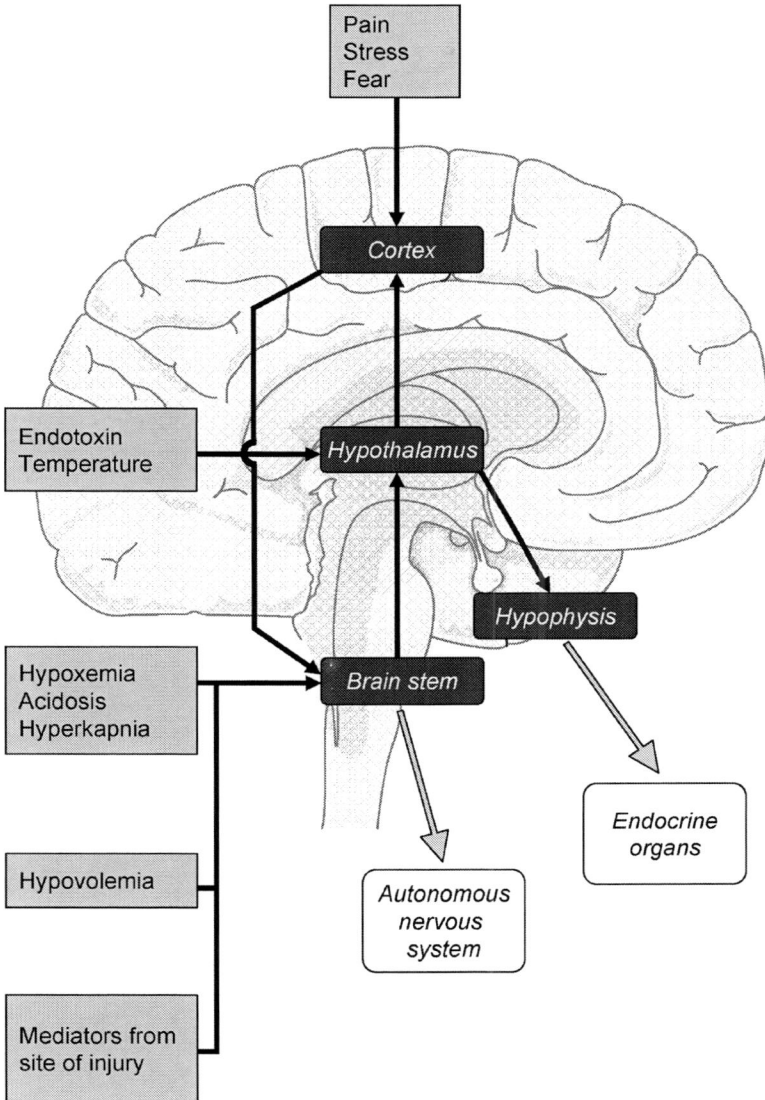

Fig. 5.1 Neuroendocine axis: The sequelae of trauma lead to activation of several brain regions and their interaction. Pituitary hormones and activation of vegetative centers in turn lead to the systemic acute phase response to trauma

maintaining the cardiovascular and metabolic homeostasis, leading to the metabolic (acute phase response) as well as the immunologic reaction to trauma. In that regard, the original notion of the immunologically privileged CNS has become overturned during the last decade in the context of trauma, since it has been shown that there is ample exchange between resident immunocompetent cells of the CNS (astrocytes, microglia, and neurons) and the systemic immune system.

5.3.2   Inflammatory Response

Mechanical trauma induces an unspecific humoral immune response in which the wound and its bacterial contamination play an important role. Activation of the xanthine oxidase pathway with consecutive accumulation of oxygen free radicals as well as of the complement cascade through the alternative pathway comprise the important first steps during the early phases of immune activation following trauma. This leads to recruitment of leukocytes through chemotaxis and to activation of granulocytes within the first 24 h after trauma, followed by the activation of monocytes and macrophages later on. Induction of the oxidative burst in granulocytes with release of oxygen radicals and proteases through metabolites of complement activation, leads to lipidperoxidation of cell membranes, which together with vasoactive substances such as histamine, increases membrane permeability (capillary-leak syndrome), facilitates in turn the invasion of the tissue by granulocytes. This may also affect the integrity of the Blood Brain Barrier (BBB). Other products of complement activation induce the systemic acute-phase-response, leading to hepatic induction of proinflammatory mediators. Proinflammatory cytokines such as tumor necrosis factor (TNF)-α, Interleukin (IL)-1β, IL-6, and IL-8 are released by activated leukocytes locally as well as systemically. Excessive stimulation of these proinflammatory pathways may lead to the progression of local inflammation to the whole organism, causing a systemic inflammation (Systemic Inflammatory Response Syndrome, SIRS). The ensuing generalized capillary leakage leads to fluid shifts into the interstitial space ("third compartment"), causing dysfunction of various organs, especially of the lungs, the liver, and the brain. In a large trauma registry study on more than 1,200 patients, Ertel and co-workers showed that the extent of SIRS correlates with the severity of MODS and Adult Respiratory Distress Syndrome (ARDS) as well as with the mortality following major trauma [6].

The lungs appear to be particularly prone to reacting to this hyperinflammatory state. The expression of proinflammatory cytokines, such as IL-6 and IL-8 as well as of the anti-inflammatory IL-10, has been shown to be higher within the lungs of multiply-injured patients than within the peripheral blood [7]. Therefore,blunt trauma itself and pulmonary contusion have also been identified as independent risk factors for the development of the ARDS [8]. Increased IL-10 production and HLA-DR suppression in the lungs of multitrauma patients have been shown to precede the development of nosocomial pneumonia [9]. Furthermore, local IL-10 production in the lungs has been linked to a suppression of alveolar effector cell apoptosis, leading to clinically significant pulmonary dysfunction [10]. Taken together, these data suggest an important role of the lung tissue as an immunologic organ in the development of post injury systemic inflammation (Fig. 5.2).

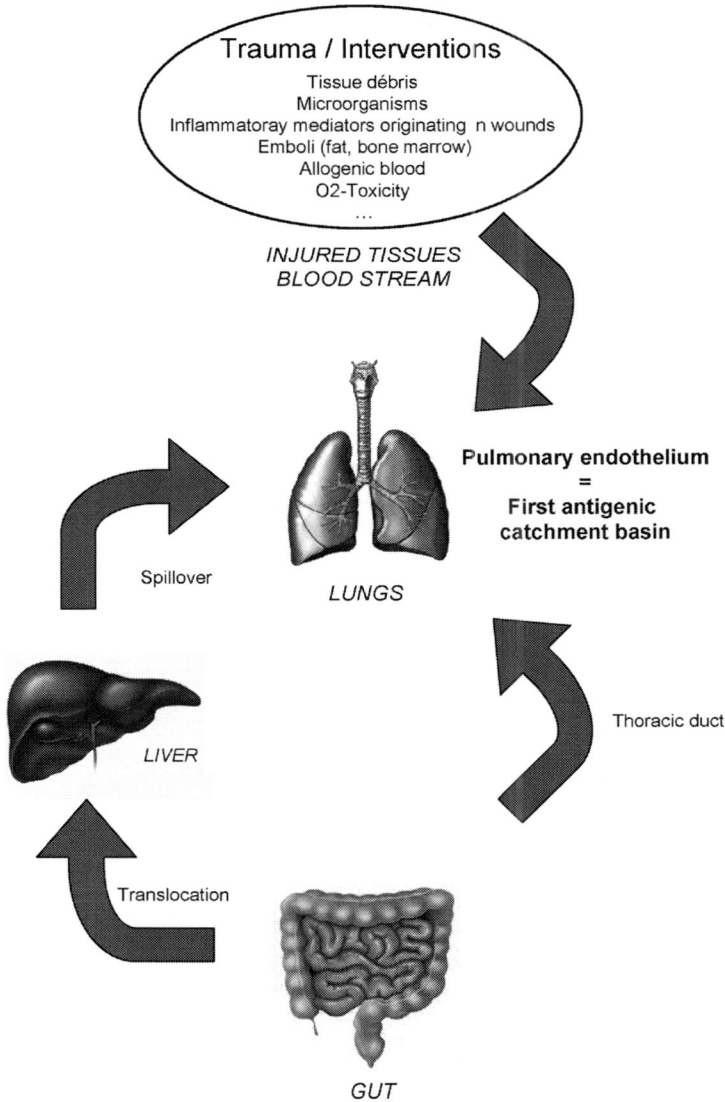

Fig. 5.2 The lung as a target organ: The antigenic load following trauma concentrates on the pulmonary endothelium, which serves as the initial immunologic point of contact

The phase of profound inflammation may progress into a phase of compensatory immunosuppression, marked by the release of anti-inflammatory cytokines such as IL-4 and IL-10 and a suppression of T-cell function, resulting in an elevated susceptibility of the trauma patient to infectious complications. This Compensatory Anti-inflammatory Response Syndrome (CARS) carries the risk of delayed MODS due to sepsis.

5.4   Secondary Brain Damage Following TBI

The extent of brain damage following trauma is determined on the one hand by the degree of immediate mechanical disruption of brain tissue due to the initial impact and deceleration (primary injury), and on the other hand by the incidence of pathophysiological changes leading to further damage of brain tissue (secondary injury). Secondary mechanisms involve such diverse pathways as a hypoxemia and hypotension [11–13] as well as a profound inflammatory response, excitatory amino acid, and calcium associated cytotoxicity, all of which may lead to acute as well as chronic cell destruction [14].

Apart from neurosurgical interventions for decompression and evacuation of intracranial mass lesions, treatment of the patient with severe TBI aims at maintaining adequate cerebral perfusion and oxygenation through circulatory and ventilatory support as well as through control of Intracranial Pressure (ICP).

5.4.1   Neuroinflammation

TBI leads to a profound but variable swelling of brain tissue. This swelling results in elevated ICP and reduced Cerebral Perfusion Pressure (CPP) and is generally believed to be one of the leading causes of unfavorable outcome following TBI [15]. The post-traumatic edema formation is due to complex cytotoxic events and vascular leakage following the breakdown of the BBB [16–18]. A profound disruption of the BBB has been observed in both experimental and clinical TBI [18–24].

Infiltration and accumulation of Polymorphonuclear Leukocytes (PMNs) into brain parenchyma have been observed in the early post-traumatic period [25]. Zhuang and colleagues [26] have suggested a relationship between cortical PMN accumulation and secondary brain injury, including lowered Cerebral Blood Flow (CBF), increased edema, and elevated ICP. The migration of leukocytes into damaged tissue typically requires the adhesion of these cells to the endothelium, which is mediated by the expression of the intercellular adhesion molecule (ICAM-1), a member of the immunoglobulin super gene family. An upregulation of ICAM-1 has, in fact, been described in experimental TBI [27–30], suggesting a role for leukocyte adhesion in the pathobiology of post-traumatic cell infiltration in the brain.

In humans, soluble ICAM-1 (sICAM-1) in Cerebrospinal Fluid (CSF) has been associated with the breakdown of the BBB after severe isolated TBI [24]. Immunocytochemical studies have further demonstrated the presence of macrophages, Natural Killer (NK) cells, helper T-cells, and T-cytotoxic suppressor cells as early as 2 days postinjury [31, 32]. The entry of macrophages into brain parenchyma following brain injury has been shown to be maximal by 24–48 h after TBI [25, 31, 32].

The specific cytokines and growth factors that have been implicated in the post-traumatic inflammatory cascade include TNF and the interleukin family of peptides, as well as Nerve Growth Factor (NGF) and Transforming Growth Factor-β (TGF-β) [33–36].

The traumatized brain, therefore, shows the classic hallmarks of inflammation: edema formation and swelling, activation of resident immune cells as well as cerebral infiltration by blood-borne immunocompetent cells, and impaired function. CNS inflammation was long believed to be a catastrophic event leading to sustained functional impairment and even death, as observed in other neuropathologies such as bacterial meningitis. However, there is increasing evidence that, in the setting of brain trauma, inflammatory pathways may be of vital importance for initiation of a regenerative response [37].

5.5 Systemic Effects of Brain Trauma

TBI is associated with a considerable rate of non-neurologic organ dysfunction. Most commonly, the respiratory system is affected, followed by cardiovascular dysfunction. Other disturbances observed affect renal and hepathologic as well as hematologic and endocrine functions. Furthermore, there is increasing evidence that the inflammatory response to brain trauma has significant systemic immunologic sequelae.

5.5.1 Respiratory Dysfunction

Acute Lung Injury (ALI), defined as a bilateral pathologic chest X-ray and a PaO_2/FiO_2 ratio of less than 300, has been found in 20–30% of patients with isolated TBI [38, 39]. In these studies, the development of ALI was associated with a twofold higher mortality rate and with a worse neurologic outcome. Neurogenic Pulmonary Edema (NPE) has been proposed as the cause for ALI following TBI [40]. The diagnosis of NPE is essentially one of exclusion, defined as bilateral pulmonary edema associated with normal left ventricular function, in the absence of any other cause for hypoxia or volume overload. However, a recent study exploring cardiac function in patients with NPE following TBI suggested a high incidence of clinically silent myocardial dysfunction in these patients [41]. Two different mechanisms appear to exist in the pathogenesis of NPE, both triggered by a sudden rise in ICP or localized ischemic damage in specific brain trigger zones in the hypothalamus, the medulla oblongata, and the area postrema, among others [42]:

The first mechanism: A hemodynamic mechanism secondary to intense pulmonary vasoconstriction due to the adrenergic response to CNS trauma, which results in an increase in pulmonary hydrostatic pressure, followed by an increase in the permeability of pulmonary vessels.

The second mechanism: An inflammatory mechanism following the neuroinflammatory response to trauma (see earlier discussion), ultimately leading to a pulmonary capillary leak as well (for a review see ref. [43]).

Recently, experimental TBI has been shown to cause extensive migration of inflammatory cells into the major airways [44].

Infection is a further major contributor to pulmonary dysfunction in patients suffering from TBI. In a study based on the Traumatic Coma Data Bank, over 40% of patients developed nosocomial pneumonia [45]. Although pneumonia is common among patients undergoing mechanical ventilation, there may be important differences in patients suffering from TBI. For instance, onset of pneumonia has been reported to occur earlier in TBI patients (day 3–4) compared to other ICU patients [46]. While there is evidence of systemic immunosuppression caused by TBI itself, specific therapies aimed at controlling intracranial hypertension, such as barbiturate coma and controlled hypothermia, may facilitate the development of pneumonia [47–49].

5.5.2 Cardiac Dysfunction

Because of the devastating effects of hypotension on neurologic outcome, cardiac dysfunction remains a challenging problem in the care of severely brain-injured patients. Although hemodynamic instability is a problem encountered daily in TBI patients, surprisingly little is known about the specific etiology of myocardial dysfunction following TBI. Echocardiographic evidence of myocardial dysfunction has been found in 41% of brain dead patients following severe TBI [50]. Massive catecholamine release, leading to myocytolysis and contraction-band necrosis, may be an explanation for these cardiologic abnormalities [51]. Furthermore, ischemic injury to specific brain trigger zones may play a role in cardiac dysfunction following severe TBI.

5.5.3 Coagulopathy

The reported incidence of blood clotting disturbances varies widely after brain trauma [52], but coagulopathy has been associated with poor outcome following TBI [53]. The brain tissue contains large amounts of thromboplastin, which is released into the blood stream after trauma to the brain parenchyma, causing disruption of coagulation homeostasis. In addition, damaged cerebral endothelium activates platelets as well as clotting cascades to produce intravascular thrombosis and depletion of coagulation factors, leading to Disseminated Intravascular Coagulation (DIC).

5.5.4 Immunologic Alterations

Markers for the activation of the cellular immune response have been found to be elevated following severe isolated TBI in serum as well as in the CSF, suggesting an important role of cellular immune activity in this context [54]. However, functional impairment of T-cells has been described in the same patient population [55–57].

Alterations in systemic concentrations of cytokines such as IL-1, IL-6, IL-8, IL-10, IL-12, and TNF-α as well as TGF-β have been reported to occur in human patients following severe head injury [22, 33, 35, 58–62]. This suggests that isolated brain trauma is capable of inducing a systemic inflammatory response. This is also supported by an extensive systemic acute phase response following isolated TBI [60]. Similar to the systemic CARS, it has been suggested that the injured CNS may cause a systemic anti-inflammatory syndrome, leading to immunosuppression. One mechanism being proposed is the inhibition of monocytes/macrophages by IL-10 [63], which has been shown to be elevated in the CSF and the serum of TBI patients [22]. In summary, it appears that isolated brain injury is capable of evoking many if not most of the immunologic and pro- and anti-inflammatory responses known to occur following blunt injury to the torso and extremities, leading to SIRS and the often lethal MODS.

5.6 Systemic Effects of Chest Injury

Outcome from survivable blunt thoracic trauma depends mainly on adequate management of acute complications affecting ventilation and gas exchange, as well as acute cardiovascular disturbances, i.e., pneumo- and hematothorax, tension pneumothorax, and cardiac tamponade. During the subacute phase in the days following trauma, systemic complications, such as the incidence of pneumonia, ARDS, and multiple organ failure, determine the time course of recovery.

Apart from rib fractures and associated complications (hemato-/pneumothorax), lung contusions are the most common sequelae of blunt thoracic injury, affecting about 10% of chest trauma patients [64]. Blunt chest injury significantly increases the need for mechanical ventilation and the duration of stay in ICU compared to trauma patients without thoracic trauma [1].

Chest injury, furthermore, predisposes the patient to the development of pneumonia, ARDS, and MODS [65]. A retrospective study by Pape and colleagues demonstrated that unilateral lung contusion carries a mortality of about 25%, increasing to 38% when both sides are affected and to over 50% if pneumothorax is present [66]. It has been shown that the severity of pulmonary contusion as measured by percentage of total lung volume correlates with the incidence of ARDS, with a sharp increase, if more than 20% of lung volume is affected [67].

Post-traumatic pneumonia has an incidence of 5–40% [68, 69], and the presence of blunt thoracic injuries significantly increases the risk of pneumonia in the polytrauma patient [65]. This may be due to a pain-induced hypoventilation, and adequate analgesia may reduce the risk of pneumonia [65] (Fig. 5.3). Furthermore, local immunologic mechanisms may also play a role in local organ infection [7, 9, 10, 70–72]. Experimental and clinical data suggest that the lungs of injured patients experience a proinflammatory cytokine response to trauma more intense than that of the systemic circulation [7] and that the traumatized lung parenchyma is a potent source of proinflammatory mediators: In a mouse model of blunt chest injury, IL-6 was not only elevated in serum following trauma, but IL-6 and other proinflammatory mediators were also shown to accumulate in bronchoalveolar lavage fluid and in lung tissue [72]. However, it is difficult to distinguish between the immunologic sequelae of blunt trauma in general and the specific consequences of lung trauma, since there is early involvement of the lungs following unspecific blunt major trauma also and since the responses may differ only subtly. The intense inflammatory response of the lungs to direct and systemic trauma makes the lung parenchyma a central player in local and systemic inflammation and infectious complication (Fig. 5.3).

Last but not least, trauma significantly impairs the fundamental function of the lungs: pulmonary gas exchange. Trauma leads to an early and extensive breakdown of the pulmonary endothelial barrier [72]. This increases the interstitial diffusion distance and affects gas exchange negatively. This and pulmonary contusions increase the amount of blood flowing through the lungs, which does not participate in gas exchange, i.e., pulmonary shunt volume [73]. The consequent decrease of oxygen in the blood (SaO_2) greatly contributes to and aggravates a profound oxygen debt caused by a reduced cardiac output and anemia as well as an increased oxygen demand (oxidative burst) during the flow phase of the systemic response to shock [74] (Fig. 5.3). As a result of this, the presence of thoracic injuries in a polytraumatized patient significantly increases the risk of systemic complications and death [65, 75–77].

5.7   Summary and Conclusion

TBI, together with thoracic trauma, is the foremost killer of multiply-injured patients. Both are present in almost half of the severely injured, and often the injuries are combined. The CNS as well as the lungs play an important role in the host

Blunt Chest Trauma

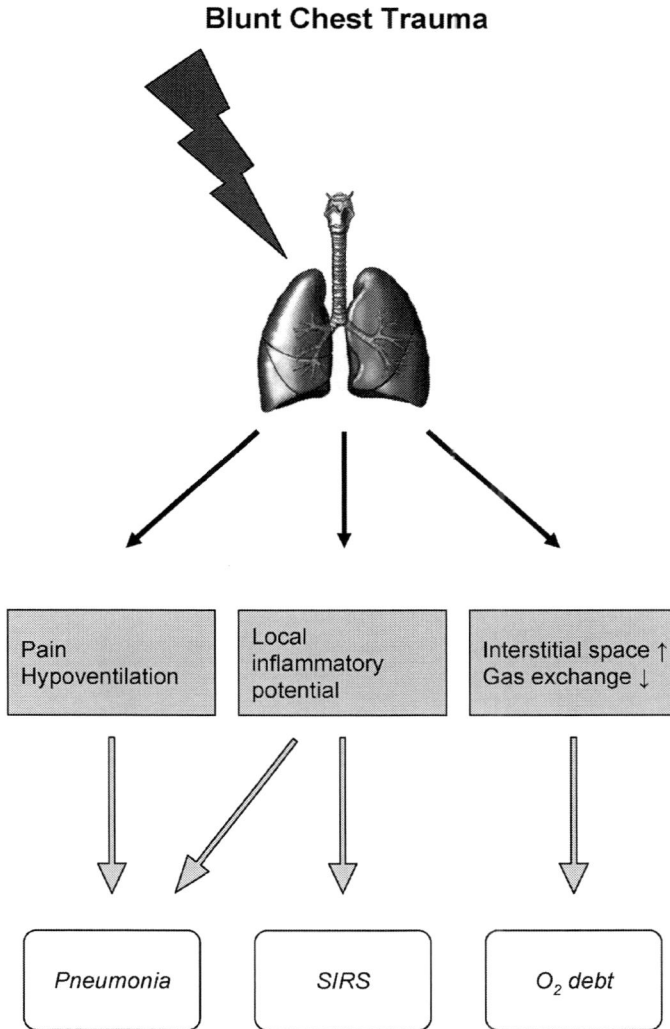

| Pain Hypoventilation | Local inflammatory potential | Interstitial space ↑ Gas exchange ↓ |

| *Pneumonia* | *SIRS* | *O₂ debt* |

Fig. 5.3 Consequences of lung trauma: Pain and consequent hypoventilation increase the risk of pulmonary infection. The high susceptibility of lung tissue to pro- and anti-inflammatory processes may lead to pneumonia locally and accounts for the major role of the lungs in the systemic inflammatory response. As a result of this inflammation, the interstitial space increases, greatly leading to a decrease of gas exchange in the alveoli

defense response to trauma. Interestingly, isolated brain injury is able to elicit a similar systemic reaction to trauma, as does trauma to the torso, including the metabolic changes and a profound inflammatory reaction, both within the CNS and in the systemic circulation. The lungs appear to be crucial in the SIRS, even if they have not been primarily injured. Additional mechanic injury to the lungs further increases the risk of the development of ARDS and multiple organ dysfunction syndrome.

In conclusion, both the brain and the lungs are important players – as target and as effector organs – in the systemic reaction to major trauma. Understanding their role in the pathophysiology of polytrauma, therefore, is the key to making correct decisions about treatment options and their timing in the care of multiply-injured patients.

References

1. Bardenheuer M, Obertacke U, Waydhas C, Nast-Kolb D. [Epidemiology of the severely injured patient. A prospective assessment of preclinical and clinical management. AG Polytrauma of DGU]. *Unfallchirurg* 2000;103(5):355–63.
2. Taeger G, Ruchholtz S, Waydhas C, Lewan U, Schmidt B, Nast-Kolb D. Damage control orthopedics in patients with multiple injuries is effective, time saving, and safe. *J Trauma* 2005;59(2):409–16.
3. Lehmann U, Rickels E, Krettek C. [Multiple trauma with craniocerebral trauma. Early definitive surgical management of long bone fractures?]. *Unfallchirurg* 2001;104(3):196–209.
4. Lehmann U, Krettek C. [Multiple trauma with craniocerebral trauma]. *Unfallchirurg* 2001;104(3):195.
5. Hildebrand F, Giannoudis PV, Griensven M, Zelle B, Ulmer B, Krettek C, Bellamy M, Pape H-C. Management of polytraumatized patients with associated blunt chest trauma: a comparison of two European countries. *Injury* 2005;36(2):293–302.
6. Ertel W, Keel M, Marty D, Hoop R, Safret A, Stocker R, Trentz O. [Significance of systemic inflammation in 1,278 trauma patients]. *Unfallchirurg* 1998;101(7):520–6.
7. Muehlstedt SG, Richardson CJ, Lyte M, Rodriguez JL. Systemic and pulmonary effector cell function after injury. *Crit Care Med* 2002;30(6):1322–6.
8. Miller PR, Croce MA, Kilgo PD, Scott J, Fabian TC. Acute respiratory distress syndrome in blunt trauma: identification of independent risk factors. *Am Surg* 2002;68(10):845–50.
9. Muehlstedt SG, Lyte M, Rodriguez JL. Increased IL-10 production and HLA-DR suppression in the lungs of injured patients precede the development of nosocomial pneumonia. *Shock* 2002;17(6):443–50.
10. Hoth JJ, Scott MJ, Owens RK, Stassen NA, Franklin GA, Cheadle WG, Rodriguez JL. Trauma alters alveolar effector cell apoptosis. *Surgery* 2003;134(4):631–7.
11. Stocchetti N, Furlan A, Volta F. Hypoxemia and arterial hypotension at the accident scene in head injury. *J Trauma* 1996;40(5):764–7.
12. Cooke RS, McNicholl BP, Byrnes DP. Early management of severe head injury in Northern Ireland. *Injury* 1995;26(6):395–7.
13. Fearnside MR, Cook RJ, McDougall P, McNeil RJ. The Westmead Head Injury Project outcome in severe head injury. A comparative analysis of pre-hospital, clinical and CT variables. *Br J Neurosurg* 1993;7(3):267–79.
14. McIntosh TK, Saatman KE, Raghupathi R, Graham DI, Smith DH, Lee VM, Trojanowski JQ. The Dorothy Russell Memorial Lecture. The molecular and cellular sequelae of experimental traumatic brain injury: pathogenetic mechanisms. *Neuropathol Appl Neurobiol* 1998;24(4):251–67.
15. Marmarou A, Anderson RL, Ward JD, Choi SC, Young HF. Impact of ICP instability and hypotension on outcome in patients with severe head trauma. *J Neurosurg* 1991;75:S59–S66.

16. Holmin S, Mathiesen T. Biphasic Edema development after experimental brain contusion in rat. *Neurosci Lett* 1995;194(1–2):97–100.
17. Unterberg AW, Stover J, Kress B, Kiening KL. Edema and brain trauma. *Neuroscience* 2004;129(4):1021–9.
18. Baskaya MK, Rao AM, Dogan A, Donaldson D, Dempsey RJ. The biphasic opening of the blood-brain barrier in the cortex and hippocampus after traumatic brain injury in rats. *Neurosci Lett* 1997;226(1):33–6.
19. Hicks RR, Baldwin SA, Scheff SW. Serum extravasation and cytoskeletal alterations following traumatic brain injury in rats – Comparison of lateral fluid percussion and cortical impact models. *Mol Chem Neuropathol* 1997;32(1–3):1–16.
20. Barzo P, Marmarou A, Fatouros P, Corwin F, Dunbar J. Magnetic resonance imaging monitored acute blood-brain barrier changes in experimental traumatic brain injury. *J Neurosurg* 1996;85(6):1113–21.
21. Fukuda K, Tanno H, Okimura Y, Nakamura M, Yamaura A. The blood-brain-barrier disruption to circulating proteins in the early period after fluid percussion brain injury in rats. *J Neurotrauma* 1995;12(3):315–24.
22. Csuka E, Morganti-Kossmann MC, Lenzlinger PM, Joller H, Trentz O, Kossmann T. IL-10 levels in cerebrospinal fluid and serum of patients with severe traumatic brain injury: relationship to IL-6, TNF-alpha, TGF-beta1 and blood-brain barrier function. *J Neuroimmunol* 1999;101(2):211–21.
23. Morganti-Kossmann MC, Hans VHJ, Lenzlinger PM, Dubs R, Ludwig F, Trentz O, Kossmann T. TGF-beta is elevated in the CSF of patients with severe traumatic brain injuries and parallels blood-brain barrier function. *J Neurotrauma* 1999;16(7):617–28.
24. Pleines UE, Stover JF, Kossmann T, Trentz O, Morganti-Kossmann MC. Soluble ICAM-1 in CSF coincides with the extent of cerebral damage in patients with severe traumatic brain injury. *J Neurotrauma* 1998;15(6):399.
25. Soares HD, Hicks RR, Smith D, McIntosh TK. Inflammatory leukocytic recruitment and diffuse neuronal degeneration are separate pathological processes resulting from traumatic brain injury. *J Neurosci* 1995;15(12):8223–33.
26. Zhuang J, Shackford SR, Schmoker JD, Anderson ML. The association of leukocytes with secondary brain injury. *J Trauma* 1993;35(3):415–22.
27. Carlos TM, Clark RSB, FranicolaHiggins D, Schiding JK, Kochanekt PM. Expression of endothelial adhesion molecules and recruitment of neutrophils after traumatic brain injury in rats. *J Leukoc Biol* 1997;61(3):279–85.
28. Isaksson J, Lewen A, Hillered L, Olsson Y. Up-regulation of intercellular adhesion molecule 1 in cerebral microvessels after cortical contusion trauma in a rat model. *Acta Neuropathol* 1997;94(1):16–20.
29. Shibayama M, Kuchiwaki H, Inao S, Yoshida K, Ito M. Intercellular adhesion molecule-1 expression on glia following brain injury: participation of interleukin-1 beta. *J Neurotrauma* 1996;13(12):801–8.
30. Rancan M, Otto VI, Hans VH, Gerlach I, Jork R, Trentz O, Kossmann T, Morganti-Kossmann MC. Upregulation of ICAM-1 and MCP-1 but not of MIP-2 and sensorimotor deficit in response to traumatic axonal injury in rats. *J Neurosci Res* 2001;63(5):438–46.
31. Holmin S, Soderlund J, Biberfeld P, Mathiesen T. Intracerebral inflammation after human brain contusion. *Neurosurgery* 1998;42(2):291–8.
32. Holmin S, Mathiesen T, Shetye J, Biberfeld P. Intracerebral inflammatory response to experimental brain contusion. *Acta Neurochir (Wien)* 1995;132(1–3):110–9.
33. Morganti-Kossman MC, Lenzlinger PM, Hans V, Stahel P, Csuka E, Ammann E, Stocker R, Trentz O, Kossmann T. Production of cytokines following brain injury: beneficial and deleterious for the damaged tissue. *Mol Psychiatry* 1997;2(2):133–6.
34. Hans VH, Kossmann T, Lenzlinger PM, Probstmeier R, Imhof HG, Trentz O & Morganti-Kossmann MC. Experimental axonal injury triggers interleukin-6 mRNA, protein synthesis and release into cerebrospinal fluid. *J Cereb Blood Flow Metab* 1999;19(2):184–94.

35. Ott L, McClain CJ, Gillespie M, Young B. Cytokines and metabolic dysfunction after severe head-injury. *J Neurotrauma* 1994;11(5):447–72.
36. Rothwell NJ, Hopkins SJ. Cytokines and the nervous-system. 2. Actions and mechanisms of action. *Trends Neurosci* 1995;18(3):130–6.
37. Lenzlinger PM, Morganti-Kossmann MC, Laurer HL, McIntosh TK. The duality of the inflammatory response to traumatic brain injury. *Mol Neurobiol* 2001;24(1–3):169–81.
38. Bratton SL, Davis RL. Acute lung injury in isolated traumatic brain injury. *Neurosurgery* 1997;40(4):707–12.
39. Holland MC, Mackersie RC, Morabito D, Campbell AR, Kivett VA, Patel R, Erickson VR, Pittet JF. The development of acute lung injury is associated with worse neurologic outcome in patients with severe traumatic brain injury. *J Trauma* 2003;55(1):106–11.
40. Berthiaume L, Zygun D. Non-neurologic organ dysfunction in acute brain injury. *Crit Care Clin* 2006;22(4):753–66.
41. Bahloul M, Chaari AN, Kallel H, Khabir A, Ayadi A, Charfeddine H, Hergafi L, Chaari AD, Chelly HE, Ben Hamida C, Rekik N, Bouaziz M. Neurogenic pulmonary edema due to traumatic brain injury: evidence of cardiac dysfunction. *Am J Crit Care* 2006;15(5):462–70.
42. Simon RP. Neurogenic pulmonary-edema. *Neurol Clin* 1993;11(2):309–23.
43. Baumann A, Audibert G, McDonnell J, Mertes PM. Neurogenic pulmonary edema. *Acta Anaesthesiol Scand* 2007;51(4):447–55.
44. Kalsotra A, Zhao J, Anakk S, Dash PK, Strobel HW. Brain trauma leads to enhanced lung inflammation and injury: evidence for role of P4504Fs in resolution. *J Cereb Blood Flow Metab* 2007;27(5):963–74.
45. Piek J, Chesnut RM, Marshall LF, van Berkum-Clark M, Klauber MR, Blunt BA, Eisenberg HM, Jane JA, Marmarou A, Foulkes MA. Extracranial complications of severe head-injury. *J Neurosurg* 1992;77(6):901–7.
46. Cazzadori A, DiPerri G, Vento S, Bonora S, Fendt D, Rossi M. Aetiology of pneumonia following isolated closed head injury. *Respir Med* 1997;91(4):193–9.
47. Loop T. The immune system: basic principles and modulation by anaesthetics. *Anasthesiol & Intensivmed* 2003;44(1):53–65.
48. Loop T, Humar M, Pischke S, Hoetzel A, Schmidt R, Pahl HL, Geiger KK, Pannen BH. Thiopental inhibits tumor necrosis factor alpha-induced activation of nuclear factor kappa B through suppression of I kappa B kinase activity. *Anesthesiology* 2003;99(2):360–7.
49. Harris OA, Colford JM, Good MC, Matz PG. The role of hypothermia in the management of severe brain injury. A meta-analysis. *Arch Neurol* 2002;59(7):1077–83.
50. Dujardin KS, McCully RB, Wijdicks EFM, Tazelaar HD Seward JB, McGregor CGA, Olson LJ. Myocardial dysfunction associated with brain death: clinical, echocardiographic, and pathologic features. *J Heart Lung Transplant* 2001;20(3):350–7.
51. Connor RCR. Myocardial damage secondary to brain lesions. *Am Heart J* 1969;78(2):145–8.
52. Stein SC, Smith DH. Coagulopathy in traumatic brain injury. *Neurocrit Care* 2004;1(4):479–88.
53. Kearney TJ, Bentt L, Grode M, Lee S, Hiatt JR, Shabot MM. Coagulopathy and catecholamines in severe head-injury. *J Trauma* 1992;32(5):608–12.
54. Lenzlinger PM, Hans VH, Joller-Jemelka HI, Trentz O, Morganti-Kossmann MC, Kossmann T. Markers for cell-mediated immune response are elevated in cerebrospinal fluid and serum after severe traumatic brain injury in humans. *J Neurotrauma* 2001;18(5):479–89.
55. Quattrocchi KB, Frank EH, Miller CH, Amin A, Issel BW, Wagner FC. Impairment of helper T-cell function and lymphokine-activated killer cytotoxicity following severe head-injury. *J Neurosurg* 1991;75(5):766–73.
56. Quattrocchi KB, Issel BW, Miller CH, Frank EH, Wagner FC. Impairment of helper T-cell function following severe head-injury. *J Neurotrauma* 1992;9(1):1–9.
57. Quattrocchi KB, Miller CH, Wagner FC, DeNardo SJ, DeNardo GL, Ovodov K, Frank EH. Cell-mediated-immunity in severely head-injured patients – the role of suppressor lymphocytes and serum factors. *J Neurosurg* 1992;77(5):694–9.

58. Hans VH, Kossmann T, Joller H, Otto V, Morganti-Kossmann MC. Interleukin-6 and its soluble receptor in serum and cerebrospinal fluid after cerebral trauma. *Neuroreport* 1999;10(2): 409–12.
59. Bell MJ, Kochanek PM, Doughty LA, Carcillo JA, Adelson PD, Clark RS, Wisniewski SR, Whalen MJ, DeKosky ST. Interleukin-6 and interleukin-10 in cerebrospinal fluid after severe traumatic brain injury in children. *J Neurotrauma* 1997;14(7):451–7.
60. Kossmann T, Hans VH, Imhof HG, Stocker R, Grob P, Trentz O, Morganti-Kossmann C. Intrathecal and serum interleukin-6 and the acute-phase response in patients with severe traumatic brain injuries. *Shock* 1995;4(5):311–7.
61. Kossmann T, Stahel PF, Lenzlinger PM, Redl H, Dubs RW, Trentz O, Schlag G, Morganti-Kossmann MC. Interleukin-8 released into the cerebrospinal fluid after brain injury is associated with blood-brain barrier dysfunction and nerve growth factor production. *J Cereb Blood Flow Metab* 1997;17(3):280–9.
62. Whalen MJ, Carlos TM, Kochanek PM, Wisniewski SR, Bell MJ, Clark RS, DeKosky ST, Marion DW, Adelson PD. Interleukin-8 is increased in cerebrospinal fluid of children with severe head injury. *Crit Care Med* 2000;28(4):929–34.
63. Woiciechowsky C, Schoning B, Lanksch WR, Volk HD, Docke WD. Mechanisms of brain-mediated systemic anti-inflammatory syndrome causing immunodepression. *J Mol Med* 1999;77(11):769–80.
64. Kulshrestha P, Munshi I, Wait R. Profile of chest trauma in a Level I trauma center. *J Trauma* 2004;57(3):576–81.
65. Trupka A, Nast-Kolb D, Schweiberer L. Blunt chest trauma. *Unfallchirurg* 1998;101(4): 244–58.
66. Pape HC, Remmers D, Rice J, Ebisch M, Krettek C, Tscherne H. Appraisal of early evaluation of blunt chest trauma: development of a standardized scoring system for initial clinical decision making. *J Trauma* 2000;49(3):496–504.
67. Miller PR, Croce MA, Bee TK, Qaisi WG, Smith CP, Collins GL, Fabian TC. ARDS after pulmonary contusion: accurate measurement of contusion volume identifies high-risk patients. *J Trauma* 2001;51(2):223–30.
68. Segers P, Van Schil P, Jorens P, Van Den Brande F. Thoracic trauma: an analysis of 187 patients. *Acta Chir Belg* 2001;101(6):277–82.
69. Sariego J, Brown JL, Matsumoto T, Kerstein MD. Predictors of pulmonary complications in blunt chest trauma. *Int Surg* 1993;78(4):320–3.
70. Muehlstedt SG, Richardson CJ, West MA, Lyte M, Rodriguez JL. Cytokines and the pathogenesis of nosocomial pneumonia. *Surgery* 2001;130(4):602–9.
71. Perl M, Gebhard F, Bruckner UB, Ayala A, Braumuller S, Buttner C, Kinzl L, Knoferl MW. Pulmonary contusion causes impairment of macrophage and lymphocyte immune functions and increases mortality associated with a subsequent septic challenge. *Crit Care Med* 2005;33(6):1351–8.
72. Perl M, Gebhard F, Braumuller S, Tauchmann B, Bruckner UB, Kinzl L, Knoferl MW. The pulmonary and hepatic immune microenvironment and its contribution to the early systemic inflammation following blunt chest trauma. *Crit Care Med* 2006;34(4):1152–9.
73. Michaels AJ. Management of post traumatic respiratory failure. *Crit Care Clin* 2004;20(1): 83–99.
74. Cuthbertson DP. Post-shock metabolic response. *Lancet* 1942;1:433–7.
75. Bosse MJ, MacKenzie EJ, Riemer BL, Brumback RJ, McCarthy ML, Burgess AR, Gens DR, Yasui Y. Adult respiratory distress syndrome, pneumonia, and mortality following thoracic injury and a femoral fracture treated either with intramedullary nailing with reaming or with a plate – A comparative study. *J Bone Joint Surg Am* 1997;79A(6): 799–809.
76. Clark GC, Schecter WP, Trunkey DD. Variables affecting outcome in blunt chest trauma – flail chest vs pulmonary contusion. *J Trauma* 1988;28(3):298–304.
77. Johnson JA, Cogbill TH, Winga ER. Determinants of outcome after pulmonary contusion. *J Trauma* 1986;26(8):695–7.

Chapter 6
Patient Selection: Orthopedic Approach in Isolated Injuries

Brad A. Prather and Craig S. Roberts

6.1 Introduction

In an era of hand transplantation, the Lower Extremity Assessment Project (LEAP) study data have created increased pressure for limb salvage rather than immediate amputation for complex lower extremity injury. Limb salvage is performed frequently using limb damage control (LDC). LDC is the specific application of the principles of damage control orthopedics to the complex lower extremity injury. Like damage control orthopedics for the polytrauma patient with long bone fractures, LDC uses initial damage control spanning external fixation and adjunctive soft tissue techniques (antibiotic bead pouches and negative pressure dressings), antibiotic nails after prolonged external fixation as a bridge to intramedullary nailing, and staged definitive osteosynthesis.

Although overall patient survival is usually expected with isolated lower extremity injuries, survival of the leg is often still tenuous. And even if the limb survives, there is no guarantee that the ultimate functional outcome will be optimal. In addition, heroic acute limb surgeries such as immediate extensive open plating procedures are generally not safe in these situations because they create additional soft tissue trauma on the limb analogous to the second hit phenomenon of acute femoral nailing described by Giannoudis and colleagues [1].

LDC includes the assessment of perfusion, limb oxygenation, limb metabolism (e.g., pH), soft tissue injury, limb temperature, limb hemostasis, compartment swelling, and skeletal stability. The various interventions of LDC include re-establishing perfusion, decreasing the metabolic burden from the soft tissue damage (e.g., lactic acid, nonviable tissue, and contamination), cavity decompression with fasciotomies, limb warming, hemostasis, protecting the wound from the hospital environment, and re-establishing limb alignment and stability.

C.S. Robert (✉)
Department of Orthopedic Surgery, University of Louisville, 210 E. Gray Street, Suite 1003, Louisville, KY, 40202, USA
e-mail: craig.roberts@louisville.edu

H.-C. Pape et al. (eds.), *Damage Control Management in the Polytrauma Patient*, DOI 10.1007/978-0-387-89508-6_6, © Springer Science+Business Media, LLC 2010

```
                        ┌─────────────────────────────┐
                        │  Complex Lower Extremity Injury │
                        └─────────────────────────────┘
```

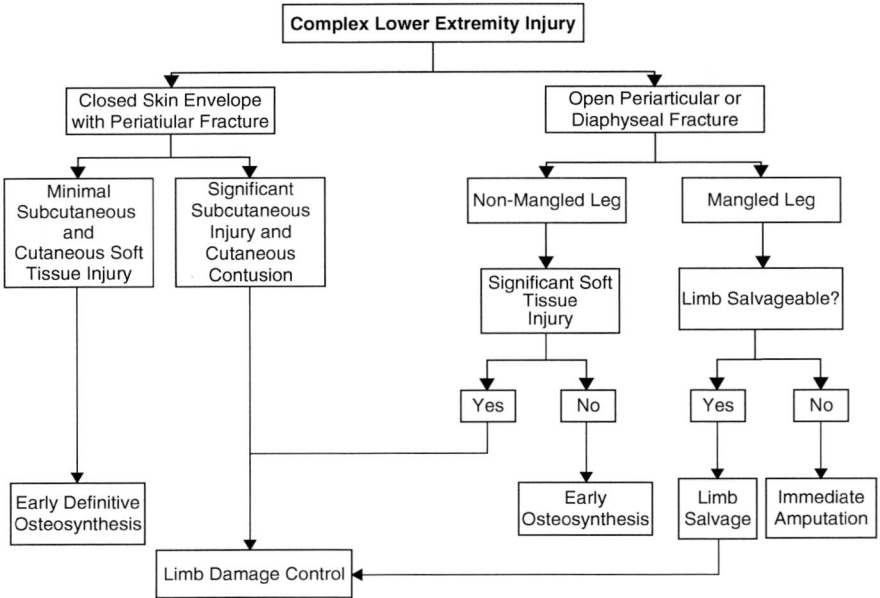

Fig. 6.1 Common lower extremity injury flowchart

Three types of injury complexes may benefit from LDC: complex periarticular/articular injuries, isolated diaphyseal fractures with significant soft tissue injury with either open or closed fracture, and the mangled leg (Fig. 6.1). The isolated high-energy lower extremity injury is less common than polytrauma complex extremity injuries, but the treatment of these complex extremities is similar. Limb salvage versus amputation is often the initial decision. Complex periarticular/articular injuries can have elements of the mangled extremity. More commonly, the soft tissue component of the injury dictates the timing of definitive osteosynthesis.

Damage control external fixation is the platform for LDC. Damage control frames maintain length, provide bony stability, and allow wound access – all with minimal risk. Pin placement away from the area of future surgical incisions, good soft-tissue handling techniques, and bicortical pin placement permit maximum benefits from LDC frames and decreases pin track complications.

This chapter will review the use of LDC with spanning external fixation of isolated lower extremity injuries and adjunctive techniques (negative-pressure dressings, antibiotic bead pouches, and antibiotic nails).

6.2 Specific Applications of Limb Damage Control by Fracture Type

6.2.1 Pilon Fractures

Pilon fracture management has been fraught with complications when there is underappreciation of the extent of the soft tissue injury and immediate plating. Temporary transarticular external fixation in combination with reconstruction of the articular surface using ligamentotaxis or minimally invasive osteosynthesis has a low infection rate [2, 3].

External fixation protocols consist of initial placement of an external fixator, which spans the ankle joint. Concomitant open reduction and fixation of the fibula is no longer automatically performed and is only performed on a case-by-case basis. Following initial stabilization, patients with isolated injuries can often be discharged and readmitted for definitive reconstruction. Polytrauma patients and patients who require frequent wound assessment are kept hospitalized for observation and treatment [4].

Classification of the concomitant soft tissue injury improves decision making for appropriate fracture treatment, decreases complications, and may be of prognostic value [5]. The Gustilo and Anderson classification of open fractures and the original Tscherne classification of soft tissue injury with closed fractures are no longer thought to be sufficient for classifying many complicated injuries [5]. The use of more sophisticated grading systems (e.g., Hannover fracture scale or the AO soft-tissue grading system) for classification of a fracture with a concomitant soft tissue injury may provide a better method of stratifying these injuries in order to make better decisions about treatment. In addition, future methods such as bioelectrical impedance may provide a more precise way to assess soft tissue injury and post-traumatic swelling [6].

LDC is an excellent option for pilon fracture management when there is a concomitant open fracture wound, an extensive closed soft tissue injury, or gross skeletal instability with a loss of alignment. In these cases, an LDC approach with sequential steps is an excellent option. The options for the first step include a temporary ankle joint spanning fixator without fibular fixation or a temporary ankle joint spanning fixator with fibular fixation. Our preferred ankle spanning damage control fixator uses two 5-mm half-pins in the tibia, two 4-mm half-pins in the calcaneus, and two 4-mm half-pins in the forefoot (one pin in the first metatarsal and one pin in the fifth metatarsal). The hindfoot pins are connected with a stop sign type partial hexagonal ring parallel to the plane of the sole of the foot, and the forefoot pins are connected with a second stop sign type partial hexagonal ring perpendicular to the first ring. These two rings are attached to each other with short bars. With this construct, the pilon fracture can be realigned and easily controlled.

The condition of the soft tissues dictates the time interval between spanning external fixation and definitive osteosynthesis. An interval of 7–21 days is usually necessary.

Following soft tissue recovery, secondary definitive osteosynthesis can usually be safely performed. In studies comparing Type IIIC fractures, results consistently reveal improved outcome with a two-stage treatment compared to early definitive plate fixation or definitive external fixation [7].

Nearly all patients presenting with pilon fractures can be treated with LDC except for the low-energy spiral extension fracture described by Maale and Seligson [8]. These injuries can sometimes be safely treated with early, initial ORIF.

6.2.2   Diaphyseal Tibia/Fibula Fractures

Grade III open tibial fractures require specialized orthopedic care, and injuries greater than a Gustilo IIIB often require combined orthopedic and plastic surgical care [9] and are often an excellent indication for LDC.

Soft tissue condition, vascular status, and neurological status need to be carefully evaluated. However, initial plantar sensation is not prognostic of long-term plantar sensory status or functional outcomes, and, therefore, should not be included in initial decision of LDC or amputation [10].

An important consideration is the technique of external fixation. Overdistraction of the limb ought to be avoided because it can tighten fascia and lead to increased compartment pressures. Placement of joints in neutral position if possible is recommended. Options for LDC external fixation montages for the tibia include uniplanar frames for midshaft fractures with minimal comminution, and multiplanar frames for comminuted midshaft fractures. The anteromedial quadrant of the tibia is best suited for 5-mm half-pins [11].

An open soft tissue injury can be easily managed around spanning external fixation. If free flaps are necessary and external fixation is chosen as definitive fixation of a tibial fracture, there is an increased rate of complications [12]. In cases in which external fixation of the tibia is prolonged (2 weeks), an antibiotic nail can be used as an intermediate step between external fixation and intramedullary nailing with a locked, metallic nail. The use of an antibiotic nail as a bridging step is described later in this chapter. If adjunctive wound treatment is necessary (vacuum-assisted dressings, antibiotic bead pouches, antibiotic nails), the completion of wound healing is necessary prior to definitive fracture fixation.

6.2.3   Tibial Plateau Fractures

Tibial plateau fractures are really combination injuries to the bone and the soft tissues. Soft tissue injury with tibial plateau fractures includes a complex array ranging from skin contusions to complex ligamentous, meniscal, and capsular pathology [13, 14]. Immediate, definitive surgical treatment particularly with multiple plates and screws has traditionally been associated with substantial complications such as infection, knee stiffness, malunion, loss of fixation, osteomyelitis, wound break-down, and amputation. The LDC approach is particularly useful for high-energy injuries (Schatzker Type IV, V, and VI injuries).

LDC consisting of temporary joint-spanning external fixation allows osseous stabilization, access to the soft tissues, and prevention of further articular damage. External fixators, specifically those with MRI-compatible/safe components, also allow a greater degree of injury assessment by allowing for MRI evaluation of knee ligaments and menisci prior to definitive osteosynthesis.

LDC involves the use of initial spanning external fixation across the knee with two or three 5-mm half-pins in the anteromedial tibia and two or three 5-mm half-pins in the anterolateral distal thigh connected by a large diameter bar or multiple smaller diameter bars. In instances of patient body weight greater than 250 pounds, 6-mm half-pins can be used. The soft tissue injury can easily be reassessed and managed around the fixator. When the condition of the soft tissues is optimized, generally 7–14 days, the fixator can be removed and definitive osteosynthesis performed.

One especially sinister variant of plateau fractures is the knee fracture-dislocation, generally Schatzker type IV V, or VI, or AO type C injuries. Vascular evaluation is especially important in these cases. A vascular-compromised limb is best treated with LDC. An externally fixed leg provides a stable platform for the vascular surgeon. Once major soft tissue injuries have been treated, definitive fracture treatment and ligament repair can be planned in conjunction with the vascular surgeon.

Blast injuries have a degree of contamination and soft tissue injury that often precludes definitive osteosynthesis using plates and screws. In these cases, the spanning external fixator can be converted to fine wire fixation with all-ring constructs or hybrid constructs. Hybrid fixation methods (combined percutaneous fixation and external fixation or fine wire ring fixators) for definitive treatment are another option encompassed in the LDC approach. This approach has been shown to give results similar to spanning external fixation converted to open reduction internal fixation [15–17].

6.2.4 Femoral Diaphyseal Fractures

Much of the damage control orthopedic literature stems from the treatment of femoral shaft fractures in polytrauma patients [18, 19]. Isolated femoral diaphyseal fractures, which are good indicators for the LDC model, are relatively rare. LDC ought to be considered when there are concomitant head injuries, severe fat embolism, low arterial oxygenation, and suspected spine fractures.

Early external fixation within the initial 24 h decreases pulmonary morbidity and respiratory insufficiency [20, 21]. LDC is also an excellent option with a femur fracture with compartment syndrome.

Other additional specific indications for LDC for femoral fractures include concomitant vascular surgery and large skin defects and degloving injuries that will

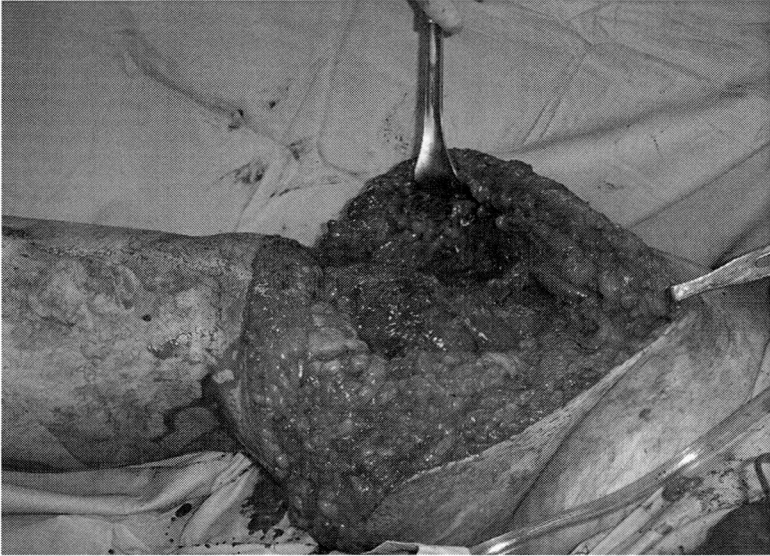

Fig. 6.2 Injury photograph of an isolated open femoral diaphyseal fracture with degloving injury

ultimately require regional or free-flap coverage [22]. The large muscular envelope of the thigh can be a forgiving environment providing an excellent muscular surface for skin grafting and a thick barrier to infection. Treatment of these large injuries with LDC does not add an additional risk of infection as rates are comparable to those after primary intramedullary fixation [23]. Even in the worst case scenarios in which prolonged external fixation (>2 weeks) is required, an antibiotic nail can be used as an intermediate step after external fixator removal prior to intramedullary nailing with a locked, metal nail. Therefore, the implementation of a damage control approach for patients with femoral shaft fracture can be based on the complexity of the soft tissue injury and the time it takes until definitive fixation (Figs. 6.2–6.8).

6.3 The Mangled Extremity

Mangled limbs are leg or arm injuries in which limb viability is questionable, limb loss is a possibility, and immediate amputation is an option. Data from the LEAP study have noted that the criteria for limb salvage or amputation are not clear cut, and decision making cannot be made based on an injury grading scale [24]. Previously held tenets of an insensate foot being an absolute indication for amputation have changed as well [10]. The LEAP study provides support for limb salvage and, therefore, the LDC approach to lower extremity injury. However, many factors

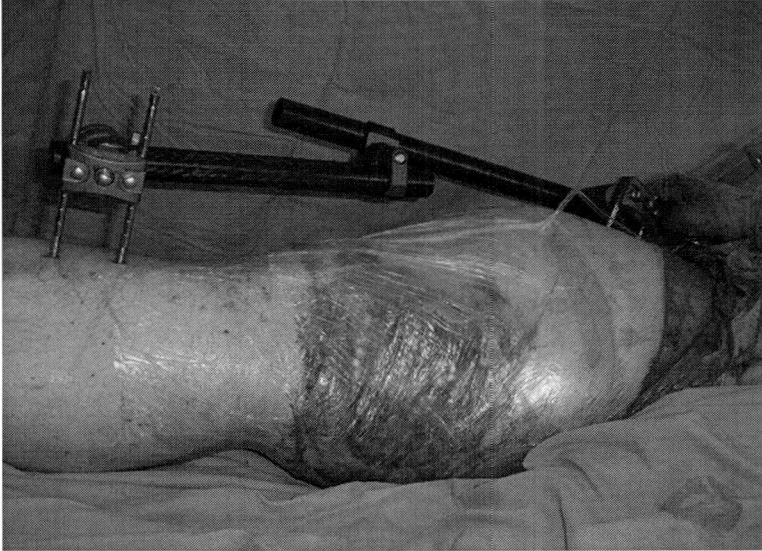

Fig. 6.3 Initial surgery involved debridement, spanning external fixator, and antibiotic bead pouch

must be considered as salvaged limbs incur longer hospital stays, more complications, multiple surgeries, and often equivalent outcomes to amputation [24]. Instances of vascular injury, tibial nerve disruption, or sepsis may present a picture for which limb salvage is unlikely to be successful, and, in these patients, careful consideration of amputation should be made [25].

The blunt, nonpenetrating, or crush component of a lower extremity injury is potentially limb-threatening. The associated crush injury can include myoglobinuria, renal failure, and multiple organ system failure [26]. Similar to polytrauma resuscitation and monitoring, the mangled extremity patient in the immediate postinjury period must be carefully reassessed and monitored.

Recently, data on hindfoot injuries have brought to question nearly all aspects of the LDC method. Open hindfoot injuries in particular illustrate the goals of DCO of the mangled extremity: timely coverage/closure of wounds, restoration of overall alignment with soft tissue coverage, anatomic reduction, and selection of patients who may benefit from early/primary amputation [25]. Open fractures of the talus are more common than calcaneal fractures and are less likely to involve amputation. However, talar fractures or fracture dislocations often have large soft tissue defects that often require flap coverage. Flap coverage of this rather distal area requires a free flap and, hence, plastic surgery involvement [27, 28]. These open injuries, whether treated with percutaneous fixation or delayed osteosynthesis, are often

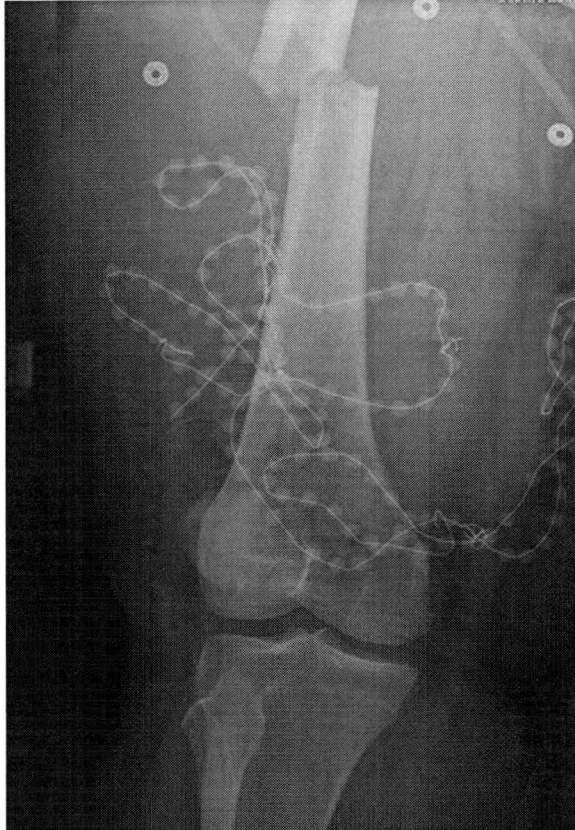

Fig. 6.4 Postoperative radiograph after initial surgery

associated with long-term pain, ambulatory dysfunction and psychosocial impairment, and frequently requires below-the-knee amputation [25, 29]. In the authors' own series (unpublished data), it has been noted that multilevel injuries to the foot and ankle in which more than two adjacent segments are injured have a risk of toe amputation of more than 20%.

6.4 Adjunctive Measures

Advanced soft tissue management is crucial in LDC. Open injuries greater than Gustilo grade II open fracture often necessitate a staged approach to soft tissue management. Wound management objectives includes eliminating nonviable tissue,

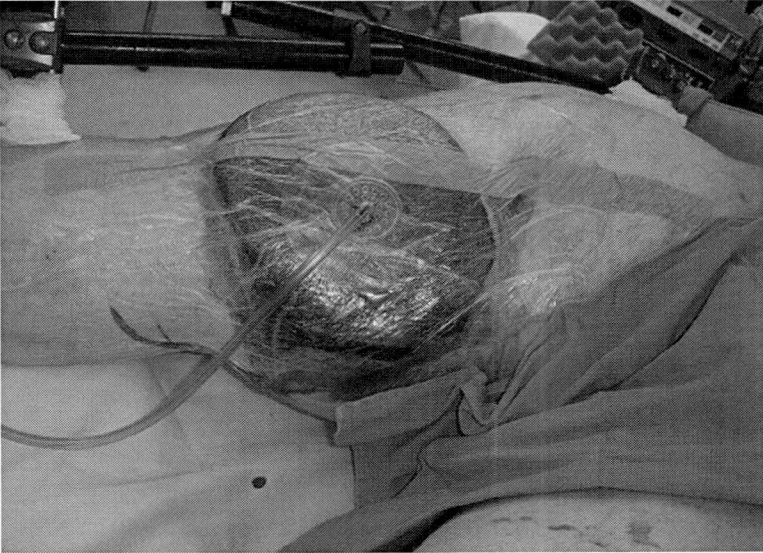

Fig. 6.5 Second look surgery with repeat debridement and VAC was performed on post-op day 3

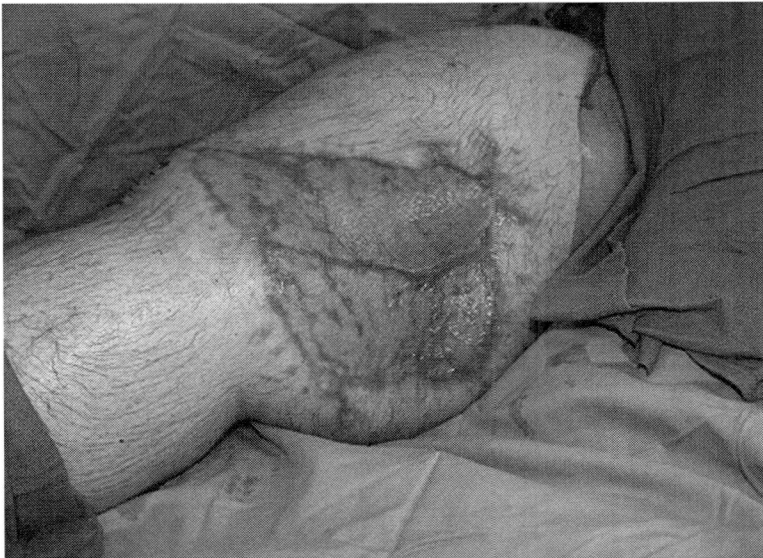

Fig. 6.6 Wound at the time of antibiotic nail insertion several weeks after split thickness skin graft

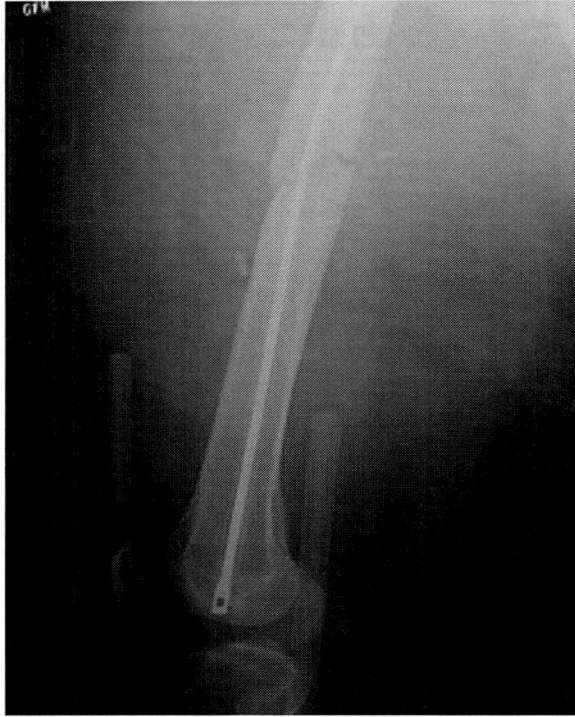

Fig. 6.7 Antibiotic nailing was performed at postinjury day 35

decreasing injury wound contamination, preventing nosocomial infection, improving soft tissue viability, and sealing the wound from direct communication with the environment. To achieve these objectives, three adjunctive measures are useful: the antibiotic bead pouch, vacuum-assisted dressings, and the antibiotic nail.

Antibiotic bead pouches consist of a porous plastic film placed over the soft tissue defect with antibiotic-impregnated PMMA beads establishing a "closed" bead hematoma. The fracture environment thus contains high local levels of antibiotics [30, 31]. A drain is brought out of the pouch; rather than being attached to suction, it is attached for overflow only, thus preventing unwanted pressure. The use of systemic antibiotics consisting of second-generation systemic cephalosporins and aminogylcosides is continued in addition to the antibiotic beads. Normal sequential debridement of open fractures coincides with bead pouch changes, which maintain the high concentration of local antibiotics. Therefore, the potential advantages seen are isolation of a wound from the hospital environment and avoidance of systemic toxicity of antibiotics. The bead pouch technique creates a favorable local environment for earlier wound closure [32].

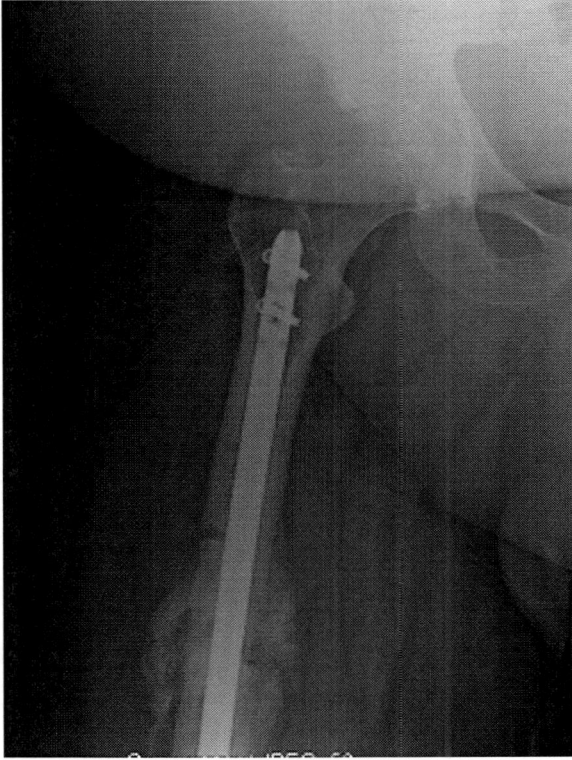

Fig. 6.8 Follow-up radiograph at 3 months after injury. Exchange nailing with removal of antibiotic nail and locked nailing was performed at postinjury day 50

Vacuum-assisted (VAC) or negative pressure wound therapy has become a common modality for treatment of open fracture wounds, particularly when the wound has been treated with serial debridements and antibiotic bead pouches and is being prepared for soft tissue coverage (e.g., skin grafts, free flaps, etc.). The VAC can be easily applied around external fixators and is available as a portable device that can facilitate patient mobilization.

The benefits of VAC wound therapy are the conversion of an open wound to a closed controlled wound. Although not considered a sterile environment, it does provide a barrier that can be easily changed much less frequently than conventional gauze dressings. Vacuum devices have been shown to decrease the bacterial count of wound beds [33]. There are no data that they decrease infection rates. The amount to which bacterial load is decreased has been debated; however, it has been shown that nonfermentative Gram-negative bacteria are decreased. It may be that vacuum dressings predispose to different organisms [34]. The device works by continuously evacuating wound effluent. The result is an improvement of microcirculation, enhanced granulation tissue formation, and vastly improved wound healing parameters [35]. Overall, the VAC is a promising technique that provides a bridge from the large open wounds after several debridements and antibiotic bead pouches to the staged soft tissue coverage procedure. Empiric observations suggest that the VAC is a powerful tool, but level I or II studies are pending.

A third adjunctive measure employed with LDC is the antibiotic nail. Often, conversion to intramedullary fixation from an external fixator must be delayed for an extended period of time due to the management of the soft tissue injury or the management of the chest injury. Whether this is wound contamination or contaminated pin sites, the risk of infectious complications on conversion to intramedullary fixation after two or three weeks of external fixation is more likely to occur [23]. In the past, staged conversion to intramedullary nails was performed, following fixator removal after an interim period of antibiotics and splinting [36]. The use of an antibiotic nail can replace this step. Antibiotic nails are used to maintain fracture alignment, deliver local antibiotics, and treat or prophylax against medullary infection. Like antibiotic beads, they deliver a high concentration of antibiotics to a local environment and produce an improved environment for definitive fixation.

Antibiotic nails for long bone fractures previously treated with external fixation are made intraoperatively using 40 French chest tube, standard PMMA cement; vancomycin, tobramycin, or gentamycin antibiotic powder; and flexible Ender's nails [37, 38]. In the operative setting, intramedullary reaming is performed, cultures are taken, and definitive fixation is staged based on optimized injury factors.

Although there is no level I or II evidence available to support the use of antibiotic nails, empirical evidence is promising. Antibiotic nails provide a bridge between the diaphyseal femur or tibial fracture that has required prolonged external fixation with a relatively long (>2–3 weeks) period before definitive intramedullary nailing with conventional, intramedullary nails.

6.5 Summary and Conclusions

LDC is an approach that applies damage control orthopedics to isolated extremity injuries. LDC emphasizes limb salvage, spanning external fixation, and delayed definitive osteosynthesis. LDC is a method of expediting soft tissue recovery and optimizing the timing and conditions for future definitive osteosynthesis. Various external fixation montages may be applied for lower extremity injuries with re-establishment of limb length and alignment, stabilization of soft tissue envelopes, and creation of a stable skeletal platform for soft tissue management and staged definitive osteosynthesis. Although the focus here has been on the lower extremity, LDC can be considered for complex, upper extremity injuries as well. Future studies are needed to clarify basic treatment protocols and generate level I and II evidence. The very nature of these complex extremity injuries requires flexibility, imagination, and careful decision making to optimize the chances of a good functional outcome.

References

1. Giannoudis PV, Smith RM, Bellamy MC, Morrison JF, Dickson RA, Guillou PJ. Stimulation of the inflammatory system by reamed and unreamed nailing of femoral fractures. An analysis of the second hit. *J Bone Joint Surg Br* 1999; 81(2):356–61.
2. Bonar SK, Marsh JL. Unilateral external fixation for severe pilon fractures. *Foot Ankle* 1993; 14:57–64.
3. Scheck M. Treatment of comminuted distal tibial fractures by combined dual-pin fixation and limited open reduction. *J Bone Joint Surg Am* 1965; 47:1537–1553.
4. Sirkin M, Sanders R, DiPasquale T, Herscovici D. A staged protocol for soft tissue management in the treatment of complex pilon fractures. *J Orthop Trauma* 2004; 18(8 Suppl):S32–8.
5. Südkamp NP. Soft tissue injury: Pathophysiology and its influence on fracture management. In: Rüedi TP, Murphy WM, eds. *AO Principles of Fracture Management.* New York, NY: Thieme; 2000:59–77.
6. King RJ, Clamp JA, Hutchinson JW, Moran CG . Bioelectrical impedance: A new method for measuring post-traumatic swelling. *J Orthop Trauma* 2007; 21(7):462–468.
7. Blauth M, Bastian L, Krettek C, Knop C, Evans S. Surgical options for the treatment of severe tibial pilon fractures: A study of three techniques. *J Orthop Trauma* 2001; 15(3):153–60.
8. Maale G, Seligson D. Fractures through the distal weight-bearing surface of the tibia. *Orthop* 1980; 3:517–21.
9. Naique SB, Pearse M, Nanchahal J. Management of severe open tibial fractures: The need for combined orthopaedic and plastic surgical treatment in specialist centres. *J Bone Joint Surg Br* 2006; 88(3):351–7.
10. Bosse MJ, McCarthy ML, Jones AL, Webb LX, Sims SH, Sanders RW, MacKenzie EJ, the Lower Extremity Assessment Project. The insensate foot following severe lower extremity trauma: An indication for amputation? *J Bone Joint Surg Am* 2005; 87(12):2601-8.
11. Ziran BH, Smith WR, Anglen JO, Tornetta III P. External fixation: How to make it work. *J Bone Joint Surg* 2007; 89:1620–32.
12. Webb LX, Bosse MJ, Castillo RC, MacKenzie EJ, the Lower Extremity Assessment Project . Analysis of surgeon-controlled variables in the treatment of limb-threatening type-III open tibial diaphyseal fractures. *J Bone Joint Surg* 2007; 89:923–928.
13. Gardner MJ, Yacoubian S, Geller D, Pode M, Mintz D, Helfet DL, Lorich DG. Prediction of soft-tissue injuries in Schatzker II tibial plateau fractures based on measurements of plain radiographs. *J Trauma* 2006; 60(2):319–23; discussion 324.
14. Bennett WF, Browner B. Tibial plateau fractures: A study of associated soft tissue injuries. *J Orthop Trauma* 1994; 8(3):183–8.
15. Egol KA, Tejwani NC, Capla EL, Wolinsky PL, Koval KJ. Staged management of high-energy proximal tibia fractures (OTA types 41): The results of a prospective, standardized protocol. *J Orthop Trauma* 2005; 19(7):448–55; discussion 456.
16. Watson JT, Ripple S, Hoshaw SJ, Fyhrie D. Hybrid external fixation for tibial plateau fractures: Clinical and biomechanical correlation. *Orthop Clin North Am* 2002; 33:199–209, ix.
17. Marsh JL, Smith ST, Do TT. External fixation and limited internal fixation for complex fractures of the tibial plateau. *J Bone Joint Surg Am* 1995; 77:661–73.
18. Nowotarski PJ, Turen CH, Brumback RJ, Scarboro JM.Conversion of external fixation to intramedullary nailing for fractures of the shaft of the femur in multiply injured patients. *J Bone Joint Surg Am* 2000; 82:781–8.
19. Scalea TM, Boswell SA, Scott JD, Mitchell KA, Kramer ME, Pollak, AN. External fixation as a bridge to intramedullary nailing for patients with multiple injuries and with femur fractures: Damage control orthopedics. *J Trauma* 2000; 48: 61–21.
20. Johnson KD, Cadambi A, Seibert GB. Incidence of adult respiratory distress syndrome in patients with multiple musculoskeletal injuries: Effect of early operative stabilization of fractures. *J Trauma* 1985; 25:375–84.

21. Riska EB, Myllynen P. Fat embolism in patients with multiple injuries. *J Trauma* 1982; 22:891–94.
22. Giannoudis PV, Papakostidis C, Roberts CS. A review of the management of open fractures of the tibia and femur. *J Bone Joint Surg Br* 2006; 88(3):281–9.
23. Harwood PJ, Giannoudis PV, Probst C, Krettek C, Pape H-C. The risk of local infective complications after damage control procedures for femoral shaft fracture. *J Orthop Trauma* 2006; 20(3):181–9.
24. Cannada LK, Jones AL. Demographic, social and economic variables that affect lower extremity injury outcomes. *Injury* 2006; 37(12):1109–16.
25. Lawrence SJ, Singhal M. Open hindfoot injuries. *J Am Acad Ortho Surg* 2007; 15:367–76.
26. Mubarak SJ, Owen CA. Compartmental syndrome and its relation to the crush syndrome: A spectrum of disease. A review of 11 cases of prolonged limb compression. *Clin Orthop* 1975; 113:81–9.
27. Attinger C. Soft tissue coverage for lower-extremity trauma. *Orthop Clin North AM* 1995; 26:295–334.
28. Baumeister S, Germann G. Soft tissue cover of the extremely traumatized foot and ankle. *Foot Ankle Clin* 2001; 6:867–903.
29. Montoli C, Depietri M, Barbieri S, D'Angelo F. Total extrusion of the talus: A case report. *J Foot Ankle Surg* 2004; 43:321–6.
30. Ostermann PA, Henry SL, Seligson D. Treatment of 2d and 3d degree complicated tibial shaft fractures with the PMMA bead pouch technic. *Unfallchirurg* 1989; 92(11):523–30.
31. Henry SL, Ostermann PA, Seligson D. The prophylactic use of antibiotic impregnated beads in open fractures. *J Trauma* 1990; 30(10):1231–8.
32. Ostermann PA, Henry SL, Seligson D. Timing of wound closure in severe compound fractures. *Orthopedics* 1994; 17(5):397–9.
33. Weed T, Ratliff C, Drake DB. Quantifying bacterial bioburden during negative pressure wound therapy: Does the wound VAC enhance bacterial clearance? *Ann Plast Surg* 2004; 52(3):276–9; discussion 279–80.
34. Mouës CM, Vos MC, van den Bemd GJ, Stijnen T, Hovius SER. Bacterial load in relation to vacuum-assisted closure wound therapy: A prospective randomized trial. *Wound Repair Regen* 2004; 12(1):11–7.
35. Banwell PE, Musgrave M. Topical negative pressure therapy: Mechanisms and indications. *Int Wound J* 2004; 1(2):95–106.
36. Della Rocca GJ, Crist BD. External fixation versus conversion to intramedullary nailing for definitive management of closed fractures of the femoral and tibial shaft. *J Am Acad Orthop Surg* 2006; 14(10 Suppl):S131–5.
37. Madanagopal SG, Seligson D, Roberts CS. The antibiotic cement nail for infection after tibial nailing. *Orthopaedics* 2004; 27(7):709–12.
38. Paley D, Herzenberg. Intramedullary infections treated with antibiotic cement rods: Preliminary results in nine cases. *J Orthop Trauma* 2002;16(10):723–9.

Chapter 7
Patient Selection: Orthopedic Approach in Polytrauma

Hans-Christoph Pape, Christopher C. Tzioupis, and Peter V. Giannoudis

7.1 Introduction

The development of the "two hit" theory has been helpful in understanding why certain patients may deteriorate unexpectedly after a major trauma and subsequent major surgery [1, 2]. Both the type and the severity of injury, the rescue conditions, and the individual patient's response are given facts at the time of patient's admission, representing the "first hit" in a trauma patient [1]. The subsequent treatment and unexpected complications can modify the clinical course substantially [3–7]. Thus, during the hospital stay, volume replacement, ventilatory support, and the surgical strategy are important variables [8] that may be modified by the hospital physician and thus regulate the degree of the impact of the second hit [9].

An individualized selection process determines which patients undergo a primary-definitive procedure and which patients benefit from temporary stabilization of their major extremity fractures to minimize the impact of surgery, also known as condition-tailored damage control orthopedic surgery.

For decades, assessment of the patient's clinical status relied on systolic blood pressure alone or in combination with other cardiovascular parameters [10]. The first criteria for appraising blunt trauma patients for orthopedic surgery were published in 1978 and suggested the use of systolic blood pressure, heart rate, central venous pressure, and hematocrit for essential evaluation. In addition, cardiac index, pulmonary arterial pressure, coagulation status, and acid-base parameters were also found to be of value for the early period after trauma [11]. Threshold levels for decision making, however, had not yet been developed at this stage.

Later, Asensio and colleagues [12] described the use of intraoperative parameters for predicting outcome and providing guidelines as to when to institute the damage control approach. These parameters include body temperature of $\leq 34°C$, $pH \leq 7.2$, serum bicarbonate ≤ 15 mEq/L, transfusion volume of

H.-C. Pape FACS (✉)
Department of Orthopaedic Surgery, University of Pittsburgh, 3471 Fifth Avenue, #1010, Pittsburgh, PA, 15213, USA
e-mail: papeHC@aol.com

H.-C. Pape et al. (eds.), *Damage Control Management in the Polytrauma Patient*, DOI 10.1007/978-0-387-89508-6_7, © Springer Science+Business Media, LLC 2010

RBC ≥ 34,000 mL (12–14 units of RBCs), total blood replacement (including RBCs and whole blood) of ≥5,000 mL, or total intraoperative fluid replacement, including crystalloid, blood, and blood products, ≥12,000 mL.

Blood pressure has also been included in scoring systems for patient assessment. Allgöwer's group [13] developed a simple score (shock index) that uses the ratio between the systolic blood pressure and the heart rate. If this ratio drops below a value of one, the patient is defined as in shock. Although the shock index has been questioned in the past, it has recently been shown to be effective in predicting late adverse outcome in blunt trauma patients [14].

The Revised Trauma Score (RTS) has been widely used and summarizes information on the respiration, the circulation, and the neurological status [15]. In a similar fashion, the criteria proposed by the Advanced Trauma Life Support program (ATLS®) also include four different stages of hemorrhage [16].

All the scores mentioned above have been mainly designed for prehospital evaluation. As time passes after trauma, it is evident that hemorrhagic shock and cardio respiratory parameters are not the only important variables for determining outcome. Several cascades are stimulated that could be of value for the evaluation of polytrauma patient.

The initiation of cascade pathways by hemorrhagic shock includes the hemostatic response (eventually leading to DIC) and the inflammatory response, which causes an imbalance of pro- and anti-inflammatory reactions [17–22]. Immunologic reactions may also be stimulated by a drop in body temperature [23]. Therefore, based on their experience with gunshot wounds, general surgeons have utilized the laboratory parameters associated with hemorrhagic shock to describe a patient's critical condition [24].

These parameters express the degrees of hypothermia, acidosis, and coagulopathy induced by hemorrhagic shock and have been summarized by the term "triad of death." [25–27] It has been confirmed that the triad of death is relevant for evaluating patients with penetrating trauma and viable for decision making in the emergency room [23, 28]. Blunt trauma patients undergo different pathogenetic changes: blood loss is usually slower, and the soft tissue extremity and thoracic injuries are often more severe [29–31].

The inclusion of "soft-tissue injuries," i.e., all muscular and subcutaneous injuries of the extremities, lung, abdomen, and pelvis, has been advocated [32, 33]. As outlined earlier, the integration of soft tissue injuries into the assessment of the determination of the patient's clinical classification helps define relevant markers of clinical grading.

Subsequently, all these parameters that have been discussed have been extrapolated beyond the abdominal cavity to the clinical setting for polytrauma patients with sustained extremity injuries.

The four pathophysiological entities – hemorrhagic shock, coagulopathy, hypothermia, soft tissue injuries and inflammation – defined as the "four pathophysiological cycles of blunt polytrauma" are relevant to the clinical course of the polytrauma patient.

7.2 The Four Pathophysiological Cycles of Blunt Polytrauma

7.2.1 *Hemorrhagic Shock*

Hemorrhagic shock is usually diagnosed through classic clinical parameters, although in young patients a sustained physiological reserve may delay changes in pulse and blood pressure and, subsequently, the diagnosis of shock. Border and colleagues [34] defined a patient being in a state of shock when there was a loss of 1–2 L of blood volume. Most investigators agree that a systolic BP < 90 mmHg can effectively identify the presence of hemorrhagic shock [35–39]. In contrast, other authors have proposed that the duration of malperfusion is a more important factor than the initial value, with a critical interval of 70 min defined as the threshold [1, 39].

The filling pressure on the right side may be measured using sub-clavian or jugular central venous catheters. The Central Venous Pressure (CVP) is likely to rise when there is an increase in the intra-thoracic pressure, e.g., in thoracic trauma, mechanical ventilation with Positive End-Expiratory Pressure (PEEP), and is often of little value when initially assessing shock. The use of a pulmonary arterial catheter (Swan–Ganz catheter) allows much more accurate and reliable estimation of cardiac function.

For the determination of blood loss from parenchymal organs, an estimated overall blood loss of more than 2,000 cc (class III and IV) has been used for classification of hemodynamic instability [40]. In order to estimate the degree of blood loss, some authors have advocated the requirement of mass transfusion (10 units/12 h) for guiding surgical strategy [41]. Sauaia and colleagues [42] described an excess of 6 units of blood as associated with a higher risk of organ failure and death and used this threshold value as a predictive parameter.

Urinary output may also be used as a parameter to determine volume depletion, provided that the urinary production is not altered by an injury to the genitourinary system. Urinary output < 25 mL/½ h in the emergency room has been determined to represent an indicator for urgent increase in volume therapy [43].

Laboratory parameters provide further information for evaluating shock status and may be especially useful in assessing response to therapy. In particular, the arterial pH, base excess, and plasma lactate levels reflect ongoing tissue ischemia, and various clinical and experimental studies have shown a correlation between these parameters and the degree of shock [44, 45]. Furthermore, their failure to normalize following therapy has been shown to correlate with poor outcome [46, 47].

Acidosis on admission was shown to be a significant marker of outcome, with a general consensus of pH < 7.2 as a cut off [12]. However, a low pH level alone should not be used as an indication to withdraw or withhold treatment [48]. To increase the diagnostic sensitivity of this parameter, the combined parameters of shock, defined by a blood loss of 4–5 L, hypothermia (core temperature < 34°C), and acidosis (pH < 7.25) have been advocated as threshold levels for the triad of death [49].

Likewise, base deficit is used as a marker of abnormal tissue perfusion, and an abnormal base excess was found to be associated with increases in mortality rates [31]. It has been proposed that the time taken to normalize base excess is more important than the absolute value, in terms of being a marker of the patient's response to resuscitation and correction of their state of shock [41, 50].

Lactate levels appear to have a slightly different relevance, as they have been used as a marker of ongoing tissue hypoperfusion. Because lactate is not normalized by the body's buffer systems, it may be more representative of the current overall state of tissue perfusion. Lactate clearance times of >24 h have been reported to better correlate with outcome than admission values. Blow and colleagues [46] used lactate levels to guide resuscitation. Claridge and colleagues [47] later confirmed these results: when lactate levels >2.5 did not respond to fluid challenge, invasive monitoring (PA catheter) and aggressive resuscitation including (vasopressor and inotropic agents) were performed and demonstrated improved survival rates [34].

In addition to the physiologic parameters described above, transfusion requirements have been used as endpoints and were shown to predict outcome [51, 52]. A significant increase in mortality was described when >9 units were received [52] versus >6 units [39, 53] or >2 units [14].

Other authors argued that the overall transfusion requirements may not be the best clinical parameters to predict outcome. Failure of hemostasis and ongoing blood loss may affect outcome rather than absolute transfusion requirements. Nonetheless, transfusion requirements have been identified as an independent risk factor for late adverse outcome such as multiple organ failure [53].

In summary, the diagnosis of volume depletion can be based on several parameters, including the systolic BP, the need for blood transfusions, acid base changes, and urine output. More invasive monitoring is required for the calculation of stroke volumes [54, 55].

7.2.2   Coagulopathy

Coagulopathy occurs as a result of hypothermia, platelet and coagulation factor dysfunction, activation of the fibrinolytic system, and hemodilution following massive resuscitation.

Repeated investigations have demonstrated that platelet counts are a stable and reliable parameter to measure the consumption of platelets. A decreased systemic platelet count on day 1 (<80,000 μl) [56] was associated with Multiple Organ Failure (MOF) and death, as was decreased platelet function and increased activation [57]. Abnormal values of the Partial Thromboplastin Time (PTT) and the Prothrombin Time (PT) were studied. An admission, PT > 15 s or a PTT > 50 [32] and PT > 19 or a PTT > 60 [58] were found to be predictors of adverse outcome [59]. Demsar and colleagues [60] used computer modeling with 174 variables and found a PTT > 78.8 (worst value after admission) to be the second most important predictor of MOF and death. Other investigators have demonstrated that coagulation parameters are significantly altered in patients who developed complications or died [9].

More recently, it has been suggested that the serum levels of D-dimers are valuable screening markers for perioperative complications, such as ARDS and MOF [27, 34]. Furthermore, D-dimer concentrations have also been described as markers for the extent of the soft tissue injury [61, 62].

In summary, the best screening marker for coagulopathy and adverse outcomes is the platelet count, with initial platelet values < 90,000 being a sign of impending Disseminated Intravascular Coagulopathy (DIC) if no other cause of coagulopathy can be identified.

7.2.3   Hypothermia

In contrast to the perceived benefits of hypothermia in elective surgery, clinical experience in trauma patients has identified hypothermia as an independent factor for morbidity and mortality [63, 64].

There are several important causes of hypothermia in the trauma patient such as blood loss, environmental exposure, prolonged rescue times, and metabolic changes. Heat production for maintenance of euthermia in the presence of surrounding low temperatures increases oxygen requirements. If tissue oxygen consumption is limited due to hemorrhagic shock, heat production cannot offset ongoing losses, resulting in hypothermia. Hypothermia may be also be induced by anesthetic agents, leading to a decrease in heat production by as much as one third [62].

The consequences of decreased body temperature for the other cascade systems are best described for the coagulatory response. Hypothermic coagulopathy rises significantly whenever the core temperature drops below 34°C [65].

The effect of low admission temperatures had been studied in numerous publications in the available literature. Threshold values for the development of complications ranged between 32 and 36°C [53]. Rewarming time has also been associated with outcome. In a randomized controlled trial investigating the effect of arteriovenous re-warming, a mortality rate of 100% was found in patients failing to re-warm [66].

In summary, hypothermia is a well described cause for further complications in blunt trauma patients. There is a close connection with the other cascade systems described in this chapter.

7.2.4   Soft Tissue Injuries and Inflammation (Extremity Soft Tissue Damage, Lung Contusion)

It is common sense that severe abdominal trauma and other injuries to the trunk implicate sustained shock states and severe soft tissue trauma [67, 68].

In contrast, the quantification of chest trauma in the polytrauma patient presents a distinct problem, as the AIS only gives a crude estimate of the degree of pulmonary damage [69, 70]. Thus a new score, the Thoracic Trauma Score (TTS), was developed on the basis of the chest x-ray findings and physiological parameters (Table 7.1) [71]. Due to the wide range of injury patterns in patients with blunt trauma, it is useful to identify the clinical parameters that appear to be associated with adverse outcomes. Recently, an increased awareness of the importance of chest injuries has been recognized [72]. It is of note that a lung contusion has been judged to be more relevant to the development of complications in the patient's clinical course than the bony lesion [30].

While it is well understood that isolated soft tissue lesions are a concern for orthopedic surgeons due to their local complications, these injuries may be even more relevant in the polytrauma situation in terms of their systemic effects. Local tissue hypoxia and necrosis may systemically spread, and changes induced by fractures and other injuries may have additive effects. Non-extremity soft tissue injuries can induce further systemic insults in addition to those already induced by extremity trauma [73].

Some systemic sequelae deriving from major fractures or surgical procedures are well described. After long bone fractures, intramedullary contents enter the bloodstream [74] and may induce the formation of thrombi due to high thromboplastin content [59]. Among the sequelae known to occur after torso trauma and major fractures associated with severe soft tissue injuries are necrosis, inflammation, and systemic acidosis [75]. However, quantification of the influence of severe soft tissue injuries with regard to the clinical course is difficult [17].

In addition to the factors described here, it has been argued that a close relationship between extremity injuries and lung function exists, as debris from open wounds and the fracture site enters the venous circulation and the lungs. The lung has been called a "filter organ" that prevents these substances from entering the arterial bloodstream [76]. A trauma-induced hemorrhage causes an increase in microvascular permeability that occurs in all organs including the lung [56], although it has an extraordinary ability to clear interstitial fluid via the lymphatic systems [77].

Table 7.1 Thoracic Trauma Severity Score. For calculation of the total score, all categories are summed up. A minimum value of 0 points and a maximum value of 25 points can be achieved

Grade	$P80_2/F10_2$	Rib fracture	Contusion	Pleural involvement	Age (v)	Points
0	>400	0	None	None	<30	0
I	300–400	1–3	1 lobe, unilateral	PT	30–41	1
II	200–300	3–6	1 lobe, bilateral or 2 lobes unilateral	HT/HPT unilateral	42–54	2
III	150–200	>3 bilateral	<2 lobes bilateral	HT/HPT bilateral	55–70	3
IV	<150	Flail chest	≥2 lobes bilateral	TPT	>70	5

Reprinted with permission of Wolters Kluwer from [71]

The lung contains the largest micro-vascular bed in the body. Therefore, an increase in interstitial edema and a reduction of oxygenation capacity may occur [78].

7.3 Determination of the Patient's Condition

In order to assess the clinical condition more precisely, a new patient category has been added to the three existing classes (stable, unstable, in extremis) [79]. The term "borderline" has been coined to describe a patient who is in apparently stable condition preoperatively, but who deteriorates unexpectedly and may develop organ dysfunction [79]. Once initial assessment and intervention is complete, patients can be separated into one of these four categories in order to guide the subsequent approach to their care.

This assessment is done on the basis of overall injury severity, the presence of specific injuries, and current hemodynamic status as detailed above [79]. Any deterioration in the clinical state or physiological parameters should prompt rapid reassessment and adjustment of management approach as appropriate [8].

Achieving end points of resuscitation is of paramount importance for the classification of the patient into the appropriate category. End points of resuscitation include: stable hemodynamics, stable oxygen saturation, lactate level <2 mmol/L, no coagulation disturbances, normal temperature, urinary output >1 mL kg/h, and no requirement for inotropic support.

7.3.1 Stable Condition

Stable patients have no life-threatening injuries, respond to initial therapy, and are hemodynamically stable without inotropic support. There is no evidence of coagulopathy, ongoing occult hypoperfusion, abnormalities of acid base status, or hypothermia.

7.3.2 Borderline Condition

Factors identifying the borderline patient have been defined as follows:

- Injury Severity Score > 40
- Multiple injuries (ISS > 20) in association with thoracic trauma (AIS > 2)
- Multiple injuries in association with severe abdominal or pelvic injury and hemorrhagic shock at presentation (systolic BP < 90 mmHg)
- Patients with bilateral femoral fractures
- Radiographic evidence of pulmonary contusion

- Hypothermia below 35°C
- Patients with additional moderate or severe head injuries (AIS 3 or greater)
- Initial mean pulmonary arterial pressure > 24 mmHg (if available)

As indicated by this list, the borderline condition does not involve the physiologic changes described in the four cascades. These factors represent an increased risk for mortality and are independent of the basic parameters that may or may not be normal.

7.3.3 Unstable Condition

Patients who remain hemodynamically unstable despite initial intervention are at greatly increased risk of rapid deterioration, subsequent multiple organ failure, and death [80, 81].

7.3.4 In Extremis

Patients in extremis have been well-classified by general surgeons (early blood loss of 4–5 L, a core temperature of 34 C, and a pH of less than 7.25) [49].

These patients are in acute life-threatening condition and often have ongoing uncontrollable blood loss. They remain severely unstable despite continuing resuscitative efforts and are usually suffering the effects of the "deadly triad" of hypothermia, acidosis, and coagulopathy (Table 7.2).

7.4 Value of Scoring Systems in Polytrauma Patients

Many trauma scoring systems (e.g., the abbreviated injury scale [82], the injury severity score [83, 84], the revised trauma score [85], the anatomic profile [86], and the Glasgow coma scale [87]) have been developed in an attempt to describe the overall condition of the trauma patient. However, Bosse and colleagues [88] noted that "there is no score that assists in decision-making during the acute resuscitation phase." This may be due to the fact that these scores were developed for the use at the accident scene, or focused on one specific organ system only.

The authors' earlier recommendations were based on the observation that patients with blunt trauma injuries had a higher incidence of ARDS after being submitted to a nailing procedure for a femur shaft fracture in the presence of chest trauma [89]. The authors therefore tried to limit the degree of surgical impact by advocating an unreamed femoral nailing procedure for patients with a thoracic

Table 7.2 A patient may be categorized into one of the four different classes (stable, borderline, unstable, in extremis) if he/she meets the criteria in at least three out of the four categories

	Parameter	Stable (grade I)	Borderline (grade II)	Unstable (grade III)	In extremis (grade IV)
Shock	Blood pressure (mmHg)	100 or more	80–100	60–90	50–60
	Blood units (2 h)	0–2	2–8	5–15	>15
	Lactate levels	Normal range	Approximately 2.5	>2.5	Severe acidosis
	Base deficit (mmol/L)	Normal range	No data	No data	>6–18
	ATLS classification	I	II–III	III–IV	IV
	Urine output (mL/h)	>150	50–150	<100	<50
Coagulation	Platelet count (µg/mL)	>110,000	90,000–110,000	<70,000–90,000	<70,000
	Factor II and V (%)	90–100	70–80	50–70	<50
	Fibrinogen (g/dL)	>1	Approximately 1	<1	DIC
	D-Dimer	Normal range	Abnormal	Abnormal	DIC
Temperature		>34°C	33–35°C	30–32°C	30°C or less
Soft-tissue injuries	Ling function; PaO_2/FiO_2	>350	300	200–300	<200
	Chest trauma scores; AIS	AIS I or II	AIS 2 or more	AIS 2 or more	AIS 3 or more
	Thoracic trauma score; TTS	0	I–II	II–III	IV
	Abdominal trauma (Moore)	≤II	≤III	III	III or >III
	Pelvic trauma (AO class)	A type (AO)	B or C	C	C (crush, rollover adb.)
	Extremities	AIS I–II	AIS II–III	AIS III–IV	Cursh, rollover extreme
Surgical Strategy	Damage control (DCO) or		DCO if uncertain		
	Definitive surgery (ETC)	ETC	ETC if stable	DCO	DCO

Reprinted with permission of Wolters Kluwer from [32]

trauma AIS of 2–4 points. At this stage, there was no easy access to Pulmonary Arterial (PA) catheterization. High PA and wedge pressures have been associated with adverse pulmonary reactions [90]. The authors therefore recommended PA catheter monitoring for certain cases. Finally, for patients in critical condition (hemodynamically unstable) or with associated thoracic trauma (AIS > 4 points), the authors proposed avoiding intramedullary stabilization and instead

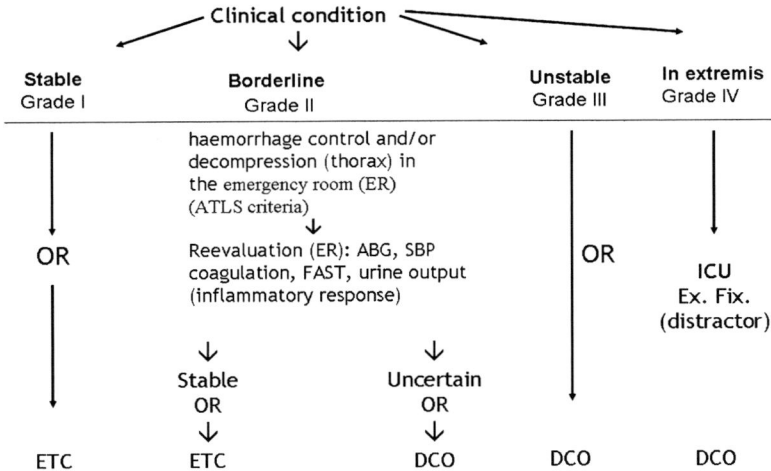

Fig. 7.1 General recommendations for the fixation of major extremity and pelvic fractures in polytrauma patient (Reprinted with permission from Pape H-C. Giannoudis P, Krettek C. The timing of fracture treatment in polytrauma patients: relevance of damage control orthopaedic surgery. *Am J Surg* 2002, 183:622–629. With permission from Elsevier.)

recommended applying a temporary external fixator until the pulmonary situation stabilizes [91].

Subsequently, other authors have added further clinical criteria to describe when the damage control orthopedic approach is appropriate. These criteria include a pH of <7.24, a temperature of <35°C, operative times of greater than ninety minutes, coagulopathy, and transfusion of more than ten units of packed red blood cells. Furthermore, certain specific orthopedic injury patterns appear to be more amenable to damage control orthopedics; these include, for example, femoral fractures in a multiply injured patient, pelvic ring injuries with exsanguinating hemorrhage, and poly-trauma in a geriatric patient [92].

Based on the current understanding of pathophysiological principles, the authors feel that the initial polytrauma patient assessment can be structured according to the "four pathophysiological cycles of polytrauma" described earlier. A patient may be categorized into one of the four different classes (stable, borderline, unstable, in extremis), if he or she meets the criteria in at least three out of the four categories. However, it is important to note that individual variations exist (Fig. 7.1).

As outlined earlier, the existence of a femur fracture represents a special entity, and the indication for the type of fixation has been widely discussed in the past. It is understood that the femur shaft fracture should be initially stabilized if a patient is stable. In the patient who is not stable, the algorithm described in Fig. 7.2 is recommended. A staged approach appears to adequately adapt the degree of surgical treatment to the condition of the patient.

The critical parameters can be summarized as follows: Soft tissue injuries (major extremity fractures, crush injuries, severe pelvic fractures, lung contusions

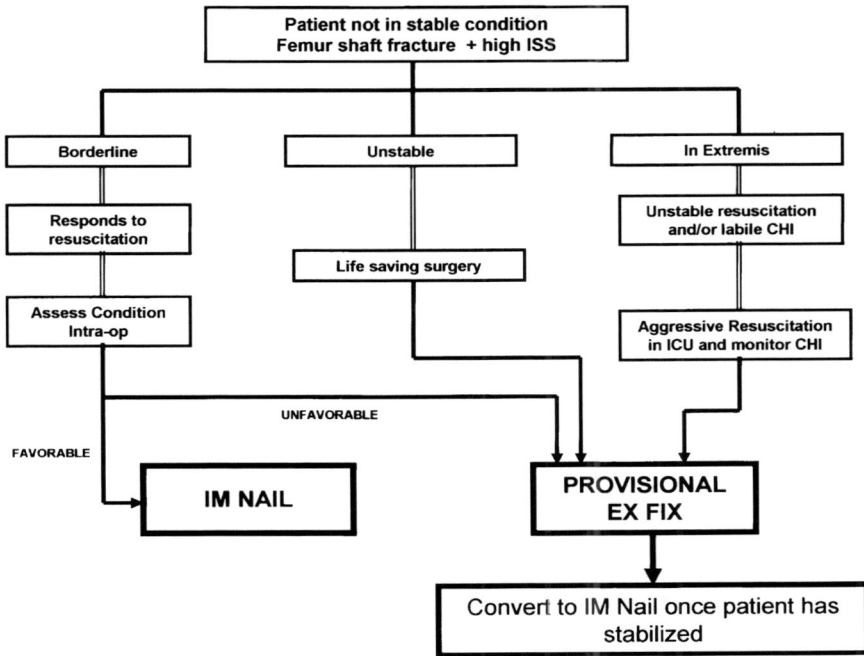

Fig. 7.2 Exemplary algorithm for the fixation of a femur shaft fracture in polytrauma with high ISS

AIS > 2), coagulopathy (platelets < 90,000), and shock (systolic BP < 90 mmHg, requirement of vasopressors) contribute to hypothermia (core temp < 33°C) and are dangerous.

Given these recommendations for extremity injuries, it is understood that these suggestions must be integrated into the general distribution and severity pattern of all injuries. In patients with severe head injuries or those with life-threatening hemorrhages, the algorithm in Fig. 7.2 should be interrupted whenever an acute change in the clinical condition occurs. The dynamic nature of events in the polytrauma patient, rather than any score or algorithm, often dictates the sequence of interventions.

7.5 Summary and Conclusion

The clinical assessment of patients with multiple injuries is complex. In addition to the severity of the injuries sustained, the presence or absence of a borderline status is the major decision-making factor. More than a single parameter should be used to judge the status. In addition to the assessment of shock, coagulopathy, and hypothermia, judgment on the soft tissue injuries and hidden hypoxemia is required. Rapid changes also can occur, thus requiring reassessment preoperatively or intraoperatively.

References

1. Giannoudis PV, Smith RM, Bellamy MC, Morrison JF, Dickson RA, Guillou PJ. Stimulation of the inflammatory system by reamed and unreamed nailing of femoral fractures. An analysis of the second hit. *J Bone Joint Surg Br* 1999;81:356-61.
2. Pape HC, Schmidt RE, Rice J, van Griensven M, das Gupta R, Krettek C, Tscherne H. Biochemical changes after trauma and skeletal surgery of the lower extremity: quantification of the operative burden. *Crit Care Med* 2000;28:3441-8.
3. Giannoudis PV, Veysi VT, Pape HC, Krettek C, Smith MR. When should we operate on major fractures in patients with severe head injuries? Am J Surg 2002 ;183:261-7.
4. Giannoudis PV. When is the safest time to undertake secondary definitive fracture stabilization procedures in multiply injured patients who were initially managed using a strategy of primary temporary skeletal fixation. *J Trauma.* 2002;52:811-2.
5. Pape HC, van Griensven M, Rice J, Gansslen A, Hildebrand F, Zech S, Winny M, Lichtinghagen R, Krettek C. Major secondary surgery in blunt trauma patients and perioperative cytokine liberation: determination of the clinical relevance of biochemical markers. *J Trauma* 2001;50:989-1000.
6. Bone LB, Johnson KD, Weigelt J, Scheinberg R. Early versus delayed stabilization of femoral fractures: a prospective randomized study. *J Bone Joint Surg* 1989 ;71:336-40.
7. Pape HC, Grimme K, Van Griensven M, Sott AH, Giannoudis P, Morley J, Roise O, Ellingsen E, Hildebrand F, Wiese B, Krettek C; EPOFF Study Group. Impact of intramedullary instrumentation versus damage control for femoral fractures on immunoinflammatory parameters: prospective randomized analysis by the EPOFF Study Group. *J Trauma* 2003;55:7-13.
8. Giannoudis PV. Surgical priorities in damage control in polytrauma. *J Bone Joint Surg* 2003;85:478-83.
9. Giannoudis PV, Smith RM, Perry SL, Windsor AJ, Dickson RA, Bellamy MC. Immediate IL-10 expression following major orthopaedic trauma: relationship to anti-inflammatory response and subsequent development of sepsis. *Intensive Care Med* 2000;26:1076-81.
10. Smith RM, Giannoudis PV. Trauma and the immune response. *J R Soc Med* 1998; 91:417-20.
11. Trentz O, Oestern HJ, Hempelmann G, Kolbow H, Sturm J, Trentz OA, Tscherne H. Criteria for the operability of patients with multiple injuries. *Unfallheilkunde* 1978;81:451-8.
12. Asensio JA, McDuffie L, Petrone P, Roldan G, Forno W, Gambaro E, Salim A, Demetriades D, Murray J, Velmahos G, Shoemaker W, Berne T.V, Ramicone E, Chan L. Reliable variables in the exsanguinated patient which indicate damage control and predict outcome. *Am J Surg* 2001;182:743-51.
13. Burri C, Henkemeyer H, Pässler HH, Allgöwer M. Evaluation of acute blood loss by means of simple hemodynamic parameters. *Prog Surg* 1973;11:109-27.
14. Pape HC, Erhardtsen E, Meyer C, Leppäniemi AK. Recombinant factor VIIa for life-threatening hemorrhage in trauma patients: review of the literature. *Eur J Trauma* 2006;32:439-48.
15. Champion HR, Copes WS, Sacco WJ, Gann DS, Gennarelli TA, Flanagan ME. A revision of the Trauma Score. *J Trauma* 1989;29(5):623-9.
16. American College of Surgeons Committee on Trauma. *ATLS® student course Manual,* sixth edition. Chicago: American College of Surgeons 1997, pp. 89-109.

17. Giannoudis PV. Current concepts of the inflammatory response after major trauma: an update. *Injury* 2003;34:397–404.
18. Giannoudis PV, Pape HC, Cohen AP, Krettek C, Smith RM. Review: systemic effects of femoral nailing: from Kuntscher to the immune reactivity era. *Clin Orthop Relat Res* 2002; 378–86.
19. Giannoudis PV, Hildebrand F, Pape HC. Inflammatory serum markers in patients with multiple trauma. Can they predict outcome? *J Bone Joint Surg Br* 2004;86:313–23.
20. Pape HC, Hildebrand F, Krettek C. Decision making and and priorities for surgical treatment during and after shock trauma room treatment. *Unfallchirurg* 2004 ;107:927–36.
21. Pape HC, Zelle BA, Hildebrand F, Giannoudis PV, Krettek C, van Griensven M.Reamed femoral nailing in sheep: does irrigation and aspiration of intramedullary contents alter the systemic response? *J Bone Joint Surg Am* 2005;87:2515–22.
22. Pape HC. Immediate fracture fixation – which method? Comments on the John Border Memorial Lecture, Ottawa, 2005. *J Orthop Trauma* 2006;20:341–50.
23. Hildebrand F, van Griensven M, Giannoudis P, Schreiber T, Frink M, Probst C, Grotz M, Krettek C, Pape HC. Impact of hypothermia on the immunologic response after trauma and elective surgery. *Surg Technol Int* 2005;14:41–50.
24. Bone RC. Toward a theory regarding the pathogenesis of the systemic inflammatory response syndrome: what we do and do not know about cytokine regulation. *Crit Care Med* 1996;24: 162–72.
25. Asensio JA, Petrone P, O'Shanahan G, Kuncir EJ. Managing exsanguination: what we know about damage control/bailout is not enough. *Proc (Bayl Univ Med Cent)* 2003;16: 294–6.
26. Rotondo MF, Schwab CW, McGonigal MD, Phillips GR 3rd, Fruchterman TM, Kauder DR, Latenser BA, Angood PA. "Damage control": an approach for improved survival in exsanguinating penetrating abdominal injury. *J Trauma* 1993;35:375–82.
27. Moore EE, Thomas G. Orr Memorial Lecture: staged laparotomy for the hypothermia, acidosis, and coagulopathy syndrome. *Am J Surg* 1996;172:405–10.
28. Johnson JW, Gracias VH, Schwab CW, Reilly PM, Kauder DR, Shapiro MB, Dabrowski GP, Rotondo MF. Evolution in damage control for exsanguinating penetrating abdominal injury. *J Trauma* 2001;51:261–71.
29. Seibel R, LaDuca J, Hassett JM, Babikian G, Mills B, Border DO, Border JR. Blunt multiple trauma (ISS 36), femur traction and the pulmonary failure septic state. *Ann Surg* 1985;202:283.
30. Pelias ME, Townsend MC, Flancbaum L. Long bone fractures predispose to pulmonary dysfunction in blunt chest trauma despite early operative fixation. *Surgery* 1992;111:576–9.
31. Hauser CJ, Zhou X, Joshi P, Cuchens MA, Kregor P. Devidas M, Kennedy RJ, Poole GV, Hughe JL. The immune microenvironment of human fracture/soft-tissue hematomas and its relationship to systemic immunity. *J Trauma* 1997;42:895–903.
32. Pape H-C, Giannoudis PV, Krettek C, Trentz O. Timing of fixation of major fractures in blunt polytrauma: Role of conventional indicators in clinical decision making. *J Orthop Trauma* 2005;19:551–62.
33. Allami MK, Partenheimer A, Sommer K, Jamil W, Gerich T, Krettek C, Pape HC. Complete aortic rupture in a polytrauma patient: damage control orthopaedics. *J Trauma.* 2008;64(2):E24–8.
34. Border JR, La Duca J, Seibel R. Priorities in the management of the patient with polytrauma. *Prog Surg* 1975;14:84–120.
35. Gruen GS, Leit ME, Gruen RJ, Peitzman AB. The acute management of hemodynamically unstable patients with pelvic ring fractures. *J Trauma* 1994;36:706–13.
36. Eberhard LW, Morabito DJ, Matthay MA, Mackersie RC, Campbell AC, Marks JD, Alonso JA, Pittet JF. Initial severity of metabolic acidosis predicts the development of acute lung injury in severely traumatized patients. *Crit Care Med* 2000;28:125–31.
37. Siegel JH, Rivkind AI, Dalal S, Goodarzi S. Early physiologic predictors of injury severity and death in blunt multiple trauma. *Arch Surg* 1990;125:498–508.

38. Cinat ME, Wallace WC, Nastanski F, West J, Sloan S, Ocariz J, Wilson SE. Improved survival following massive transfusion in patients who have undergone trauma. *Arch Surg* 1999;134:964–9.
39. Garrison JR, Richardson JD, Hilakos AS, Spain DA, Wilson MA, Miller FB, Fulton RL. Predicting the need to pack early for severe intra-abdominal hemorrhage. *J Trauma* 1996;40:923–7.
40. Moore FA, Moore EE, Jones TN, McCroskey BL, Peterson VM. TEN versus TPN following major abdominal trauma – reduced septic morbidity. *J Trauma* 1989;29:916–22.
41. Oestern HJ, Regel G. Clinical care of the polytrauma patient. In Tscherne H. Regel G (eds): *Polytrauma management*. New York: Springer 1997, Chapter 9, pp 225–238.
42. Sauaia A, Moore FA, Moore EE, Haenel J, Read RA, Lezotte DC. Early predictors of postinjury MOF. *Arch Surg* 1994;129:39–45.
43. Regel G, Lobenhoffer P, Tscherne H. Acute management of the polytrauma patient. In Tscherne H. Regel G (eds): *Polytrauma management*. New York: Springer 1997, Chapter 11, pp 257–297.
44. Rixen D, Siegel JH. Metabolic correlates of oxygen debt predict posttrauma early acute respiratory distress syndrome and the related cytokine response. *J Trauma* 2000;49(3):392–403.
45. Rixen D, Raum M, Holzgraefe B, Sauerland S, Nagelschmidt M, Neugebauer EA, Group SaTS. A pig haemorrhagic shock model: oxygen debt and metabolic acidemia as indicators of severity. *Shock* 2001;16(3):239–44.
46. Blow O, Magliore L, Claridge JA, Butler K, Young JS. The golden hour and the silver day: detection and correction of occult hypoperfusion within 24 hours improves outcome from major trauma. *J Trauma* 1999;47(5):964–9.
47. Claridge JA, Crabtree TD, Pelletier SJ, Butler K, Sawyer RG, Young JS. Persistent occult hypoperfusion is associated with a significant increase in infection rate and mortality in major trauma patients. *J Trauma* 2000;48(1):8–14.
48. Ferrara A, MacArthur JD, Wright HK, Modlin IM, McMillen MA. Hypothermia and acidosis worsen coagulopathy in the patient requiring massive transfusion. *Am J Surg* 1990;160:515–8.
49. Carillo C, Fogler RJ, Shaftan GW. Delayed gastrointestinal reconstruction following massive abdominal trauma. *J Trauma* 1993;34:233–5.
50. Husain FA, Martin MJ, Mullenix PS, Steele SR, Elliott DC. Serum lactate and base deficit as predictors of mortality and morbidity. *Am J Surg* 2003;185(5):485–91.
51. Tran DD, Cuesta MA, van Leeuwen PA, Nauta JJ, Wesdorp RI. Risk factors for multiple organ system failure and death in critically injured patients. *Surgery* 1993;114–1:21–30.
52. Riska EB, Bostman O, von Bonsdorff H, Hakkinen S, Jaroma H, Kiviluoto O, Paavilainen T. Outcome of closed injuries exceeding 20-unit blood transfusion need. *Injury* 1988;19:273–6.
53. Bernard GR, Artigas A, Brigham KL, Carlet J, Falke K. The American-European Consensus Conference on ARDS. Consensus conference on ARDS. *Am J Respir Crit Care Med* 1994;149:818–24.
54. Gando S, Nanzaki S, Kemmotsu O. Disseminated intravascular coagulation and sustained systemic inflammatory response syndrome predict organ dysfunctions after trauma: application of clinical decision analysis. *Ann Surg* 1999;229:121–7.
55. Malone DL, Kuhls D, Napolitano LM, McCarter R, Scalea T. Back to basics: validation of the admission systemic inflammatory response syndrome score in predicting outcome in trauma. *J Trauma* 2001;51:458–63.
56. Nuytinck JK, Goris JA, Redl H, Schlag G, van Munster PJ. Posttraumatic complications and inflammatory mediators. *Arch Surg* 1986;121–8:886–90.
57. Jacoby RC, Owings JT, Holmes J, Battistella FD, Gosselin RC, Paglieroni TG. Platelet activation and function after trauma. *J Trauma* 2001;51:639–47.
58. Varani J, Ward RA. Mechanisms of endothelial cell injury in acute inflammation. *Shock* 1994;2:311–9.
59. Moore EE, Shackford SR, Pachter HL. McAninch JW, Browner BD, Champion HR, Flint LM, Gennarelli TA, Malangoni MA, Ramenofsky ML. Organ injury scaling: Spleen, liver and kidney. *J Trauma* 1989;29:439.

60. Demsar J, Zupan B, Aoki N, Wall MJ, Granchi TH, Robert Beck J. Feature mining and predictive model construction from severe trauma patient's data. *Int J Med Inf* 2001;63:41–50.
61. Kwan HC. Role of fibrinolysis in disease processes. Semin Thromb Haemost 1984;10:71–9.
62. Meyer DM, Horton JW. Effect of different degrees of hypothermia on myocardium in treatment of hemorrhagic shock. *J Surg Res* 1990;48:61–7.
63. Tsuei BJ, Kearney PA. Hypothermia in the trauma patient. *Injury* 2004;35:7–15.
64. Kirkpatrick AW, Chun R, Brown R, Simons RK. Hypothermia and the trauma patient. *Can J Surg* 1999;42-5:333–43.
65. McInerney JJ, Breakell A, Madira W, Davies TG, Evans PA. Accidental hypothermia: the metabolic and inflammatory changes observed above and below 32°C. *Emerg Med J* 2002;19:219–23.
66. Gentilello LM, Jurkovich GJ, Stark MS, Hassantash SA, O'Keefe GE. Is hypothermia in the victim of major trauma protective or harmful? A randomized, prospective study. *Ann Surg* 1997;226–4:439–47.
67. Wojcik K, Gazdzik TS, Jaworski JM, Kaleta M. The influence of body injuries on bone union of femoral shaft fractures treated by different operative methods. *Chir Narzadow Ruchu Ortop Pol* 2004;69:19–22.
68. Anwar IA, Battistella FD, Neiman R, Olson SA, Chapman MW, Moehring HD. Femur fractures and lung complications: a prospective randomized study of reaming. *Clin Orthop Relat Res* 2004;422:71–6.
69. Baker SP, O'Neill B, Haddon W, Long WB. The injury severity score: A method for describing atients with multiple injuries and evaluating emergency care. *J Trauma* 1974;14:187–196.
70. Wagner RB, Crawford WO Jr, Schimpf PP, Jamieson PM, Rao KC. Quantification and pattern of parenchymal lung injury in blunt chest trauma: diagnostic and therapeutic implications. *J Comput Tomogr* 1988;12:270–81.
71. Pape H-C, Remmers D, Rice J, Ebisch M, Krettek C, Tscherne H. Appraisal of early evaluation of blunt chest trauma: Development of a standardized scoring system for initial clinical decision making. *J Trauma* 2000;49:496–504.
72. Rotondo MF, Bard MR. Damage control surgery for thoracic injuries. *Injury* 2004;35:649–54.
73. Adams JM, Hauser CJ, Livingston DH, Fekete Z, Hasko G, Forsythe RM, Deitch EA. The immunomodulatory effects of damage control abdominal packing on local and systemic neutrophil activity. *J Trauma* 2001;50–5:792–800.
74. Gossling HR, Pellegrini VD. Fat embolism syndrome – a review of the pathophysiology and physiological basis of treatment. *Clin Orthop Relat Res* 1982;165:68–72.
75. Patrick DA, Moore EE, Moore FA, Biffl WL, Barnet CC. Release of anti-inflammatory mediators after major torso trauma correlates with the development of post injury multiple organ failure. *Am J Surg* 1999;178:564–8.
76. Meek RN, Woodruff B, Allardyce DB. Source of fat macroglobules in fractures of the lower extremity. *J Trauma* 1972;12:432–4.
77. Staub NC. Pulmonary edema. Physiol Rev 1974;54:678.
78. Sturm JA, Wisner DH, Oestern HJ, Kant CJ, Tscherne H. Creutzig H. Increased lung capillary permeability after trauma: a prospective clinical study. *J Trauma* 1986;26:409–18.
79. Pape H-C, Auf'm'Kolck M, Paffrath T, Regel G, Sturm JA, Tscherne H. Primary intramedullary femur fixation in multiple trauma patients with associated lung contusion – a cause of posttraumatic ARDS? *J Trauma* 1993;34(4):540–4.
80. Shapiro MB, Jenkins DH, Schwab CW, Rotondo MF. Damage control: collective review. *J Trauma* 2000;49:969–78.
81. Meregalli A, Oliveira RP, Friedman G. Occult hypoperfusion is associated with increased mortality in hemodynamically stable, high risk, surgical patients. *Crit Care* 2004;8–2:R60–5.
82. Association for the Advancement of Automotive Medicine. *The abbreviated injury scale.* 1990 revision. Des Plaines, IL: Association for the Advancement of Automotive Medicine, 1990.

83. Baker SP, O'Neill B, Haddon W Jr, Long WB. The injury severity score: a method for describing patients with multiple injuries and evaluating emergency care. *J Trauma* 1974;14:187–96.
84. Copes WS, Champion HR, Sacco WJ, Lawnick MM, Keast SL, Bain LW. The Injury Severity Score revisited. *J Trauma* 1988;28:69–77.
85. Champion HR, Sacco WJ, Copes WS, Gann DS, Gennarelli TA, Flanagan ME. A revision of the Trauma Score. *J Trauma* 1989;29:623–9.
86. Copes WS, Champion HR, Sacco WJ, Lawnick MM, Gann DS, Gennarelli T, MacKenzie E, Schwaitzberg S. Progress in characterizing anatomic injury. *J Trauma* 1990;30:1200–7.
87. Teasdale G, Jennett B. Assessment of coma and impaired consciousness. A practical scale. *Lancet* 1974;2:81–4.
88. Bosse MJ, MacKenzie EJ, Riemer BL, Brumback RJ, McCarthy ML, Burgess R, Gens DR, Yasui Y. Adult respiratory distress syndrome, pneumonia, and mortality following thoracic injury and a femoral fracture treated either with intramedullary nailing with reaming or with a plate. A comparative study. *J Bone Joint Surg Am* 1997;79:799–809.
89. Pape HC, Tscherne H. Early definitive fracture fixation, pulmonary function and systemic effects. In Baue AE, Faist E, Fry M (eds): *Multiple organ failure.* New York: Springer 2000, pp 279–90.
90. Sturm JA, Lewis FR Jr, Trentz O, Oestern HJ, Hempelman G, Tscherne H. Cardiopulmonary parameters and prognosis after severe multiple trauma. *J Trauma* 1979 ;19:305–18.
91. Pape HC, Hildebrand F, Pertschy S, Zelle B, Garapati R, Grimme K, Krettek C, Reed RL 2nd. Changes in the management of femoral shaft fractures in polytrauma patients: from early total care to damage control orthopedic surgery. *J Trauma* 2002;53:452–61.
92. Roberts CS, Pape HC, Jones AL, Malkani AL, Rodriguez JL, Giannoudis PV. Damage control orthopaedics: evolving concepts in the treatment of patients who have sustained orthopaedic trauma. *Instr Course Lect* 2005;54:447–62.

Part II
Phases of Damage Control

Chapter 8
Phase 0: Damage Control Resuscitation in the Pre-hospital and Emergency Department Settings

Andrew B. Peitzman and Babak Sarani

8.1 Introduction

Pre-hospital trauma care was first formalized into a trauma course for ambulance personnel in 1962 by Drs. J.D. Farrington and Sam Banks [1]. The Emergency Medical System (EMS) has evolved significantly since then, with the expansion of the 911 system to include most of the United States and the development of a multi-tiered training system for emergency medical responders. At the basic level, the emergency medical responder may be a "first responder" who is trained in advanced first aid. The highest level ground-based emergency responder in the United States is usually a paramedic, who works under the auspices of a regional medical director and is trained in the use of various medications, intravenous fluid therapy, and procedures (e.g., intubation, needle thoracostomy) to stabilize patients en route to the hospital. Conversely, many European countries utilize physicians as the highest level ground-based EMS responder. Most rotary-wing aeromedical transport providers utilize flight nurses as the highest level medical emergency responder, while many fixed-wing aeromedical transport companies utilize physicians for long-range transfers.

While the EMS system was shown to decrease the mortality following cardiac arrest in the 1960s [2], the need for advanced life support measures, such as those provided by paramedics, for trauma patients remains controversial. Some studies have found that exsanguinating trauma patients, especially in urban settings, have lower mortality if they are rapidly transported to an appropriate trauma center with little to no pre-hospital therapy administered, while other studies have refuted this finding [3]. However, this debate may only be germane following penetrating trauma in an urban setting where definitive care is readily available, and its extrapolation to patients who have sustained severe Traumatic Brain Injury (TBI) or who have been injured in the rural community is controversial. Patients who are injured

A.B. Peitzman (✉)
Department of Surgery, University of Pittsburgh, F-1281 UPMC-Presbyterian,
Pittsburgh, PA, 15213, USA
e-mail: peitzmanab@upmc.edu

H.-C. Pape et al. (eds.), *Damage Control Management in the Polytrauma Patient*,
DOI 10.1007/978-0-387-89508-6_8, © Springer Science+Business Media, LLC 2010

in rural areas, which inherently implies longer time from injury to EMS activation and EMS scene arrival to definitive care, may benefit from advanced maneuvers to minimize prolonged hypoperfusion and shock.

Abbreviated laparotomy, "damage control," was introduced into trauma surgery as a concept in the early 1990s. Since then, damage control has become an accepted approach in many surgical disciplines and has been shown to lower mortality [4]. Briefly, this concept involves treating all life-threatening injuries without definitive repair (i.e., control of hemorrhage, shunting severed blood vessels temporarily, and stopping bowel contamination) to allow for an ongoing resuscitation prior to definitive repair. The planning for damage control generally begins in the trauma bay or emergency department following evaluation of the patient by the trauma surgeon, but should ideally start in the pre-hospital setting based on the EMS personnel's report to the trauma center. A system-wide approach to the exsanguinating patient optimizes the chance for survival. The pre-hospital providers should recognize the patient who needs urgent control of bleeding and expedite transport, and focus treatment on only essential interventions. In the emergency department, factors that are critical in determining whether or not to utilize this strategy include the magnitude of the base deficit, lactate, coagulopathy, hypothermia, or systemic acidosis on arrival at the Emergency Department (ED) or the magnitude of the multi-system/multi-cavitary injury. The specific injuries are not factored into this decision as much as the patient's physiologic status. The previously noted factors are directly related to the severity of injury and time to definitive care. The triad of hypothermia, acidosis, and coagulopathy is a predictor of mortality following injury, and patients who present with these factors either in the field or on arrival at the trauma center should undergo damage control resuscitation.

This chapter will review resuscitation strategies for severely injured patients in the pre-hospital and ED settings. These settings represent a continuum of care in the initial triage, evaluation, and management of the patient, and the initial plan of care is best created in this arena. The patient's ultimate outcome depends, largely, on strategies developed and therapies instituted in the pre-hospital and ED settings. Each section is organized in the "ABCD" primary survey format taught in the Advanced Trauma Life Support Course of the American College of Surgeons [5], and it is assumed that the reader has a solid understanding of the fundamental principles involved in assessing and resuscitating the injured patient.

8.2 Pre-hospital Resuscitation

8.2.1 Rural Versus Urban Environment

The models of instituting therapeutic measures in the field prior to arrival at the hospital have been dubbed "scoop and run" or "stay and play." However, there is another model that involves instituting therapy en route to the hospital without delaying scene departure. This model is colloquially called "scoop and play." The choice of method employed depends on the setting in which the injury has occurred, the probable injuries sustained, and the patient's physiologic status.

Furthermore, the particular approach utilized must factor in the pre-hospital concepts of damage control, such as abbreviated scene time and aeromedical transport.

Rural trauma differs greatly from urban trauma, both in injury mechanism and also in probability of survival. Most injuries in the rural setting result from blunt mechanism of injury, and the few penetrating injuries that occur result mainly from suicide and hunting accidents as opposed to homicide. Furthermore, the chances of dying following injury are at least three to four times higher in the rural setting [6, 7]. The major reason for this difference is a relative lack of access to the EMS and healthcare systems, and lack of resources.

The timing of trauma resuscitation has traditionally been divided into two intervals: the "platinum 10 minutes" and the "golden hour." The platinum ten minutes involves transporting a patient from the scene of injury within 10 min of the EMS crews' arrival, and the golden hour describes the time interval for defining all injuries and treating all life-threatening injuries. However, these concepts do not apply readily to the rural setting. In this environment, the patient may not be discovered for many hours (or days) following injury. Furthermore, rescue from the scene may require complicated extrication and a prolonged transport time. The time from a motor vehicle crash to arrival in the hospital exceeds 1 h in 30% of rural collisions as opposed to 7% in urban settings [8]. Moreover, the nearest facility may not be a trauma center. Whereas EMS crews are routinely instructed to bypass non-trauma designated facilities for a trauma center in the urban setting, this may not be possible in the rural environment, where the nearest trauma center may be a long distance from the nearest hospital. Because of these factors, patients who have injuries that may not be life-threatening in the urban setting may present in extremis following injury in rural areas.

Damage control should start in the pre-hospital setting with the goal of minimizing or alleviating shock in these patients with utilization of aeromedical transport to decrease the time to definitive care and institution of the therapies that are discussed in the subsequent sections. These patients are best served with a "scoop and play" model. These factors should govern the procedures, if any, performed prior to transport of the patient, considering that 60% of severe TBI patients have injuries outside of the brain and require multiple interventions [9].

8.2.2   Airway and Breathing

One of the biggest controversies in the pre-hospital care of the injured patient involves airway management. Endotracheal intubation remains the gold standard to secure the airway in the pre-hospital setting, and is successful in 80–90% of cases [10, 11]. Proponents of early intubation cite studies show worsened mortality from delayed intubation, whereas opponents of pre-hospital intubation point out that these studies were carried out in hospitalized patients and that the most common cause of early mortality in injured patients is exsanguination, not loss of airway [12–15]. Therefore, they argue that transport of the patient to the trauma center should not be delayed for intubation. A retrospective review of the national trauma data bank involving 7,452 patients found an association between pre-hospital intubation, hypotension, and worsened survival [16].

Despite these arguments, there are groups of patients who benefit from early intubation. The question should not be whether to intubate *any* injured patient, but rather *which* patients should be intubated en route to the hospital. As noted above, one such group is patients injured in the rural setting where the transport time is long. Other urban groups include those with traumatic brain injury, airway compromise/impending obstruction, inhalation injury, direct airway trauma, and severe hypoxemia that cannot be corrected with non-invasive ventilation. It has been shown that even transient episodes of hypoxemia worsen the neurologic outcome after TBI [17]. A retrospective study in San Diego showed that mortality improved in patients with TBI who underwent pre-hospital intubation [18], but this finding was refuted in a subsequent prospective study. The latter study, however, has been faulted for an excessive rate of hyperventilation following intubation, a known risk factor for worsened outcome following TBI [19]. A study of TBI patients transported by rotary wing aircraft showed that pre-hospital intubation with end-tidal pCO_2 monitoring improved mortality outcomes [20]. More recently, a prospective study of 492 patients found that pre-hospital intubation of TBI patients improved mortality if the pCO_2 on arrival at the hospital was 30–35 mmHg, but that mortality worsened if the pCO_2 was outside of these limits [21]. This finding persisted even after controlling the severity of injury. Caution is needed in the interpretation and comparison of studies of pre-hospital versus hospital intubation since many pre-hospital providers are restricted from using neuromuscular blocking agents, whereas physicians routinely use these drugs as part of the rapid sequence induction. This suggests that patients who are successfully intubated by paramedics have a worse initial neurologic examination and may be more severely injured than those intubated in the ED.

Paramedics should be trained to deal with the consequences of inability to intubate. Patients can be temporized with Bag-Valve-Mask (BVM) ventilation and quickly transported to the hospital or a procedure other than orotracheal intubation can be attempted. Nasotracheal intubation is often not feasible in trauma patients due to possible facial or skull fracture. Other invasive airway measures that can be considered if BVM ventilation is not efficacious or a prolonged period of transport is required include: use of a supraglottic airway (e.g., laryngeal mask airway, LMA), Combitube® (Tyco-Kendall, Mansfield, MA) insertion, or needle or surgical cricothyroidotomy. The incidence of successful supraglottic airway insertion by paramedics has been shown to be 88–93% under optimal circumstances [22, 23], but it may be lower in the trauma setting in which patient access may be restricted. Furthermore, these devices do not protect the airway from aspiration. Combitube® insertion by paramedics is successful in 70–95% of cases when used either as a rescue device or as a primary means of invasive airway control [24, 25]. Because of the uncertain success rate of invasive rescue airway adjuncts and the concern regarding a delay in diagnosis and treatment of other possible life-threatening injuries, rapid transport with ongoing BVM ventilation of patients who cannot be intubated is appropriate in the urban setting where transport times are short: the "scoop and run" model. A final and least often utilized option involves cricothyroidotomy. Needle cricothyroidotomy is a paramedic skill, but most regions restrict open (or surgical) cricothyroidotomy to flight nurses or physicians. Needle cricothyroidotomy with jet ventilation can be an effective means of oxygenation but has been shown to be ineffective for ventilation and pCO_2 exchange. Therefore, it may not be as beneficial as expected in TBI patients, in whom a rise in pCO_2 is associated with an increase in the intracranial pressure due to cerebral vasodilation. Nonetheless, cricothyroidotomy may be life-saving in the patient who cannot be oxygenated using any modality and presents with hypoxemia in extremis: a rare situation in which "scoop and run" may not be ideal.

Paramedics also need to be ready to address the consequences of successful intubation. Other injuries, such as TBI or pneumothorax, can be exacerbated as a result of intubation. As previously noted, it has been shown that neurologic outcome following TBI is worsened if the patient is hyperventilated due to the vasoconstrictive effect of hypocapnea [26]. An end-tidal capnograph should be used in all trauma patients following intubation, particularly if prolonged transport is anticipated; the ventilation rate should be titrated to maintain a pCO_2 of 30–35 mmHg. A simple pneumothorax can quickly convert to a tension pneumothorax after intubation and positive pressure ventilation. Patients who become hypotensive or have worsening hypoxemia after intubation should have needle thoracostomy performed with an expected 30–60% incidence of improvement in vital signs [27]. The thoracostomy can be directed initially to the hemithorax in which decreased breath sounds are noted. Decompression of both sides of the chest should be carried out in cases in which the breath sounds are symmetric or decompression of one hemithorax does not result in a favorable change in the vital signs. Of note, a sampling of chest CT scans in medical and surgical patients in a military facility in Texas showed that the mean chest wall thickness at the second intercostal space in the mid-clavicular line of this group was 4.24 cm (4.9 cm in women and 4.2 cm in men), and 25% of the group had a chest wall thickness greater than 5 cm [28]. Based on these results, decompressive needle thoracostomy should be carried out using angiocatheters that are at least 5 cm long to optimize chances that the catheter penetrates into the pleural space. Another option is to place the needle thoracostomy in the anterior axillary line at the fourth or fifth interspace, where the chest wall is thinner. Hypotension following intubation may also be due to impaired venous return and cardiac output due to institution of positive pressure ventilation. This is particularly common in volume depleted patients, such as patients with ongoing hemorrhage. The hypotension can be overcome by the administration of intravenous fluid and by ensuring that the respiratory rate is slow enough to allow time for exhalation and to prevent breath-stacking (or auto-PEEP).

Patients who are intubated in the field or in the emergency department frequently do not receive adequate analgesia or sedation. Although this may not be as germane to the ground-based EMS provider who is intubating an obtunded patient, it is relevant to aeromedical crews or ground-crews who use sedatives and paralytics to intubate patients who may have a depressed level of consciousness but can still perceive pain and fear. Hypotension should not be used as a criterion to withhold all sedatives and analgesics, but rather should be used as a guide to determine the amount of each agent given.

8.2.3   Circulation

Assessment of adequate circulation in the injured patient in the pre-hospital setting involves measuring blood pressure and heart rate, assessment of mental status, and control of hemorrhage. Of note, the presence of truncal hemorrhage cannot be easily determined and hence cannot be treated in this setting. Patients in whom hemorrhage is suspected or who are hypotensive without a defined reason should be emergently transported to a trauma center since definitive therapy is not possible in the field, and transport should not be delayed for institution of therapy, including intravenous fluids: the "scoop and run" or "scoop and play" models. Patients who are exsanguinating from extremity wounds can be temporized using a tourniquet to stop bleeding and then rapidly transported to a trauma center to minimize the resultant limb ischemic time. Controversy remains in this area regarding the patients who should be given intravenous fluids, the composition of intravenous fluids to be used, and the quantity to be administered. Novel topical hemostatic agents may also provide a means to slow or stop external hemorrhage en route to the hospital. This topic is discussed in detail in the next section.

Several studies have shown that delay of transport in attempting to institute fluid therapy worsens mortality following severe trauma in urban settings [29–31]. Most of these patients are hypotensive due to hemorrhage, and infusion of large volumes of intravenous fluid only serves to induce a dilutional coagulopathy and hypothermia, and may also result in a transient increase in systemic blood pressure, which may disrupt the clot and worsen the hemorrhage [30, 32]. This concept was first put forth in 1918 by Cannon, who stated that "inaccessible or uncontrolled sources of blood loss should not be treated with intravenous fluids until the time of surgical control" [33]. Whereas intravenous access can be obtained en route to the trauma center, transport of the patient should not be delayed for this procedure. The possible exceptions include patients who have a prolonged transport time, in whom judicious administration of intravenous fluids may be beneficial, and TBI patients, in whom hypotension has been shown to worsen the neurologic outcome.

Accepted and traditional teaching for the resuscitation of injured patients calls for rapid infusion of 2 L of crystalloid for hypotensive patients. However, as noted above, this therapy may worsen the hemorrhage and the overall outcome in victims of penetrating trauma [29, 30]. The concept of "permissive hypotension," in which therapy is titrated to keep the systolic blood pressure (SBP) approximately 80 mmHg until operative control of hemorrhage has been achieved, is becoming an accepted endpoint to resuscitation [32]. However, as stated previously, whereas this approach may be beneficial to the patient with vascular or solid abdominal organ injury, it may be harmful to someone with TBI and intracranial hypertension. Its applicability to patients sustaining blunt force injury has not been demonstrated. Because the ability to diagnose specific injury (e.g., TBI) in the field is uncertain and difficult, rapid transport of potentially brain injured or hemorrhaging patients is the best intervention in urban settings. This point was demonstrated in the study of Demetriades and colleagues, which showed that patients transported by private vehicle following wounding had a better outcome than those transported by ambulance after controlling for injury severity and confounding variables [34]. The authors suggested that delay in transport to institute therapy, such as intravenous fluid administration, factored into the mortality difference.

In rural settings, administration of intravenous fluids seems more logical, since the transport time is inherently longer and patients frequently have had a longer "down-time" prior to EMS arrival. Furthermore, it is not clear how long patients can be allowed to remain hypotensive without negative sequelae. Retrospective studies have found that patients with a systolic blood pressure greater than 110 mmHg have significantly lower mortality than those with a SBP of 90–109 mmHg [35, 36]. However, caution should still be taken in normalizing the blood pressure or rapidly infusing fluids for the previously mentioned reasons. Currently, the best endpoints to pre-hospital resuscitation following penetrating trauma are a SBP greater than 80–90 mmHg and proper mental status. This policy has most recently been adopted by the United States armed forces in the Iraq and Afghanistan conflicts [37]. Patients with blunt force trauma may benefit from a higher SBP.

Although most injured patients receive either normal saline or lactated ringers solution en route to the hospital, other fluids are available and may be beneficial. These include hypertonic saline and solutions that exert an osmotic pressure, such as hetastarch. Currently, use of these solutions is restricted to the ED setting. Blood transfusion is available with some aeromedical services, but not routinely used during the pre-hospital resuscitation of civilian injuries due to many reasons, including the need for refrigeration and storage, and the possibility of transfusion reaction.

Clinical use of hypertonic saline (HTS) was first described in 1980s in a series of trials that showed that an infusion of 250 mL of 7.5% saline resulted in a net less fluid required to resuscitate trauma patients. This is because the hypertonic solution draws fluid from the intracellular and interstitial compartments into the intravascular compartment, thereby resulting in a ratio of volume retained in the intravascular space to the volume infused that is greater than 1. However, survival advantage from this modality has not been consistently demonstrated due to multiple shortcomings in various study designs [3, 37, 38]. Of note, the studies that suggested a survival advantage in patients who received HTS showed that patients with TBI and cerebral edema, hemorrhagic shock, victims of penetrating trauma, and patients who needed either immediate surgery or emergency blood transfusion were most likely to respond to HTS [3]. More recently, investigators have described favorable anti-inflammatory properties associated with HTS and are now investigating whether infusion of HTS can have a delayed impact on survival by ameliorating the systemic inflammatory response associated with trauma [37, 38]. Although HTS is not currently used routinely in pre-hospital care, its use may be most beneficial in rural trauma, where infusion of small aliquots can ameliorate intracranial hypertension while simultaneously treating hypotension. Further clinical studies are needed to better understand the HTS administration.

8.3 Emergency Department Resuscitation

Ideally, the ED should represent a continuation of care in the resuscitation of the patient, with the added benefit of providing a controlled environment with advanced diagnostic modalities and therapeutics. At times, the ED is also a starting point for the resuscitation of severely injured patients. This is the case for patients who are transported to the hospital by private vehicle or non-EMS personnel, such as the police. As a common starting point, the principles discussed in this section apply to such circumstances and assume that a patient arrives with little pre-hospital intervention. Lastly, for all but the most minor injuries, the ED should not represent a phase of definitive treatment; this is best deferred to other areas of the hospital, such as the operating theater, interventional radiology, or the in-patient areas.

Resuscitation in the ED can be performed using either a horizontal or vertical model. In the latter model, the resuscitator and the team leader are the same person, and must perform most (if not all) interventions while also diagnosing the patient's injuries and leading the overall plan of care. This model is frequently used in rural settings, where there are few practitioners. In the horizontal resuscitation model, a cadre of practitioners performs numerous tasks simultaneously, while the team leader oversees the plan of care. This model is more efficient, but it requires substantially more resources.

8.3.1 Airway

The resources and controlled environment of the ED provide an opportunity to expeditiously control the airway and stabilize a patient's respiratory status. In accordance with the general principle of preparation, prior to arrival of an injured patient, protocols directing how the intubation should proceed should be well established. Decisions such as which medications should be used to facilitate intubation, who should attempt to intubate, and how this procedure should be performed should be defined a priori.

The resources of a hospital, however, can also lead to unnecessary delay in resuscitation. For example, in instances in which orotracheal intubation is not possible, there is little role for fiberoptic intubation of trauma patients, even in patients who are otherwise stable. Whereas careful fiberoptic intubation requiring a prolonged effort may be seen as a success in patients with known isolated respiratory failure, trauma patients have the potential for severe concomitant injuries that cannot be assessed and treated until the airway is secure. Factors that should be considered in the decision to abandon further attempts at orotracheal intubation and proceed with cricothyroidotomy include both the patient's physiologic status and the time spent in attempting orotracheal intubation.

Protocols should be in place to direct the trauma team in the care of patients who arrive with "rescue" airway devices, such as the Combitube®. This tube and other obturator tubes are not definitive airways and should be changed in the controlled hospital setting. However, this change may be best undertaken after the patient has been evaluated and urgent diagnostic tests have been performed. This tube change is precarious since the presence of the rescue device implies a difficult airway, and the person most experienced with airway management (including possibly an anesthesiologist) should be responsible for changing the tube.

Patients who arrive agitated or combative should be assumed to have a head injury until proven otherwise. (Hypoxemia and hypoperfusion are also common causes of agitation and combativeness). Because of this, it is imperative that their oxygen saturation and blood pressure be optimized to prevent secondary brain injury. Furthermore, emergent brain CT scanning is needed to determine if the patient has diffuse axonal injury or a mass lesion requiring craniotiomy. Frequently, these patients will need to be urgently intubated to ensure that these goals are met. The induction regimen used to facilitate intubation should have a low risk of hypotension and maximize the chances of expedient, successful intubation. Commonly, etomidate is used to induce unconsciousness, and succinylcholine is also given to relax the patient and facilitate direct laryngoscopy. Agitated patients should not be sedated with benzodiazepine/neuroleptic medications until the presence of brain injury has been determined because this may increase the likelihood of airway compromise, aspiration, or secondary brain injury.

8.3.2   Breathing

The principles of ventilation discussed earlier also apply to the patient in the ED. In particular, it is critical that patients have end-tidal pCO_2 monitoring to ensure that the pCO_2 is kept between 30 and 35 mmHg in order to minimize the risk of secondary brain injury due to hyperventilation.

Damage control resuscitation of trauma patients in the ED requires expeditious diagnostic testing and decision making. In instances where immediate diagnostic capability is not available, definitive intervention that can be both diagnostic and therapeutic is indicated. For example, the diagnosis of pneumothorax can be made based on physical examination alone. The presence of subcutaneous emphysema should be considered a hallmark of tension pneumothorax and should prompt immediate chest tube insertion. In instances where hard signs of pneumothorax are not present but the patient remains hypoxic, tube thoracostomy can be diagnostic, therapeutic, and potentially life-saving. However, an effective, rapid diagnostic modality that can also be used in this situation is surgeon-performed ultrasound. This modality has been shown to be accurate and more rapid than supine chest X-ray for diagnosing pneumothorax following injury [39, 40].

Breathing may also be impaired hours after injury due to pain or worsening pulmonary contusion. These injuries are associated with the transmission of significant force to the chest wall, and are frequently found in association with flail chest. Patients require aggressive pain control, often supplemented by epidural analgesia to optimize minute ventilation, and many will require intubation and mechanical ventilation. The role of epidural analgesia to treat the pain associated with multiple rib fractures is discussed further on [41].

Patients with rapidly expanding pulmonary contusion may become hypoxic despite institution of early mechanical ventilation. Once pneumothorax has been excluded by CT scan of the chest, such patients should undergo immediate recruitment maneuvers in the ED to reverse (or recruit) atelectactic alveoli. A recruitment maneuver is performed by serially increasing the expiratory resistance to 30–40 cm H_2O and maintaining it for 30–40 s (or less if the patient's blood pressure decreases). Recruitment maneuver is associated with impaired venous drainage from the head, and therefore is relatively contraindicated in TBI patients. However, the risk for transient increase in the intracranial pressure must be weighed against the known detrimental effect of hypoxia following TBI.

8.3.3   Circulation

The strategy governing fluid resuscitation in the ED should follow the same principles as discussed earlier for pre-hospital care. As already discussed, patients with penetrating injury should not be resuscitated to systolic blood pressure greater than 80–90 mmHg until definitive control of bleeding is obtained. This section will discuss various resuscitative and hemostatic strategies for exsanguinating patients, but the clinician should recall that a tourniquet may represent the best therapeutic intervention for a bleeding patient with an extremity injury until surgical control is obtained.

The options for the type of fluid(s) that can be used for resuscitation in the hospital setting are numerous. Lactated ringers solution is the traditional fluid used for resuscitation of trauma patient; but it has been shown to be pro-inflammatory and possibly detrimental in large quantities [42, 43]. Infusion of large quantities of normal saline is associated with hyperchloremic acidosis. The patient may not be able to tolerate this exogenous acid load if there is pre-existing severe acidosis due to injury. Use of HTS has been discussed earlier. Non-biologic colloid solutions, such as hetastarch, are three times more efficacious than crystalloid solutions for expansion of plasma volume, although this has not been shown to result in a survival benefit.

Of note, albumin is not recommended for use in trauma patients based on post-hoc analysis of the SAFE trial, which showed that its use may worsen mortality in injured patients, especially following TBI [44]. Finally, blood products can serve as robust colloid volume expanders and also replete hematologic deficits resulting from exsanguination.

Based on experiences from recent wars, early use of blood and blood products may be associated with improved outcome following injury, particularly in severely injured, coagulopathic patients. Severely injured patients who are coagulopathic on arrival at the ED have been described to have a condition termed "the coagulopathy of trauma." This coagulopathy is the result of hemorrhage with consumption of coagulation factors and severe tissue disruption, and is worsened by the dilutional effects of infusion of crystalloid solutions. Preliminary reports from the military suggest that aggressive use of fresh frozen Plasma and Red Blood Cell transfusion (PRBC) in a 1:1 ratio in exsanguinating patients may impart survival benefit [45]. However, studies of civilian trauma patients show that blood products, especially plasma, are routinely under-dosed [46]. Transfusion of equal parts of blood, plasma, and platelets is recommended in patients who require more than 8 units of blood in the first 24 h of resuscitation.

Plasma is commonly frozen to prevent degradation of the clotting factors. It takes approximately 30 min to thaw Fresh Frozen Plasma (FFP) because it must be thawed slowly to prevent degradation of proteins; it has a shelf-life of 5–7 days once thawed. Each 30 min delay in administration of the first unit of plasma decreases the odds of correction of warfarin-induced coagulopathy by 20% in patients with intracerebral bleeding [47]. Because of this, centers that use FFP frequently store several thawed units of plasma for use in emergencies. When available, early use of thawed plasma as a part of the exsanguinating patient's overall resuscitation is advised.

Blood should be immediately available for transfusion in the ED. Type O blood can be safely transfused to all patients, although females of child-bearing age should be transfused O− if possible. Furthermore, massive transfusion (defined as 8–10 units of blood within 24 h) of non-type specific blood is rarely associated with a transfusion reaction in trauma patients [48]. An in-line blood warmer system should be used when patients are being emergently transfused with non-reconstituted PRBC to prevent worsening hypothermia from administration of a large volume of cold blood. However, caution is needed when using rapid infusion systems in the trauma bay/emergency department because patients who need rapid infusion of blood have a source of bleeding that needs to be controlled either in the operating room or in the angiography suite. Rapid infusion of fluids in these instances may dislodge the clot, thereby increasing the rate of hemorrhage worsening mortality [49].

Controversy persists regarding the need for transfusion in critically ill and injured patients. Many studies in trauma patients have found an association between transfusion of blood and increased morbidity or mortality [50–54]. However, these studies refer to resuscitated patients whose source of bleeding has been controlled. A restrictive transfusion strategy may be beneficial in this cohort, but it is detrimental in actively bleeding patients. Studies of Jehovah's Witnesses found a significant increase in mortality when the perioperative hemoglobin is 6–8 g/dL [55, 56].

Studies recommending a transfusion strategy for platelet repletion are inconclusive, although maintenance of a level greater than 100,000 cells/μL in bleeding patients appears to be appropriate. As noted earlier, based on expert opinion, empiric platelet transfusion as a part of a massive transfusion protocol should be started after 8 units of PRBC have been transfused and should continue at a ratio of 1:1:1 for each unit of PRBC and plasma transfused until hemorrhage is controlled [57]. In addition, use of aspirin may worsen the intracranial hemorrhage following traumatic brain injury [58], and many trauma centers utilize empiric platelet transfusion in patients who were prescribed anti-platelet medications, including non-steroidal anti-inflammatory agents. Platelet transfusion has been shown to reverse the platelet dysfunction caused by clopidogrel specifically [59].

Commonly measured endpoints for resuscitation using intravenous fluids include blood pressure, heart rate, and urine output. However, other endpoints, such as serum lactate concentration and base deficit, are also predictive of the need for transfusion and survival [60, 61]. Over 85% of injured patients with a significant base deficit on arrival at the hospital will require a blood transfusion [62], and a base deficit less than 6 or lactate greater than 22 mg/dL after 12 h is associated with increased mortality. Although not proven, early transfusion based on base deficit rather than overt physiologic changes (e.g., hypotension) may result in less morbidity from prolonged occult end-organ ischemia. These serum markers should be tested on arrival in all severely injured patients.

Protocols facilitating rapid mobilization of blood bank resources for severely injured patients requiring massive transfusion should be established and rehearsed regularly. The trauma exsanguination protocol at each of the authors' institutions requires one phone call to initiate and includes immediate release of: 10 units of type O+ PRBC, 6 units of platelets, and 4 units of thawed plasma. Recombinant Factor VIIa is also dispensed in accordance with an established protocol.

Two intravenous hemostatic agents, Factor VIIa and Prothrombin Complex (PCC), have been shown to decrease the hemorrhage and the need for blood transfusion in injured and coagulopathic patients. Factor VIIa may decrease the overall transfusion needs of injured patients (especially following blunt mechanism of injury), but it has not been shown to impact mortality [63–67]. However, factor VIIa is of limited efficacy once the patient is profoundly acidemic (pH < 7.1 or lactate > 14), thrombocytopenic (platelet count < 50,000 cells/μL), or coagulopathic (prothrombin time > 18 s), and its administration prior to transfusion of 8 units of PRBC may be more beneficial than later administration, assuming that surgical control of bleeding has been obtained [68]. Because of the latter caveat, Factor VIIa is rarely administered in the trauma bay or emergency department, but it should be considered as a part of the patient's overall hemostatic plan early during the course of resuscitation. Conversely, PCC may be of significant benefit in the emergency department as a part of the initial resuscitation in patients with warfarin-induced coagulopathy. Prothrombin complex consists of pooled clotting factor concentrates and is available in a variety of brands. The exact clotting factors present and percent composition may vary based on the product used. However, PCC has been shown to be the most rapid and lasting method to reverse the warfarin-induced coagulopathy [69–74]. Furthermore, PCC does not carry the risk of transfusion-associated volume overload, commonly seen following administration of large volume of FFP.

A variety of novel, topical hemostatic agents are now used by the military in the pre-hospital setting and by civilian trauma centers in the emergency department and operating theater. These compounds include QuikClot® (Z-Medica, Wallingford, CT) and HemCon® (HemCon Medical Technologies, Portland, OR), in addition to others. These agents have various mechanisms of action, but all of them induce a hypercoagulable state locally and have been shown to decrease the hemorrhage significantly in high grade solid organ and vascular injury [75, 76]. These products are especially useful in the emergency department for exsanguinating wounds that are not amenable to immediate control using a tourniquet.

Resuscitative Thoracotomy (RT) represents the most invasive and extreme method to obtain temporary control of hemorrhage and attempt fluid resuscitation. The decision to utilize this extreme measure must be made with a firm understanding of the cost and risk-to-benefit ratio associated with the procedure and only when immediate operative intervention following RT is possible. Fewer than 1% of patients with a blunt mechanism of injury survive following RT, whereas the survival following penetrating injury is 5–50%, depending upon specific organ injury [77]. The highest odds of survival are with isolated cardiac injuries, particularly stab wounds, which have at least a 50% survival rate [78]. However, in all patient populations, it has been shown that patients who present with a wide QRS complex rhythm or electrical cardiac activity with a rate less than 40 beats per minute do not survive following RT regardless of the injury mechanism [79]. Furthermore, RT carries a significant risk of iatrogenic injury to the medical team due to the hurried nature of the procedure, lack of a surgical technician to facilitate safe and quick passage of instruments to the surgeon, and frequent lack of experience on the part of the house-staff and nurses involved in the procedure. The incidence of HIV, viral hepatitis, and other blood-borne diseases can be as high as 20% in trauma patients requiring RT [78], and the risk of harm to the medical team must be weighed against the possibility of benefit to the patient when deciding whether or not to perform this procedure. The exact technique of RT and methods for repair of possible injuries are beyond the scope of this chapter, and the reader is directed to other sources for a discussion on these points.

8.3.4   Disability

A quick neurologic examination is a key part of the primary survey, but this should also include pain control and sedation as needed. The examination includes parameters to determine the Glasgow Coma Score, ability to move all extremities, and pupillary function. However, this category should also include ensuring proper analgesia and sedation, particularly in patients who arrive having received neuromuscular blocking agents to facilitate intubation. Frequently, these patients do not receive adequate pain control and anti-anxiety therapy, despite being pharmacologically paralyzed [80].

As already noted, patients with possible TBI require aggressive intervention to prevent secondary brain injury. In addition to other factors, any episode of hypoxemia, hypercapnea, or hypotension directly correlates with worsened recovery and survival following TBI. Therefore, patients with a Glasgow Coma Score ≤ 8 should be intubated, both for airway protection and prevention of aspiration, and to prevent sudden desaturation or hypercapnea. Furthermore, reversal of potential coagulopathy in patients with a history of anti-platelet or warfarin therapy should not be delayed until this history is verified or radiographic evidence of TBI is obtained. In patients who present with signs or symptoms of elevated intracranial pressure, such as posturing, unilateral mydriasis, or hypertension with bradycardia, measures to decrease the ICP should not be delayed until radiographic confirmation is obtained. These patients should have an end-tidal pCO_2 monitoring to allow for slight hyperventilation to a pCO_2 of 30–35 mmHg, and should receive 1 g/kg of mannitol intravenously if they are not hypotensive. Also, the stretcher should be placed in reverse trendelenburg position to facilitate venous outflow from the cranium. A CT scan of the brain is imperative to define the pathology and determine the type of neurosurgical intervention possible. If the patient cannot be taken to the intensive care unit immediately, an intracranial pressure monitor should be placed in the emergency department. There is no role for intravenous steroid therapy for TBI [81].

There is significant controversy regarding the use of high-dose methylprednisolone for Spinal Cord Injury (SCI). A series of studies in the 1990s suggested that a high dose of steroid therapy may improve the neurologic recovery following blunt, incomplete SCI [82]. However, these studies had significant shortcomings and also documented a high incidence of nosocomial infection following administration of steroids. Currently, trauma centers, in concert with their spine specialists, are individually determining whether or not the risk-benefit ratio of steroids justifies their use following SCI, and a firm recommendation of their utility cannot be made. When used, the steroid regimen needed is methylprednisolone 30 mg/kg over 15 min followed by 5.4 mg/kg/h for 23 h if the regimen is started within 3 h of injury or for 47 h if it is started between 3 and 8 h of injury. There is no role for steroid therapy following complete SCI, SCI due to penetrating trauma, or SCI that is diagnosed greater than 8 h from the time of injury.

8.4 Special Populations

8.4.1 Geriatric Patients

Mortality following trauma starts to increase after age 40 years [83]. However, this increased risk can be impacted by early transfer to trauma centers, invasive monitoring, and appropriate Intensive Care Unit (ICU) care. Early use of pulmonary artery catheters to direct resuscitation in elderly patients is associated with improved mortality, especially following severe injury [84, 85]. One reason for this observation may be that the elderly patients do not have the ability to augment their cardiac output either due to pharmacologic blockade of the sympathetic nervous system or pre-existing disease. Therefore, they may not present with the classic symptoms of impending shock, such as tachycardia, and may have occult shock that is detectable initially only with blood test or invasive hemodynamic monitoring. Injured elderly patients requiring admission to the ICU should have admission expedited to shorten the time course to placement of invasive monitors. In cases in which this is not possible, serum markers of shock should be measured in the emergency department and invasive hemodynamic monitors should be placed as needed while waiting for ICU transfer.

Elderly patients also have a significantly higher incidence of rib fractures [86]. Moreover, such injuries are associated with a significantly higher morbidity and mortality in those over 60 years of age [87]. Aggressive, immediate analgesia along with intensive care monitoring are needed to decrease the potential morbidity. Many centers utilize epidural analgesia or paravertebral blocks in patients with multiple rib fractures and in those who have a limited vital capacity due to pain. Epidural analgesia allows optimal pain control without the adverse effects of respiratory and mental status depression or ileus, and has been shown to decrease mortality by at least 50% in patients over 60 years of age [41, 88–90]. Because of this, epidural analgesia should be started in the emergency department in this patient population if there are no contraindications to its use.

Oral anticoagulation is common in the elderly population. These medications greatly increase the morbidity associated with any injury, particularly head injury. Because of this, urgent CT scan evaluation is needed in any patient suspected of or confirmed to be using warfarin. However, often the trauma team does not know whether or not a patient is using warfarin, and frequent tests for coagulopathy require at least 30 min to process. In these instances, the trauma team must decide whether empiric therapy with plasma should be administered or if the presence of hemorrhage and use of anticoagulants should be confirmed before plasma is prescribed. Reversal of coagulopathy can require many units of plasma, depending upon the degree of coagulopathy present and the patient's ideal body mass index. Large volume plasma transfusion carries a significant risk of volume overload, heart failure, and myocardial infarction in the elderly population. This risk must be weighed against the possibility of unremitting hemorrhage. Once the decision to transfuse plasma is made, the transfusion should begin quickly in the emergency department setting.

8.4.2   The Pregnant Patient

Five percent of pregnant women are injured annually [91]. The most common mechanism of injury involves motor vehicle collisions, and factors associated with fetal demise include the injury severity score, base deficit, and abnormal uterine activity [92]. Fetal loss following trauma frequently follows prolonged maternal hemorrhage, hypotension, hypoxemia, or uterine trauma. Maternal shock is associated with 80% risk of fetal demise [93]. In general, aggressive resuscitation of the mother is associated with improved outcomes in the fetus, and neither diagnostic testing (i.e., radiographs) nor any specific treatment (e.g., interventional radiology) should be withheld or altered due to pregnancy. However, protocol driven tests (e.g., pelvic x-ray) can often be omitted based on the patient's injury mechanism, physiologic status, and physical examination. Uncrossmatched, type O− blood can be transfused to a pregnant patient for the same indications that apply to the non-pregnant patient.

Evaluation and treatment of the injured pregnant patient require the attention of the trauma team, emergency department staff, and obstetrical team. Ideally, the obstetrical team should be present in the emergency department at the time of patient's arrival. The trauma team should direct the mother's resuscitation and evaluation, while the obstetrical team can monitor the uterine and fetal activity for signs of distress or pre-term labor. Fetal and uterine monitoring should be instituted as soon as possible in those with a gestational age greater than 24 weeks. This can be estimated by determining if the uterus is between the umbilicus and the xiphoid [91]. A vaginal examination should be performed as part of the secondary survey to assess for bleeding that may signify pre-term labor or uterine/placental trauma. The Focused Abdominal Sonography for Trauma (FAST) has been shown to have 83% sensitivity for detecting free intraperitoneal fluid during pregnancy, although this depends largely on the user's experience [94].

With a few caveats, the evaluation of the injured pregnant patient proceeds in the same fashion as that of any other patient. Initially, the mother should be placed at a 15° tilt to the left to move the gravid uterus off the inferior vena cava. All patients should be placed on supplemental oxygen because resting oxygen consumption is increased during pregnancy. Furthermore, patients who are intubated should have their end-tidal pCO_2 monitored and adjusted to 30 mmHg because this is the normal resting pCO_2 of pregnancy. Large-bore intravenous access should be established, and the patient should be fluid resuscitated. One of the earliest signs of maternal hemorrhage is fetal distress because maternal blood flow will shunt away from the placenta during early shock [93]. Furthermore, the physiologic expansion of intravascular volume that occurs with pregnancy makes maternal hypotension a late finding of shock.

Peri-mortem cesarean section represents the most invasive and drastic measure that can be performed on a pregnant patient. This procedure should only be considered if the fetus gestation is greater than 24 weeks old. Fetal outcomes are best if the mother has had less than 5 min of cardiopulmonary resuscitation; fetal survival has been reported as long as 15 min after maternal demise [93]. In cases in which the mother has also undergone a resuscitative thoracotomy prior to cardiac arrest, the ischemic time to the fetus starts from the time the maternal aorta is cross-clamped. As opposed to peri-mortem cesarean section, emergency cesarean section for indications other than maternal demise (e.g., uterine rupture, DIC, uterine injury) is associated with 45% fetal survival and 72% maternal survival [95].

8.5   Future Trends

There are many promising research projects currently underway to address pre-hospital and emergency department resuscitation. Such projects include novel crystalloid solutions, such as ethyl pyruvate, which can both resuscitate patients and also modulate the inflammatory response that frequently leads to multi-organ dysfunction following trauma. Also, research is ongoing to find a blood substitute that is stable at room temperature. This would allow paramedics to initiate transfusion to hemorrhaging patients prior to arrival at the hospital and would allow hospital personnel to continue this therapy without the known risks of allogenic blood transfusion. Improvements in intravenous and topical hemostatic agents will allow rapid control of hemorrhage. Finally, "smart" technology is being developed to prevent iatrogenic injury. An example of this is the Smart Bag® (O-Two Medical Tech, Ontario). This is a bag-valve-mask system that senses the flow rate of air generated by squeezing the bag and limits both the pressure and flow generated to minimize the risk of gastric distention and excessive ventilation.

References

1. McSwain NE Jr. Pre-hospital care. In Feliciano DV, Moore EE, Mattox KL (eds.) Trauma 3rd ed. Stamford, CT: Appleton & Lange, 1996.
2. Pantridge J, Adgey A. Pre-hospital coronary care: the mobile coronary care unit. *Am J Cardiol* 1969;24(5):666.
3. Bulger EM, Maier RV. Pre-hospital care of the injured: what's new. *Surg Clin North Am* 2007;87(1):37–53.
4. Johnson JW, Gracias VH, Schwab CW, Reilly PM, Kauder DR, Dabrowski GP, Shapiro MB, Rotondo MF. Evolution in damage control for exsanguinating penetrating abdominal injury. *J Trauma* 2001;51(2):261–9; discussion 9–71.
5. http://www.facs.org/trauma/atls/about.html.
6. Maio RF, Green PE, Becker MP, Burney RE, Compton C. Rural motor vehicle crash mortality: the role of crash severity and medical resources. *Accid Anal Prev* 1992;24(6):631–42.
7. Muelleman RL, Walker RA, Edney JA. Motor vehicle deaths: a rural epidemic. J *Trauma* 1993;35(5):717–9.
8. Champion HR, Copes WS, Sacco WJ, Lawnick MM, Keast SL, Frey CF. The Major Trauma Outcome Study: establishing national norms for trauma care. *J Trauma* 1990;30(11):1356–65.
9. Siegel JH. The effect of associated injuries, blood loss, and oxygen debt on death and disability in blunt traumatic brain injury: the need for early physiologic predictors of severity. *J Neurotrauma* 1995;12(4):579–90.
10. Doran JV, Tortella BJ, Drivet WJ, Lavery RF. Factors influencing successful intubation in the pre-hospital setting. *Prehosp Disaster Med* 1995;10(4):259–64.
11. Wang HE, Kupas DF, Paris PM, Bates RR, Yealy DM. Preliminary experience with a prospective, multi-centered evaluation of out-of-hospital endotracheal intubation. *Resuscitation* 2003;58(1):49–58.
12. Esposito TJ, Sanddal ND, Hansen JD, Reynolds S. Analysis of preventable trauma deaths and inappropriate trauma care in a rural state. *J Trauma* 1995;39(5):955–62.
13. Rivara FP, Maier RV, Mueller BA, Luna GA, Dicker BG, Herman CN, Kenagy JW, Copass MK, Carrico CJ. Evaluation of potentially preventable deaths among pedestrian and bicyclist fatalities. *JAMA* 1989;261(4):566–70.

14. Acosta JA, Yang JC, Winchell RJ, Simons RK, Fortlage DA, Hollingsworth-Fridlund P, Hoyt DB. Lethal injuries and time to death in a level I trauma center. *J Am Coll Surg* 1998;186(5):528–33.
15. Sauaia A, Moore FA, Moore EE, Moser, KS, Brennan R, Read RA, Pons PT. Epidemiology of trauma deaths: a reassessment. *J Trauma* 1995;38(2):185–93.
16. Shafi S, Gentilello L. Pre-hospital endotracheal intubation and positive pressure ventilation is associated with hypotension and decreased survival in hypovolemic trauma patients: an analysis of the National Trauma Data Bank. *J Trauma* 2005;59(5):1140–5; discussion 5–7.
17. Chesnut RM, Marshall LF, Klauber MR, Blunt BA, Baldwin N, Eisenberg HM, Jane JA, Marmarou A, Foulkes MA. The role of secondary brain injury in determining outcome from severe head injury. *J Trauma* 1993;34(2):216–22.
18. Winchell RJ, Hoyt DB. Endotracheal intubation in the field improves survival in patients with severe head injury. Trauma Research and Education Foundation of San Diego. *Arch Surg* 1997;132(6):592–7.
19. Davis DP, Peay J, Sise MJ, et al. The impact of pre-hospital endotracheal intubation on outcome in moderate to severe traumatic brain injury. *J Trauma* 2005;58(5):933–9.
20. Poste JC, Davis DP, Ochs M, Vilke GM, Castillo EM, Stern J, Hoyt DB. Air medical transport of severely head-injured patients undergoing paramedic rapid sequence intubation. *Air Med J* 2004;23(4):36–40.
21. Warner KJ, Cuschieri J, Copass MK, Jurkovich GJ, Bulger EM. The impact of pre-hospital ventilation on outcome after severe traumatic brain injury. *J Trauma* 2007;62(6):1330–6; discussion 6–8.
22. Cook TM, Hommers C. New airways for resuscitation? *Resuscitation* 2006;69(3):371–87
23. Young B. The intubating laryngeal-mask airway may be an ideal device for airway control in the rural trauma patient. *Am J Emerg Med* 2003;21(1):80–5.
24. Atherton GL, Johnson JC. Ability of paramedics to use the Combitube in pre-hospital cardiac arrest. *Ann Emerg Med* 1993;22(8):1263–8.
25. Davis DP, Valentine C, Ochs M, Vilke GM, Hoyt DB. The Combitube as a salvage airway device for paramedic rapid sequence intubation. *Ann Emerg Med* 2003;42(5):697–704.
26. Davis DP, Dunford JV, Poste JC, Ochs M, Holbrook T, Fortlage D, Size MJ, Kennedy F, Hoyt DB. The impact of hypoxia and hyperventilation on outcome after paramedic rapid sequence intubation of severely head-injured patients. *J Trauma* 2004;57(1):1–8; discussion 8–10.
27. Davis DP, Pettit K, Rom CD, Poste JC, Sise MJ, Hoyt DB, Vilke GM. The safety and efficacy of pre-hospital needle and tube thoracostomy by aeromedical personnel. *Prehosp Emerg Care* 2005;9(2):191–7.
28. Givens ML, Ayotte K, Manifold C. Needle thoracostomy: implications of computed tomography chest wall thickness. *Acad Emerg Med* 2004;11(2):211–3.
29. Bickell WH, Wall MJ, Jr, Pepe PE, Martin RR, Ginger VF, Allen MK, Mattox KL. Immediate versus delayed fluid resuscitation for hypotensive patients with penetrating torso injuries. *N Engl J Med* 1994;331(17):1105–9.
30. Kwan I, Bunn F, Roberts I. Timing and volume of fluid administration for patients with bleeding following trauma. *Cochrane Database Syst Rev* 2001(1):CD002245.
31. Sampalis JS, Tamim H, Denis R, Boukas B, Ruest S-A, Nikolis A, Lavoie A, Fleiszer D, Brown R, Mulder D, Williams JI. Ineffectiveness of on-site intravenous lines: is pre-hospital time the culprit? *J Trauma* 1997;43(4):608–15; discussion 15–7.
32. Revell M, Greaves I, Porter K. Endpoints for fluid resuscitation in hemorrhagic shock. *J Trauma* 2003;54(5 Suppl):S63–7.
33. Alam H, Rhee P. New developments in fluid resuscitation. *Surg Clin North Am* 2007;87(1):55–72.
34. Demetriades D, Chan L, Cornwell E, Belzberg H, Berne TV, Asensio J, Chan D, Eckstein M, Alo K. Paramedic vs private transportation of trauma patients. Effect on outcome. *Arch Surg* 1996;131(2):133–8.
35. Eastridge BJ, Salinas J, McManus JG, Blackburn L, Bugler EM, Cooke WH, Concertino VA, Wade CE, Holcomb JB. Hypotension begins at 110 mm Hg: redefining "hypotension" with data. *J Trauma* 2007;63(2):291–7; discussion 7–9.

36. Edelman DA, White MT, Tyburski JG, Wilson RF. Post-traumatic hypotension: should systolic blood pressure of 90–109 mmHg be included? *Shock* 2007;27(2):134–8.
37. Alam HB, Rhee P. New developments in fluid resuscitation. *Surg Clin North Am* 2007;87(1):55–72.
38. Kramer GC. Hypertonic resuscitation: physiologic mechanisms and recommendations for trauma care. *J Trauma* 2003;54(5 Suppl):S89–99.
39. Blaivas M, Lyon M, Duggal S. A prospective comparison of supine chest radiography and bedside ultrasound for the diagnosis of traumatic pneumothorax. *Acad Emerg Med* 2005;12(9):844–9.
40. Dente CJ, Ustin J, Feliciano DV, Rozycki GS, Wyrzykowski AD, Nicholas JM, Salomone JP, Ingram WL. The accuracy of thoracic ultrasound for detection of pneumothorax is not sustained over time: a preliminary study. *J Trauma* 2007;62(6):1384–9.
41. Mackersie RC, Karagianes TG, Hoyt DB, Davis JW. Prospective evaluation of epidural and intravenous administration of fentanyl for pain control and restoration of ventilatory function following multiple rib fractures. *J Trauma* 1991;31(4):443–9; discussion 9–51.
42. Cotton BA, Guy JS, Morris JA, Jr., Abumrad NN. The cellular, metabolic, and systemic consequences of aggressive fluid resuscitation strategies. *Shock* 2006;26(2):115–21.
43. Rhee P, Wang D, Ruff P, Austin B, DeBraux S, Wolcott K, Burris D, Ling G, Sun L. Human neutrophil activation and increased adhesion by various resuscitation fluids. *Crit Care Med* 2000;28(1):74–8.
44. Myburgh J, Cooper J, Finfer S, Bellomo R, Norton R, Bishop N, Kai Lo S, Vallance S. Saline or albumin for fluid resuscitation in patients with traumatic brain injury. *N Engl J Med* 2007;357(9):874–84.
45. Holcomb JB, Jenkins D, Rhee P, Johannigman J, Mahoney P, Mehta S, Cox ED, Gehrke MJ, Beilman GJ, Schreiber M, Flaherty SF, Grathwohl KW, Spinella PS, Perkins JG, Beekley AC, McMullin NR, Park MS, Gonzalez EA, Wade CE, Dubick MA, Schwab CW, Moore FA, Champion HR, Hoyt DB, Hess JR. Damage control resuscitation: directly addressing the early coagulopathy of trauma. *J Trauma* 2007;62(2):307–10.
46. Geeraedts LM, Jr, Demiral H, Schaap NP, Kamphuisen PW, Pompe JC, Frolke JP. "Blind" transfusion of blood products in exsanguinating trauma patients. *Resuscitation* 2007;73(3):382–8.
47. Goldstein JN, Thomas SH, Frontiero V, Joseph A, Engel C, Snider R, Smith EE, Greenberg SM, Rosand J. Timing of fresh frozen plasma administration and rapid correction of coagulopathy in warfarin-related intracerebral hemorrhage. *Stroke* 2006;37(1):151–5.
48. Dutton RP, Shih D, Edelman BB, Hess J, Scalea TM. Safety of uncrossmatched type-O red cells for resuscitation from hemorrhagic shock. *J Trauma* 2005;59(6):1445–9.
49. Hambly PR, Dutton RP. Excess mortality associated with the use of a rapid infusion system at a level 1 trauma center. *Resuscitation* 1996;31(2):127–33.
50. Beale E, Zhu J, Chan L, Shulman I, Harwood R, Demetriades D. Blood transfusion in critically injured patients: a prospective study. *Injury* 2006;37(5):455–65.
51. Charles A, Shaikh AA, Walters M, Huehl S, Pomerantz R. Blood transfusion is an independent predictor of mortality after blunt trauma. *Am Surg* 2007;73(1):1–5.
52. Dunne JR, Riddle MS, Danko J, Hayden R, Petersen K. Blood transfusion is associated with infection and increased resource utilization in combat casualties. *Am Surg* 2006;72(7):619–25; discussion 25–6.
53. Malone DL, Dunne J, Tracy JK, Putnam AT, Scalea TM, Napolitano LM. Blood transfusion, independent of shock severity, is associated with worse outcome in trauma. *J Trauma* 2003;54(5):898–905; discussion 905–7.
54. Moore FA, Moore EE, Sauaia A. Blood transfusion. An independent risk factor for postinjury multiple organ failure. *Arch Surg* 1997;132(6):620–4; discussion 624–5.
55. Carson JL, Duff A, Poses RM, Berlin JA, Spence RK, Trout R, Noveck H, Strom BL. Effect of anaemia and cardiovascular disease on surgical mortality and morbidity. *Lancet* 1996; 348(9034):1055–60.
56. Carson JL, Noveck H, Berlin JA, Gould SA. Mortality and morbidity in patients with very low postoperative Hb levels who decline blood transfusion. *Transfusion* 2002;42(7):812–8.

57. Ketchum L, Hess JR, Hiippala S. Indications for early fresh frozen plasma, cryoprecipitate, and platelet transfusion in trauma. *J Trauma* 2006;60(6 Suppl):S51–8.
58. Sakr M, Wilson L. Best evidence topic report. Aspirin and the risk of intracranial complications following head injury. *Emerg Med J* 2005;22(12):891–2.
59. Vilahur G, Choi BG, Zafar MU, Viles-Gonzalez JF, Vorchheimert DA, Fuster V, Badimon JJ. Normalization of platelet reactivity in clopidogrel-treated subjects. *J Thromb Haemost* 2007;5(1):82–90.
60. Davis J, Kaups K. Base deficit in the elderly: a marker of severe injury and death. *J Trauma* 1998;45:873–7.
61. McNelis J, Marini CP, Jurkiewicz A, Szomstein S, Simms HH, Ritter G, Nathan IM. Prolonged lactate clearance is associated with increased mortality in the surgical intensive care unit. *Am J Surg* 2001;182(5):481–5.
62. Davis JW, Parks SN, Kaups KL, Gladen HE, O'Donnell-Nicol S. Admission base deficit predicts transfusion requirements and risk of complications. *J Trauma* 1996;41(5):769–74.
63. Boffard KD, Riou B, Warren B, Choong PI, Rizoli S, Rossaint R, Axelsen M, Kluger Y, NovoSeven Trauma Study Group. Recombinant factor VIIa as adjunctive therapy for bleeding control in severely injured trauma patients: two parallel randomized, placebo-controlled, double-blind clinical trials. *J Trauma* 2005;59(1):8–15; discussion 15–8.
64. Dutton RP, McCunn M, Hyder M, D'Angelo M, O'Connor J, Hess J, Scalea TM. Factor VIIa for correction of traumatic coagulopathy. *J Trauma* 2004;57(4):709–18; discussion 18–9.
65. Geeraedts LM, Jr., Kamphuisen PW, Kaasjager HA, Verwiel JM, van Vugt AB, Frolke JP. The role of recombinant factor VIIa in the treatment of life-threatening haemorrhage in blunt trauma. *Injury* 2005;36(4):495–500.
66. Mohr AM, Holcomb JB, Dutton RP, Duranteau J. Recombinant activated factor VIIa and hemostasis in critical care: a focus on trauma. *Crit Care* 2005;9(Suppl 5):S37–42
67. Rizoli SB, Nascimento B, Jr., Osman F, Netto FS, Kiss A, Callum J, Brenneman FD, Tremblay L, Tien HC. Recombinant activated coagulation factor VII and bleeding trauma patients. *J Trauma* 2006;61(6):1419–25.
68. Perkins JG, Schreiber MA, Wade CE, Holcomb JB. Early versus late recombinant factor VIIa in combat trauma patients requiring massive transfusion. *J Trauma* 2007;62(5):1095–9; discussion 9–101.
69. Lavenne-Pardonge E, Itegwa MA, Kalaai M, Klinkenberg G, Loncke JL, Pelgrims K, Strengers PF. Emergency reversal of oral anticoagulation through PPSB-SD: the fastest procedure in Belgium. *Acta Anaesthesiol Belg* 2006;57(2):121–5.
70. Strengers PF, Drenth JC. PPSB as first choice treatment in the reversal of oral anticoagulant therapy. *Acta Anaesthesiol Belg* 2002;53(3):183–6.
71. Makris M, Greaves M, Phillips WS, Kitchen S, Rosendaal FR, Preston EF. Emergency oral anticoagulant reversal: the relative efficacy of infusions of fresh frozen plasma and clotting factor concentrate on correction of the coagulopathy. *Thromb Haemost* 1997;77(3):477–80.
72. Yasaka M, Sakata T, Minematsu K, Naritomi H. Correction of INR by prothrombin complex concentrate and vitamin K in patients with warfarin related hemorrhagic complication. *Thromb Res* 2002;108(1):25–30.
73. Baker RI, Coughlin PB, Gallus AS, Harper PL, Salem HH, Wood EM. Warfarin reversal: consensus guidelines, on behalf of the Australasian Society of Thrombosis and Haemostasis. *Med J Aust* 2004;181(9):492–7.
74. Cartmill M, Dolan G, Byrne JL, Byrne PO. Prothrombin complex concentrate for oral anticoagulant reversal in neurosurgical emergencies. *Br J Neurosurg* 2000;14(5):458–61.
75. Pusateri AE, Holcomb JB, Kheirabadi BS, Alam HB, Wade CE, Ryan KL. Making sense of the preclinical literature on advanced hemostatic products. *J Trauma* 2006;60(3):674–82.
76. Ward KR, Tiba MH, Holbert WH, Blocher CR, Draucker GT, Proffitt EK, Bowlin. GL, Ivatury RR, Diegelmann RF. Comparison of a new hemostatic agent to current combat hemostatic agents in a Swine model of lethal extremity arterial hemorrhage. *J Trauma* 2007;63(2):276–83; discussion 83–4.

77. Mazzorana V, Smith RS, Morabito DJ, Brar HS. Limited utility of emergency department thoracotomy. *Am Surg* 1994;60(7):516–20; discussion 20–1.
78. Hunt PA, Greaves I, Owens WA. Emergency thoracotomy in thoracic trauma-a review. *Injury* 2006;37(1):1–19
79. Battistella FD, Nugent W, Owings JT, Anderson JT. Field triage of the pulseless trauma patient. *Arch Surg* 1999;134(7):742–5; discussion 5–6.
80. Chao A, Huang CH, Pryor JP, Reilly PM, Schwab CW. Analgesic use in intubated patients during acute resuscitation. *J Trauma* 2006;60(3):579–82.
81. Roberts I, Yates D, Sandercock P, Farrell B, Wasserberg J, Lomas G, Cottingham R, Svoboda P, Brayley N, Mazairac G, Laloë V, Muñoz-Sánchez A, Arango M, Hartzenberg B, Khamis H, Yutthakasemsunt S, Komolafe E, Olldashi F, Yadav Y, Murillo-Cabezas F, Shakur H, Edwards P, CRASH trial collaborators. Effect of intravenous corticosteroids on death within 14 days in 10008 adults with clinically significant head injury (MRC CRASH trial): randomised placebo-controlled trial. *Lancet* 2004;364(9442):1321–8.
82. Bracken M. Steroids for acute spinal cord injury. *Cochrane Database Syst Rev* 2002;(2): CD001046.
83. Morris JA, Jr., MacKenzie EJ, Damiano AM, Bass SM. Mortality in trauma patients: the interaction between host factors and severity. *J Trauma* 1990;30(12):1476–82.
84. Schultz RJ, Whitfield GF, LaMura JJ, Raciti A, Krishnamurthy S. The role of physiologic monitoring in patients with fractures of the hip. *J Trauma* 1985;25(4):309–16.
85. Victorino GP, Chong TJ, Pal JD. Trauma in the elderly patient. *Arch Surg* 2003;138(10):1093–8.
86. Battistella FD, Din AM, Perez L. Trauma patients 75 years and older: long-term follow-up results justify aggressive management. *J Trauma* 1998;44(4):618–23; discussion 23.
87. Bulger EM, Arneson MA, Mock CN, Jurkovich GJ. Rib fractures in the elderly. *J Trauma* 2000;48(6):1040–6; discussion 6–7.
88. Bulger EM, Edwards T, Klotz P, Jurkovich GJ. Epidural analgesia improves outcome after multiple rib fractures. *Surgery* 2004;136(2):426–30.
89. Moon MR, Luchette FA, Gibson SW, Crews J, Sudarshan G, Hurst JM, Davis K Jr, Johannigman JA, Frame SB, Fischer JE. Prospective, randomized comparison of epidural versus parenteral opioid analgesia in thoracic trauma. *Ann Surg* 1999;229(5):684–91; discussion 91–2.
90. Wisner DH. A stepwise logistic regression analysis of factors affecting morbidity and mortality after thoracic trauma: effect of epidural analgesia. *J Trauma* 1990;30(7):799–804; discussion 804–5.
91. Mattox KL, Goetzl L. Trauma in pregnancy. *Crit Care Med* 2005;33(10 Suppl):S385–9.
92. Shah KH, Simons RK, Holbrook T, Fortlage D, Winchell RJ, Hoyt DB. Trauma in pregnancy: maternal and fetal outcomes. *J Trauma* 1998;45(1):83–6.
93. Henderson SO, Mallon WK. Trauma in pregnancy. *Emerg Med Clin North Am* 1998;16(1):209–28.
94. Goodwin H, Holmes J, Wisner DH. Abdominal ultrasound examination in pregnant trauma patients. *J Trauma* 2001;50:689.
95. Morris JA, Jr, Rosenbower TJ, Jurkovich GJ, Hoyt DB, Harviel JD, Knudson, MM, Miller RS, Burch JM, Meredith JW, Ross SE, Jenkins JM, Bass, JG. Infant survival after cesarean section for trauma. *Ann Surg* 1996;223(5):481–8; discussion 8–91.

Chapter 9
Phase I: Abbreviated Surgery

General

Gary Lombardo and John P. Pryor

The damage control concept is most often applied to injuries of the abdomen and chest. The goals of this Phase I are rapid control of hemorrhage, followed by control of contamination and removal of frankly necrotic tissue if necessary. As stated clearly in previous chapters, the extent of the procedure is limited by time and the patient's ongoing physiological status. Many traditional surgical techniques are significantly modified during damage control, especially within the abdominal cavity.

9.1 Damage Control Laparotomy

To prepare for acute massive bleeding, the following preoperative precautions are undertaken: An aortic occluder or clamp is held by the first assistant, and two functioning suction catheters are readied. If available, a cell salvage device is set up and primed. Adequate blood products must be in the operating room prior to skin incision. The scrub team prepares a generous supply of opened lap pads and a large bowl to catch the evacuated clot.

Abdominal damage control procedures generally start with a generous midline incision to allow adequate access and exposure of the intra-abdominal and pelvic viscera. If the particular injury is known before the laparotomy is begun, a few modifications are considered. In patients with an isolated liver injury from a penetrating injury, the incision may be spared in the superior aspect to allow coverage of the eventual hepatic packing. However, in most cases, additional injuries have to be considered and evaluated during the laparotomy.

Similarly, if a large pelvic hematoma is suspected, truncating the incision to leave the suprapubic muscles intact will help the tamponade effect after packing. In all cases, it is most important to have adequate visualization of the injuries. Thus, if needed, one can quickly abort these modifications and extend the incision as far

G. Lombardo (✉) and J.P. Pryor
Department of Trauma, Surgical Critical Care, and Emergency Surgery, Westchester Medical
Center, New York Medical College, Valhalla, NY, 10595, USA

H.-C. Pape et al. (eds.), *Damage Control Management in the Polytrauma Patient*,
DOI 10.1007/978-0-387-89508-6_9, © Springer Science+Business Media, LLC 2010

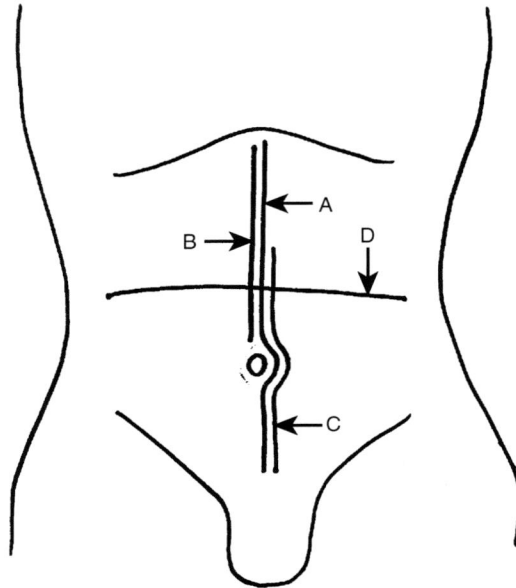

Fig. 9.1 Incisions used in damage control surgery (**a**) long midline, (**b**) upper abdominal sparing, (**c**) lower abdominal sparing, and (**d**) transverse

as required to gain control of injuries. A difficult operation should never be made more challenging by inadequate operative exposure.

Rarely, patients will present in extremis with a previous abdominal midline scar. In these cases, consider a transverse incision to quickly access the peritoneum on either side of the midline (Fig. 9.1). Avoid the use of a classic bilateral chevron since this incision does not afford adequate visualization of the lower abdomen and pelvis.

The skin and fascia are cut with a knife, and the peritoneum is inspected. If bulging and purple colored, massive intraperitoneal bleeding has occurred. The anesthesia team prepares for an acute drop in the blood pressure when the peritoneal tamponade is released and, if possible, has active resuscitation in progress.

The peritoneum is opened by making a small hole superiorly and then running a semiclosed scissor inferiorly down the midline to splay the peritoneum open. Blood and clot are evacuated, taking care to salvage as much as possible into a cell saver if feasible. With the majority of the clot evacuated, one must decide if there is localized bleeding, such as often seen in penetrating injury, or diffuse bleeding, seen more often in blunt mechanisms. If an individual bleeding source is seen, move to *control that source first*. This is most often a bleeding spleen, kidney, or retroperitoneal vessel. If there is diffuse bleeding with an unclear source, pack all four quadrants with open laparotomy pads to gain temporary tamponade. Once the identified source is controlled or once the quadrants are packed with diffuse bleeding control, the procedure is temporarily halted. The surgeon and the anesthesiologist confer at this point, and the team is allowed to "catch up" with the resuscitation. This pause in the procedure should not be more than a few minutes, but often it is enough time to begin reestablishing hemodynamic stability before continuing with the operation. If packs have been placed, they are removed one quadrant at a time, starting with the quadrants least likely to contain the bleeding source. The remainder of the damage control laparotomy is organ specific and will be described subsequently.

The principles of hypothermia, acidosis, and coagulopathy as the indications to perform a damage control laparotomy have a firm physiological foundation. The decision regarding how much surgery to perform and regarding the timing of when the operation is aborted is more an art than a science. In general, once the decision is made to perform damage control surgery, the operation should be stopped as soon as possible. To that end, there are a few goals that must be accomplished before ending the operation, including control of surgical bleeding, control of all bowel injuries, and removal of frankly necrotic tissue.

Foremost, all surgical bleeding must be controlled before leaving the operating room. *Surgical bleeding* is distinguished from *coagulopathic bleeding* in that the former is controllable with a stitch or tie, whereas the latter is only controllable with packing, hemostatic dressings, or correction of the coagulation cascade. The differentiation is not always straightforward, such as in the case of bleeding that continues to well up from a retroperitoneal wound. However, it is an axiom that if surgically correctable bleeding is not controlled before leaving the operating room, there will be a high likelihood of treatment failure and the need to return to the operating room prematurely.

One must make an assertive effort to fully explore the abdomen for bowel injuries. A missed bowel injury that allows continuing contamination will add a septic response to the patient's physiological burden and increase the mortality. If there is a significant pancreatic injury that cannot be resected, one must provide wide drainage, as the free pancreatic fluid will also cause a severe inflammatory response. This is less of an issue with bile and urine, but drainage of these sources is also recommended.

Finally, inspect for grossly necrotic tissue that must be resected prior to concluding the procedure. Frankly dead tissue will exacerbate the inflammatory cascade, and, if it involves a hollow viscus, a subsequent perforation is possible before the next operation is performed. Once these goals are met, the operation is ended and the patient is moved to damage control Phase II.

9.2 Liver

Massive injury to the hepatic parenchyma is one of the most common indications for damage control surgery. Emergency hepatic resection performed by nonhepatobiliary surgeons is associated with a high mortality. Therefore, truncated procedures incorporating limited, if any, initial hepatic parenchymal resections are the basis for treatment of severe liver trauma. Techniques focus on control of surgical hemorrhage, tamponade of small vessel bleeding, and the use of angiographic embolization as an adjunct to hemorrhage control. The steps of hepatic control are summarized by the 4 "Ps": pressure, packing, Pringle, and pictures (angiography).

Active hemorrhage is initially controlled with manual compression. This temporizing measure will stop the majority of venous bleeding and allow the anesthesia team to replace volume loss and continue aggressive resuscitation. Perihepatic packing provides hemostasis via compression of the underlying hepatic parenchyma while the patient is actively resuscitated and hemodynamically optimized. If at all possible, the ligamentous attachments of the liver, including the falciform ligament, are *not* mobilized. This will allow the abdominal wall and the liver to be held in tension when superior packs are placed, increasing the effectiveness of the tamponade. Dry, folded lap pads are placed under direct visualization, providing compression tamponade between the anterior abdominal/chest wall, the diaphragm, and the retroperitoneum (Fig. 9.2). As an adjunct to packing, direct en masse suturing acts to reapproximate the liver tissue and may help provide compression and tamponade. It is performed with a blunt-tipped 0 chromic suture situated in deep, full-thickness

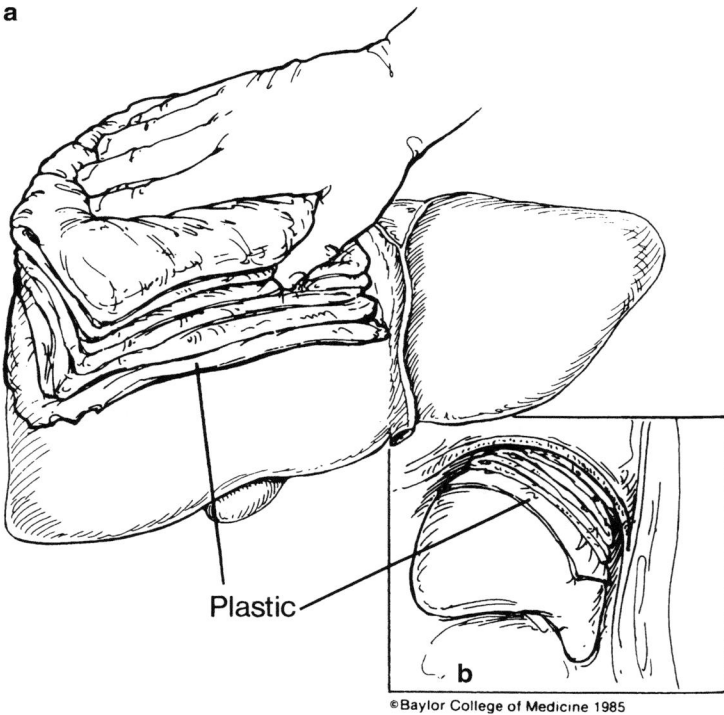

© Baylor College of Medicine 1985

Fig. 9.2 Liver packing (Reprinted with permission of Elsevier from Feliciano DV, Pachter HL. Hepatic trauma revisited. *Curr Probl Surg* 1989;26:453. Copyright © Baylor College of Medicine, 1985.)

throws either in a mattress or in a continuous fashion. This technique is especially helpful when there is a stellate laceration, with tissue fractured in several planes.

Continued bleeding postmanual compression should be followed with inflow control of the porta hepatis (Pringle maneuver). The porta is identified and isolated by placing the fingers into the foramen of winslow, the thumb across the ventral surface of the portal vein, and then pinching the lesser omentum to create a window around the structures (Fig. 9.3). Control of the porta hepatis is best achieved with a Rummel tourniquet or a vessel loop. The use of a formal clamp is discouraged due to the possible damage to the bile duct and, more important, the bile duct arterial supply during the clamping period.

Controversy surrounds the length of time of acceptable "clamp" time and therefore hepatic warm ischemia time to avoid postprocedure sequela. Studies cite acceptable clamp times extending from 20 to 75 min of continuous hepatic warm ischemia [1–3]. A reasonable practice pattern would include a continuous warm ischemia time of 20 min with a 5 min reperfusion time prior to reapplication of the inflow clamp.

If there is a large parenchymal disruption, the wound is inspected for actively bleeding larger vessels that can be directly controlled and ligated. Tangential injuries to large veins are best managed with repair using fine (5-0 or 6-0) non-absorbable suture in a venorrhaphy manner. Free ends of vessels can be clamped and tied.

Injuries of the parenchyma forming a deep, narrow tract pose both a diagnostic and therapeutic challenge as the bleeding source is not directly visualized. Examples include tracts resulting from stab wounds, fragments, or gunshot wounds missiles. Attempts to "plug the holes" may be ineffective since the bleeding source is not

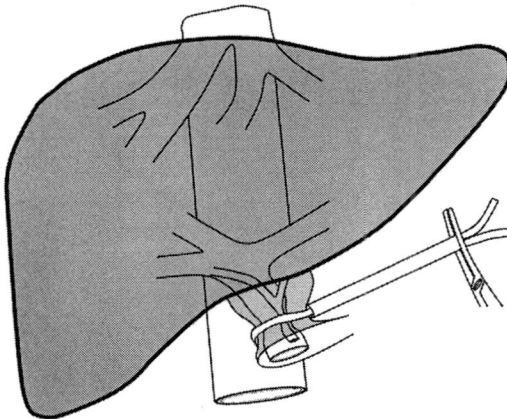

Fig. 9.3 The Pringle maneuver (Reprinted with permission of Elsevier from Abdalla EK, Noun R, Belghiti J. Hepatic vascular occlusion: Which technique? In Khatri VP, Schneider PD (eds) Surgical Clinics of North America: Liver Surgery: Modern Concepts and Techniques 2004;84(2):566.)

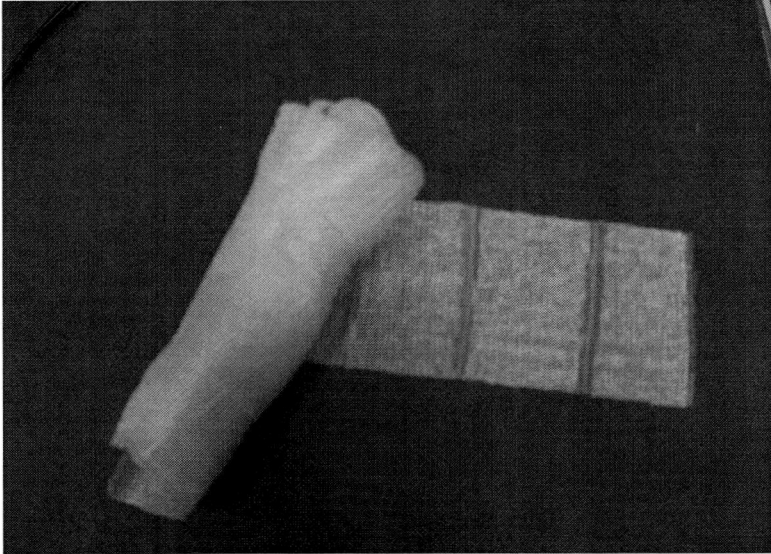

Fig. 9.4 The Kauder tampon

directly controlled. In these cases, consider providing tamponade throughout the tract by inserting hemostatic material filling the entire tract. One example is the "Kauder tampon," which consists of long pieces of gel foam wrapped in surgicell to form a long hemostatic tube (Fig. 9.4). This is introduced into the tract with long tissue forceps.

Another technique for long narrow tracts is application of balloon catheter tamponade using either a Fogarty or a foley catheter inserted into the injury tract, with subsequent inflation and examination for tamponade [4–7] (Fig. 9.5). The uninflated catheter is inserted all the way into the tract. Then, it is slowly withdrawn and inflated sequentially until the bleeding point is controlled. The proximal end of the tube is then brought through a separate stab incision in the anterior abdominal wall, and secured in position and inflated for later deflation and removal during reexploration. There are also now commercially available balloon catheters that work in a similar fashion.

For injury involving a large disruption of Glisson's capsule, as well as for major hepatic lobar disruptions, wrapping the liver with absorbable mesh provides tamponade by way of circumferential compression. The theory is to restore basic hepatic architecture and provide hemostasis, thus avoiding a major hepatic resection in the initial operative procedure [4, 8, 9]. Care must be taken to fashion the wrap in such a way as to not occlude the portal vessels or hepatic venous outflow.

Omental packing of parenchymal defects and capsular tears is a useful adjunct in obtaining hemostasis with the added benefit of controlling postprocedure biliary leaks. Viable omentum is mobilized on a pedicle, filling dead space with viable

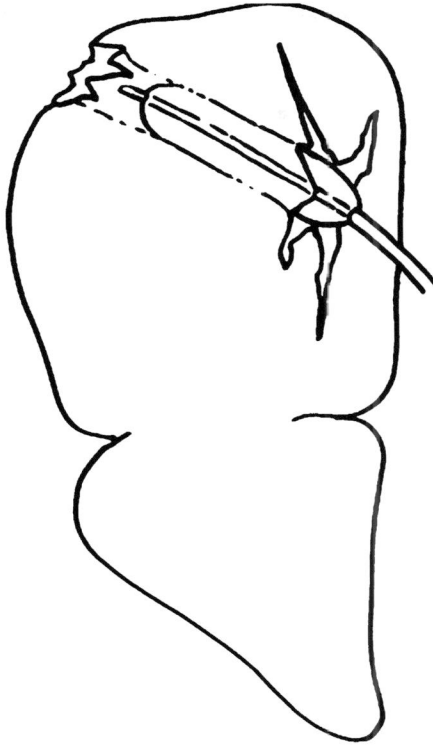

Fig. 9.5 Balloon tamponade of the liver

tissue and providing a conduit for macrophage egress into the site of injury. Often, this technique is reserved for the second damage control operation since the omentum, once placed, should not be disturbed in subsequent operations to allow it to heal into the liver injury site.

The techniques that have been described are successful in halting significant hemorrhage in the vast majority of cases and are to be used as first-line therapy. The goal of Phase I is hemostasis, not the reestablishment of normal anatomy or architecture. Thus, when hemostasis is achieved, the procedure should be ended. Rarely, bleeding continues from continued *surgical bleeding*. In these rare cases, further attempt must be made to identify and control large vessel bleeding by selective vascular ligation or resectional debridement. Hepatotomy and debridement are performed with in-flow control using the Pringle maneuver. The liver parenchyma is then divided using a standard finger fracture technique with direct visualization and ligation of identified bleeding vessels [10–12]. The gastrointestinal anastomosis (GIA) stapler can also be used to rapidly divide liver tissue and gain access to major bleeding sites. Resectional debridement without selective vascular ligation is performed in the situation of a significant coagulopathy in which parenchymal bleeding is intense and vessel identification would prove an exercise in futility. A Pringle maneuver is performed, and the hepatic tissue surrounding the injured segment is clamped between two large clamps such as Kelly clamps. The devitalized tissue within the clamps is then sharply divided and deep horizontal mattress sutures are placed at the periphery of the debrided laceration site. The clamps are removed and the dead space is filled with viable omentum.

Anatomical resections, once popular in hepatic trauma, have been associated with a prohibitively high mortality rate and are currently not considered during a damage control procedure. Hepatic artery ligation has also been described for emergent vascular control of life-threatening hepatic hemorrhage. If the bleeding rate is decreased or controlled with application of the Pringle maneuver intraoperatively, control may be obtained via ligation of the hepatic artery. Today, this approach has largely been replaced with a multimodality approach including hepatic angiography and embolization. In fact, overzealous hepatic artery ligation leaves no access for subsequent selective angiography and embolization. Also, one must recall that there are several common variations of hepatic arterial blood supply that may not be controlled at the porta hepatis, such as a replaced right hepatic artery arising from the superior mesenteric artery (SMA).

9.2.1 Hepatic Vein and Retrohepatic Vena Caval Injury

Severe hepatic traumatic injuries may involve extension to, or primarily involve, the hepatic veins or the vena cava. Management of such injury has plagued surgeons as they are rare and challenging. Intrinsic to the dilemma is that attempted mobilization and visualization of the injury may facilitate life-threatening hemorrhage by releasing the tamponade of the suspending ligaments of the liver. Methods of repair described include direct repair with and without vascular isolation and tamponade with containment.

First, one must determine that there is a real need to explore and repair a caval injury. There are many caval injuries causing retrohepatic hematomas that will resolve without any management. Mobilization of the liver with these retrohepatic hematomas is indicated only if there is active bleeding from a rent in the retroperitoneum causing ongoing blood loss or if there is an extensive hematoma causing caval compression [13–15]. Direct repair (transhepatic) without shunting includes occlusion of the portal triad, and mobilization of the liver with finger fracture dissection to the site of injury with direct repair of the injury [16].

If the cava is approached in an extrahepatic plane, there must be some way to control bleeding and allow blood return to the right atrium. Unlike all other veins in the body, if the suprarenal caval blood flow is interrupted for a matter of minutes, cardiac arrest often occurs from inadequate preload to the right heart. Control of caval bleeding may be performed with an atriocaval shunt, which is often constructed at the time of surgery from an endotracheal tube or chest tube. It is a complex procedure that takes forethought and access to the atrium, necessitating a sternotomy (Fig. 9.6). The preferred method in institutions with the capability would be total hepatic exclusion,

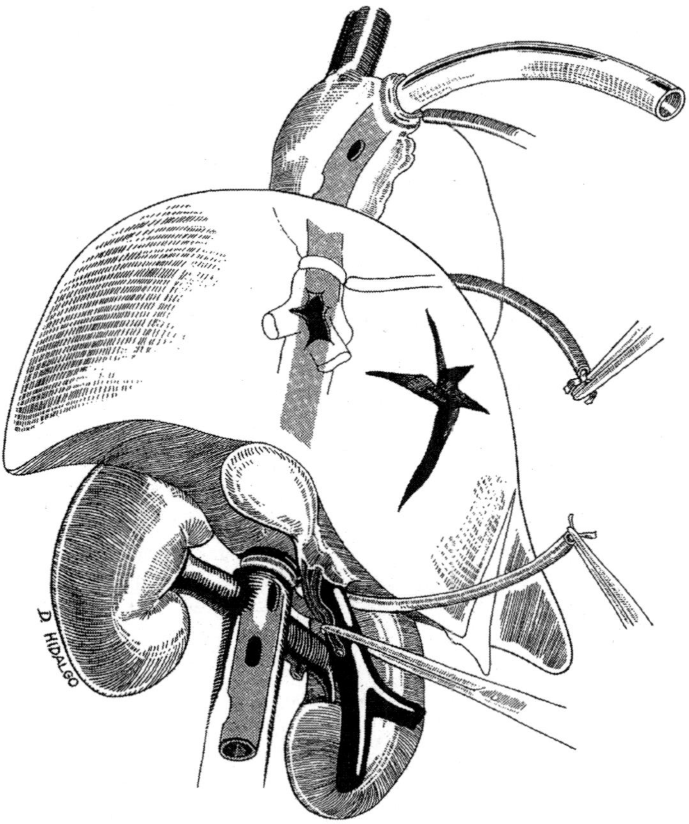

Fig. 9.6 Atriocaval shunt (Reprinted with permission of The McGraw-Hill Companies from Pachter HL, Liang HG, Hofstetter SR. Liver and Biliary Tract Trauma. In Feliciano DV, Moore EE, Mattox KL (eds) Trauma, Third Edition. Stamford, CT: Appleton & Lange, 1996.)

in which a veno-venous bypass circuit is used to shunt venous blood from the lower half of the body back to the right atrium via superior vena cava (Fig. 9.7). With veno-venous bypass, the cava can be safely occluded proximal and distally for repair to occur. As with anatomic resection, direct repair with and without shunting has reported mortality rates from 70% to 80% [17–20].

9.2.2   *Extrahepatic Biliary and Portal Triad Injury*

Extrahepatic biliary and portal triad injury represents a rare injury complex. These injuries are reported as involving 0.07–0.21% of all trauma admissions [10, 11]. Trauma to the gallbladder should be managed with a cholecystectomy. Injury involving the portal vein should be managed with lateral venorrhaphy, with or without

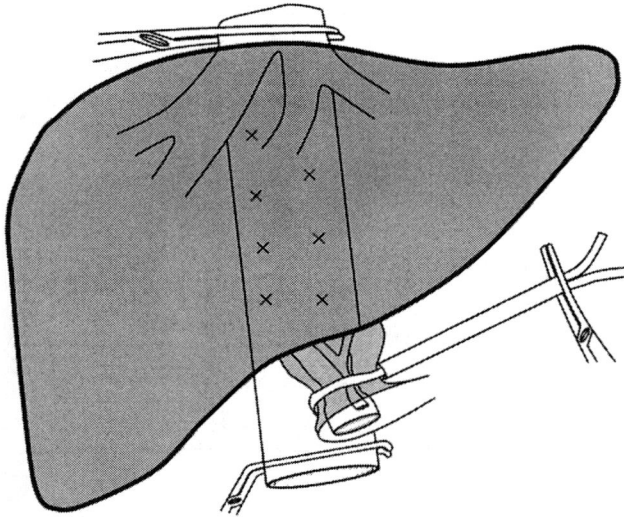

Fig. 9.7 Total hepatic occlusion (Reprinted with permission of Elsevier from Abdalla EK, Noun R, Belghiti J. Hepatic vascular occlusion: Which technique? In Khatri VP, Schneider PD (eds) Surgical Clinics of North America: Liver Surgery: Modern Concepts and Techniques 2004;84(2):566.)

a vein patch. In the face of life-threatening exsanguination, ligation of the portal vein is acceptable. Reported survival rates in the literature after portal vein ligation cite survival ranging from 10% to 80% [10, 21]. Anecdotal reports of temporary shunting of the portal vein have been reported [22]. Survival with these injuries relies on rapid identification of injury, damage control maneuvers (including rapid determination of the necessity of vascular ligation as opposed to repair), early termination of the operative intervention, and aggressive postoperative resuscitation. With injury involving the hepatic artery, attempted primary repair is acceptable but ligation in the face of impending metabolic failure is the procedure of choice. Bile duct injury in the patient with hemodynamic instability requires nothing but packing and wide drainage. Definitive repair is delayed for the planned second exploration postresuscitation.

9.3   Spleen

Damage control surgical principles necessitate a rapid, yet safe operative procedure to control hemorrhage. In the face of hemodynamic instability and metabolic failure, splenectomy remains the safest choice of surgical procedure. However, in patients found with an American Association for the Surgery of Trauma (AAST) grade 1 or 2 injury, topical application of microfibrillar collagen, topical hemostatic agents, fibrin glue, or rapid suture repair may be attempted to avoid splenectomy and potential retroperitoneal bleeding in a coagulopathic patient. In patients with AAST grade 3–5 injury, splenectomy remains the procedure of choice.

9.4   Intestinal Injury

Traumatic injury involving the GI tract is common: Gunshot wounds that penetrate the peritoneum are associated with GI tract injury in over 80% of cases, and stab wounds have an associated 30% incidence of hollow viscus injury [23]. The high incidence of reported GI tract involvement often necessitates damage control techniques for hemostasis and contamination containment. Injury may involve contusion, intramural hematoma, full-thickness perforation, or mesenteric bleeding and avulsion.

Techniques to control bleeding and contamination differ depending on the site of intestinal injury. In general, all sites of intestinal leak need to be controlled during the first damage control procedure to decrease the risk of a systemic inflammatory reaction from spilled intestinal contents during the resuscitative phase of damage control Phase II.

9.4.1   Stomach

In the case of penetrating injury with a single identified defect, mobilization of the stomach is necessary for complete exposure and thorough evaluation. Several areas known to hide injury include greater and lesser gastric curvatures, proximal posterior gastric wall, fundus, and posterior cardia. Injury complex involving intramural hematoma, small partial thickness, or full-thickness lacerations of the stomach (grade 1–3) can be managed with a rapidly placed continuous suture or a stapling device. Larger lacerations or injuries with significant tissue devascularization (grade 4 and 5) are controlled in a damage control fashion with staple diversion, with or without tube gastrostomy.

Devastating injury to the gastroesophageal junction can be temporized with stapling across the distal esophagus and proximal stomach, with a nasogastric tube placed into the esophagus. Severe, large injuries to the stomach wall, such as high-velocity firearm injuries, can be treated with gastric resection, with delayed anastomosis.

9.4.2   Duodenum

Mortality rates for pancreatoduodenal injuries range from 6% to 34%. The anatomical location of these organs - deep, central, and retroperitoneal - presents a diagnostic challenge in the hemodynamically unstable patient. Complication rates from injury of these structures have been reported between 30% and 63% [24–29].

The proximity of the pancreas and duodenum to several vital structures makes the possibility of an associated vascular injury likely. Patients who die from injury involving the pancreas and duodenum usually have an injury complex involving a major vascular structure, the liver, or spleen. As such, the need to incorporate these organs and their potential injuries into a damage control procedure is clear. Fortunately, pancreatoduodenal injury remains relatively rare, with reported estimate between 0.2% and 5% of all abdominal trauma [27, 30–33].

Simple lacerations of the duodenum should be repaired with a rapidly placed continuous suture utilizing an omental or serosal buttress. Transected ends of the duodenum should be rapidly closed using suture or a stapling device, and definitive repair should be delayed until a subsequent operation. Complex lacerations of the duodenum can be closed around a T-tube as a temporizing maneuver. This allows closure and decompression at the same time.

Pyloric exclusion and diverticulization with antecolic gastrojejunostomy are important parts of complex duodenal injury management. However, these should not be performed during the first operation since they are involved procedures that will add unnecessary time to the operation. Care is made to drain the injury well, both internally and externally. A nasogastric tube placed near the duodenal repair is often used along with a Jackson-Pratt drain close to, but not up against, the duodenum externally.

Particular vigilance must be maintained when evaluating the retroperitoneal duodenum. In blunt and semiurgent situations, retroperitoneal injuries are often detected on preprocedure imaging. Intraoperative findings necessitating thorough retroperitoneal and pancreatic evaluation include central retroperitoneal hematoma, edema of the lesser sac, and peripancreatic structures as well as retroperitoneal bile staining. If there is a concern for a retroperitoneal duodenal injury, it is imperative to mobilize the entire duodenum and repair any injury found.

9.4.3 Pancreas

The pancreas is one of the most complex organs for application of damage control techniques. Similar to duodenal injury, pancreatic injury is often associated with vascular injury, and, unlike simple bowel injuries, the pancreatic secretion causes a significant systemic inflammatory response if not controlled early. The pancreas is assumed injured in any case when a retroperitoneal hematoma, swelling, or extensive edema at the base of the mesentery is found. In all cases, the full extent of the gland must be inspected for injury. Access to the pancreas is best through the lesser omentum for the body and tail, whereas the head is best inspected via a Kocher maneuver. A key principle is visual inspection and bimanual palpation of the entire pancreas.

Injury to the gland anywhere to the left of the mesenteric vessels is considered a distal injury and is best managed by distal pancreatectomy, with splenectomy. Although a spleen-sparing pancreatectomy could be considered, this often adds time and blood loss to the procedure, and thus this is often abandoned in most damage control operations. In desperate cases with many other injuries, the distal pancreatic injury may be temporized with transection of the body on either side of the injury only, leaving formal distal resection for another operation.

Injury to the head and neck of the pancreas poses a special challenge. Even a "temporizing" resection would be a time-consuming procedure. Thus, for most head and neck injuries, the recommendation is to widely drain the injury without an attempt at resection during the first operation. This allows resuscitation to better prepare the patient for an extensive second operation and also allows time to determine if there is a major pancreatic duct injury using either endoscopic retrograde cholangiopancreatography (ERCP) or magnetic resonance cholangiopancreatography (MRCP).

9.4.4 Combined Pancreatoduodenal Injury

Treatment of combined injury to both the duodenum and pancreas is based on the integrity of the distal bile duct, ampulla, and the severity of the duodenal injury. On the basis of potential injury to these vital structures, required investigation includes cholangiogram, pancreatography, and ampulla evaluation. In the patient with proven metabolic and hemodynamic compromise, these studies are usually not feasible. As with the majority of duodenal trauma, an attempt at primary repair is advised, with wide closed drainage of the pancreatic injury. If the integrity of the duodenal repair is in question, a lateral duodenostomy, or an antegrade and retrograde jejunostomy, act as useful adjuncts to avoid leak or duodenal blow out.

Severe injury to the duodenal pancreatic head complex may eventually necessitate gastric diversion via a pyloric exclusion procedure for contamination control, although this should not be considered during the initial procedure.

In situations in which there is severe, nonreconstructable injury to both the head of the pancreas and the duodenum, the *trauma Whipple* procedure will be the only option to control all injuries. Unlike traditional pancreaticoduodenectomy, the *trauma Whipple* is a staged procedure. As mentioned, if the patient remains hypotensive, acidotic, and cold, the only procedure performed during the first operation is wide drainage. If time and hemodynamics allow, the resection part of the Whipple is performed, but none of the anastomoses are completed. The patient should subsequently be resuscitated, with reanastomosis performed in 24–48 h.

9.4.5 Small Bowel

Evaluation of the small bowel follows standard practice of complete evisceration and careful, yet rapid, inspection of the entire length starting at the ligament of Treitz and ending at the cecum. Individual enterotomies are amenable to rapid, single-layer, full-thickness, transverse closure using a continuous nonabsorbable suture. Multiple or large perforations within a short segment of bowel should be managed with segmental resection of all injuries with a stapling device. Alternatively, umbilical tape may be used to ligate bowel segments on either side of an injury with no further resection needed. The ligated or stapled bowel is then returned to the peritoneal cavity without ostomy creation or anastomosis.

Mesenteric hematomas must be evaluated. If small and nonexpanding, they are left alone and reevaluated at the time of definitive repair. If significant bleeding is noted from the mesentery, the hemorrhage should be controlled with suture ligature. Mesenteric defects are not closed during the initial procedure, with formal repair delayed to the reexploration. Nonsurgical bleeding is controlled, or at least temporized, via abdominal packing.

While the primary focus of the damage control procedure is the rapid control of hemorrhage and contamination, added benefit of bowel "second look" is found in the mandatory second exploration. Bowel of questionable viability may be left intact and reevaluated after the patient is resuscitated rather than proceeding with initial resection. Bowel anastomosis and abdominal closure may also be facilitated at second exploration by allowing initial edema to regress.

9.4.6 Colon

Colonic injury resulting from a blunt traumatic force is uncommon, reported between 2% and 5% [34]. The injuries occur with equal frequency throughout the colon [34–37]. They may present as avulsion injury resulting from mesenteric stripping or as seromuscular disruptions. Blunt trauma to the colon may also present as large defects in the colonic wall, resulting in luminal blowout.

In cases of penetrating injury, the colon is the second most frequently injured organ behind the small bowel [34, 38–42]. Firearm injury accounts for 75–80% of colonic penetrating injury, with stab wounds accounting for the remaining 20–25%. Among the blunt injuries, open book pelvic fractures from straddling on a motorcycle tank are most frequent [34, 42–47].

Injuries to the colon should be dealt with in a rapid fashion as time for definitive repair is not available. Preventing fecal contamination from small colotomies can be obtained with a rapid, full-thickness, continuous suture. When multiple colotomies are noted in a single segment of colon or a large defect is noted, control of fecal contamination can expeditiously be obtained using transversely placed linear stapling device or bowel ligation with umbilical tape both proximal and distal to the perforation. The ligated bowel is then returned to the abdominal cavity without anastomosis or ostomy formation. In the case of an adjacent acetabular fracture, the colostomy should be placed as far away from the future inguinal incision (for the orthopedic approach) as tolerable. Definitive repair is delayed for 24–48 h until the end points of resuscitation are met.

The most pressing decision to make in colonic injury is whether to perform a primary anastomosis or diversion. In the vast majority of damage control procedures, the colon is left stapled or sewn off with neither an anastomosis nor a diversion during the first operation. If multiple injuries are noted in different sections of colon, it is acceptable to staple or tie off sections, leaving a "closed loop" intervening segment as long as the second operation can be accomplished within 24–48 h. If there will be a significant delay in the formation of an anastomosis or formal diversion, a distal temporary decompression can be accomplished using a malecot catheter sewn into the distal orifice and brought out the abdomen to a drainage bag. This will at least decompress the air in the colon and perhaps decrease the swelling encountered during the second operation.

9.4.7 Rectum

Firearms account for approximately 80% of all rectal injuries. Among the blunt injuries to the rectum are pelvic disruptions that usually occur in conjunction with severe internal hemorrhage. Stab wounds are a rare mechanism of rectal injury and have been reported to be responsible for 3% of injuries, while transanal injuries, including iatrogenic injury, account for 6% of reported cases [34, 48–59].

The majority of the morbidity and mortality from rectal injury is due to the resulting sepsis and multiorgan failure relating to inadequate drainage or missed injury. The unique anatomical position of the rectum, with two-thirds of the rectal wall not visible from within the abdomen at laparotomy, causes the surgeon a dilemma in diagnosis in many cases. If a rectal injury is either confirmed or *highly suggested* by the trajectory of findings of a retroperitoneal hematoma in the pelvic floor, rectal diversion is indicated. Rectal fecal diversion is accomplished via either an end sigmoid colostomy, with Hartman's segment left in place, or a loop colostomy with distal segment stapled off. Rectal injury is one potential exception to the rule that formal ostomies are not created at the first operation, since immediate diversion may halt ongoing fecal contamination of the perirectal space.

Two adjuncts to diversion of rectal injuries are distal segment washout and presacral drainage. Each has potential benefits and disadvantages that will be covered in subsequent chapters. Neither should be performed at the time of the first damage control operation.

9.5 Abdominal Vasculature

The incidence of major abdominal vascular injury associated with blunt abdominal trauma is reported at 5–10%. In patients with penetrating abdominal trauma, stab wounds are associated with a 10% incidence of major vascular injury, while gunshot wounds to the abdomen have a major abdominal vascular injury in 20–25% of patients [60–63]. The crux of damage control techniques for abdominal vessels is understanding which arteries can be ligated, which can be shunted, and which need definitive repair during the first operation. Many arteries of the abdomen can be ligated in desperate situations (renal, branches of the celiac, proximal SMA, and internal iliac arteries), whereas others cannot be ligated (aorta, proximal celiac, distal SMA, and external iliac arteries). The development of intravascular shunts championed by both civilian and military use has provided surgeons with a damage control option for many of the main vessels of the body. Shunts can be placed to restore flow, delaying definitive repair for later operations. Some situations will call for immediate repair (periceliac aorta).

Injuries to vascular structures found in the abdomen have classically been divided into five distinct zones (Fig. 9.8): the classic retroperitoneal zones (1–3), the portal area, and the retrohepatic area. Zone 1 refers to the midline retroperitoneum and has a supramesocolic and an inframesocolic area. The supramesocolic area contains the suprarenal abdominal aorta, celiac axis, proximal SMA, proximal renal arteries, and the superior mesenteric vein. The inframesocolic area contains the infrarenal abdominal aorta and the infrahepatic inferior vena cava. Zone 2 describes the area of the upper lateral retroperitoneum and contains the renal arteries and veins. Zone 3 refers to the pelvic retroperitoneum and contains the iliac arteries and veins. The portal area contains the portal vein and hepatic artery. In a damage control exploration of the trauma patient with active hemorrhage from the abdominal cavity, hemorrhage control must be obtained prior to any other intraoperative maneuvers. As previously described, solid organ bleeding is initially controlled with direct pressure and abdominal packing. Vascular control is accomplished with direct pressure via sponge sticks or lap pads until proximal and distal control is obtained with vascular clamps.

9.5.1 Zone 1: Supramesocolic Injury

Hemorrhage or hematoma in the midline supramesocolic area may result from injury to the suprarenal aorta, celiac axis, proximal SMA, or proximal renal artery. In the case of a supramesocolic zone 1 aortic injury, survival has been reported in the literature to vary between 8.3% and 34.8%. [64–75]. Proximal vascular control of the aorta at this level is obtained with immediate manual compression of the aorta against the vertebral column at the diaphragmatic hiatus. Exposure is rapidly obtained by dividing the lesser omentum with gastric and esophageal retraction to the left. The muscle fibers of the crura are bluntly dissected from the aorta, and the supra celiac aortic cross clamp can be placed. If this dissection is not possible, an aortic occluder device may be used to hold pressure against the aorta on the spine until a formal clamp can be applied. If control is still not possible, especially for injuries just at the diaphragmatic hiatus, one should consider performing a left thoracotomy and clamping the distal thoracic aorta for inflow control.

Distal control of the aorta at this location can be difficult and may require control of the celiac axis. With inflow control, one should perform a medial visceral rotation by opening the retroperitoneum above the left kidney and rotating everything above

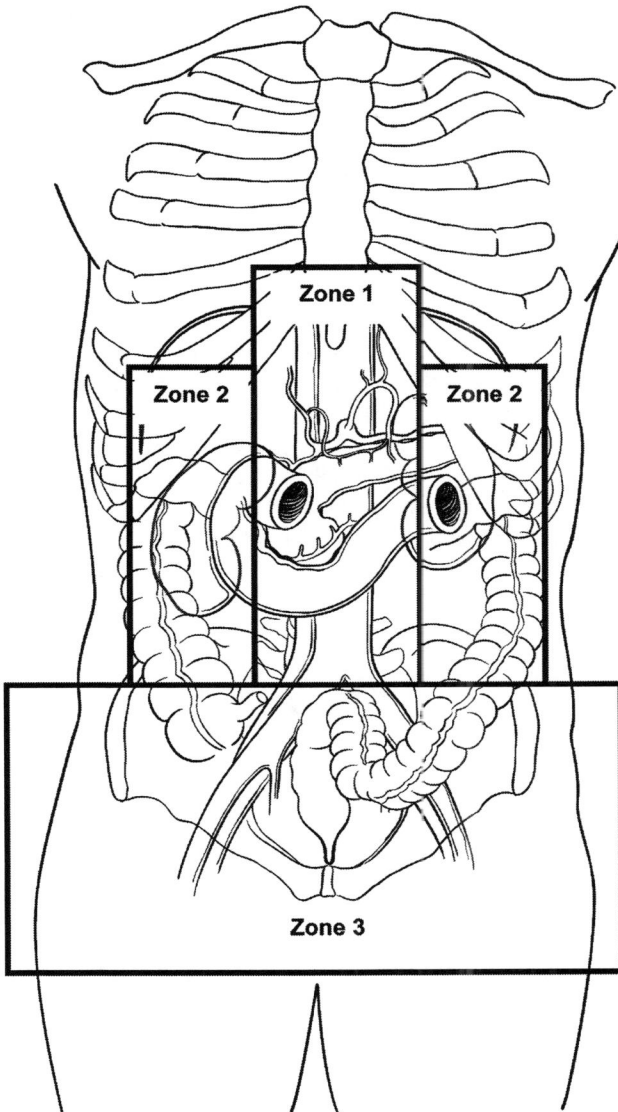

Fig. 9.8 The zones of the retroperitoneum (Adapted from [30])

the kidney to the right. Then one should follow the renal artery to the aorta as a landmark. Small perforating wounds to the aorta are repaired rapidly with lateral aortorrhaphy with 3-*O*-polypropylene suture. If primary suture repair will result in significant narrowing of the vessel lumen, repair should be performed with polytetrafluoroethylene (PTFE) patch aortoplasty. In the situation of extensive injury or significant loss of the aortic wall, incorporation of a synthetic vascular conduit, that is, Dacron, albumin coated Dacron, or PTFE, may have to be incorporated. Although a concern exists regarding the use of synthetic graft material and associated gastrointestinal injury, and classical teaching describes the use of the extra-anatomical bypass, this is not practical in the damage control setting. Interposition grafts that become contaminated can be removed in subsequent operations with or without the use of an extra-anatomical bypass.

Ligation of the vessels for injury involving the celiac axis and its branches applies to both the nondamage and damage control procedures. The diffuse collateralization of the vessels between the celiac axis and the SMA branches will provide sufficient blood flow following ligation. Ligation of the celiac axis should not result in any short term sequela other than possible necrosis of the gallbladder, which should be addressed at the definitive procedure with cholecystectomy.

Injury involving the SMA has a survival rate reported in the literature reported between 22% and 58.7% [62–65, 71, 74–80]. SMA injuries are classified using the Fuller classification (Fig. 9.9). This classification describes the level of the vessel injury extending from Fuller zone 1 located directly beneath the pancreas and continuing distally to Fuller zone 4 located at the level of the enteric branches [81]. Traditionally, ligation of the proximal SMA is tolerated because of collateral blood flow to the midgut from the pancreaticoduodenal and middle colic vessels. However, in the unstable patient with exsanguinating hemorrhage, vasoconstriction

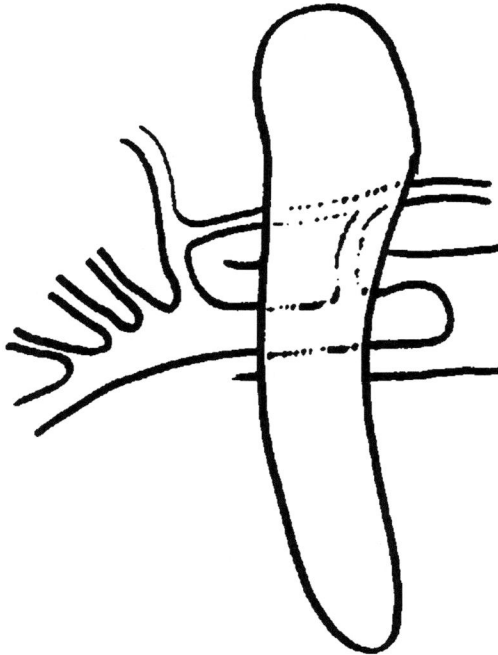

Fig. 9.9 The Fuller zones of the superior mesenteric artery

will prove inadequate to support the distal midgut, resulting in ischemia and necrosis of the bowel [82]. Thus, rapid insertion of a temporary intraluminal shunt should be employed in *any type of SMA injury.*

Proximal superior mesenteric *vein* injury may also present with a supramesocolic zone 1 hematoma. This injury is safely dealt with via ligation in a damage control procedure. A review of the literature concerning superior mesenteric venous injury revealed an 85% survival in patients treated with ligation as opposed to a 64% survival in patients treated with venous repair. Reported mean survival rates of patients with superior mesenteric venous injury range from 58.3% to 72.1% [62, 64, 65, 71, 74, 75, 78, 80, 83–85]. The inferior mesenteric artery and vein can both be ligated with impunity.

9.5.2   Zone 1: Inframesocolic Injury

Injuries in the inframesocolic area of zone 1 involve the infrarenal aorta or the infrahepatic vena cava. Survival for patients sustaining infrarenal aortic injury has been reported ranging between 34.2% and 46.2% [62, 65, 68, 70–73, 86]. Exposure of the aorta in the inframesocolic area is obtained by reflecting the transverse mesocolon upward toward the stomach, eviscerating the small bowel to the patient's right, and opening the midline retroperitoneum. Proximal control is obtained by placing an aortic cross clamp just below the left renal vein as it crosses the midline over the aorta. Distal control is obtained at the aortic bifurcation. During exploration, if a large inframesocolic zone 1 hematoma is identified, an alternate approach is a direct dissection over the apex of the hematoma directly down to the level of the injury, with proximal and distal control of the aorta obtained at the level of the vascular rent.

Injury of the aorta at this level is usually successfully repaired via lateral aortorrhaphy using 3-0 or 4-0 polypropylene suture. If repair results in luminal narrowing or if the defect is large, the repair may require patch aortoplasty, end-to-end anastomosis, or the use of a Dacron or PTFE graft. Aortic shunting has been accomplished with some success. A large chest tube is used with double ligatures on each side to prevent displacement. Care is taken not to introduce the distal end down in an iliac artery, causing untoward ischemia of the nonperfused limb. Depending on the duration of the limb ischemia and the associated soft tissue injury, an emergent amputation to prevent ischemia reperfusion injury can be lifesaving.

Survival rates for patients with infrahepatic inferior vena cava injury reported in the literature depend on the location of the injury. The survival rate ranges from 29.9% to 76.1%, with an average of 72.2% when suprahepatic and retrohepatic caval injuries are excluded. The average survival increases to 76.1% when only infrarenal inferior vena cava injuries are included [62, 64, 71, 73, 87–93]. Injury involving the infrahepatic inferior vena cava necessitates adequate exposure for both identification and repair. While a midline retroperitoneal incision and dissection incorporating visualization of both the aorta and the inferior vena cava have been described, most trauma surgeons agree that excellent exposure of the inferior vena cava from the infrahepatic area to the confluence of the iliac veins is obtained via a right medial visceral rotation, leaving the right kidney in place with complete mobilization of the descending colon and the second and third portions of the duodenum. If an anterior wall perforation is identified, direct partial occlusion is obtained using a Satinsky vascular clamp with direct transverse venorrhaphy using 4-0 or 5-0 polypropylene sutures. In the situation of inadequate hemorrhage control using partial occlusion, or if the injury is extensive, near complete occlusion of the inferior vena cava can be obtained via sponge stick compression or using DeBakey aortic clamps both proximal and distal to the injury site. It is recommended to perform simultaneous aortic cross clamping, as near total occlusion will severely limit venous return to the heart in a previously hemodynamically compromised patient. Routine attempts to place vascular clamps on the vena cava are discouraged because this can lead to vessel damage from the clamp or the attempt to dissect the back wall with the vessel tethered by lumbar veins.

Injury involving the posterior wall of the inferior vena cava visualized through an anterior defect can be approached by extending the anterior defect, suture repair of the posterior wall from inside the lumen, with subsequent repair of the anterior defect. If the injury is not amenable to this repair or if the injury involves the posterior wall of the suprarenal inferior vena cava, incorporation of the right kidney with the medial visceral rotation will allow access to the posterior wall. Caution must be utilized in performing this maneuver to ensure ligation of the first lumbar vein, as it typically enters at the right renal vein/ inferior vena cava junction.

An area of the inferior vena cava notorious for difficult exposure and repair is the inferior vena cava/right renal vein junction. As with other complex venous injury patterns, proximal and distal control is obtained via sponge stick compression. As described for posterior wall injury, medial rotation of the kidney after bowel rotation will bring the short right renal vein into view and allow access to the vena cava at this level. Venous injury is repaired using transverse venorrhaphy, composite vein interposition graft, or Dacron or PTFE interposition graft.

In the case of the exsanguinating patient with noted or impending metabolic failure who would not tolerate prolonged repair, ligation of the inferior vena cava may be necessary. Ligation of the *infrarenal* inferior vena cava below the renal vessels is usually well tolerated. Strict attention to postoperative volume status to maintain the patient's circulating volume as well as 5–7 days of bilateral lower extremity wrapping with elastic wraps and elevation are imperative adjuncts [91]. Lower extremity compartment syndromes are possible, and, occasionally, patients may require bilateral four-compartment fasciotomy. Ligation of the *suprarenal* inferior vena cava is usually accompanied by acute renal failure as well as massive edema of the lower half of the body. This should only be performed in the face of terminal shock. A method to allow later reconstruction in the patient with metabolic failure involves the insertion of a temporizing intraluminal shunt as a damage control measure.

9.5.3   Zone 2

Hematoma or hemorrhage in the upper lateral/peri-renal area may involve injury to the renal artery, the renal vein, both the renal artery and renal vein, or the renal parenchyma. If active bleeding is noted from the retroperitoneum overlying the renal vessels or from Gerota's fascia, the retroperitoneum lateral to the kidney is incised, and the kidney is delivered into the wound. Vascular control is obtained with a large vascular clamp placed proximal to the renal hilum. Small perforations in the artery or vein can be repaired via suture repair, resection of the injured vascular segment with end-to-end anastomosis, interposition graft, or, as with the left renal vein, ligation. In the situation of impending metabolic failure and the institution of damage control technique, it is best to perform a nephrectomy, after palpation of a normal-sized contralateral kidney, as opposed to complex vascular repair or revascularization. Overall survival rates reported in the literature for patients with renal artery injury range from 65.1% to 87%, with renal salvage reported in only 30–40%. A reported survival rate of 42–88% has been reported for patients with renal vein injuries [62, 64, 65, 80, 92, 94, 95].

9.5.4   Zone 3

Hematoma or hemorrhage in the pelvic area may result from injury to the iliac artery, the iliac vein, or both the iliac artery and the iliac vein. This is one of the most technically challenging areas of the body in which to obtain vascular control of injuries. The survival rate among patients with iliac artery injury in the literature has varied based on reported concomitant injury, ranging from 45% to 81%. Survival rates reported in the literature among patients with iliac vein injury is reported as 58.6–95% [62, 64, 65, 78, 80, 81, 96–98].

Exposure of the proximal iliac vessels is obtained by eviscerating the small bowel to the right and dividing the midline retroperitoneum over the aortic bifurcation. Proximal vascular control on the distal abdominal aorta is obtained via this exposure. Distal vascular control is obtained at the external iliac vessel as it emerges from the pelvis just proximal to the inguinal ligament. Exposure and control of the internal iliac artery are obtained via continued division of the retroperitoneum of the pelvis, with combined elevation of the proximal common iliac and distal external iliac artery using vessel loops.

The *internal* iliac artery can be ligated with impunity unilaterally. Bilateral internal iliac artery ligation has a high risk of gluteal necrosis, especially in patients with concomitant shock. Injury involving the common or external iliac artery must be shunted or repaired since ligation of these vessels will result in progressive ischemia of the ipsilateral lower extremity. Shunting should be the first option, and care must be taken to choose a shunt that is large enough to allow continuation of the normal, fluid-filled caliber of the artery. Repair options include lateral arteriorrhaphy, end-to-end anastomosis, and interposition venous or PTFE graft.

Mobilization of the ipsilateral internal iliac artery to the ipsilateral injured external iliac artery or transposition of one iliac artery to the side of the contralateral iliac artery for bifurcation injury have been described, but these constitute too much surgery during the first case [99–101].

Injuries involving the common or external iliac vein are much more difficult to control and manage than iliac artery injury. Control is first attempted with sponge sticks forced down on the tissue to occlude blood flow from the low pressure venous system. One must recall that arterial inflow control will decrease the venous outflow with isolated venous injuries, and this should always be completed first. Although one may think to get inflow occlusion at the groin for venous injuries, the collateralization is so great in the pelvis that this will not decrease forward venous bleeding appreciably. In rare cases of an injury at the inguinal ligament or very proximal thigh, an abdominoinguinal incision may provide access to the entire pelvic sidewall and all vasculature (Fig. 9.10). At the level of the iliac vein confluence, visualization is hindered via the overlying aortic bifurcation. Rapid access may be obtained by temporary division of the right common iliac artery and mobilization of the aortic bifurcation to the left. The artery is then repaired or shunted after repair or ligation of the vein [62, 102].

In the situation of a damage control procedure, all iliac veins, both internal and external, can be ligated safely with similar precautions as described for ligation of the inferior vena cava. At times, it may be logistically easier to get control with 5.0 prolene in a venorrhaphy manner then attempting to get control around the vessel with a clamp.

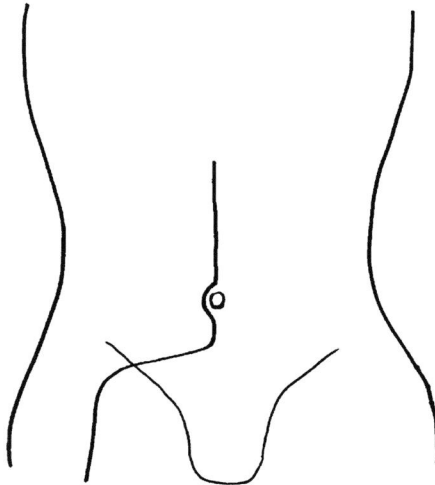

Fig. 9.10 The abdominal-inguinal incision

9.5.5   *Porta Hepatis*

Injury to the portal vein and hepatic artery, as discussed earlier in the *Liver* section of this chapter, will present with hematoma or hemorrhage from the right upper quadrant and area of the porta hepatis. Control of the proximal hepatoduodenal ligament should be obtained using the Pringle maneuver and direct control of the hemorrhage site with finger pressure. Distal control is obtained via placement of a vascular clamp or with forceps control. Prior to suture placement, the vascular injury should be precisely defined due to the proximity of the common bile duct. Hepatic artery injury is managed with ligation and is usually very well tolerated. Injury to the portal vein should be repaired or bypassed depending on the stability of the patient. If extensive injury is encountered or if damage control technique is necessary for patient survival, the portal vein may be ligated as previously discussed.

9.6   Genitourinary Tract

Damage control techniques for injury involving the structures of the genitourinary tract involve intentionally delaying surgical intervention for injury not immediately life threatening. Virtually all urological injury with the exception of active hemorrhage from the kidney or renal pedicle can be managed in a delayed fashion. When the patient stabilizes, imaging may characterize injury amenable to nonoperative therapy, subsequently avoiding potential morbidity and mortality of operative management. In patients with renal injury, if hemostasis is obtained or if minimal bleeding is noted, the kidney and perinephric area can be packed for continued hemostasis, with renal reconstruction deferred to a second laparotomy. Damage control techniques for active renal hemorrhage include nephrectomy as the procedure of choice. Ureteral injury may be managed with ligation or may be left in situ for delayed repair, but this risks urinary obstruction or infection. Another option is an externalized stent passed through the injury and into the renal pelvis with the proximal end brought out through a stab incision. In the case of severe uncontrolled bleeding from the urinary bladder or if a large amount of necrotic tissue is present requiring extensive debridement, the ureters should be externalized and the pelvis aggressively packed for tamponade for delayed reconstruction/repair. Injuries of the urethra and external genitalia should be managed with suprapubic catheter drainage of the urinary bladder and occlusive dressing, with later reconstruction when stabilized [103].

9.7   Temporary Abdominal Closure

Abbreviated closures provide simple, rapid, temporary closure of an incision to the thoracic or abdominal incision. The simplest method involves towel clip or suture closure of the skin only. The towel clips or continuous suture are placed 1 cm from the skin edge and 1 cm distal to the previously placed suture or clip. This method requires the skin edges to be reapproximated, thus controlling fluid loss and preventing evisceration.

When the skin edges are not able to be reapproximated or if reapproximation would result in intracavitary hypertension with subsequent development of a compartment syndrome, the abdomen can be packed open with laparotomy pads and moist sterile gaze or with the creation of a temporary silo. This will allow coverage of the viscera and prevent evisceration. The temporary silo can be formed from plastic wound drapes (Bogota Bag) or other commercially available products. These devices are sutured to the skin edges, bridging the gap of the open abdomen.

Vacuum-assisted wound closure incorporates sterile, radio-opaque towels placed over a sterile plastic barrier, which keeps the bowel in the abdominal cavity and protected from the towel. Jackson-Pratt drains are placed over the towel and covered with a second sterile plastic sheet, then placed to suction (Fig. 9.11). Institutional variations as well as commercially available systems all function in a similar fashion: visceral coverage preventing desiccation, removal of peritoneal fluid, and medial force on the fascial and skin edge to prevent loss of domain.

9.8   Thoracic

The concept of abbreviated or damage control surgery, when applied to thoracic injury, follows the principles outlined previously: a truncated operative procedure to control hemorrhage and contamination. An anterolateral thoracotomy is the incision

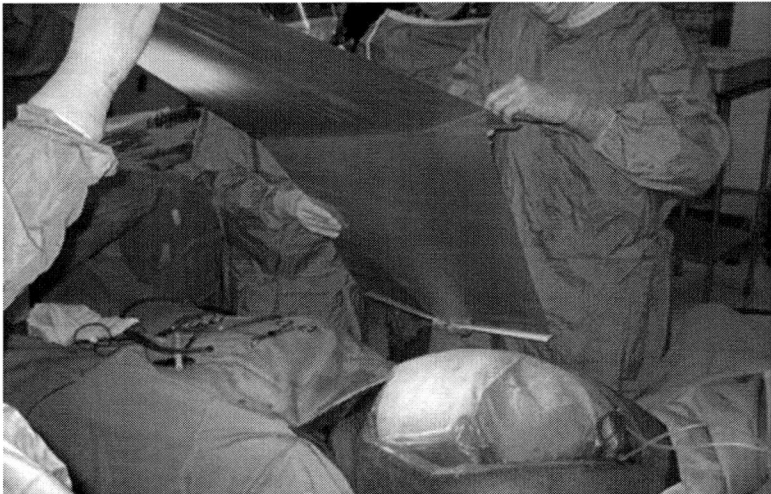

Fig. 9.11 A damage control temporary abdominal dressing

of choice for the patient in extremis with suspected intrathoracic injury. It provides rapid and emergent exposure to injured structures including the heart and pericardium, as well as the descending aorta and pulmonary structures.

9.8.1   Pulmonary

Injuries involving the lung parenchyma are dealt with in rapid fashion by performing nonanatomically stapled resections of injured tissue, thus providing rapid hemostasis and control of injury [104]. Deeper lobar injuries resulting from penetrating missiles, stab wounds, or deep penetrating wounds not amenable to nonanatomic staple resection may be managed with *tractotomy* and selective vascular ligation of bleeding tissue/vessels [104–107]. For larger areas of tissue destruction and uncontrolled bleeding, en masse lobectomy or pneumonectomy may be necessary.

In cases of exsanguinating hemorrhage with signs of metabolic failure, a vascular clamp can be placed across the hilum of the lung as a damage control procedure [108]. A technique termed the pulmonary hilar twist can be done by division of the inferior pulmonary ligament and subsequent 180° rotation of the lung using the hilum as the center point of rotation. This maneuver rapidly controls hilar exsanguination and additionally prevents air embolism [109].

9.8.2   Thoracic Vasculature

When hemodynamic compromise results from intrathoracic vascular injury, techniques incorporating ligation, prosthetic graft repair, and intravascular shunting have been described. Limited experience has been reported in recent literature with damage control techniques of thoracic vasculature injury, as patients in extremis with this injury complex usually do not survive the initial insult or present to the hospital in a clinical picture amenable to surgical therapy. Shunting has been described for subclavian injury, common carotid injury, and aortic injury. The innominate vein can be ligated with impunity. The innominate artery can be ligated with a significant degree of morbidity, but this may potentially be lifesaving.

9.8.3   Esophageal

Thoracic esophageal injury in the hemodynamically unstable patient with proven or impending metabolic failure is managed with abbreviated/damage control surgical procedure. Hemostasis is secured and contamination is controlled with wide drainage and staple diversion of the injured segment of esophagus. The patient is admitted to the ICU for continued resuscitation, with a deferred formal resection/repair to be performed after metabolic endpoints of resuscitation have been reached.

9.8.4 Cardiac

Injuries to the heart present as a unique injury complex. The patient most commonly presents in hemodynamic shock. Small injuries can usually be controlled with finger compression, with subsequent suture repair of the injury as both the damage control and definitive repair procedure. Hand stapling of such injuries has also been reported in the literature [110, 111].

In larger injuries of the cardiac chamber walls, initial control of hemorrhage not amenable to finger compression has been reported using a clamped foley catheter, with the inflated balloon filling the ventricular wall rent. The tissue can then be reapproximated using sutures over the inflated balloon; in one experience, this has created a larger hole if excess pull is placed on the foley catheter [112].

In cases of significant rupture with a large defect of the chamber wall, a technique for rapid repair utilizes occlusion of the superior vena cava and inferior vena cava to obtain inflow control. This is followed by horizontal mattress stay sutures on both sides of the defect. The sutures are then crossed over the midline, acting to approximate the two sides of the injury. A continuous suture is then employed to repair the closely approximated defect, with subsequent removal of the inflow occlusion and rapid incision closure with continued resuscitation in the ICU [113, 114].

9.8.5 Chest Wall Closure

At the conclusion of the initial operative damage control procedure, the thoracic wall should be closed in an en masse fashion using a large single continuous suture. Closure may be accomplished with the aid of prosthetic material such as a large IV bag, mesh patch, or plastic sheets if there has been significant tissue loss or if attempted closure resulted in additional hemodynamic compromise. The median sternotomy may be left open with an Ioban® (3M, St. Paul, MN) type dressing if there is significant thoracic space swelling or if there is heart dysfunction with attempted closure.

9.9 Summary and Conclusion

Certain precautions have to be taken prior to performing a damage control laparotomy, such as aortic occluder or clamp held by the first assistant, two functioning suction catheters, a cell salvage device primed, and adequate blood products in the operating room.

Abdominal damage control procedures generally start with a generous midline incision to allow for adequate access to and exposure of the intra-abdominal and pelvic viscera. If a large pelvic hematoma is present, the incision leaves the suprapubic muscles intact to help the tamponade effect after packing. If an individual bleeding source is seen, move to *control that source first*. The procedure requires frequent reevaluation and cooperation between the surgeon and the anesthesiologist. Packing is done, and the triad of death has to be respected.

In conclusion, a damage control laparotomy is entirely different from a regular laparotomy and requires frequent precautions regarding blood loss and drop of blood pressure.

References

1. Pachter HL, Spencer FC, Hofstetter SR, Liang HG, Coppa GF. Significant trends in the treatment of hepatic trauma: Experience with 411 injuries. Ann Surg 1992;215: 492–502.
2. Sheldon G, Rutledge R. Hepatic trauma. Adv Surg 1989;22: 179.
3. Man K, Fan ST, Ng IO, Lo CM, Liu CL, Wong J. Prospective evaluation of Pringle maneuver in hepatectomy for liver tumors by a randomized study. Ann Surg 1997;226: 704–713.
4. Fabian TC, Bee TK. Liver and biliary tract trauma. In Feliciano DV, Moore EE, Mattox KL (eds) Trauma, Fifth ed. New York: McGraw-Hill, 2004, pp.637–662.
5. Demetriades D. Balloon tamponade for bleeding control in penetrating liver injuries. J Trauma 1998;44: 538539.
6. Wilson RF, Walt AJ. Management of Trauma: Pitfalls and Practice, Second ed. Baltimore: Williams & Wilkins, 1996, p.476.
7. Erb RE, Mirvis SE, Shanmuganathan K. Gallbladder injury secondary to blunt trauma: CT findings. J Comput Assist Tomogr 1994;18: 778784.
8. McFadden D, Lawelor B, Ali I. Portal vein injury. Can J Surg 1987;30: 91.
9. Sheldon G, Lim R, Yee E, Petersen S. Management of injuries to the porta hepatis. Ann Surg 1985;202: 539–545.
10. Jurkovich GJ, Hoyt DB, Moore FA, Ney AL, Morris JA, Scalea TM, Pachter HL, Davis JW, Bulger E, Simons RK, Moore EE, McGill JW, Miles WS. Portal triad injuries – A multicenter study. J Trauma 1995;39: 426–434.
11. Dawson DL, Johansen KH, Jurkovich GJ. Injuries to the portal triad. Am J Surg 1991;161: 545–551.
12. Sharma O. Blunt gallbladder injuries: Presentation of 22 cases with review of the literature. J Trauma 1995;39: 576–580.
13. Beal SL. Fatal hepatic hemorrhage: An unresolved problem in the management of complex liver injury. J Trauma 1990;30: 163–169.
14. Fabian TC, Croce MA, Stanford GG, Payne LW, Margiante EC, Voeller GR, Kudsk KA. Factors affecting morbidity following hepatic trauma. A prospective analysis of 482 injuries. Ann Surg 1991;213: 540–548,
15. Cue JI, Cryer HG, Miller FB, Richardson JD, Polk HC Jr. Packing and planned reexploration for hepatic and retroperitoneal hemorrhage: Critical refinements of a useful technique. J Trauma 1990;30:1007–1011.
16. Pachter HL, Feliciano DV. Complex hepatic trauma. Surg Clin North Am 1996;76: 763–782.
17. Richardson JD, Franklin GA, Lukan JK, Carrillo EH, Spain DA, Miller FB, Wilson MA, Polk HC Jr, Flint LM. Evolution in the management of hepatic trauma: A 25 year perspective. Ann Surg 2000;232: 324–330.
18. Schrock T, Blaisdell W, Mathewson C. Management of blunt trauma to the liver and hepatic veins. Arch Surg 1968;96: 698–704.
19. Pilcher DB, Harman PK, Moore EE. Retrohepatic vena cava balloon shunt introduced via the sapheno-femoral junction. J Trauma 1977;17: 837–841.

20. Baumgartner F, Scudamore C, Nair C, Karusseit O, Hemming A. Venovenous bypass for major hepatic and caval trauma. J Trauma 1995;39: 671–673.
21. Stone HH, Fabian TC, Turkelson M. Wounds of the portal venous system. World J Surg 1982;6: 335–341.
22. Fish JC. Reconstruction of the portal vein. Case reports and literature review. Am J Surg 1966;32: 472–478.
23. Diebel LN. Stomach and small bowel. In Feliciano DV, Moore EE, Mattox KL (eds) Trauma, Fifth ed. New York: McGraw-Hill, 2004, pp.687–708.
24. Wilson R, Moorehead R. Current management of trauma to the pancreas. Br J Surg 1991;78(10): 1196–1202.
25. Ivatury R, Nallathambi M, Gaudino J, Rohman M, Stahl WM. Penetrating duodenal injuries: An analysis of 100 consecutive cases. Ann Surg 1985;202 (2): 154–158.
26. Martin T, Feliciano DV, Mattox KL, Jordan GL Jr. Severe duodenal injuries: Treatment with pyloric exclusion and gastrojejunostomy. Arch Surg 1983;118: 631–635.
27. Jurkovich GJ, Bulger EM. Duodenum and Pancreas. In Feliciano DV, Moore EE, Mattox KL (eds) Trauma, Fifth ed. New York: McGraw-Hill, 2004, pp.709–734.
28. Ivatury RR, Nallathambi M, Rao P, Stahl WM. Penetrating pancreatic injuries. Analysis of 103 consecutive cases. Am Surg 1990;56 (2): 90–95.
29. Snyder W, Weigelt JA, Watkins WL, Bietz DS. The surgical management of duodenal trauma. Arch Surg 1980;115: 422–429.
30. Blaisdell F, Trunkey D. Abdominal trauma. In Trauma Management. New York: Thieme-Stratton, 1982.
31. Cuddington G, Rusnak CH, Cameron RD, Carter J. Management of duodenal injuries. Can J Surg 1990;33 (1): 41–44.
32. Sukul K, Lont H, Johannes E. Management of pancreatic injuries. Hepatogastroenterology 1992;39: 447–450.
33. Cook D, Walsh JW, Vick CW, Brewer WH. Upper abdominal trauma: Pitfalls in CT diagnosis. Radiology 1986;159(4): 65–69.
34. Burch JM, Brock JC, Gevirtzman L, Feliciano DV, Mattox KL, Jordan GL Jr, DeBakey ME. The injured colon. Ann Surg 1986;203: 701–711.
35. Burch JM. Injury to the colon and rectum. In Feliciano DV, Moore EE, Mattox KL (eds) Trauma, Fifth ed. New York: McGraw-Hill, 2004, pp.735–753.
36. Howell HS, Bartizal JF, Freeark RJ. Blunt trauma involving the colon and rectum. J Trauma 1976;16: 624–632.
37. Duaterive AH, Flancbaum L, Cox EF. Blunt intestinal trauma: A modern day review. Ann Surg 1985;201: 198–203.
38. Schrock TR, Christensen N. Management of perforating injuries of the colon. Surg Gynecol Obstet 1972;1: 135, 65–68.
39. Abcarian H, Lowe R. Colon and rectal trauma: Surg Clin North Am 1978;58: 519–537.
40. Stone HH, Fabian TC. Management of perforating colon trauma: Randomization between primary closure and exteriorization. Am Surg 1979;190: 430436.
41. Orsay CP, Merlotti G, Abcarian H, Pearl RK, Nanda M, Barrett J. Colorectal trauma. Dis Colon Rect 1989;32: 188–190.
42. Levinson MA, Thomas DD, Wiencek RG, Wilson RF. Management of the injured colon: Evolving practice at an urban trauma center. J Trauma 1990;30: 247253.
43. Nallathambi MN, Ivatury RR, Shah PM, Gaudino J, Stahl WM. Aggressive definitive management of penetrating colon injuries: 136 cases with 3.7 percent mortality. J Trauma 1984;24: 500–505.
44. Shannon FL, Moore EE. Primary repair of the colon: When is it a safe alternative? Surgery 1985;98: 851–860.
45. George SM, Fabian TC, Voeller GR, Kudsk KA, Mangiante EC, Britt LG. Primary repair of colon wounds: A prospective trial in nonselected patients. Ann Surg 1989;209: 728–734.
46. Chappuis CW, Frey DJ, Dietzen CD, Panetta TP, Buechter KJ, Cohn I Jr. Management of penetrating colon injuries: A prospective randomized trial. Ann Surg 1991;213: 492.

47. Burch JM, Martin RR, Richardson RJ, Muldowny DS, Mattow KL, Jordan GL, Morgenstern L. Evolution of the treatment of injured colon in the 1980s. Arch Surg 1991;126: 979–984.
48. Grasberger RC, Hirsch EF. Rectal trauma – A retrospective analysis and guidelines for therapy. Am J Surg 1983;145: 795–799.
49. Vitale GC, Richardson JD, Flint LM. Successful management of injuries to the extraperitoneal rectum. Am J Surg 1983;49: 159–162.
50. Tuggle D, Huber PJ. Management of rectal trauma. Am J Surg 1984;148: 806.
51. Mangiante EC, Graham AD, Fabian TC. Rectal gunshot wounds - Management of civilian injuries. Am J Surg 1986;52: 37–40.
52. Shannon FL, Moore EE, Moore FA, McCroskey BL. Value of distal colon washout in civilian rectal trauma - Reducing gut bacterial translocation. J Trauma 1988;28: 989–994.
53. Burch JM, Feliciano DV, Mattox KL. Colostomy and drainage of civilian rectal injuries: Is that all? Ann Surg 1989;209: 600–611.
54. Thomas DD, Levison MA, Dyskstra B, Bender JS. Management of rectal injuries – Dogma versus practice. Am Surg 1990;56: 507–510.
55. Ivatury RR, Licata J, Gunduz Y, Rao P, Stahl WM. Management options in penetrating rectal injuries. Am Surg 1991;57: 50–55.
56. Barone JE, Sohn N, Nealon TG. Perforations and foreign bodies of the rectum: Report of 28 cases. Ann Surg 1976;184: 601–604.
57. Haas PA, Fox TA. Civilian injuries of the rectum and anus. Dis Colon Rectum 1979;22: 17–23.
58. Robertson HD, Ray JE, Ferrari BTR, Gathright JB Jr. Management of rectal trauma. Surg Gynecol Obstet 1982;154:161–164.
59. Marti MC, Morel P, Rohner A. Traumatic lesions of the rectum. Int J Colorectal Dis 1986;1:152–154.
60. Fischer RP, Miller-Crotchett P, Reed RL 2nd. Gastrointestinal disruption: The hazard of non-operative management in adults with blunt abdominal injury. J Trauma 1988;28: 1445–1449.
61. Cox CF. Blunt abdominal trauma. A 5-year analysis of 870 patients requiring celiotomy. Ann Surg 1984;199: 467–474.
62. Feliciano DV. Abdominal vascular injury. In Feliciano DV, Moore EE, Mattox KL (eds) Trauma, Fifth ed. New York: McGraw-Hill, 2004, pp.755–777.
63. Feliciano DV, Burch JM, Spjut- Patrinely V, Mattox KL, Jordon GL. Abdominal gunshot wounds: An urban trauma center's experience with 300 consecutive patients. Ann Surg 1988;208: 362–364.
64. Asensio JA, Chahwan S, Hanpeter D, Demetriades D, Forno W, Gambaro E, Murray J, Velmahos G, Marengo J, Shoemaker WC, Berne TV. Operative management and outcome of 302 abdominal vascular injuries. Am J Surg 2001;180: 528–533.
65. Tyburski JG, Wilson RF, Dente C, Steffes C, Carlin AM. Factors affecting mortality rates in patients with abdominal vascular injuries. J Trauma 2001;50:1020–1026.
66. Mattox KL, McCollum WB, Jordan GL Jr, Beall AC Jr, DeBakey ME. Management of upper abdominal vascular trauma. Am J Surg 1974;128: 823–828.
67. Accola KD, Feliciano DV, Mattox KL, Bitondo CG, Burch JM, Beall AC Jr, Jordan GL Jr. Management of injuries to the suprarenal aorta. Am J Surg 1987;154:613–618.
68. Lim RC Jr, Trunkey DD, Blaisdell FW. Acute abdominal aortic injury. An analysis of operative and post operative management. Arch Surg 1974;109: 706–711.
69. Buchness MP, LoGerfo FW, Mason GR. Gunshot wounds of the suprarenal abdominal aorta. Ann Surg 1976;42:1–7.
70. Brinton M, Miller SE, Lim RC Jr, Trunkey DD. Acute abdominal aortic injuries. J Trauma 1982;22:481–486.
71. Kashuk JL, Moore EE, Millikan JS, Scott J, Moore JB. Major abdominal vascular trauma – A unified approach. J Trauma 1982;22: 672–679.
72. Millikan JS, Moore EE. Critical factors in determining mortality from abdominal aortic trauma. Surg Gynecol Obstet 1987;160: 313–316.

73. Jackson MR, Olson DW, Beckett WC, Olsen SB, Robertson FM. Abdominal vascular trauma. Am Surg 1992;58: 622–626.
74. Accola KD, Feliciano DV, Mattox KL, Burch JM, Beall AC Jr, Jordan GL Jr. Management of injuries to the superior mesenteric artery. J Trauma 1986;26:313–319.
75. Fullen WD, Hunt J, Altemeier WA. The clinical spectrum of penetrating injury to the superior mesenteric arterial circulation. J Trauma 1972;12: 656–666.
76. Graham JM, Mattox KL, Beall AC Jr, DeBakey ME. Injuries to the visceral arteries. Surgery 1978;84: 835–839.
77. Lucas AE, Richardson JD, Flint LM, Polk HC Jr. Traumatic injury of the proximal superior mesenteric artery. Ann Surg 1981;193: 30–34.
78. Sirinek KR, Gaskill HV 3rd, Root HD, Levine BA. Truncal vascular injury – Factors influencing survival. J Trauma 1983;23: 372–377.
79. Asensio JA, Britt LD, Borzotta A, Peitzman A, Miller FB, Mackersie RC, Pasquale MD, Pachter HL, Hoyt DB, Rodriguez JL, Falcone R, Davis K, Anderson JT, Ali J, Chan L. Multi-institutional experience with the management of superior mesenteric artery injuries. J Am Coll Surg 2001;193: 354–365.
80. Davis TP, Feliciano DV, Rozycki GS, Bush JB, Ingram WL, Salomone JP, Ansley, JD, Span DA, Davis TP. Results with abdominal vascular trauma in the modern era. Am Surg 2001;67: 565–571.
81. Millikan JS, Moore EE, Van Way CW 3rd, Kelly GL. Vascular trauma in the groin: Contrast between iliac and femoral injuries. Am J Surg 1981; 142: 695–698.
82. Reilly PM, Rotondo MF, Carpenter JP, Sherr SA, Schwab CW. Temporary vascular continuity during damage control: Intraluminal shunting for proximal superior mesenteric artery injury. J Trauma 1995;39: 757–760.
83. Donahue TK, Strauch GO. Ligation as definitive management of injury to the superior mesenteric vein. J Trauma 1988;28: 541–543.
84. Graham JM, Mattox KL, Beall AC Jr. Portal venous system injuries. J Trauma 1978;18: 419–422.
85. Stone HH, Fabian TC, Turkleson ML. Wounds of the portal venous system. World J Surg 1982;6: 335–341.
86. Cheek RC, Pope JC, Smith HF, Britt LG, Pate JW. Diagnosis and management of major vascular injuries: A review of 200 operative cases. Am Surg 1975;41: 755–760.
87. Oldhafer KJ, Frerker M, Winkler M, Schmidt, U. Complex inferior vena cava and renal vein reconstruction after abdominal gunshot injury. J Trauma 1999;46: 721–723.
88. Burch JM, Feliciano DV, Mattox KL, Edelman M. Injuries of the inferior vena cava. Am J Surg 1988;156: 549–551.
89. Frezza EE, Valenziano CP. Blunt traumatic avulsion of the inferior vena cava. J Trauma 1997;42: 141–143.
90. Graham JM, Mattox KL, Beall AC Jr, DeBakey ME. Traumatic injuries of the inferior vena cava. Arch Surg 1978;113: 413–418
91. Kudsk KA, Bongard F, Lim RC Jr. Determinants of survival after vena caval injury: Analysis of a 14-year experience. Arch Surg 1984;119: 1009–1012.
92. Wiencek RG, Wilson RF. Abdominal venous injuries. J Trauma 1986;26: 771–778.
93. Klein SR, Baumgartner FJ, Bongard FS. Contemporary management strategy for major inferior vena caval injuries. J Trauma 1994;37: 35–42.
94. Brown MF, Graham JM, Mattox KL, Feliciano DV, DeBakey ME. Renovascular trauma. Am J Surg 1980;140: 802–805.
95. McAninch JW, Carroll PR. Renal trauma: Kidney preservation through improved vascular control. J Trauma 1985; 22: 285–290.
96. Ryan W, Synder III W, Bell T, Hunt T. Penetrating injuries of the iliac vessels. Am J Surg 1982;144: 642–645.
97. Burch JM, Richardson RJ, Martin RR, Mattox KL. Penetrating iliac vascular injuries: Experience with 233 consecutive patients. J Trauma 1990;30:1450–1459.

98. Wilson RF, Wiencek RG, Balog M. Factors affecting mortality rate with iliac vein injuries. J Trauma 1990;30: 320–323.
99. Feliciano DV, Mattox KL, Graham JM, Bitondo CG. Five year experience with PTFE grafts in vascular wounds. J Trauma 1985;25:71.
100. Landercasper RJ, Lewis DM, Snyder WH. Complex iliac arterial trauma: Autologous or prosthetic vascular repair. Surgery 1993;114: 9–12.
101. Landreneau RJ, Mitchum P, Fry WJ. Iliac artery transposition. Arch Surg 1989;124: 978–981.
102. Salam AA, Stewart MT. New approach to wounds of the aortic bifurcation and inferior vena cava. Surgery 1985;98: 105–108.
103. Coburn M. Damage control for urologic injuries. Surg Clin North Am 1987;77: 821–834.
104. Velmahos G, Baker C, Demetriades D, Goodman J, Murray JA, Asensio JA. Lung sparing surgery after penetrating trauma using tractotomy, partial lobectomy and pneumonorraphy. Arch Surg 1999;134: 186–189.
105. Asensio JA, Demetriades D, Berne JD, Velmahos G, Cornwell EE, Murray J, Gomez H, Falabella AA, Chahwan S, Shoemaker W, Berne TV. Stapled pulmonary tractotomy: A rapid way to control hemorrhage in penetrating pulmonary injuries. J Am Coll Surg 1997;185: 486–487.
106. Karmy-Jones R, Jurkovich G, Shatz D, Brundage S, Wall MJ Jr, Engelhardt S, Hoyt DB, Holcroft J, Knudson MM, Management of traumatic lung injury: A western trauma association multicenter review. J Trauma 2001;51: 1049–1053.
107. Wall MJ Jr, Villavicencio RT, Miller CC, Aucar JA, Granchi TA, Liscum KR, Shi D, Mattox KL. Pulmonary tractotomy as an abbreviated thoracotomy technique. J Trauma 1998;45: 1015–1023.
108. Wall MJ Jr, Soltero E. Damage control for thoracic injuries. Surg Clin North Am 1997;77(4): 863–878.
109. Feliciano, DV, Mattox KL. Indications, technique and pitfalls of emergency center thoracotomy. Surg Rounds 1981;4: 32–40.
110. Macho JR, Markison RE, Schecter WP. Cardiac stapling in the management of penetrating injuries of the heart: Rapid control of hemorrhage and decreased risk of personal contamination. J Trauma 1993;34:711–716.
111. Bowman MR, King RM. Comparison of staples and sutures for cardiorrhaphy in traumatic puncture wounds of the heart. J Emerg Med 1996;14:615–618.
112. Feliciano DV, Burch JM, Mattox KL, Bitondo CG, Fields G. Balloon catheter tamponade in cardiovascular wounds. Am J Surg 1990;160: 583–587.
113. Trinkle JK, Toon RS, Franz JL, Arom KV, Grover FL. Affairs of the wounded heart: Penetrating cardiac wounds. J Trauma 1979;19: 467–472.
114. Wall MJ Jr, Mattox KL, Chen C, Baldwin JC. Acute management of complex cardiac injuries. J Trauma 1997;42(5): 905–912.

Orthopedics

Dieter Nast-Kolb, Christian Waydhas, Steffen Ruchholtz, and Georg Taeger

9.1 Introduction

In the management of multiply injured patients, the concept of Damage Control Orthopedics (DCO) is being developed. The work of various authors has demonstrated the impact of injury severity on the clinical immunoinflammatory response and its prognostic relevance regarding organ dysfunction or organ failure and clinical outcome. Data published by the authors and other investigators have clearly demonstrated an additive inflammatory response caused by surgical trauma [18, 23, 25, 40]; this additive inflammatory response is assumed to be significantly higher after primary definitive fracture treatment for major extremity fractures when compared with external fixation. Three retrospective cohort-studies have reported a possible reduction in organ dysfunction and an improvement in survival using the DCO approach [29, 30, 32]. These studies could also demonstrate that primary external fracture fixation and secondary conversion to definite osteosynthesis are not associated with an increased rate of local and systemic complications.

Advocates of DCO claim that multiply injured patients with severe brain and chest injuries as well as those with an unstable cardiopulmonary or circulatory condition are at high risk for developing a severe systemic immunoinflammatory reaction during early total fracture care. Therefore, to avoid additive surgical trauma, they recommend primary external fracture fixation for these patients. Following improvement of medical conditions due to intensive care treatment, definitive fracture care should be performed at the earliest possible time.

D. Nast-Kolb, C. Waydhas, S. Ruchholtz, and G. Taeger (✉)
Deparment of Trauma Surgery, Hufelandstr. 55, Essen, 45147, Germany
e-mail: georg.taeger@uk-essen.de

9.2 Fixation of Major Extremity Fractures

Primary stabilization of major fractures in multiply injured patients is known to be one of the important principles of treatment and has been shown to reduce the incidence of posttraumatic complications as well as organ failure [1–5]. In a recent study, Brundage et al. reviewed their registry data of patients with multiple injuries since 1985 and identified 1362 patients with fractures of the femoral shaft. They differentiated patients with respect to timing of surgical fracture fixation into four cohorts (less than 24, 24–48, 48–102 h, and greater than 102 h following trauma). According to this study, early fracture fixation is associated with improved outcome, even with concomitant head and chest injury [6].

With the implementation of standardized procedures for operative fracture treatment more than three decades ago, however, immediate overall fracture stabilization was also found to be associated with an increased rate of concomitant complications, secondary multiple organ failure (MOF), and even mortality [1, 7]. These findings led to the hypothesis that step-by-step procedures in those critically ill patients could be safer and thus result in a better prognosis. These concepts were reflected in early algorithms for diagnostics and treatment of multiply injured patients published by Schweiberer et al. and Trentz et al. [8, 9]. These authors described three phases: lifesaving and immediate surgery within the first hour, early surgery within 24 h, and (secondary) surgery delayed subsequent to the vulnerable proinflammatory phase that is estimated to last for 3–5 days after trauma [10]. At that time, the concept of Damage Control Surgery was developed; it addressed only major injuries responsible for significant blood loss at initial laparotomy [11]. It was found that by using this approach on patients with devastating abdominal injuries, mortality could be reduced significantly [12, 13].

9.2.1 Effects on Pulmonary Function and Head Trauma

Whereas DCS is accepted worldwide, the strategy of early fracture treatment still remains a controversial issue, especially with regard to the stabilization of diaphyseal fractures of the femur [14]. There is indeed no doubt that primary fracture fixation in the early stage significantly reduces the incidence of pulmonary complications as well as organ failure and does improve survival in comparison to initial nonoperative fracture management [1–3, 5, 15]. However, there is evidence indicating that complete and definitive fracture care in the initial phase of multiply injured patients with concomitant thoracic, abdominal, or severe traumatic brain injury may be associated with increased pulmonary complications, acute respiratory distress syndrome, or deterioration of outcome [1, 7].

Several authors have reported marked alterations in pulmonary function caused by intramedullary femoral nailing in experimental sheep models. Stürmer and Schuchardt described a greatly increased intramedullary pressure during the reaming process when performing reamed intramedullary nailing [16]. Furthermore, Wenda et al. could clearly demonstrate by ultrasound that reaming of the femoral canal leads to pulmonary embolism [17]. In addition to this result, Pape et al. investigated effects on pulmonary function caused by intramedullary reaming and nailing in an animal model. They found the effects associated with intramedullary nailing to be comparable to those effects seen in lung contusion and hemorrhagic shock [18].

In 1997, Jaicks et al. reported greater amounts of fluid administration in patients with severe head injuries when early and definitive fracture was executed [7]. Patients with moderate or severe brain injury and femoral fractures were found eight times more likely to become hypotensive when primary fracture treatment was performed within the first 2 h, regardless of the surgical technique [19]. Other authors did not find any difference regarding mortality and outcome when comparing patients who had severe brain injury and femoral fracture treated with intramedullary nailing to patients who had severe brain injury but no femoral fracture [20].

However, the clinical observation of severe MOF and even death following primary femoral nailing in certain patients contributed to a critical reflection on initial and complete fracture treatment, although such cases are published only sporadically [21].

9.2.2   Immunological Changes After Trauma and Major Extremity Surgery

Clinical and experimental research focused on the potential immunological impact of early fracture stabilization in multiply injured patients in terms of an additional trauma related to surgery. Key publications are summarized here to illustrate how the strategy of initial and complete fracture (Early Total Care, ETC) has changed in favor of a more tailored approach that comprises primary external fracture fixation and secondary definitive osteosynthesis. This concept has been named DCO, analogous to the DCS-strategy. Data from the German Trauma Registry (German Society of Trauma Surgery, DGU) demonstrate a rise in the number of early external fixations of femoral and tibial fractures performed, from 35% between 1993 and 1996 to 46% between 2002 and 2005 (Fig. 9.12) [33].

It is well known that SIRS (systemic inflammatory response syndrome) and MOF are caused by an early increase of pro- and anti-inflammatory cytokines. It has been shown that a large variety of mediators and indicators of inflammatory responses are elevated in severely injured patients [22].

The authors developed a prospective study of severely injured patients between 1985 and 1990 to evaluate the correlation of early inflammation and the rate of organ failure and organ-failure-related death. The authors could clearly demonstrate that, in addition to many other mediators of coagulation and fibrinolysis, plasma concentrations of neutrophil elastase, lactate, antithrombin III, interleukin-6, and interleukin-8 differed significantly at the time of admittance to the trauma room for patients with lethal outcome caused by MOF as compared to those patients who survived organ failure and those who had an uneventful recovery (Fig. 9.13) [23]. Corresponding results have been published by Ertel et al. [24].

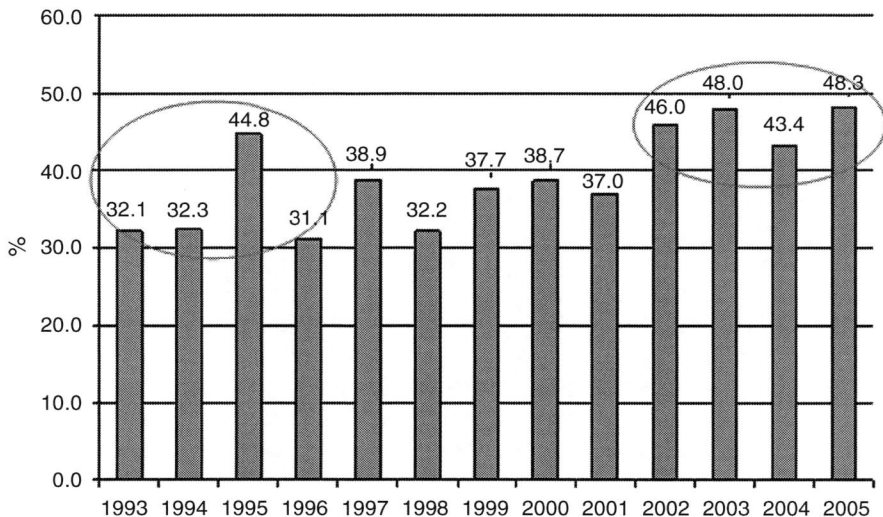

Fig. 9.12 Increasing rate of external fixation of femoral and tibial fractures, documented in the German Trauma Registry of the Polytrauma Study Group of the German Trauma Society (Data from [33])

In a comparative analysis of accidental trauma and surgery-related trauma, it could be shown that the intensity of the secondary inflammatory response after 19 femoral intramedullary nailings and eight plate-osteosyntheses of the pelvis was comparable to the intensity observed in patients with mild and moderate accidental trauma [25] (Fig. 9.14).

These results were confirmed in another analysis of patients [40] who underwent reamed femoral nailing that was not associated with multiple injury and patients who had undergone a total hip replacement. Both surgical procedures caused a mean postoperative PMN-elastase release of 300 ng/ml, which was comparable to the release found in patients with moderate multiple injuries (ISS 16–24). Interestingly, reamed nailing of the tibia as well as plate-fixation of ankle fractures did not cause any relevant inflammatory response.

The potential clinical relevance of these findings is illustrated in Fig. 9.15, which displays a multiply injured patient with an ISS (Injury Severity Score) of 26 points. The patient has a moderate inflammatory response with an IL-6 level of 390 pg/ml at the time of hospital admittance. He suffered from primary respiratory failure during the first week, but then recovered well with corresponding normalization of cytokine levels. At day 9 after trauma, femoral and tibial fractures were treated by reamed intramedullary nailing. Subsequently, the patient again suffered from respiratory failure with a similar inflammatory response as during the initial posttraumatic period.

Similar results were found in eight patients following secondary spine surgery [25]. Albeit of lesser magnitude, changes in the blood levels of inflammation indicators and mediators showed a similar pattern to those in patients after severe accidental

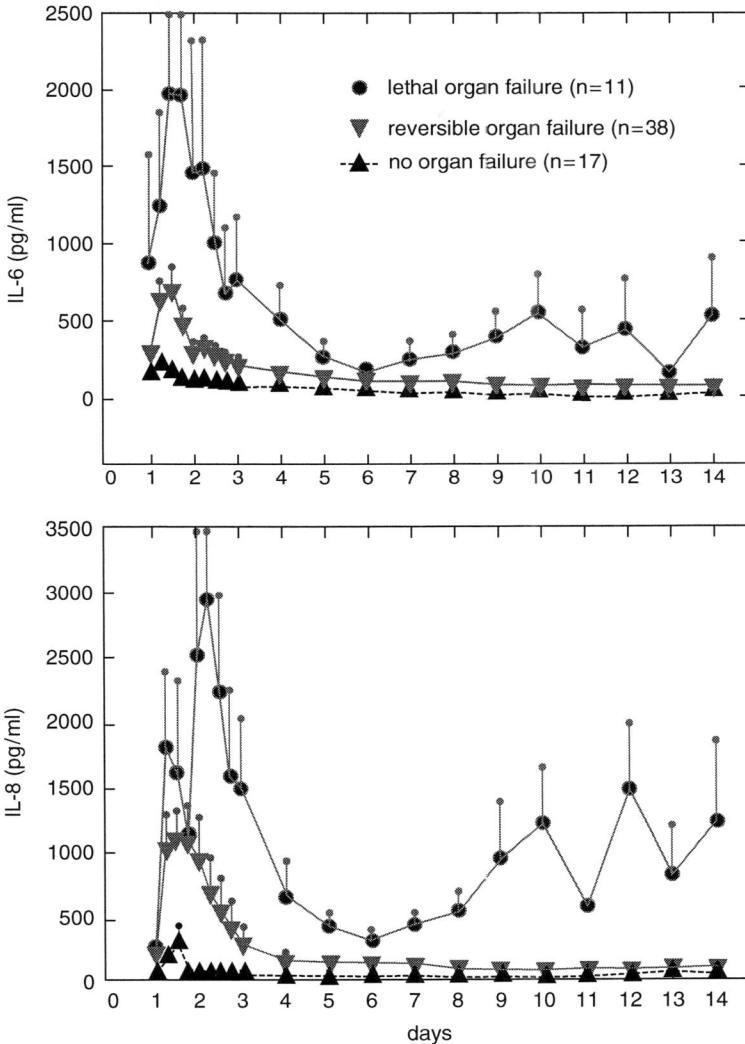

Fig. 9.13 Time course of plasma concentrates of interleukin-6 (IL-6) and interleukin-8 (IL-8) in patients with MOF-related lethal organ failure (*red dotted line*, $n = 11$), reversible organ failure (*blue triangular lines*, $n = 38$), and uneventful recovery (*green barred lines*, $n = 17$) (Modified with permission of Wolters Kluwer from [40].)

trauma. These changes impacted the clinical course in the form of significant respiratory dysfunction with an average drop in the pO_2/FiO_2 ratio from 361 to 260.

Although the benefit of immediate fracture stabilization in multiply injured patients is not disputed [2] and ETC has been proven beneficial in some patients, a group of severely injured individuals may be endangered by the additional burden,

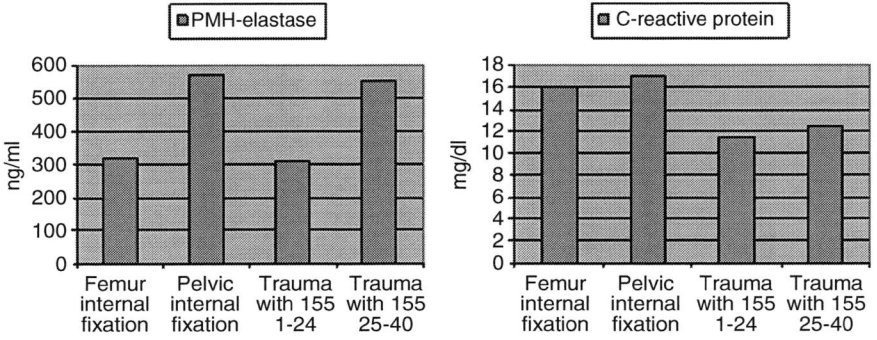

Fig. 9.14 Comparison of indicators of the posttraumatic and postoperative inflammatory response after different orthopaedic operations and varying degrees of injury severity (Data from [42].)

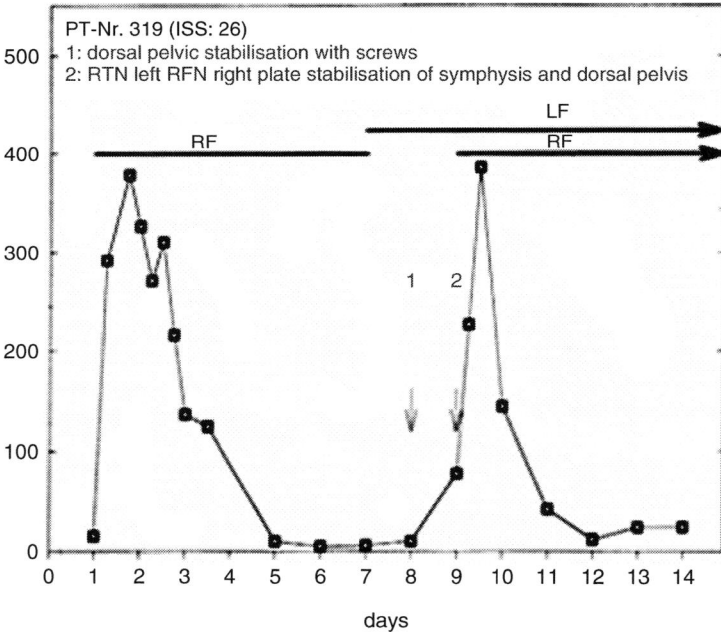

Fig. 9.15 Inflammatory response of a male patient (ISS: 26) with trauma-related primary and operative-related secondary respiratory failure

which seems to be associated with ETC procedures (blood loss, coagulopathy, acidosis, hypothermia, and tissue injury).

Pape et al. evaluated the effect of different types of fracture stabilization on the systemic release of cytokines in a prospective multicenter study [26]. Thirty five patients with multiple injuries were included. Seventeen patients (ISS 22) received early intramedullary nailing for femoral fractures, whereas the fractures in 18 patients (ISS 23) were stabilized by external fixation. Concentrations of IL-6 and IL-8 were significantly elevated in the clinical course following intramedullary nailing, but not in patients who underwent initial external fixation and secondary conversion to an intramedullary osteosynthesis. The authors concluded that these findings may become clinically relevant in patients who are at high risk for developing complications due to severe injuries.

These results were recently confirmed by Harwood et al., who reported on the alterations in the systemic inflammatory response when comparing ETC and DCO for femoral fractures [27]. In this retrospective study, the authors evaluated 174 patients with a modified ISS (New Injury Severity Score, NISS) of more than 20 points who required surgical fixation of diaphyseal fractures of the femur. Patients who did not survive at least 3 days and those who were younger than 16 years were excluded. Of the 174 patients included, DCO was performed in 97 individuals who had more severe injuries and a NISS-score of 36.2, while, for the other 77 individuals with a NISS-score of 25.4, ETC was the initial fracture treatment. Although the decision whether to stabilize the fracture by DCO- cr ETC-procedure was based on the assessment of the current trauma leader, the groups did not differ in terms of demographic or comorbidity-related patterns.

Despite the fact that patients of the DCO group had considerably more severe injuries (severe head and chest injuries), the SIRS-score was significantly higher for ETC patients during the observation period (12–72 h postoperatively). Similarly, the intensity of the postoperative inflammatory response related to the procedure of intramedullary nailing (initial in ETC, delayed in DCO) was found to be significantly higher in patients who underwent early and definitive fracture stabilization (ETC) compared to patients with DCO. On average, DCO-patients had shorter postoperative SIRS and did have less incidence of organ failure [27].

Interestingly, DCO patients who still had an elevated SIRS-score when they underwent secondary conversion suffered longer and more profoundly from SIRS and MODS. In addition to the conclusion that DCO is useful in multiply and severely injured patients, the authors recommend postponing conversion osteosynthesis until the patients' inflammatory response has subsided to maximize the benefit of DCO [27].

Another attempt to better understand the mechanisms endangering multiply injured patients requiring immediate surgical intervention for fracture fixation was conducted by Pape et al. [28]. In this study, they investigated the clinical outcome with respect to the duration of surgical procedures for fracture fixation within the first 24 h after trauma. Data were extracted from the prospective multicenter database of the German Trauma Registry. Patients were allocated to groups: those who underwent surgery for 1–3 h, those who underwent surgery for 3–6 h, and those who underwent surgery for more than 6 h. These groups showed no differences with respect to demographic data, severity, and pattern of injury (AIS (Abbreviated Injury Scale) and ISS) or the incidence and location of fractures that required surgery. There were also no detectable differences in initial prehospital treatment, or parameters of respiration, circulation, and coagulation. In addition, topography and type of surgical interventions did not differ between these groups. By multivariate analysis,

Table 9.1 Comparison of outcome of severely injured patients dependent on the total duration of the initial surgical intervention(s) (Data from [28])

Duration of surgery (h)	1–3	3–6	>6
Patients (n)	103	189	66
Injury severity score	26,3	26,9	25,4
Glasgow Coma Scale	9,8	10,3	9,4
Days of ventilation	9,5	11	15
Mortality	11%	11%	22.7%*

*$p < 0.05$

surgical interventions that lasted more than 6 h were found to have a significant and severe impact on postoperative pulmonary dysfunction and mortality (Table 9.1).

Pape et al. categorized severely injured patients who seemed to be in stable condition prior to surgery but who may subsequently have deteriorated unexpectedly as "borderline patients." He judged DCO to be the treatment of choice for initial fracture stabilization in this subgroup of patients.

All these reports led to a more critical consideration of early total care and a growing interest into the concept of DCO for patients with multiple injuries and fractures requiring immediate stabilization. Some of the most important studies evaluating time savings, complications, and effectiveness will be reviewed in next.

Scalea et al. were among the first who reported on applying DCS-patterns outside the abdomen for treatment in orthopedic trauma in terms of initial fracture stabilization [29]. In their retrospective review on 324 patients with femoral fractures, 43 patients were treated according to DCO by external fracture stabilization, whereas 281 had initial intramedullary nailing. Patients with external fixation had significantly higher injuries (ISS 26.8 vs 16.8) and required significantly more nonorthopedic major surgical interventions. External fracture fixation was used as a bridge to secondary and definite osteosynthesis to allow resuscitation and intensive care treatment at the earliest time possible. Sufficient fracture stabilization took only 35 min without causing any further surgical trauma. Conversion to secondary osteosynthesis was performed as soon as organ functions were restored. On average, conversion took place within 4 days. With such a short time period until conversion, the authors did not find an increased rate of relevant complications related to the initial external fracture fixation [29]. From the same institution, Nowotarski et al. reported an infection rate of 1.7% in 59 fractures of the femur stabilized by initial external fixation and secondary osteosynthesis within 7 days following trauma [30].

9.2.3   Results Obtained from Clinical Studies

In a survey of multiply injured individuals treated between 1981 and 2000, most of the patients treated in the first cohort between 1981 and 1992 underwent early total fracture care, whereas just 17% of 225 femoral fractures were stabilized by external fixation. In contrast, from 1993 to 2000, more than 35% of those patients had their fractures initially stabilized by external fixation followed by secondary conversion osteosynthesis. This study clearly demonstrates an increasing number of primary external fracture fixations in severely injured patients in which primary nailing could be detrimental [31]. But this study as well as most of the other retrospective studies could not satisfy the objections raised by advocates of early total care who asserted hypothetical burdens derived from external fracture fixation.

It is the data from the prospective study on DCO published by Taeger et al., executed in the authors' own trauma center, that provides sufficient information on that issue [32]. In that study, severely injured patients were differentiated for primary external fracture fixation according to formal criteria (for instance ISS > 16). The study intended to clarify whether these criteria are safe to use in terms of DCO-concept-related complications. Furthermore, prospective data are needed to assess the amount of time saved and the reduction of blood loss in terms of early resuscitation/intensive care treatment when DCO procedures are performed instead of ETC. Therefore, in the same patient, the duration of the initial external fixation (DCO) was compared to the duration of the secondary definitive osteosynthesis, which was considered to be ETC (cons-ETC). In doing so, inter-individual factors (such as ASA, fracture type, experience of surgeon, etc.), which might influence the rate of complications as well as time saved, could be ruled out. This study of 75 patients (ISS 37.7) clearly demonstrated a major reduction in operation time when using DCO, which was more than fourfold compared to ETC (Fig. 9.16). Another relevant

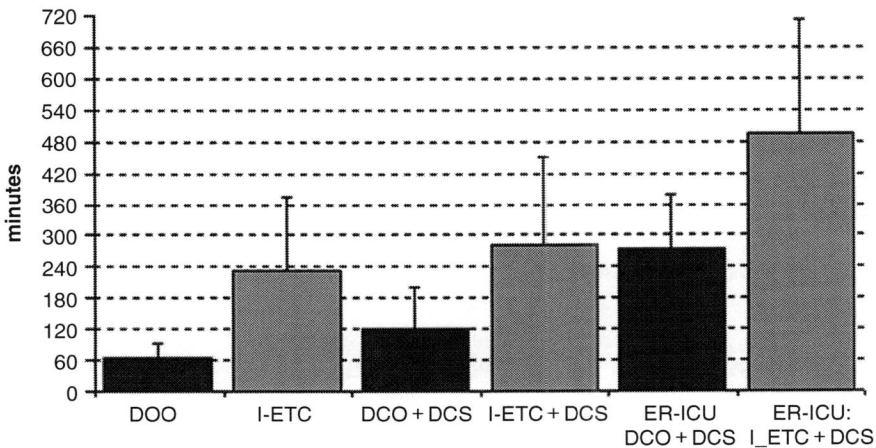

Fig. 9.16 Comparison of operation times (mean, SD) for Damage Control Orthopaedics (DCO), Damage Control Surgery (DCS) for all other locations, and for the hypothetical early total care (h-ETC) of the orthopedic lesions, which was equivalent to the actual operation time needed for definitive fracture stabilization during the delayed operation after initial DCO management. First pair of columns: DCO and h-ETC for all fractures/patient; second pair of columns: DCO and h-ETC plus all emergency operations (DCS); third pair of columns: time interval between ER-admission and ICU for DCO + DCS and h-ETC and DCS (Data from [32].)

piece of information from the figure is illustrated by the plots representing the time span between admission to the trauma room and admission to ICU. By summarizing the time required for initial trauma-management as well as all types of required surgical interventions (including DCS, etc.) and diagnostics, it could be shown that ETC would significantly delay adequate treatment in ICU. Additionally, DCO was associated with a significantly lower blood loss. DCO was not associated with an increased number of procedure-related local complications, i.e., pin-tract infections, osteitis, and pseudarthrosis. Nor did DCO and secondary single stage conversion osteosynthesis cause a measurable delay in rehabilitation or discharge of patients. Because in DCO patients, the expected mortality using the TRISS methodology was 39.3%, the actual observed mortality in this study was 20%.

Finally, the highly significant reduction of almost 20% in the expected hospital mortality of DCO-patients compared to patients with similar injury severity patterns but without required fracture stabilization indicates the potential advantages of this concept regarding reduction of systemic inflammatory response, organ dysfunction, and mortality [32]. Thus far, this prospective study does prove that in contradiction to the claims of advocates of ETC, the DCO approach does not lead to an increased rate of local complications. But this study did not intend to answer and thus does not contribute to the still unsolved question as to which severely patients require DCO instead of early total care.

Rixen et al. published a meta-analytical review and registry analysis of the treatment modalities in severely injured patients with femoral fractures [33]. Up to this point, the literature mostly consisted of a moderate level of evidence (only three with evidence-level 1b), which revealed that initial fracture fixation is advantageous; even considering subgroups, it was impossible to suggest a better approach due to insufficient data, insufficient evidence, and contradictory results. Results from the registry analysis clearly showed an increased use of the DCO approach during the last three decades. Furthermore, the analysis demonstrated the nonexistence of valid or reliable criteria for deciding whether to use DCO versus ETC.

Although some evidence has accumulated in favor of DCO over early total care, in many situations it remains unclear for which patients this is the case and for which patients early total care may be a better choice. There appears to be a less severely injured population that may benefit from ETC and for whom DCO may unnecessarily prolong treatment. On the other hand, very heavily traumatized subjects may require DCO because any other option could be life-endangering. Between these two groups there exists a subset in which the decision toward one or the other modality is less clearly defined. Patients in this group have been termed "borderline" patients [18, 28, 34, 35].

Among the major determinants for this decision are the following factors: the severity of injury, the physiologic state of the patient, and the type and duration of surgery. However, there is no available scientific data other than from retrospective observational studies or expert opinions.

A generally accepted criterium for performing ETC is an ISS below 16 points, and there is virtually no exception, unless an obviously life-endangering comorbidity or a contraindication for surgery for reasons not related to the acute trauma itself is present. It less clear where a line should be drawn above which DCO is unambiguously preferred to ETC. Many authors advise against ETC when oxygen transport is impaired or hypoxia is present [1, 15,29,30], when coagulopathy prevails [1, 15, 29, 30, 36], when the patient has severe intracranial injury or solid-organ injuries that require emergency operation (e.g., DCS) [1, 29,30,37], or when the patient is hemodynamically unstable [6, 29, 30, 36, 38] or is in extremis [38, 39].

A number of more specific conditions have been suggested that indicate a severity of condition that might deter using ETC (Table 9.2).

The heterogeneity of the DCO criteria and the gap between the agreed ETC and the proposed DCO criteria leave a considerable group of patients in an indeterminate situation. Pape and Tscherne as well as Pape and Krettek [34, 35] have suggested the term "borderline patients" for these subjects. They comprise individuals with:

- ISS > 20 and additional chest trauma
- Multiply injured patient including a pelvic or abdominal injury leading to hemorrhagic shock (initial systolic blood pressure < 90 mmHg)
- ISS > 40

Table 9.2 Recommendations from the literature when to perform ETC or DCO

ETC favored	Indeterminate?	DCO favored
ISS < 16 [32]		ISS > 40 [43]
		Severe coagulopathy, DIC [15, 29, 30, 37]
		Platelet count < 90,000–100,000/μl [9, 36, 38]
		Fibrinogen < 100 mg/dl [9]
		Prothrombin time > 25 s [9]
		Hemodynamic instability [6, 9, 29, 30]
		Severe base deficit [37], base deficit < −6 [9]
		Excess lactate [37]
		Shock with mass transfusion [38]
		Catecholamine treatment [36]
		SvO_2 < 65% [9]
		Impaired oxygenation [15, 29, 30, 37]
		pO_2/FiO_2 < 200 [37] to <300 [9]
		Hypothermia [37]
		Admission temperature ≤32°C [38]
		Emergency surgery for other injuries or prolonged surgery [29, 30, 37]
		Surgery > 6 h [38]
		Injury patterns: concomitant
		Severe chest injury (e.g., pulmonary contusion, AISthorax ≥ 3 [37, 44, 45]
		Severe traumatic brain injury (e.g., GCS < 8, increased intracranial pressure. AIShead ≥ 3) [44, 29, 30, 37]
		Severe abdominal injury (e.g., thoracoabdominal, solid organ injuries requiring emergency surgery [29, 30, 37]
		Multiple long bone fractures or severe pelvic fracture [44, 37, 38]

- Bilateral pulmonary contusion
- Mean pulmonary artery pressure > 24 mmHg

They have proposed reevaluation of these patients at the end of the resuscitation period in the emergency department. If their circulation and coagulation have been stabilized, they may proceed to undergo ETC. If not or if the stabilization is doubtful, then DCO is recommended.

However, the assessment of these borderline patients can be difficult and may depend on the expertise of the surgeon.

A more conservative strategy (toward DCO) may result in a larger proportion of patients treated with external fixation who would have tolerated or may even have benefited from ETC. On the other hand, the secondary definitive care during day time might result in increased safety of the procedure and appears not to be associated with an increased local risk [32]. A definitive recommendation based on high-quality scientific data cannot be given at the present time.

9.2.4 Timing of Definitive Stabilization Following DCO

If DCO is accepted as a safe method for initial fracture treatment in multiple trauma patients, another unresolved question in the decision-making process for those patients arises. A therapy regimen following the DCO concept with external fixateurs necessitates a secondary surgical procedure for definitive fracture stabilization. Timing these secondary operations in severely injured patients is also difficult and has not yet been specified. As mentioned earlier, the surgical trauma itself causes immune responses that are very similar to those observed after the accidental trauma. Therefore, a vulnerable phase of persisting immune deterioration has been postulated to occur after trauma. In this phase, an additional "second hit" in form of a surgical trauma should be avoided because an exaggerated pro- and/or anti-inflammatory response is expected to occur. However, an exact characterization based on clinical or immunological parameters for this "vulnerable phase" is missing. Therefore, the decision-making process in terms of the timing of secondary operations in multiple trauma patients after initial DCO therapy is mainly based on the experience of the responsible surgeon and intensive care physician. Only a few studies so far have addressed this question with a more systematic approach.

Retrospective analysis revealed a higher incidence of MOF in patients treated between days 2 and 4 after trauma (46.6%), compared to patients who underwent secondary surgery between days 5 and 8 (15.7%) [28, 38]. In the early treated group from this study, IL-6 serum levels above 500 pg/ml correlated with postoperative organ failure. An earlier study showed that the rate of postoperative organ function deterioration after surgery on days 2 and 3 after trauma correlated with pulmonary function [40]. Patients with good respiratory function as indicated by a pO_2/FiO_2-ratio of more than 280 mmHg presented with an uneventful postoperative course in 89% of cases, whereas those with a worse pulmonary function at the time of surgery (day 2 or 3) developed postoperative organ function deterioration 70% of the time.

Waydhas et al. reported a cohort of prospectively monitored severely injured patients who were primarily treated by external fixateur for fracture treatment followed by secondary definitive treatment [40]. Timing of the secondary operation was decided on the basis of pulmonary, liver, and renal organ function. The mean time point for the secondary operation was 7 days after trauma. After the secondary operation, 38% of patients developed MOF, while 62% had an uneventful course. The two groups did not differ in terms of age, sex, ISS, pattern of injury, or duration of surgery. However, analysis of organ functions and laboratory parameter at the time point of secondary surgery revealed significant differences between these two groups in terms of platelet counts, inflammatory status, and pulmonary function. Patients who did not have postoperative MOF had lower C-reactive protein (CRP) values, higher platelet counts, and better pulmonary functions preoperatively (Table 9.3). The predictive role of pulmonary function, platelet count, and the degree of the inflammatory response has been confirmed by another study [38]. This analysis also included fluid input/output ratio as another parameter of value (Table 9.3).

The findings of these two studies and some expert opinion suggest the following criteria for the timing of secondary operations in multiple trauma patients:

- $paO_2/FiO_2 > 250–280$
- CRP < 11 mg/dl
- Platelet > 100,000–150,000/μl
- Normalized or negative I/O ratio
- Intracranial pressure below 20 mmHg

Further parameters may include the absence of new or progressive infiltrates on the chest X-ray, progressive renal failure, and progressive liver dysfunction (increasing or elevated bilirubin serum levels).

The inflammatory status reflected by CRP obviously seems to be involved in the development of postoperative MOF. This fact supports the existence of a vulnerable phase of the immune system after multiple trauma. The earlier mentioned criteria

Table 9.3 Comparison of the preoperative condition before secondary operations after day 3 in two independent studies of patients who did or did not develop postoperative multiple organ failure

	From Waydas et al. [40]	From Waydas et al. [40]	From Pape et al. [38]	From Pape et al. [38]
	+MOF	−MOF	+MOF	−MOF
ISS	36,0	41,5	36,1	32,3
pO2/FiO2-ratio	305	351	210	350
Platelet count (×10³ μl)	118	236	95	140
I/O-ratio (l/24 h)			6,8	2,2
C-reactive protein (mg/dl)	12,4	7,6		
Elastase (ng/ml)	92,2	61,3		
Interleukin-6 (pg/dl)			1,620	910

Only variables with significant differences are shown

may be thought of as "safe" factors to consider in the timing of secondary surgery in multiply injured patients. However, on the basis of these criteria, definitive fracture treatment in multiply injured patients does not occur within the first 12 days after injury, as shown in two further prospective trials of primary DCOS therapy and timing of secondary surgery. In one trial, the mean time point of secondary surgery was 13.7 days [32]; in the other trial, the secondary operations were performed 17 days after trauma [41]. Although both trials did not reveal any serious infectious complications, there exists a variety of concerns with a more delayed definitive fracture treatment. Besides possible pin track infections caused by external fixators, delayed fracture treatment may also complicate surgical treatment due to factors such as organizing hematoma or beginning fracture consolidation in extra anatomical positions. However, the surgical concern against delayed fracture treatment and the assumption that organ failure, e.g., caused by ventilator-associated pneumonia, occurs irrespectively of a "second hit" due to surgical trauma, forces the implementation of strategies with earlier secondary surgery in many trauma centers. It remains to be elucidated by how much inflammatory or anti-inflammatory response can be tolerated in terms of the "second" surgical hit.

9.3   Summary and Conclusion

Patients with multiple injuries are at high risk for developing posttraumatic systemic immunoinflammatory responses with organ dysfunction, organ failure, and death. Despite formal parameters (ISS, AIS, GCS, etc.) indicating the severity of injury, there are currently no reliable parameters to exactly assess the trauma load and predict its potential effect on the immune responses or its impact on the further clinical course.

Early total care is obviously the optimal treatment strategy for orthopedic fracture treatment. But what is uncertain is the impact of the surgical trauma caused by ETC on the multiply injured individual. There is consensus that ETC should not be applied in multiply injured patients with high injury severity score and signs of hemorrhage, coagulopathy, hypothermia, acidosis with base excess, and metabolic and organ-related disorders. Also, the complexity of fracture care by intramedullary nailing must be taken into account when deciding the course of fracture treatment.

DCO has been proven to save time, prevent additional blood loss, and avoid local complications in the later course. The simplicity of external fixation might also influence the decision. It seems clear that patients with moderate injuries and stable conditions should undergo ETC.

For the large group of patients with severe injury to the brain, chest, or abdomen but in whom physiological parameters are not or only slightly affected, it is of greatest importance that neither ETC nor DCO is considered a strictly followed model. As long as the lack of evidence persists, an individual assessment must be performed on the basis of the parameters mentioned in this chapter to select the most appropriate approach for each patient.

The multicenter study that has just recently been launched in German Trauma centers [33] could provide data in the future to aid decision making in this problematic subgroup of multiply injured patients.

References

1. Behrmann S, Fabrian T, Kudsk K, Taylor J. Improved outcome with femur fractures: early vs. delayed fixation. J Trauma 1990;30: 792–797.
2. Bone LB, Johnson KD, Weigelt J, Scheinberg R. Early versus delayed stabilization of femoral fractures: a prospective randomized study. J Bone Joint Surg Am 1989;71: 336–340.
3. Broos P, Stappaerts K, Luiten E, Gruwez K. The importance of early internal fixation in multiply injured patients to prevent late death due to sepsis. Injury 1987;18: 235–237.
4. Goris RJA, Gimbrere JSF, van Niekerk JLM, Schoots FJ, Booy LHD. Early osteosynthesis and prophylactic mechanical ventilation in the multitrauma patient. J Trauma 1982;22: 895–902.
5. Johnson KD, Cadambi A, Seibert GB. Incidence of adult respiratory distress syndrome in patients with multiple musculoskeletal injuries: effect of early operative stabilization of fractures. J Trauma 1985;25: 375–383.
6. Brundage SI, McGhan R, Jurkovich GJ, Mack CD, Maier RV. Timing of femur fracture fixation: effect on outcome in patients with thoracic and head injuries. J Trauma 2002;52: 299–307.
7. Jaicks R, Cohn S, Moller B. Early fracture fixation may be deleterious after head injury. J Trauma 1997;42: 1–6.
8. Schweiberer L, Dambe LT, Klapp F. [Multiple injuries: severity and therapeutic measures]. Chirurg 1978;49(10): 608–614.
9. Trentz O, Oestern HJ, Hempelmann G, Kolbow H, Sturm J, Trentz O, Tscherne H. Criteria for the operability of patients with multiple injuries. Unfallheilkunde 1978;81: 451–458.
10. Schweiberer L, Nast-Kolb D, Duswald KH, Waydhas C, Muller K. [Polytrauma - treatment by the staged diagnostic and therapeutic plan]. Unfallchirurg 1987;90(12): 529–538.
11. Rotondo M, Zonies D. "Damage control": an approach for improved survival in exsanguinating penetrating abdominal injury. J Trauma 1993;35: 375–382.
12. Rotondo M, Zonies D. The damage control sequence and underlying logic. Surg Clin North Am 1997;77: 761–777.
13. Stone H, Strom P, Mullins R. Management of the major coagulopathy with onset during laparotomy. Ann Surg 1981;197: 532–535.
14. Nast-Kolb D, Waydhas C, Jochum M, Spannagl M, Duswald KH, Schweiberer L. [Is there a favorable time for the management of femoral shaft fractures in polytrauma?]. Chirurg 1990;61: 259–265.
15. Seibel R, Laduca J, Hasset JM, Babikian G. Blunt multiple trauma (ISS 36), femur traction, and the pulmonary failure-septic state. Ann Surg 1985; 202: 283–293.
16. Stürmer KM, Schuchardt W. [New aspects of closed intramedullary nailing and marrow cavity reaming in animal experiments. II. Intramedullary pressure in marrow cavity reaming (author's transl)]. Unfallheilkunde 1980;83(7): 346–352.
17. Wenda K, Ritter G, Degreif J, Rudigier J. [Pathogenesis of pulmonary complications following intramedullary nailing osteosyntheses]. Unfallchirurg 1988;91(9): 432–435.
18. Pape HC, Dwenger A, Regel G, Jonas M, Krumm K, Schweitzer G, Sturm JA. [Does lung contusion and general injury severity have an effect on the lung following intramedullary femoral nailing? An animal model]. Unfallchirurg 1991.94: 381–389.
19. Townsend R, Lhereau T, Protetch J, Riemer B, Simon D. Timing fracture repair in patients with severe brain injury (Glasgow Coma Scale score < 9). J Trauma 1998;44: 977–983.

20. McKee MD, Schemitsch EO, Vincent LO, Sullivan I, Yoo D. The effect of a femoral fracture on concomitant closed head injury in patients with multiple injuries. J Trauma 1997;42(6): 1041–1045.
21. Giannoudis P, Stone M, Bellamy M, Smith R. Fatal systemic inflammatory response syndrome following early bilateral femoral nailing. Intensive Care Med 1998;24: 641–642.
22. Deitsch E. Multiple organ failure: pathophysiology and potential future therapy. Ann Surg 1992; 216: 117.
23. Nast-Kolb D, Waydhas C, Gipper-Steppert C, Schneider I, Trupka A, Ruchholtz S, Zettl R, Schweiberer L, Jochum M. Indicators of the posttraumatic inflammatory response correlate with organ failure in patients with multiple injuries. J Trauma 1997;42(3): 446–455.
24. Ertel W, Keel M, Bonaccio M, Steckholzer U, Gallati H, Kenney JS, Trentz O. Release of antiinflammatory mediators after mechanical trauma correlates with severity of injury and clinical outcome. J Trauma 1995;39: 879–887.
25. Waydhas C, Nast-Kolb D, Kick M, Richter-Turtur M, Trupka A, Machleidt W, Jochum M, Schweiberer L. [Operative injury in spinal surgery in the management of polytrauma patients]. Unfallchirurg 1993;96: 62–65.
26. Pape H, Grimme K, van Griensven M, Sott A, Giannoudis P, Morley J, Roise O, Ellingsen E, Hildebrand F, Wiese B, Krettek C. Impact of intramedullary instrumentation versus damage control for femoral fractures of immunoinflammatory parameters: prospective randomized analysis by the EPOFF Study Group. J Trauma 2003;55: 7–13.
27. Harwood P, Giannoudis P, van Griensven M, Krettek C, Pape H. Alterations in the systemic inflammatory response after early total care and damage control procedures for femoral shaft fracture in severely injured patients. J Trauma 2005;58: 446–454.
28. Pape H, Stalp M, Van Griensven M, Weinberg A, Dahlweit N, Tscherne H. [Optimal timing for secondary surgery in polytrauma patients: an evaluation of 4,314 serious-injury cases]. Chirurg 1999;70: 1287–1293.
29. Scalea T, Boswell S, Scott J, Mitchell KA, Kramer ME, Pollak AN. External fixation as a bridge to intramedullary nailing for patients with multiple injuries and with femur fractures: damage control orthopedics. J Trauma 2000;48: 613–623.
30. Nowotarski P, Turen C, Brumback R, Scarboro J. Conversion of external fixation to intramedullary nailing for fractures of the shaft of the femur in multiply injured patients. J Bone Joint Surg Am 2000;82-A: 781–788.
31. Pape H-C, Hildebrand F, Pertschy S, Zelle B, Garapati R, Grimme K, Krettek C. Changes in the management of femoral shaft fractures in polytrauma patients: from early total care to damage control orthopedic surgery. J Trauma 2002;53: 452–455.
32. Taeger G, Ruchholtz S, Waydhas C, Lewan U, Schmidt B, Nast-Kolb D. Damage control orthopedics in multiple injures patients is effective, time saving and safe. J Trauma 2005;59: 409–416
33. Rixen D, Grass G, Sauerland S, Lefering R, Raum MR, Yucel N, Bouillon B, Neugebauer EAM, the Polytrauma Study Group of the German Trauma Society. Evaluation of criteria for temporary external fixation in risk-adapted damage control orthopedic surgery of femur shaft fractures in multiple trauma patients: "evidence-based medicine" versus "reality" in the trauma registry of the German Trauma Society. J Trauma 2005;59: 1375–1395.
34. Pape H, Tscherne H. Early definitive fracture fixation with polytrauma: advantages versus systemic/pulmonary consequences. In Baue AE, Faist E, Fry DE (eds). Multiple Organ Failure. New York: Springer, 2000: 279–290.
35. Pape HC, Krettek C. [Management of fractures in the severely injured – influence of the principle of "damage control orthopaedic surgery"]. Unfallchirurg 2003;106: 87–96.
36. Kutscha-Lissberg F, Hopf KF, Kollig E, Muhr G. How risky is early intramedullary nailing of femoral fractures in polytraumatized patients? Injury 2001;32: 289–293.
37. Reynolds MA, Richardson JD, Spain DA. Is the timing of fracture fixation important for the patient with multiple trauma? Ann Surg 1995;222: 470–481.
38. Pape HC, van Griensven M, Rice J, Gansslen A, Hildebrand F, Zech S, Winny M, Lichtinghagen R, Krettek C. Major secondary surgery in blunt trauma patients and perioperative

cytokine liberation: determination of the clinical relevance of biochemical markers. J Trauma 2001;50: 989–1000.

39. Riska EB, Myllynen P. Fat embolism in patients with multiple injuries. J Trauma 1982;22: 891–894.

40. Waydhas C, Nast-Kolb D, Trupka A, Zettl R, Kick M, Wiesholler J, Schweiberer L, Jochum M. Posttraumatic inflammatory response, secondary operations and late multiple organ failure. J Trauma 1996;40: 624–631.

41. Flohe S, Lendemans S, Schade FU, Kreuzfelder E, Waydhas C. Influence of surgical intervention in the immune response of severely injured patients. Intensive Care Med 2004;30: 96–102.

42. Waydhas C, Nast-Kolb D, Kick M, Trupka A, Zettl R, Wiesholler R, Schmidbauer S, Jochum M, Schweiberer L. [Postoperative homeostatic imbalance after trauma surgical interventions of various degrees in polytrauma]. Unfallchirurg 1995;98: 455–463.

43. Friedl H, Stocker R, Czermak B, Schmal H, Trentz O. Primary fixation and delayed nailing of long bone fractures in severe trauma. Tech Orthop 1996;11: 59–66.

44. Nast-Kolb D, Ruchholtz S, Waydhas C, Schmidt B, Taeger G. Damage control orthopedics. Unfallchirurg 2005;108: 804–811.

45. Sturm JA, Oestern HJ, Nerlich ML, Lobenhoffer P. Early osteosynthesis of femoral fractures in multiple trauma: danger or advantage? Langenbecks Arch Chir 1984;364: 325–327.

Chapter 10
Phase II: The ICU Phase of Damage Control: Managing the Patient from Door to Door

Bryan A. Cotton and C. William Schwab

10.1 Introduction

The Intensive Care Unit (ICU) phase has been central to the concept of delayed definitive care of trauma since it was described by Stone and colleagues and later systematically defined and named by Rotondo, Schwab, and colleagues [1, 2]. The initial operative procedures are abbreviated, and temporizing measures are employed, allowing transport to the ICU for correction of metabolic and physiologic problems. When the patient is to return to the operating room for definitive surgical procedures (Phase III) is determined by the success of this phase (Phase II) of care. In addition, careful ICU management can be the difference between prompt fascial closure and rapid liberation from the ventilator and an "unclose-able" abdomen with prolonged mechanical ventilation [3–13].

The massive fluid and blood component resuscitation utilized in the emergency room and operating theater, the dramatic visual nature of large devastating wounds, and an "open abdomen" with discontinuity of bowel can be overwhelming for even the most experienced ICU staff. Such cases require the implementation of dramatic adjustments to the ICU team's time, priorities, and focus of care on a single patient. Routine progression of care and achievement of therapeutic end-points are often impossible, and "unconventional" management is often necessary. The ICU team will require a thorough and adequate understanding of all injuries and interventions from both the anesthesia and surgical team. No other patient population requires such close collaboration, communication, and repeat evaluations by all those responsible for their care.

Given the overlapping nature of the resuscitation throughout the three phases of damage control, we have chosen to approach this chapter as a "door-to-door" process and management review. The ICU phase of Damage Control (DC) is a continuation of Phase I concepts, proceeding through the initial 24–48 h of addressing a

B.A. Cotton (✉)
Department of Surgery, Vanderbilt University School of Medicine,
1211 21st Avenue South, 404 MAB, Nashville, TN, 37212, USA
e-mail: bryan.cotton@vanderbilt.edu

H.-C. Pape et al. (eds.), *Damage Control Management in the Polytrauma Patient*,
DOI 10.1007/978-0-387-89508-6_10, © Springer Science+Business Media, LLC 2010

myriad of management issues, while simultaneously assessing whether bleeding has stopped and the patient is able to return to the operating room for Phase III. The authors begin with a brief review of the key components of a successful sign-out/hand-off, followed by a discussion of how to approach the reversal of coagulopathy, acidosis, and hypothermia, which dominate the first 6–8 h in the ICU. A systemic approach to key issues such as prolonged sedation, analgesia and pharmacological paralysis, neurologic evaluation, use of anticoagulants and antibiotics, and conducting additional out-of-ICU diagnostic studies follows. The authors address special situations such as the patient who continues to hemorrhage, the patient who does not resuscitate or correct in the first 24 h, and the patient who remains or becomes hemodynamically and physiologically unfit for OR transport. Finally, we will discuss several unique issues that arise in this phase of DC, such as intravascular shunts, transport of these patients, and futile care or when to "call it quits."

10.2   In the Door

10.2.1   The "Hand-Off"

Safe and efficient transfer of care has become increasingly difficult as work-hour restrictions have been implemented and an increasing percentage of complex patients arrive in the ICUs [14, 15]. Recent changes in medical education have disrupted the traditional practice of patient hand-off and "ownership," and the delivery of a patient to the ICU by an individual not present during the entire case is increasingly common. As such, a standardized and mandatory hand-off process that follows a "checklist" should occur at the patient's bedside upon arrival to the ICU. Members of the operative team, the surgeon and/or a senior surgical resident/fellow, and the anesthesia attending or the senior resident/anesthetist should be active participants. Critical care physician(s) along with the primary nurse and other supporting staff should receive the patient as a team.

Standardized "sign-out" procedures assure transfer and centralization of information and facilitate improved information management and overall delivery of care [16–19]. Some of the key components include age, identified injuries, allergies, medications received (including anesthetic agents, neuromuscular blockers, analgesics, vasopressors, and antibiotics), co-morbid conditions and therapies, vitals sign abnormalities and trends, initial and most recent labs, crystalloid and colloid-infused blood products transfused, estimated blood loss, and urinary output. In addition, it is critical that procedures performed, indication for DC, unaddressed injuries, and injuries still requiring further work-up are discussed. Standard bedside sign-out should also include the presence and location of arterial and venous access, and drains, shunts, and indwelling catheters (Fig. 10.1).

ICU HAND-OFF REPORT

MR Number:_____

DOB: _____ **Age:** _____ **Gender:** _____

ASA: _____ **OR:** _____ **DOS:** __/__/____

ID Band Location: _____

OR Time In: _____ **Time Out:** _____

Allergies: _____

Anesthesia Attending: _____ **Anesthesia Provider:** _____

Type of Anesthesia: _____

Surgical Procedure: _____

Presenting Diagnosis: _____

Attending Surgeon: _____ **Surgical Resident:** _____

First Assist: _____

Surgical Information and Issues: _____

Pre-opVitals: BP: __/___ **HR:** ___bpm **RR:** ___/min **SPO2:** ___% **Temp:** ___ °F

Problem List/Medical History: _____

Injuries: _____

Airway Management: _____

Anesthetic Agent: _____

Paralyzed: YES   NO   **Reversed: YES   NO**

Intra-op Vital Signs BP: _____ **HR:** _____ **SPO2:** _____ **Temp:** _____

Medications Administered (Total Dose, Units, Route, Time of Last Dose):

_____   _____   _____

_____   _____   _____

_____   _____   _____

Fluids- Input: crystalloid _____ **colloid** _____

             blood products _____

        Output: _____

Invasive Monitors/ IV Arterial Lines: _____

Intra-op Labs: _____

Events/Complications: _____

Special Precautions (spine/radiation/etc): _____

Plans: _____

_____

Fig. 10.1 Standardized ICU bedside sign-out/hand-off sheet

10.2.2   Coagulopathy

Reversing coagulopathy, acidosis, and hypothermia during hemorrhagic shock resuscitation represents the foundation of damage control principles. Of the three, coagulopathy is most affected by the presence and severity of the other two. The causes of resuscitation-related coagulopathy are complex and multifactorial, including Disseminated Intravascular Coagulation (DIC), hemodilution, hypothermia, and other metabolic derangements [20].

Prevention of or attenuating the severity of coagulopathy centers on limiting ongoing tissue injuries and hypoxia, and preemptive transfusion of clotting factors and platelets [20–22]. Dilutional coagulopathy is a potentially preventable complication of massive crystalloid administration and is treated by replacing clotting factors and platelets and minimizing crystalloid-based fluids [23]. In injured patients arriving from the operating room following massive resuscitation, disturbances in coagulation may be observed as early as 35°C [24–28]. Given this, it may be warranted to address the contributing factors of coagulopathy more aggressively in an effort to minimize their additive effects until normothermia is restored [29]. Additionally, the efficiency and overall activity of most clotting factors are substantially reduced in an acidic environment (<7.40) [20, 30–32].

An increasing body of literature has demonstrated the negative impact of various crystalloids regimens on platelet function and coagulation [33–35]. As such, their use in the early post-operative period should be approached with caution, and the implementation of more aggressive and proactive blood-product regimens should be considered. However, blood products should be given under close clinical evaluation, using patient physiology, drain output, and laboratory data to guide their administration. Currently, no randomized trials exist to suggest how much and how fast these products should be given. However, there are several retrospective studies that would suggest administering packed-red blood cells and thawed plasma in a 3:2 and possibly even in a 1:1 ratio while coagulopathy is being actively addressed [36, 37]. The patient's International Normalized Ratio (INR) should be kept below 1.7 (preferably less than 1.5), and the platelet count should be kept above 50,000 (preferably greater than 80,000). Though quite expensive, recombinant factor VIIa has been shown to reduce the incidence and severity of coagulopathy in massively injured patients with ongoing transfusion requirements [38–42].

10.2.3   Metabolic Acidosis

Metabolic acidosis is the result of tissue hypo-perfusion (shock) and the subsequent oxygen debt to tissues [43]. Acidosis decreases cardiac contractility, attenuates adrenergic receptor responsiveness to inotropic agents, and impairs perfusion of the kidneys. In addition, acidosis causes a strong impairment in coagulation as measured by both time to clot and clot strength [44]. Following damage control, patients may develop metabolic acidoses from a variety of sources, most of which are not immediately life threatening. As such, these acid-base disturbances should be evaluated systematically repeatedly and not be treated with thoughtless repeated boluses of crystalloid [7, 45].

Impairment in oxygen delivery leads to anaerobic glycolysis, which results in an increase in lactate [45]. In light of this, many authors have suggested that lactate is the end-point to be used in guiding and measuring the effectiveness of resuscitation of in the acute post-operative period. While the value of lactate as a prognostic index of mortality is impressive, the data supporting its use as a resuscitation end-point are poor and, at best, often misinterpreted. Abramson, Scalea, and colleagues noted a significant decrease in survival with longer times to clear lactate [46]. What the authors also found and what is usually overlooked is that 40% of non-survivors cleared their lactate in a timely fashion and 30% of survivors never cleared their lactate. Other authors have evaluated various lab parameters (bicarbonate, base deficit, and pH) and have demonstrated their utility in quantifying hypo-perfusion and acidosis. In fact, investigators from Los Angeles have recently shown that serum bicarbonate outperformed pH, anion gap, and lactate [47, 48]. Regardless of the marker of acidosis and perfusion, it is the trend towards "normal" and not their absolute correction that best reflects successful correction of life-threatening processes (e.g., hemorrhage) and adequate restoration of cellular perfusion.

Even in the face of adequate volume resuscitation, patients may have a persistent acidosis and elevated lactate. Given the multitude of sources of elevated lactate (acute lung injury, head trauma, soft tissue injury, activation of central nociceptive sites), this is not uncommon [45]. Restoration of pH to normal or near-normal levels allows the patient's own homeostatic mechanisms of acid-base regulation to assume their vital function again. In situations of severe acidosis, some authors have advocated the use of acid buffers such as tris-hydroxymethyl-amino-methane (THAM) and sodium bicarbonate [49–51]. THAM is a weak base providing a temporary buffer to the extracellular fluid through the acceptance of hydrogen ions. Unlike sodium bicarbonate, its effects are observed even when carbon dioxide elimination is impaired. THAM is the buffer of choice in the situation in which CO_2 elimination is impaired and when faced with evolving hypernatremia (or when attempting to avoid its development) [50, 51]. In the presence of severe acidemia (pH ≤ 7.20), THAM rapidly restores pH and acid-base regulation, resulting in reversal of acidemia-related cardiac dysfunction. Sodium bicarbonate, while also effective, generates free CO_2 and paradoxically aggravates acidemia when CO_2 elimination from tissues or lungs is hindered (e.g., heart failure, hemorrhagic shock, or pulmonary failure).

10.2.4   Hypothermia

Hypothermia leads to decreased oxygen consumption and an increase in anaerobic metabolism (and acid by-products), impaired cardiac performance, and lethal arrhythmias. Factors contributing to hypothermia include hemorrhagic shock and large volume resuscitation. Gentilello demonstrated that the presence of hypothermia increases fluid requirements and independently increases acute mortality after severe injury [52]. While 28°C is usually held as the definition of severe hypothermia (and carries a 10% mortality) in non-injured patients, similar degrees of hypothermia result in devastating consequences (with almost 100% mortality) in trauma patients [53–55]. In light of this, a separate classification is reserved for trauma patients and is defined as mild hypothermia (34–36°C), moderate hypothermia (32–34°C), and severe hypothermia (<32°C) [52, 56]. Heat is lost in the trauma patient through several mechanisms, each requiring different methods to limit their cumulative effects. Cold fluids and blood products infused into these patients can dramatically lower the core body temperature. Additionally, exposure and immobilization lead to conductive, convective, and evaporative losses.

10.2.4.1 Warming Techniques

Several passive methods exist to address heat loss and reduce progression of hypothermia. Initially, wrapping the patient with warmed blankets (including coverage of the distal extremities and entire scalp) may be adequate. Forced-air warming systems efficiently provide heat directly to the skin and allow for convective transfer of heat [57–60]. Whenever possible, warmed intravenous fluids should be used and a heated ventilator circuit employed. The inspired gas should be heated to 41°C, and the ventilator should be fully humidified to increase heat conductance to lung vascular beds [61]. The rate of rewarming through such methods ranges from 1 to 2°C per hour.

There are various forms of active core rewarming that are more efficient, but they are also invasive. Peritoneal dialysis provides heat in the form of conductance through direct action on intraperitoneal structures and indirectly through the hemidiaphragms to the heart and lungs [61]. This is usually performed through a catheter that delivers heated dialysate at 40–45°C into the peritoneal cavity. Initially, 2–3 L are infused and left for approximately 30 min. The rate of rewarming through peritoneal dialysis ranges from 2 to 3°C per hour [61]. Pleural lavage with 40–45°C fluid raises core temperature approximately 2–3°C per hour. However, both this and the peritoneal dialysis are quite labor intensive and invasive, and require large-volume flow rates.

In cases in which active rewarming using extracorporeal techniques is required, Cardiopulmonary Bypass (CPB) remains the gold standard. While CPB increases core temperature by 1–2°C every 5 min, it is labor intensive, requires surgical access, and utilizes systemic heparinization [62–65]. Alternatives to bypass are Continuous Arteriovenous Rewarming (CAVR) and Continuous Venovenous Rewarming (CVVR). These techniques use closed circuit flow of the patient's own blood through a warming device, warming the core temperature at a rate of 3–5°C per hour [63, 64]. Both techniques are less labor intensive, do not require the same level of skilled personnel, and are much easier to set up than cardiopulmonary bypass. These techniques also utilize percutaneous access without systemic heparinization.

10.2.5   Neurological Management

The importance of attaining the goals of pain control and relief of anxiety and agitation cannot be over emphasized and are crucial to successful patient management throughout the ICU stay. Pain and its related components of anxiety and agitation are frequently mismanaged and poorly addressed, and the impact of these on patient satisfaction and outcomes is under-appreciated. As such, the authors have chosen to address each component below as distinct entities (pain, anxiety, and agitation) rather than as a generic management strategy (pain control and sedation). Given the devastating nature of many of these wounds, achieving adequate pain control and anxiolysis in this patient population is a difficult task.

10.2.5.1   Analgesia

Pain stimuli cause the release of numerous cytokines, augment the sympathetic nervous system response to stress and injury, increase levels of corticotropin and anti-diuretic hormone, and activate components of the renin–angiotensin–aldosterone axis [66]. In addition, immunological dysfunction, hypercoagulable states, and electrolyte disturbances are related to the perception of pain. Combined with providing humane care through analgesia, these biological sequelae require an aggressive approach to achieve adequate pain control.

In the awake patient, the level of pain reported by the patient should be considered the standard for both the initial evaluation and response to analgesia. However, in the sedated and intubated patient, one must rely on objective clinical findings. Among these are tachypnea, tachycardia, and hypertension. Unfortunately, these physiological findings do not reliably correlate with the experience of pain. In fact, less than one-third of events are associated with abnormal vital signs in post-operative patients [67]. Evaluation of both subjective "pain-related behaviors" (such as amount of body movement, facial expressions) as well as objective measures are necessary.

Opiates form the basis for analgesia in the surgical patient and remain the mainstay of therapy (Table 10.1). Their major adverse effects include respiratory depression, hypotension, and ileus. Hypotension is more common in the patients with profound hypovolemia or in those already demonstrating cardiovascular collapse; this is seen most commonly with morphine and meperidine. Morphine has a long duration of action (with a 2–6 h half-life), allowing it to be given intermittently, with peak effects generally seen within 20 min of administration. It has several active metabolites that are potent in renal failure patients. In addition, morphine is associated with histamine release, vasodilatation, and pruritus. Fentanyl has a very rapid onset (30 s) and a short duration (half-life of 1–4 h). This agent is preferred in those patients with morphine allergies, hemodynamic instability, hypovolemia, or renal insufficiency. Fentanyl lacks the active metabolites observed with morphine, but it can demonstrate tachyphylaxis and accumulation with repeated dosing

Table 10.1 Opioids employed in the damage control patients

Opioid	Initial dosing	Half-life	Renal dosing	Hepatic dosing	Adverse events
Morphine	2–10 mg I.V.q2–6 h	3–7 h	Reduce by 25–50% if CrCL < 50	Not defined	Histamine release
Fentanyl	25–100 mcg I.V.q 1–2 h	1.5–6 h	Reduce by 25–50% if CrCL<50	Not defined	Significant accumulation in fat, tachyphylaxis, rigidity with higher doses
Hydromorphone	0.2–0.6 mg I.V.q2–3 h	2–3 h	Not defined	Not defined	Pancytopenia, agranulocytosis
Remifentanil	0.025 mcg/ kg/min continuous infusion	3–10 min	Not defined	Not defined	Muscle rigidity

Adapted with permission of The McGraw Hill Companies from Cotton BA, May AK. Sedation and analgesia. In Gracias VH, McKenney M, Reilly P, Velmahos G eds: *Acute Care Surgery*. New York: McGraw-Hill, 2008

(often extending its half-life to greater than 15 h). Fentanyl and newer related agents such as sufentanil or remifentanil should be administered as a continuous infusion during Phase II of damage control.

10.2.5.2 Sedation

While several scales exist to measure sedation (Riker Sedation–Agitation Scale and Ramsay Scale), the Richmond Agitation-Sedation Scale (RASS) is the only scale demonstrated to be a valid and reliable tool for measuring the sedation–agitation levels over the patient's hospital course [68] (Table 10.2). The RASS utilizes duration of eye contact following verbal stimulation as the primary method of assessment and means of titrating sedation. However, this is often impossible when chemical paralysis is required. For this reason, some advocate the use of sedation monitoring such as Bispectral Index (BIS) and others, but these have limited accuracy in the intubated, critically ill patient [69, 70].

Several classes of medications provide a continuous sedated state (Table 10.3) [71–74]. Benzodiazepines are the most commonly used and have a significant impact on reducing opioid requirements through attenuating the anticipatory pain response. Respiratory depression and hypotension are known side effects. Midazolam is most commonly employed as a continuous infusion (initiate at 1.0 mg/h and titrate for RASS). It has a rapid onset and shorter half-life compared to other benzodiazepines, but its active metabolites may result in prolonged sedation,

Table 10.2 Richmond-Agitation Severity Scale (RASS) for assessing sedation and agitation level

+4	Combative	Combative, violent, immediate danger to staff
+3	Very Agitated	Pulls or removes tube(s) or catheter(s); aggressive
+2	Agitated	Frequent non-purposeful movement, fights ventilator
+1	Restless	Anxious, apprehensive, but movements are not aggressive or vigorous
0	Alert and Calm	
−1	Drowsy	Not fully alert, but has sustained awakening to voice (eye opening and contact >10 s)
−2	Light Sedation	Briefly awakens to voice (eye opening and contact <10 s)
−3	Moderate Sedation	Movement or eye opening to voice (but no eye contact)
−4	Deep Sedation	No response to voice, but movement or eye opening to physical stimulation
−5	Unarousable	No response to voice or physical stimulation

Adapted with permission of The McGraw-Hill Companies, Inc., from Cotton BA, May AK. Sedation and analgesia. In Gracias VH, McKenney M, Reilly P, Velmahos G eds: *Acute Care Surgery*. New York: McGraw-Hill, 2008

Table 10.3 Sedative agents for continuous administration.

	Initial dosing	Half-life	Renal dosing	Hepatic dosing	Adverse events/ comments
Lorazepam	0.5–1.0 mg I.V.q4–8 h	6–8 h	Avoid with renal failure	Avoid with hepatic failure	No active metabolites
Midazolam	1.0 mg/h I.V., titrate for desired RASS	2–3 h	Decrease dose by 50% with CrCL <10	Use with caution in hepatic failure	Hypotension, significant respiratory depression
Dexmedeto-midine	0.2 mcg/kg/h I.V., titrate for desired RASS	1.5–2 h	Decrease dose with CrCL <50	Decrease dose with any Child-Pugh class	May load with 1.0 mcg/kg I.V., but beware hypotension, bradycardia; do not exceed 24 h infusion
Propofol	5 mcg/kg/min, titrate by 5–10 mcg/kg/min for desired RASS	3–12 h	None	None	"Infusion syndrome" seen with doses >80 mcg/kg/min; hypotension, apnea; fatty tissue distribution may prolong effect

Adapted with permission of The McGraw Hill Companies, Inc., from Cotton BA, May AK. Sedation and analgesia. In Gracias VH, McKenney M, Reilly P, Velmahos G eds: *Acute Care Surgery*. New York: McGraw-Hill, 2008 especially in those with renal insufficiency. In these situations, low-doses (0.5–1.0 mg/h) of lorazepam can be used for continuous infusions. Propofol is an intravenous anesthetic agent that achieves sedation at lower doses with a rapid onset and short duration of action. Following careful bolus administration (5–10 mcg/kg, repeat at 5 min intervals), propofol is generally administered as a continuous infusion (0.02–0.75 mg/kg/min). Propofol provides similar depth and quality of sedation to midazolam, but it is associated with quicker extubation and recovery times [71, 72].Adverse events are primarily related to duration of therapy (hypertriglyceridemia, pancreatitis, hypotension, and lactic acidosis); therefore, propofol use should be limited to 48 h or less. Other sedatives include selective alpha-2 adrenergic receptor agonists, such as dexmedetomidine, which appear to maintain adequate sedation with less risk for producing hemodynamic instability. Initial dosing at 0.2 mcg/kg/h intravenously can be employed with titration to 0.7 mcg/kg/h as needed. Compared to propofol, dexmedetomidine has the added benefit of analgesia (with less opiate requirements) [73, 74]. Adverse effects with its use include hypotension, hypertension, and severe bradycardia.

Regardless of the agent chosen, a continuous infusion is preferred in the damage control population. The specific agent chosen depends on the physician comfort level and the patient's renal and liver status. The goal RASS in this population (especially with an open abdomen or chest) should be −4 to −5. In patients with an open abdomen, a deep RASS level should be achieved prior to administration of paralytics. As with other critically ill patients, daily interruption of sedation and paralysis should be performed to allow for at least a brief neurological examination.

10.2.5.3 Paralysis

The use of Neuromuscular Blockading Agents (NMBA) in the initial management of the open abdomen remains controversial, with little evidence to support or refute their use. Opponents state the concerns of sustained use of any paralytic: generalized deconditioning, skin breakdown, and prolonged muscle weakness. Proponents argue that paralysis for the further initial management of the open abdomen prevents abdominal wall contraction and "loss of domain" of the abdominal cavity.

Use of NMBA in managing the open abdomen was first advocated in 1981 by Duff and Moffat. The authors noted that in the absence of significant adhesions or a generous and intact greater omentum, NMBA were necessary to prevent bowel evisceration until closure or until adhesions become "strong enough to prevent evisceration." [75] Several authors have suggested that administration of NMBA improves abdominal wall compliance, reverses the shift of the abdominal pressure–volume curve, and thus decreases "intraabdominal" pressure for any given intra-abdominal volume [66, 76–78]. In addition, an increasing body of literature has noted a significant decrease in intra-abdominal pressures when NMBA are administered [76, 77]. Given the repercussions of sustained intra-abdominal hypertension (atelectasis, gut ischemia, impaired renal perfusion) and the benefits of reducing the intra-abdominal pressure, a 24–48 h course of NMBA appears to outweigh the risks.

If patients receive NMBA, they should be assessed both clinically and by "train-of-four" twitch monitoring, with a goal of titrating to achieve one or two twitches [66]. Before initiating NMBA, adequate analgesia and sedation (measured by RASS −4 to −5 if possible) should be achieved. Several options exist for NMBA use in this setting. Vecuronium is an intermediate-acting NMBA that produces blockade within 90 s and typically lasts 30 min. Following bolus administration (0.1 mg/kg), an infusion should be given (0.8–1.2 g/kg/min). Vecuronium is renally excreted, and other agents should be considered in patients with renal insufficiency. Cisatracurium is an intermediate-acting NMBA that is metabolized by ester hydrolysis and Hofmann elimination, so the duration of blockade should not be affected by renal or hepatic dysfunction. In addition, it produces few, if any, cardiovascular effects. Bolus doses of 0.1–0.2 mg/kg result in paralysis in approximately 2–3 min and last approximately 20–30 min. Maintenance infusions of cisatracurium are initiated at 2.5–3.0 g/kg/min and titrated accordingly.

10.2.6 Pulmonary Management

Patients undergoing damage control often present to the ICU with evidence of Acute Lung Injury (ALI) or Acute Respiratory Distress Syndrome (ARDS) from aggressive resuscitation techniques. Shock, massive resuscitation, and multiple transfusions place the remaining patients at a high risk of developing ALI and ARDS during their ICU stay [79–82]. ALI and ARDS after trauma have two distinct patterns. The first is an early phenomenon attributable to the initial insult and consequences of crystalloid resuscitation. The second, or late form of ARDS, is more commonly related to multiple organ dysfunction and sepsis [81]. Historically, the mortality associated with ARDS in trauma approached 70%. However, two recent studies in trauma patients have demonstrated that ARDS-associated mortality is decreasing with the implementation of more conservative crystalloid resuscitation, lower mean tidal volumes (V_t), and lower mean peak inspiratory pressures [81, 82].

Many damage control patients will have varying degrees of Intra-Abdominal Hypertension (IAH). Abdominal packing and elevation of the hemidiaphragms lead to decrease in chest wall compliance [79]. Large volume resuscitation worsens compliance by increasing pulmonary edema and "stiffness" of the chest wall secondary to soft tissue and muscle edema [79, 80]. Addressing these issues directly, through minimizing further fluid, administration, delivery of higher levels of positive end expiratory pressure, and aggressive and early abdominal decompression will lessen difficulties with oxygenation and ventilation.

10.2.6.1 Ventilator Strategies

The choice of ventilator mode is likely to be site-specific and more dependent on the comfort level of the ICU physician. For this reason, the exact mode chosen is less important when the principles of low V_t, permissive hypoxia–hypercarbia, and recruitment are employed [43, 79, 80]. Airway Pressure Release Ventilation (APRV), also known as Bilevel or Bi-vent, allows spontaneous breathing superimposed on top of a set rate of breaths delivered at high pressure and very high I/E ratio [79, 83, 84]. This mode offers excellent alveolar recruitment (and minimizes de-recruitment) and promotes positive effects on gas exchange. When pressure control or pressure-regulated volume control is utilized, the ventilator is initially set for a V_t goal of 5–8 mL/kg with Positive End-Expiratory Pressures (PEEP) levels initiated at 8–10 and titrated for oxygenation. With these modes, one should aim to maintain Peak Inspiratory Pressure (PIP) of less than 40 cm H_2O and plateau pressure of less than 30 cm H_2O [43].

10.2.6.2 Ventilation

The ARDS-Net and other studies have shown that smaller tidal volumes improve outcomes from ALI [85–88]. These studies suggest that the ventilator should be set to deliver V_t in the range of 5–7 mL/ideal body weight in kilograms. The physiology behind this concept is that ALI can be caused and or worsened by alveolar overdistension. Even among those presenting to the ICU without evidence of ALI/ARDS, V_t should be kept strictly within the 5–7 mL/kg range. In fact, among patients presenting without ALI, the probability of later developing this or ARDS increases with the size of V_t [85–90]. With these lower V_t, achieving adequate ventilation may require higher respiratory rates to keep the $PaCO_2$ constant. However, increasing the respiratory rates beyond 25 breaths per minute is not likely to improve CO_2 elimination, but this can lead to over-distention of alveoli and barotrauma [79]. It may be necessary to tolerate above normal $PaCO_2$ levels in the absence of contraindications to hypercapnia (elevated intra-cranial pressure, etc.) in order to obtain these lower V_t to minimize ALI.

10.2.6.3 Oxygenation

Providing adequate oxygenation and achieving set PaO_2 goals is accomplished through the delivery and adjustment of PEEP, fractional inspired oxygen (FiO_2), and the inspiratory:expiratory time ($I:E$). FiO_2 is initially set at 100% and weaned to keep the oxygenation saturation (SaO_2) greater than 92% [43]. PEEP is necessary to maintain alveolar recruitment and reduce shunting of venous blood through non-ventilated alveolar segments. When not fully recruited, alveolar "instability" may occur, leading to lung injury through mechanical stress and inflammatory activation [79, 91]. The authors prefer to initiate PEEP at 5–8 cm H_2O and titrate in increments of 2–3 cm H_2O to reduce FiO_2 to 60% or less. As PEEP levels increase and approach 20 cm H_2O, hemodynamic changes are likely. Hypotension due to impedance of venous return and a reduction in preload is common [43].

If oxygenation remains a problem after maximizing PEEP and assuming no mechanical problems [PTX (Tension Pneumothorax), IAH, ACS, etc.], the I:E ratio should be reduced (or even reversed) to improve oxygenation. The resulting permissive hypercapnia should be tolerated as long as the patient's arterial pH remains greater than 7.2. Once the I:E ratio is reversed, NMBA and deep sedation (RASS −4 or −5) should be employed if not already in place. If such efforts are unsuccessful, recruitment maneuvers are performed by adding "sigh" breaths (periodic high volume breaths at a rate of 1–3 per minute). An alternative recruitment strategy utilizes high levels of PEEP (35–40 cm H_2O) maintained for an interval of 25–30 s [79, 92]. If the patient responds to the recruitment strategy, a change to APRV should be considered. If this fails, however, and the I:E has been reversed to 3:1–4:1, a change in ventilators (oscillating, high-frequency) should be considered.

10.2.7 Cardiovascular Management

10.2.7.1 Hemodynamic Support

Patients undergoing DC procedures frequently present with severe shock and hypovolemia. During and after the early resuscitation phase, a vasodilatory state and a subsequent generalized inflammatory phase (Systemic Inflammatory Response Syndrome or SIRS) ensues. This state correlates with end-organ hypoperfusion, hypoxia, and diffuse cytokine activation [79]. While support has traditionally focused on large volume fluid resuscitation, increasing evidence demonstrates that overzealous crystalloid use may result in systemic deterioration and further injury to the pulmonary, gastrointestinal, and renal systems as well as increased risk of abdominal compartment syndrome. The current approach has evolved towards less infusion of crystalloid, more blood and components administration, and earlier vasopressor use. Support of the cardiovascular system is guided by restoration and maintenance of end-organ perfusion. Thus, early and accurate monitoring of hemodynamics and an understanding of the end-points of resuscitation are essential.

10.2.7.2 Monitoring of Cardiovascular Status and Resuscitation End-Points

Historically, resuscitation of the severely injured patient was guided by adequate urinary output, "normalization" of vital signs, and clearance of lactic acidosis. Typically, lactate (and base deficit) measurements are drawn on the patient's arrival, and these measurements are continued every 4 h until measurements are less than or equal to two (or base deficit is <5) [43]. Should the lactate fail to clear or if it rises, further fluid resuscitation is usually instituted as one reassesses for a missed or unaddressed injury, ongoing hemorrhage, or evolving ACS.

If lactate or base deficit continues to increase or fails to correct, the patient's resuscitation should be guided by the use of an oximetric or volumetric Pulmonary Artery (PA) catheter [43, 79, 93]. This method will allow guidance of volume status and oxygen delivery without unnecessary fluid resuscitation. Resuscitation efforts are then guided by volumetric catheters using SvO_2 measurements (>65%) or Right Ventricular End-Diastolic Volume Index (RVEDVI). RVEDVI has been shown to have superior correlation with left ventricular end-diastolic volume compared with PA capillary pressures [94]. When RVEDVI is <100 mL/m^2 and there is evidence of hypoperfusion, volume expansion should proceed to raise the RVEDVI into the 100–120 mL/m^2 range. If the RVEDVI is 100–120 mL/m^2, maintenance of volume status should be the goal in the absence of tissue hypoperfusion. If the RVEDVI is >100 mL/m^2 and there is evidence of hypoperfusion, transfusing red blood cells to hemoglobin of 10 g/dL and or adding vasopressor support should be considered.

If one is using a standard PA catheter, Central Venous Pressure (CVP) should be maintained between 8 and 10 mmHg, and the PA pressure should be maintained between 12 and 15 mmHg. However, the reliability of such measures for actual volume status is often disputed. Additionally, mounting concerns about the use of PA catheterization have led to renewed interest in the use of less invasive techniques for monitoring cardiac indices. The PiCCO catheter (Pulsion Medical, Munich, Germany) provides continuous cardiac output via arterial pulse contour analysis [43]. Similarly, the Lithium Dilution Cardiac Output monitor (LiDCO, LiDCO Ltd, London, UK) uses the injection of a small amount of lithium chloride into the venous circulation. These measurements of cardiac output appear to correlate well with other more invasive techniques. Trans-esophageal Echocardiography (TEE) seems to provide more accurate information on ventricular size and provides end diastolic volume, which is a better predictor of myocardial performance than PA pressures in patients with major abdominal injuries requiring elevated ventilatory pressures [79]. Finally, Friese and colleagues demonstrated that serum B-type Natriuretic Peptide (BNP) levels increase with resuscitation after injury, and levels are higher in patients who develop pulmonary edema [95]. While traditionally validated among patients with congestive heart failure, this non-simple laboratory test may provide a useful marker of excessive volume resuscitation after injury. In fact, the authors have used this serum marker, with anecdotal success, as a "cut-point" for transitioning from crystalloid based strategies to colloid and vasopressors support.

10.2.7.3 Vasopressor Support

To reach the end-points needed to "clear" lactate and base deficit, inotropic support is often required. These agents should be initiated cautiously in an attempt to address the vasodilatory state that accompanies the response to injury. Given the susceptibility of the splanchnic circulation to ischemic injury, vasoactive agents that act primarily on the blood supply to the periphery are preferred [79, 96]. The authors prefer norepinephrine, a potent alpha and beta-1 agonist in the setting of patients without significant tachycardia. In the face of profound tachycardia, the authors prefer to utilize phenylephrine as a selective alpha agonist. Dopamine is highly non-selective, and epinephrine is a more potent beta-2 agonist, thus leading to unnecessary vasodilatation [96]. Most recently, vasopressin (0.01–0.04 U/min) has been identified as a potential answer to vasodilatory states and distributive shock after injury and exaggerated inflammatory response [7, 96]. Despite achievement of adequate filling pressures and volume status, patients may demonstrate a persistent hypoperfusion related to poor cardiac output. In these instances, dobutamine or milrinone may be employed. The authors generally titrate these agents to a urine output > 30 mL/h or cardiac index > 2.5.

   In summary, support of the cardiovascular system in DC patients is crucial, and practices are quite varied. During the early phase in the ICU, monitoring trends of data and assuring physiologic improvement are important. In addition, one should have a lower threshold for: (1) starting vasopressors; (2) stopping aggressive crystalloid administration; (3) initiating blood components and colloids.

10.2.8   Gastrointestinal Management

10.2.8.1   Stress-Ulcer Prophylaxis

Given their coagulopathic states, requirement for mechanical ventilation, and severe injury, the damage control population is the "very-high risk" group for stress ulcer [97–101]. As such, these patients should receive some form of stress ulcer prophylaxis during all phases and until the "very-high risk" criteria (mechanical ventilation, coagulopathy) have resolved and normal diet has resumed. The evidence evaluating the effect of histamine H2-receptor antagonists, cytoprotective agents (sucralfate), and proton-pump inhibitors on the rate of gastrointestinal bleeding and mortality is conflicting. A gastric pH of 5.5 has been used as an end-point for successful acid suppression therapy in patients at risk for progression of stress-related mucosal damage to stress ulcers with bleeding [97–99]. Proton-pump inhibitors such as omeprazole are superior to the other agents in maintaining gastric pH of >5.5 in mechanically ventilated patients [97–99].

10.2.8.2   Feeding

Early administration of enteral nutrition with trauma patients has been clearly shown to improve outcomes related to infectious complications [102–106]. However, patients requiring an open abdomen because of damage control maneuvers may not tolerate enteral nutrition. Generalized gastrointestinal dysfunction can induce an ileus pattern, and the edematous bowel associated with an open abdomen may become more dilated with the introduction of enteral nutrition, thereby making closure of the fascia more difficult. Many clinicians still withhold enteral feedings for fear of small bowel necrosis. However, this phenomenon is quite rare, less than 1%, and even more rare in the early phases of enteral feed administration [107, 108].

Once bowel continuity is restored, withholding enteral nutrition in those patients with an open abdomen appears to be based on fear and is not supported in the literature. Although specific studies supporting this practice are lacking, several concepts can be supported when enteral feeds are provided in this extreme critically ill population. Enteral feedings attenuate the inflammatory response and may even diminish pressor requirements during the shock state by increasing intestinal blood flow [109]. At least in theory, more venous drainage from the abdominal contents provides an environment of less swelling and smaller structures, thereby allowing for safe fascial closure. Typically, the swollen abdominal contents do not allow us to close the fascial primarily in the days following the initial insult. Provision of 30–50% of goal appears to be adequate to maintain the mucosal barrier, prevent bacteria translocation, and subsequent secondary hit of sepsis [110]. More recently, critically ill patients have demonstrated less infectious outcomes and fewer mechanical ventilator days if patients are initiated with lower nutritional provision, termed permissive underfeeding [111–113].

In an attempt to answer the question about the use of early enteral feeds and the open abdomen, investigators at Vanderbilt evaluated 78 patients with an open abdomen for at least four hospital days [114]. The authors noted that the initiation of enteral nutrition within 4 days was associated with better outcomes. Specifically, patients who received early enteral nutrition were more likely to achieve fascial closure by hospital day 8, less likely to experience fistulas formation, and had less overall hospital charges. Cheatham and colleagues noted that open abdomen enteral feedings are not only plausible but perhaps beneficial [115]. Feeds should be discontinued if concern arises about bowel motility and absorption, or if physiologic indicators of a low flow state are present.

10.2.8.3 Enteral Access

Patients undergoing damage control laparotomy are commonly at risk for malnutrition, often undergo numerous operative suites "visits" with recurrent NPO (Latin: nothing by mouth) orders, and (not uncommonly) have bowel wall edema and anastomoses. As such, early consideration and placement of enteral access (and initiation of early enteral feeding) has been advocated to reduce postoperative morbidity and further nutritional decline [114]. Enteral access is usually obtained via feeding jejunostomy (or gastrojejunostomy) or nasoduodenal (nasojejunal) feeding tubes. In terms of efficacy and complications, nasojejunal access may be preferred as it does not require violation of an intact viscus nor have the added concern of an enteric leak. When a nasojejunal or nasoduodenal tube is chosen, the authors prefer to secure the tube with a vomer sling to reduce the risk of tube dislodgement.

In the presence of a concomitant head injury or when the stomach is already injured, we often utilize a gastrojejunal feeding tube. This is secured to the abdominal wall in a Stamm fashion followed by a gastropexy. The combination gastrojejunal tube offers gastric drainage in addition to post-pyloric feeding access. As with ostomy placement, gastric or jejunal tubes should be brought out lateral to the rectus muscles in order to limit fascial injury. Fascial violation will complicate future mobilization during potential component separation techniques.

10.2.8.4   Bowel Discontinuity

Given the principles of damage control, the stomach, small bowel, and colon are often left in discontinuity, with plans for creation of an anastomosis or ostomy with the next planned surgery (Phase III). In the presence of such discontinuity, no feeding (even at a "trophic" rate) or oral medications should be utilized. Exceptions to this would include those medications that are dissolving tablets absorbed through the submucosal system (such as newer anti-psychotics and anti-depressants) or those with definite absorption in the stomach. Medications that are not available intravenously and are seen as necessary during this phase of patient care may be administered rectally if available (e.g., aspirin, acetaminophen, etc.).

10.2.9   Fluid and Electrolyte Management

10.2.9.1   Fluid Choices

Several options exist for fluid resuscitation, and the choice usually lies not in the evidence but in the familiarity. Lactated Ringers solution is, by "normal" chemistry profiles, quite physiologic in its electrolyte content as well as its pH and osmolality. Normal saline (0.9% NaCl), however, is hyperchloremic and acidotic (pH 5.5). Several forms of hypertonic saline exist (3% NaCl, 7.5% NaCl, 23%, NaCl), and these are often administered in combination with dextran. These solutions not only allow less volume to be given during ongoing resuscitation and hemorrhagic shock, but they also appear to actually mobilize fluids from the tissues. Specifically, brain tissue and visceral fluid is mobilized, and edema in these areas is reduced with the administration of hypertonic saline solutions [7, 116]. Based on this data, some have used the 3% solution as maintenance fluid (30 mL/h) in lieu of standard crystalloid solutions. This may result in more rapid resolution of visceral edema (less than 48 h), allowing for early fascial closure.

When one considers the consequences associated with large volume crystalloid resuscitation, it is not surprising to see why many centers are adopting alternative strategies and solutions to resuscitate the patient during damage control. Small volume resuscitation with hypertonic saline has shown favorable results in both hemorrhagic shock and traumatic brain injury patients. Vassar and colleagues were able to demonstrate a survival advantage with hypertonic saline when compared to standard crystalloid regimen [117]. Other solutions have also been shown to be of benefit in the early hospital resuscitation phase, the most widely studied being the 7.5% NaCl/6% dextran. In addition to reducing tissue and pulmonary edema, these solutions appear to be associated with much longer lasting hemodynamic effects, including restoration of blood pressure and tissue perfusion [7, 116, 118].

10.2.9.2 Volume of Administration

Given the close association with aggressive volume resuscitation and the inability to primarily close abdominal fascia, the authors would encourage moderation in the volume of crystalloid administered to these patients. While determining and defining euvolemia is controversial, the physician should chose one of the various endpoints available (discussed earlier) and use this as a "dipstick" of volume status. Avoiding the reflexive volume boluses when the physiology is confusing or when there is worrisome vital sign reading will help to avoid using the large volumes of crystalloid that are associated with ACS and other systemic complications [119]. Initiating the patient's fluids at a lower rate and then using small boluses to address physiological evidence of poor tissue perfusion and/or hypovolemia are likely to achieve the same end-points without the consequences of the "standard" trauma resuscitation.

10.2.9.3 Electrolytes

Massive fluid resuscitation, large blood loss, generalized physiological impairment, and severe fluid shifts are all too common to this patient population. As such, significant electrolyte abnormalities should be assumed and aggressively corrected. Calcium replacement should be fairly aggressive, especially in those who have received multiple transfusions. Replacement should be initiated intravenously, and two formulations are available: calcium chloride ($CaCl_2$) 1–2 g if central access is present or calcium gluconate 2–4 g if no central access available. Magnesium replacement should also be pursued with some level of aggressiveness. The authors generally provide 2 g of magnesium sulfate over 30 min and repeat until the magnesium level is greater than 2.0 mg/dL. Similarly, phosphate is replaced in bags of 20–40 mmol until the level is greater than 2.0 mg/dL. A serum K+ of 3–4 mEq/L correlates with a 100–200 mEq K+ deficit, while a serum K+ of 2–3 mEq/L is consistent with a deficit of 200–400 mEq. Serum potassium is continuously replaced intravenously as well and may be expected to increase by ~0.25 mEq/L for each 20 mEq potassium chloride infused. The authors attempt to maintain a serum potassium level between 3.5 and 4.0 mEq/L. However, all of the above electrolytes should be replaced much more conservatively in those patients with renal failure, and caution should be used in these patients when the serum creatinine is greater than 2.0 mg/dL.

10.2.10   Renal Management

The primary objectives in maintaining the renal system are preventing volume overload, maintaining electrolytes within normal range, and avoiding oliguria. Achieving this balance may be difficult in this patient population, given historical tendencies to aggressively resuscitate patients, insensible volume losses from the open abdomen, and the not uncommon dogma that urine output is not indicative of resuscitation status.

Acute renal failure is usually defined by the presence of oliguria (urine volume output less than 400 mL/day) or anuria (200 mL/day) with a serum creatinine greater than 2.5 g/dL. Appropriate urine output is 0.5 mL/kg/h or greater (ideal body weight). Oliguria should be assumed the result of abnormal renal function and inadequate perfusion until proven otherwise. The evaluation of this renal insufficiency/failure should begin with clinical assessment of the patient. The first measure in this assessment should be the flushing of the urinary bladder catheter to assess for potential obstruction from blood clots, casts, or other plugs. Adjuncts to this include ultrasound evaluation to evaluate the bladder volume. Next, a clinical assessment and simultaneous invasive monitoring assessment of volume should be undertaken to develop a clinical gestalt of patient status (hypovolemia, euvolemia, hypervolemia).

Additional measures of etiology include the Renal Failure Index (RFI), Fractional Excretion of Sodium (Na), and Urine Na. The Renal Failure Index is calculated by the following: (urine Na)(serum Cr)/(urine Cr). A patient is considered pre-renal when the RFI is <1 and renal when the RFI is >1. Fractional Excretion of Na (FE_{Na}) is determined by the following: (urine Na)(serum Cr)/(serum Na)(urine Cr) × 100. FE_{Na} values less than 1 are considered pre-renal, whereas values greater than 1 are attributed to renal etiology. Single value checks of Urine Na are suggestive of pre-renal status when less than 10 and renal status when greater than 20. Pre-renal sources include hypovolemia, severe cardiac dysfunction, vasogenic shock with poor renal perfusion, and intra-abdominal hypertension/abdominal compartment syndrome. The primary renal source of acute renal failure is Acute Tubular Necrosis (ATN). ATN has a variety of causes including circulatory collapse with hypoperfusion and nephrotoxin exposure (aminoglycosides, IV contrast dye, and rhabdomyolysis/myoglobinuria).

Irrespective of the cause, the basic principles in management of acute renal failure are the maintenance of euvolemia and the avoidance of nephrotoxic agents. Avoiding dogmatic end-points of lactate and catheter-directed therapy and following clinical volume status while monitoring renal function may help in this struggle. Laboratory panels and central venous pressure measurements should be employed as adjuncts to guide treatment decisions. With regard to nephrotoxic agents: If alternative medications are available or the agent is not crucial to patient care, these medications should be avoided or discontinued. If intravenous contrast dye is necessary for diagnostic studies, $NaHCO_3$ should be initiated as soon as possible in the pre-study period and continued through the procedure until infusion is complete [120].

This process involves the administration of a liter of D_5W with three amps of $NaHCO_3$ at 3 mL/kg/h as a bolus, followed by infusion of the remainder of the liter bag at 1 mL/kg/h until complete. If this is not available, 1–2 L of crystalloid should be utilized to provide adequate hydration.

The indication for renal consultation in DC patients is the need for hemodialysis. Patients who develop acute renal failure require hemodialysis when one of the following indications is met: volume overload, hyperkalemia, or refractory acidosis. Until hemodialysis is available, the above issues may be temporized with a few simple interventions. $CaCl_2$ may be given (1–2 g I.V. infusion) to stabilize cardiac rhythm, as severe hyperkalemia can precipitate lethal arrhythmias. $NaHCO_3$ (1–2 amps), a β-2 agonist inhaler treatment, or 10 U of regular insulin (I.V.) with one simultaneous ampule of D_{50} may be used to temporarily lower the potassium level to safer values. To address the hyperkalemia directly (remove potassium from the body rather than re-distribute it as with the described methods), one will need to remove it via the kidneys (high-dose loop diuretic), the gastrointestinal tract (Kayexalate enema/PO solution), or the blood (hemodialysis).

10.2.11   Endocrine Management

The initial metabolic response to acute injury aims to mobilize substrates for vital organ systems and minimize catabolism. A hypermetabolic phase follows with catecholamine release, hypercortisolism, growth hormone and glucagon release, and inactivation of peripheral thyroid hormones [121]. Blunted growth hormone pulsatility and an acute decrease of dehydroepiandrosterone sulfate have been observed. Decreased levels of T3, T4, and TSH levels are seen as part of the sick euthyroid syndrome. Replacement of these individual hormones has not proven to be of benefit.

While the initial data to support aggressive replacement of relative insulin and adrenal insufficiencies were quite specific (post-cardiac bypass and septic shock patients, respectively), their use has been rather broad and without substantiation [122, 123]. In severely injured patients, evidence regarding insulin replacement for strict euglycemia has been conflicting [124–126]. While few would argue the benefits of maintaining glucose levels below 200 mg/dL, whether trauma patients should be kept between 80 and 115 mg/dL has yet to be determined. Therefore, the authors would recommend, based on currently available data, that blood glucose levels be maintained below 150 mg/dL using a continuous insulin infusion [124, 125].

During the acute phase following injury, increased serum cortisol levels have been demonstrated, along with increased concentrations of ACTH. However, relative adrenal insufficiency, in the form of low baseline cortisol (<9 mcg) or failure to "stimulate" (<9 increase from baseline), may be present following trauma and critical illness. Annane and colleagues demonstrated that a brief course of glucocorticoid and mineralocorticoid replacement improves survival in septic shock patients [122].

Risk factors for the development of a relative adrenal insufficiency in critically ill patients include hemorrhagic shock, coagulopathy, vasopressor dependence, and etomidate exposure [127]. Given these findings, several investigators have evaluated the significance of adrenal insufficiency in trauma patients. In the absence of septic shock, the literature would suggest that routine evaluation for adrenal insufficiency and supplementation with steroids are not warranted [128]. Therefore, unless there is documentation of a medical history of adrenal insufficiency or recent steroid use, the authors would not recommend routinely obtaining cortisol (or ACTH-stimulation tests) or administering adrenal replacement therapy in the acutely injured patient.

10.2.12   Infectious Disease Management

While guidelines for antibiotic choice and duration are present for intra-abdominal injury, whether the open abdominal cavity warrants more (or less) antibiotic coverage (spectrum and duration) is unclear. Sufficient data exist to recommend a single preoperative dose of prophylactic antibiotics with broad-spectrum aerobic and anaerobic coverage as a standard of care for trauma patients with severe abdominal wounds [129, 130]. Additionally, class I and class II data are present to recommend continuation of prophylactic antibiotics for 24 h in the presence of hollow viscus injury [130]. Even in patients with destructive colon injuries, there is no difference in infection rates for patients receiving 24 h or 5 days of antibiotic coverage. In fact, infections appear to be higher in those with greater duration of coverage [129]. In patients with massive blood loss, the administered dose may be increased two- or threefold and repeated after every tenth unit of blood product transfusion until hemorrhage is under control. Post-splenectomy vaccines should be held until the inflammatory state has resolved and the immune system is capable of responding to vaccinations. In general, this is after 7 days, though some suggest administration at the 14-day mark [131].

10.2.13   Orthopedic Management and Complications

Polytraumatized patients may have various reasons for secondary worsening of their general condition. The ones caused by truncal injuries are frequently in focus because the patient has just come from the operating room where a hemorrhage control has been performed for specific lesions.

It is, therefore, important to rule out other complications that may ensue from orthopedic injuries. One of the most frequent complications is an associated compartment syndrome. Multiple trauma patients are at increased risk to develop this complication because of their increased demand of fluid replacements and secondary interstitial edema. Therefore, a compartment syndrome may not just be a problem that occurs within the first few hours, but it can ensue a day later and can be clouded by the fact that the sedated patient has no pain. Thus, careful soft tissue observation and cooling of the extremity should be performed, and a low threshold towards measurement of compartment pressures should be present. Overlooked compartment syndromes are a dangerous source for a second hit phenomenon and can yield to infection, sepsis, and death.

More rare indications for acute orthopedic intervention can be incomplete arterial injuries from fracture fragments or displaced fractures. In knee dislocations, careful monitoring is required, often using digital pulse oximetry, to diagnose delayed arterial occlusion that can occur as a result of an intimal tear. More rarely, a pseudo- aneurysm can develop from a displaced fracture or a secondary hemorrhage based on Disseminated Intravascular Coagulation (DIC).

Another important complication is soft tissue breakdown from pelvic binders or sheets. Some centers therefore have a strict policy to loosen binders and sheets periodically. Others routinely apply two sheets: one in the area of the greater trochanter and one in the area of the anterior iliac spine. These are then tightened in an alternating fashion. A breakdown of soft tissues in an unstabilized pelvic fracture will most likely interfere with the orthopedic approach required to stabilize the fracture, which may then be an important source of infection.

10.2.14   Wound and Open-Abdomen Management

10.2.14.1   General Wound Care and Laceration Repair

Wounds not previously addressed should be formally evaluated, and treatment should be initiated after the patient is deemed hemodynamically stable. Wounds requiring sub-specialty consultation and/or assistance should be addressed immediately to minimize inherent delays in the consultant process. Following this, those wounds within the purview and skill set of trauma or ICU teams are evaluated and treated. Radiographs are obtained to rule-out foreign body retention in traumatic wounds. Tetanus prophylaxis is provided if not given prior to ICU arrival and a recent administration is not available in the patient's history. Patients are positioned (with spine precautions as indicated) where the lacerations are easily accessible. Wounds should be irrigated with normal saline until all visible, loose particulate matter has been removed (a minimum of 500 mL). The wounded area should be re-assessed after irrigation for nerve, vessel, and/or tendon injury, joint capsule involvement, foreign body, and extent/depth of wound. The wound is then debrided of devitalized tissue with sharp iris scissors or fine scalpel. In general, monofilament suture is used for the superficial repair, and Vicryl® suture (Ethicon, Somerville, NJ) is used for deeper closure. However, skin staples may be used to approximate long, linear lacerations involving the scalp or areas of less cosmetic importance.

Whether used to facilitate rapid wound coverage for the chest, abdomen, or extremity, the vacuum pack technique is the dressing of choice for damage control procedures at the authors' institutions. This technique allows for the rapid and efficient coverage of the damage control compartment and is simple to trouble-shoot when recurrent abdominal compartment syndrome is suspected or when there is a "leak" in the system. More recently, some have begun using the black sponge vacuum device for the first dressing change (if not for the initial operation). As opposed to the traditional towel and occlusive Ioban® dressing (3M, St. Paul, MN) with Jackson–Pratt drains, the black sponge device appears to be associated with more rapid and more likely primary fascial closure. Investigators from Houston and Wake Forest have demonstrated that utilization of Vacuum-Assisted Wound Closure Technique (VAWC) is associated with an increased likelihood of definitive fascial closure with a low incidence of complications [132].

Open abdomen dressings should be changed at least once every 48 h. The patient should receive adequate sedation [and Neuromuscular Blocker (NMB)] followed by a prepping and draping. The previous dressing and sponge should be gently removed. Any debris is cautiously removed, and the cavity is irrigated until the effluent returns clear. The surrounding area is then cleaned and dried, and the skin prep is applied. If a black sponge vacuum is elected, the new sponge is then cut and shaped to fill the wound surface. Ensure that the sponge dressing is within the edges of the wound cavity and is not in contact with the surrounding skin. An occlusive dressing—the authors utilize a separate Ioban® (3M, St. Paul, MN) for this – is applied and 1–2 cm hole is cut in the drape. The pre-packaged suction device is then applied over the hole and attached to the negative pressure device. The authors prefer to keep the suction set at −125 mmHg. The tubing should be clamped when transferring the patient or changing the device canister to prevent loss of suction and adherence.

10.2.14.2   Intra-abdominal Pressure Management

The damage control population in general is at an extremely high risk (even when fascia is left "open") of developing Intra-Abdominal Hypertension (IAH) and recurrent Abdominal Compartment Syndrome (ACS). While temporary abdominal closure methods provide the capacity to further increase the abdominal volume, continued monitoring for ACS is required. Physiologic parameters and large volume fluid resuscitation predict which patients will develop ACS [119, 133]. Regardless of these parameters, the authors recommend that continuous or frequent scheduled monitoring be utilized. The reference standard for intermittent Intra-Abdominal Pressure (IAP) measurement is via the bladder with a maximal instillation volume of 25 mL sterile saline. Measurements should be performed in the supine position, "zeroed" at the axilla, and obtained after 30–60 s to allow for detrusor relation [134]. Normal IAP is 5–7 mmHg in critically ill adults. IAH is defined by a sustained or repeated pathological elevation in IAP ≥ 12 mmHg. ACS is defined as a sustained IAP > 20 mmHg that is associated with new organ dysfunction/failure [135].

In the patient with an already open abdomen, evaluation of IAH begins with an assessment of the tension of the current abdominal dressing. Initial management often requires taking down the temporary closure and providing more room for abdominal contents (a "looser" dressing). Non-surgical approaches can be utilized to address IAH when there is no evidence of ACS. Improvement of abdominal wall compliance can be attempted with an increase in sedation and analgesia with the addition of neuromuscular blockade [134, 135]. Evacuation of intra-luminal contents can be achieved with naso-gastric decompression, rectal decompression, and addition of promotility agents. Decreasing overall volume status (restricting fluids, diuresing patient) may also assist in the "medical" reduction of intra-abdominal pressures. If these fail to alleviate the increasing IAH or evidence of ACS develops, the abdomen should be decompressed (or the current dressing taken down) immediately.

10.2.14.3 Recurrent Abdominal Compartment Syndrome

Despite attempts to eliminate intra-abdominal hypertension by maintaining an open abdomen, some patients treated with temporary abdominal closure will develop what has been recently termed recurrent abdominal compartment syndrome. Ongoing, large volume crystalloid-based resuscitations are the primary risk factor for its development. Specifically, crystalloid infusions exceeding 10 L in the first 24 h are associated with an increased risk of recurrent ACS [133]. Based on their findings, Gracias and colleagues recommend continuous monitoring of intra-abdominal pressure, base deficit, PCO_2, and lactate [133]. The authors support their use and potential to identify recurrent ACS earlier. Given that most cases in the Gracias study occurred in the first 12 h after ICU admission, such aggressive monitoring appears warranted.

10.2.15   General Care of the Patient

10.2.15.1   Oral Hygiene

Use of standardized oral/mouth care programs is associated with a reduction in ventilator associated pneumonia. Proper oral care entails frequent tooth brushing, mouth swabbing with an antiseptic agent (chlorhexidine), and frequent suctioning of the mouth and subglottic areas. Additionally, head of bed elevation to at least 30° (preferably 45°) is an important part of minimizing aspiration and ventilator-associated pneumonia risk. However, caution should be used and spine "clearance" confirmed prior to "breaking" the bed and sitting the patient upright. If spine injury is suspected or the thoraco-lumbar spine has not been radiographically cleared, the bed may be placed into reverse Trendelenburg position.

10.2.15.2   Venous Thromboembolism Prophylaxis

Unless otherwise specified, all damage control trauma patients should receive venous thromboembolism (VTE) prophylaxis. Factors placing this group at "very high risk" for VTE event include: high Injury Severity Score (ISS), blood transfusions, immobilization, and multiple injuries. The authors utilize enoxaparin at 30 mg SQ every 12 h. Alternatively, one may chose unfractionated heparin at 5,000 U every 8 h. In patients with intra-cranial hemorrhage, post-operative from craniotomy or Intra-Cranial Pressure (ICP) monitoring or post-operative from open fixation of spine fracture, the authors hold pharmacological VTE prophylaxis for 48 h. Until this time has elapsed, the authors utilize sequential compression devices. Prior to take back for damage control, the authors do not routinely hold VTE prophylaxis.

10.2.15.3   Skin Care

If not already removed, patients should be taken off spine backboards as soon as possible after arrival. Orthopedic splints and casts should be frequently inspected for skin breakdown [136]. Attempts should be made to provide continual "off-loading" of the patient's skin to avoid injury and ulcer formation. Given the immobilized status and often edematous state of these patients, the DC population is at an extremely high risk of skin breakdown. A total skin assessment should be performed at the time of admission and/or transfer, and the state of the skin should be documented with a Braden Risk Scale once every shift. The patient should be repositioned-bound at least every 2 h.

10.2.15.4   Concomitant Injury Management

Lacerations and wounds should be addressed as soon as possible after stabilization and arrival in the ICU. With regard to orthopedic injuries: Many of these will have been addressed in a similar DC method and will not require immediate intervention, with the exception of a bedside washout and a potential orthopedic hardware adjustment. However, some patients will require bedside traction or external fixator placement. This should be done in a standardized fashion per ICU protocols. Please see the section on the management of "bedside" anesthesia for how to provide adequate sedation and analgesia for these cases.

10.2.15.5   Diagnostic Studies

When possible, all radiographic studies should be performed at the bedside. In some circumstances, however, procedures and/or diagnostic studies will require leaving the ICU premises. In these situations, the ICU and surgical team (and surgical sub-specialty consultants when relevant) should discuss the risk-benefit of obtaining said studies during the Phase II of DC. If possible, the diagnostic procedures should be scheduled for a time when the patient has successfully achieved correction of the lethal triad and the patient is ready for return to the OR for DC Phase III. When diagnostic studies are deemed urgent and worth the risk of a "road trip," the patient should be accompanied by a bedside ICU nurse and a respiratory therapist, along with an ICU physician (when possible).

10.3 Transport

Management and monitoring during transport to the OR or to diagnostic procedures should mirror that delivered in the actual facility of the ICU. This echoes the sentiments and teaching at the authors' facilities that "the ICU is a concept, not a location." Patients requiring transport back to the operating theater or to diagnostic studies should be maintained on the same ventilator mode and settings as those used in the ICU [79]. This critical portion of the patient's management is sufficiently complex to require coordination by a member of the ICU or trauma team. When transporting the patient to the OR, an anesthesiologist can assist in the role, but primary responsibility lies with the ICU leadership. The ICU team leader should be in direct communication with the scheduled anesthesiologist, OR personnel, and the blood bank. During this time, the trauma team sets up the room and procedure to minimize operative time and communicates with surgical consultants about concurrent procedures and with the radiology department about the need for potential angiographic procedures [79]. Continuous cardiac and respiratory monitoring (as well as intra-cranial or intra-abdominal when present) of the patient during transport to radiology or the OR is mandatory. One member of the transport team should be assigned to monitor the patient throughout, allowing the other team members to provide the adequate personnel to move the stretcher, patient, and equipment.

10.4 Out the Door

10.4.1 The Patient Who Corrects

Correction of the lethal triad and the achievement of hemodynamic stability mark an end-point that allows scheduled reoperation. While some would argue whether there is a specific time point in hours when a patient is "ready" for take back, operating room return usually occurs within 12–48 h after a damage control laparotomy or temporary skeletal fixation [136, 137]. The amount of time that should be allowed before take back in patients with packing or bowel discontinuity is 24–48 h.

The ICU team's role in preparing the patient beyond physiologic stability is multifaceted. The intensivist should confirm that the patient has blood products available for use in the OR. If the patient is requiring advanced ventilatory techniques, a formal sign-out (and possibly transfer of the patient's ventilator to the OR) should involve the anesthesia team [136]. Prior to leaving the ICU for DC III, the critical care team should define spine status, address other diagnostics issues, and obtain consultation as necessary.

10.4.2   The Patient Who Does Not Correct

General rules to follow that indicate the need for urgent and early return to the OR are: (1) persistent bleeding/coagulopathy; (2) abdominal compartment syndrome; (3) refractory acidosis with severe metabolic derangements; (4) gross gastrointestinal soilage of abdomen cavity [136, 137]. The patient that "fails to correct" is also one in whom missed abdominal or thoracic injuries are suspected and those whose physiology fails to be "recaptured." Such physiological failure may present subtly as a persistent, refractory distributive shock with escalating systemic inflammatory response (leukopenia or leukocytosis).

Attempts at re-opening the "failure to correct" patient at the bedside should be done with great reservation. The majority of ICUs are not equipped to handle significant bleeding, have inadequate lighting and suction, and an inexperienced staff to assist and/or access appropriate instruments in a timely fashion. The primary trauma team should be involved with all steps of the management decision tree and kept continuously "in the loop." Once the decision has been made to proceed back to the OR, the team should prepare for a comprehensive transport process as outlined earlier.

Transport of the DC patient to Interventional Radiology (IR) should be predefined and well thought out ahead of time through an ICU protocol. Orchestrating this series of motions and events from the ICU to the IR suite can be move-intense and as complex as moving the patient to the operating suite. Several members of the team will be necessary for transport, including a nursing respiratory therapist and, at times, an anesthesiologist. If possible, a senior member of the ICU team should be present for transport and intervention. The angiographer should be asked to leave the arterial sheath in place in anticipation of further or re-embolization procedures if necessary.

10.4.3   Missed Injuries and the Tertiary Examination

All patients arriving to the ICU post-operatively should undergo a detailed "head-to-toe" tertiary survey examination. This evaluation should be performed under the assumption that there are undiagnosed injuries and an abbreviated examination was all that had been previously performed. The tertiary survey is a summary of a patient's injuries, the detail and completeness of which is determined by the complexity of ongoing resuscitation [138].

This examination should include, but is not limited to: a careful inspection of the scalp and back; evaluation of the eyes for injury or retained contact lenses; rectal examination for injury, blood, and tone; and a vaginal examination for lacerations or foreign bodies [136, 137]. Neuromuscular blockade should be withdrawn (at least briefly to allow for gross assessment of the patient's "best" neurological examination). All extremities should be examined for lacerations, crepitance, and bony deformities. Joints should undergo passive range of motion, as well as assessment for effusions and laxity. Any suspicious or questionable finding should be evaluated with radiographic imaging.

Missed injuries are defined as those injuries diagnosed after discharge or transfer. Delays in diagnoses are those injuries detected after the initial evaluation and disposition but prior to discharge or transfer. The most commonly missed or delayed injuries are those of the cervical spine and the distal extremities [136–138]. Additionally, injuries to the diaphragm, retroperitoneum, genitourinary system, pancreas, and posterior portions of the stomach, duodenum, and colon are also frequently overlooked during the initial evaluation and even during Phase I of DC. Repeated examinations and aggressive investigation of all suspicious findings are indicated to minimize missed diagnoses [138].

10.4.4 Procedural Sedation

Over the last decade, the frequency of "bedside" operative procedures has increased considerably. The factors behind this include: the increasing acceptance of staged (or damage control) strategies for managing severe abdominal, soft tissue, and orthopedic injury; advances in endoscopic and percutaneous techniques; increasing competition for operating room space; difficulty of transporting severely critically ill patients; As a result, a considerable number of procedures are now being performed in the ICU that historically had been reserved for the operating theater.

Protocols and safety practices for these bedside operative procedures should be in place to assure the ability to safely perform these procedures. All patients should have blood pressure, electrocardiographic monitoring, and pulse oximetry routinely monitored throughout the procedures. Adequate personnel must be present to allow performance of the procedure, monitoring of sedation/anesthesia, medication administration, manipulation of ventilation if required, and documentation. In addition to the careful development of a bedside procedure protocol, the authors have implemented the use of a designated "proceduralist" for all bedside surgical procedures. These individuals are senior critical care nurses, trained in the assistance of bedside procedures, airway management, and intravenous general anesthetic administration.

For non-abdominal procedural sedation, bolus administration of midazolam is preferred in light of its rapid onset, depth of sedation, and amnestic effect. Initial bolus administration begins with 1.0–2.0 mg doses, followed by repeat doses as the patient's respiratory and hemodynamic status permit. For analgesia, fentanyl is utilized at doses dependent on the patient's weight, tolerance, and hemodynamic status. For the deep sedation required for abdominal bedside procedures, the authors utilize propofol in larger doses than those employed for continuous sedation (10–20 mg boluses). Ketamine is also used and well tolerated for complex wound care and dressing changes. It is usually administered in these settings at 2 mg/kg intravenously. Because of its risk of emergence delirium and emesis, ketamine is usually administered with midazolam and metoclopramide. These agents are titrated to achieve preset endpoints as patient hemodynamic status allows. For paralysis, we prefer to use vecuronium at doses of 0.1–0.15 mg/kg intravenously. NMBA are employed in the majority of bronchoscopies and major bedside operative procedures and in all "open abdomen" procedures.

10.4.5   Special Problems

10.4.5.1   Thoracic Damage Control

In patients arriving with an open chest cavity from DC procedures, the same principles of restoring physiology and reversing the lethal triad should also take precedence [136, 139–141]. As with DC in the open abdomen, there is a fine balance between providing adequate oxygen delivery while avoiding overly aggressive crystalloid resuscitation. Even more tenuous than in the open abdomen is the respiratory status and "room for error" in the DC chest patient. These patients are more likely to have concomitant pulmonary contusions and air leaks, further decreasing their pulmonary reserve [139]. Trends in chest tube output should receive a considerable amount attention. While it is common for bleeding from chest tubes to initially be quite high, the trend should be a tapering off over the following few hours as coagulopathy is addressed. An abrupt cessation in chest tube output should raise suspicions of tube clotting or malfunction. As compartment syndrome and/or tamponade can quickly follow, this situation should be immediately investigated. If chest tube output remains high (>300 mL/h), the trauma team should be notified, and a decision should be made as to whether or not surgical bleeding still exists and if a return trip to the OR is warranted.

Thoracic compartment syndrome is commonly the result of the same underlying mechanisms of gross tissue injury with aggressive crystalloid resuscitation [142]. Patients will commonly present with increasing peak inspiratory pressures. Steep rises in these pressures during attempted thoracic wall closure intra-operatively may be one of the only early warnings of its impending presentation. Decompression of the chest along previous surgical planes should be performed with placement of a temporary negative pressure dressing.

10.4.5.2   Intra-vascular Shunts

In an attempt to apply damage control principles, vascular trauma (especially to the extremities) is often managed with insertion of temporary vascular shunts. Early insertion of these shunts allows the trauma team to repair these injuries in a delayed fashion when the patient's more life-threatening issues have been addressed. These shunts are typically positioned in a slightly redundant fashion to help reduce chances of dislodgement. The shunt is secured proximally and distally with sutures tied around the shunt and vessel wall at their interface [143, 144]. It is usually flushed with heparinized saline prior to securing, but routine post-operative systemic heparinization is controversial in light of the usual multisystem injuries and coagulopathic state. Serial vascular evaluations should be performed, and any change in the examination should be reported immediately to the trauma team. Movement of the involved extremity should be kept to a minimum (or to nothing) even for radiographic evaluations.

10.5   Summary and Conclusion

The ICU phase of DC is a critical crossroads for the injured patient's physiology and his/her eventual outcome. Management decisions during this period of care can mean not only the difference between a successful return for Phase III and an "unclose-able" abdomen, but also the difference between survival and death. At its most basic, the ICU phase is a continuation of Phase I of DC, proceeding through the initial resuscitation and management issues, while simultaneously assessing when the patient is to progress to Phase III. Phase II begins with a safe and efficient transfer of care as the patient enters the ICU door. Following this "hand-off," reversing coagulopathy, acidosis, and hypothermia should be the primary goals of ICU care.

Achieving adequate control of pain and its related components of anxiety and agitation is a critical, but often mismanaged, component that deserves special attention. Hemorrhagic shock, massive resuscitation, and multiple transfusions place the DC patient at a high risk of developing ALI and ARDS during the ICU stay. It is imperative that these patients be managed with lung-protective ventilator strategies and that catheter-directed resuscitation therapies are employed. Stress ulcer prophylaxis should be provided during all phases and continued until the "very-high risk" criteria (mechanical ventilation, coagulopathy) have resolved. Once bowel continuity is restored, enteral nutrition should be initiated even in the presence of an open abdomen. Management of the renal system should be directed at the prevention of volume overload, maintenance of electrolytes within normal range, and the avoidance of oliguria. In severely injured patients, evidence regarding insulin replacement for strict euglycemia and adrenal replacement (in the absence of septic shock) has been conflicting. Finally, attention should be directed at the triage and management of non-truncal injuries and soft-tissue trauma. Orthopedic injuries should be addressed as soon as possible, and priorities for interventions developed early. Wounds not previously addressed should be evaluated as soon as the patient is deemed hemodynamically stable, with sub-specialty consultation obtained immediately to minimize inherent delays in the consultant process.

References

1. Rotondo MF, Schwab CW, McGonigal MD, Phillips GR 3rd, Fruchterman TM, Kauder DR, Latenser BA, Angood PA. "Damage control": an approach for improved survival in exsanguinating penetrating abdominal injury. *J Trauma* 1993;35(3):375–82.
2. Stone HH, Strom PR, Mullins RJ. Management of the major coagulopathy with onset during laparotomy. *Ann Surg* 1983;197(5):532–5.
3. Asensio JA, Petrone P, O'Shanahan G, Kuncir EJ. Managing exsanguination: what we know about damage control/bailout is not enough. *Proc (Bayl Univ Med Cent)* 2003;16(3):294–6.
4. Balogh Z, McKinley BA, Holcomb JB, Miller CC, Cocanour CS, Kozar RA, Valdivia A, Ware DN, Moore FA. Both primary and secondary abdominal compartment syndrome can be predicted early and are harbingers of multiple organ failure. *J Trauma* 2003;54(5):848–59.
5. Boldt J, Heesen M, Welters I, Padberg W, Martin K, Hempelmann G. Does the type of volume therapy influence endothelial-related coagulation in the critically ill? *Br J Anaesth* 1995;75(6):740–6.
6. Burch JM, Ortiz VB, Richardson RJ, Martin RR, Mattox KL, Jordan GL, Jr. Abbreviated laparotomy and planned reoperation for critically injured patients. *Ann Surg* 1992;215(5):476–83.
7. Cotton BA, Guy JS, Morris JA, Jr., Abumrad NN. The cellular, metabolic, and systemic consequences of aggressive fluid resuscitation strategies. *Shock* 2006;26(2):115–21.
8. Eddy VA, Morris JA, Jr., Cullinane DC. Hypothermia, coagulopathy, and acidosis. *Surg Clin North Am* 2000;80(3):845–54.
9. Gonzalez EA, Moore FA, Holcomb JB, Miller CC, Kozar RA, Todd SR, Cocanour CS, Balldin BC, McKinley BA. Fresh frozen plasma should be given earlier to patients requiring massive transfusion. *J Trauma* 2007;62(1):112–9.
10. Gruen RL, Jurkovich GJ, McIntyre LK, Foy HM, Maier RV. Patterns of errors contributing to trauma mortality: lessons learned from 2,594 deaths. *Ann Surg* 2006;244(3):371–80.
11. McKinley BA, Valdivia A, Moore FA. Goal-oriented shock resuscitation for major torso trauma: what are we learning? *Curr Opin Crit Care* 2003;9(4):292–9.
12. Moore EE, Burch JM, Franciose RJ, Offner PJ, Biffl WL. Staged physiologic restoration and damage control surgery. *World J Surg* 1998;22(12):1184–90.
13. Raeburn CD, Moore EE, Biffl WL, Johnson JL, Meldrum DR, Offner PJ, Franciose RJ, Burch JM. The abdominal compartment syndrome is a morbid complication of postinjury damage control surgery. *Am J Surg* 2001;182(6):542–6.
14. Van Eaton EG, Horvath KD, Lober WB, Pellegrini CA. Organizing the transfer of patient care information: the development of a computerized resident sign-out system. *Surgery* 2004;136(1):5–13.
15. Rohrich RJ, Persing JA, Phillips L. Mandating shorter work hours and enhancing patient safety: a new challenge for resident education. *Plast Reconstr Surg* 2003;111(1):395–7.
16. Grogan EL, Stiles RA, France DJ, Speroff T , Morris Jr J, Nixon B, Gaffney F, Seddon R, Pinson C. The impact of aviation-based teamwork training on the attitudes of health-care professionals. *J Am Coll Surg* 2004;199(6):843–8.
17. Hoff WS, Sicoutris CP, Lee SY, Rotondo MF, Reilly PM, Schwab CW. Formalized radiology rounds: the final component of the tertiary survey. *J Trauma* 2004;56(2):291–5.
18. Van Eaton EG, Horvath KD, Lober WB, Rossini AJ, Pellegrini CA. A randomized, controlled trial evaluating the impact of a computerized rounding and sign-out system on continuity of care and resident work hours. *J Am Coll Surg* 2005;200(4):538–45.

19. Williams RG, Silverman R, Schwind C, Fortune JB, Sutyak J, Horvath KD, Van Eaton EG, Azzie G, Potts III JR, Boehler M, Dunnington GL. Surgeon information transfer and communication: factors affecting quality and efficiency of inpatient care. *Ann Surg* 2007; 245(2):159–69.
20. Ho AM, Karmakar MK, Dion PW. Are we giving enough coagulation factors during major trauma resuscitation? *Am J Surg* 2005;190(3):479–84.
21. Brohi K, Cohen MJ, Ganter MT, Matthay MA, Mackersie RC, Pittet JF. Acute traumatic coagulopathy: initiated by hypoperfusion: modulated through the protein C pathway? *Ann Surg* 2007;245(5):812–8.
22. Hoffman M. The cellular basis of traumatic bleeding. *Mil Med* 2004;169(12 Suppl):5–7, 4.
23. Cotton BA, Guy JS, Morris JA, Jr., Abumrad NN. The cellular, metabolic, and systemic consequences of aggressive fluid resuscitation strategies. *Shock* 2006;26(2):115–21.
24. Farkash U, Lynn M, Scope A et al. Does prehospital fluid administration impact core body temperature and coagulation functions in combat casualties? *Injury* 2002;33(2):103–10.
25. Gentilello LM, Moujaes S. Treatment of hypothermia in trauma victims: thermodynamic considerations. *J Intensive Care Med* 1995;10(1):5–14.
26. Gentilello LM, Jurkovich GJ, Stark MS, Hassantash SA, O'Keefe GE. Is hypothermia in the victim of major trauma protective or harmful? A randomized, prospective study. *Ann Surg* 1997;226(4):439–47.
27. Gubler KD, Gentilello LM, Hassantash SA, Maier RV. The impact of hypothermia on dilutional coagulopathy. *J Trauma* 1994;36(6):847–51.
28. Hardy JF, de Moerloose P, Samama M. Massive transfusion and coagulopathy: pathophysiology and implications for clinical management. *Can J Anaesth* 2004;51(4):293–310.
29. Danks RR. Triangle of death. How hypothermia acidosis and coagulopathy can adversely impact trauma patients. *JEMS* 2002;27(5):61–70.
30. Ho AM, Dion PW, Cheng CA, Karmakar MK, Cheng G, Peng Ng YW A mathematical model for fresh frozen plasma transfusion strategies during major trauma resuscitation with ongoing hemorrhage. *Can J Surg* 2005;48(6):470–8.
31. Kearney TJ, Bentt L, Grode M, Lee S, Hiatt JR, Shabot MM. Coagulopathy and catecholamines in severe head injury. *J Trauma* 1992;32(5):608–11.
32. Meng ZH, Wolberg AS, Monroe DM, III, Hoffman M. The effect of temperature and pH on the activity of factor VIIa: implications for the efficacy of high-dose factor VIIa in hypothermic and acidotic patients. *J Trauma* 2003;55(5):886–91.
33. Barak M, Rudin M, Vofsi O, Droyan A, Katz Y. Fluid administration during abdominal surgery influences on coagulation in the postoperative period. *Curr Surg* 2004;61(5):459–62.
34. Boldt J, Heesen M, Welters I, Padberg W, Martin K, Hempelmann G. Does the type of volume therapy influence endothelial-related coagulation in the critically ill? *Br J Anaesth* 1995;75(6):740–6.
35. Ng KF, Lam CC, Chan LC. In vivo effect of haemodilution with saline on coagulation: a randomized controlled trial. *Br J Anaesth* 2002;88(4):475–80.
36. Cotton BA, Gunter OL, Isbell J, Au BK, Robertson AM, Morris JA Jr, St Jacques P, Young PP. Damage control hematology: the impact of a trauma exsanguination protocol on survival and blood product utilization. *J Trauma* 2008;64(5):1177–82.
37. Holcomb JB, Jenkins D, Rhee P, Johannigman J, Mahoney P, Mehta S, Cox E D, Gehrke MJ, Beilman GJ, Schreiber M, Flaherty SF, Grathwohl KW, Spinella PC, Perkins JG, Beekley AC, McMullin NR, Park MS, Gonzalez EA, Wade CE, Dubick MA, Schwab CW, Moore FA, Champion HR, Hoyt DB, Hess JR. Damage control resuscitation: directly addressing the early coagulopathy of trauma. *J Trauma* 2007;62(2):307–10.
38. Clark AD, Gordon WC, Walker ID, Tait RC. "Last-ditch" use of recombinant factor VIIa in patients with massive haemorrhage is ineffective. *Vox Sang* 2004;86(2):120–4.
39. Gowers CJ, Parr MJ. Recombinant activated factor VIIa use in massive transfusion and coagulopathy unresponsive to conventional therapy. *Anaesth Intensive Care* 2005;33(2):196–200.
40. Hedner U, Erhardtsen E. Potential role of recombinant factor VIIa as a hemostatic agent. *Clin Adv Hematol Oncol* 2003;1(2):112–9.

41. Holcomb JB. Use of recombinant activated factor VII to treat the acquired coagulopathy of trauma. *J Trauma* 2005;58(6):1298–303.
42. Holcomb JB, Hoots K, Moore FA. Treatment of an acquired coagulopathy with recombinant activated factor VII in a damage-control patient. *Mil Med* 2005;170(4):287–90.
43. Sagraves SG, Toschlog EA, Rotondo MF. Damage control surgery – the intensivist's role. *J Intensive Care Med* 2006;21(1):5–16.
44. Engstrom M, Schott U, Romner B, Reinstrup P. Acidosis impairs the coagulation: a thromboelastographic study. *J Trauma* 2006;61(3):624–8.
45. Moomey CB, Jr., Melton SM, Croce MA, Fabian TC, Proctor KG. Prognostic value of blood lactate, base deficit, and oxygen-derived variables in an LD50 model of penetrating trauma. *Crit Care Med* 1999;27(1):154–61.
46. Abramson D, Scalea TM, Hitchcock R, Trooskin SZ, Henry SM, Greenspan J. Lactate clearance and survival following injury. *J Trauma* 1993;35(4):584–8.
47. Martin MJ, FitzSullivan E, Salim A, Brown CV, Demetriades D, Long W. Discordance between lactate and base deficit in the surgical intensive care unit: which one do you trust? *Am J Surg* 2006;191(5):625–30.
48. FitzSullivan E, Salim A, Demetriades D, Asensio J, Martin MJ. Serum bicarbonate may replace the arterial base deficit in the trauma intensive care unit. *Am J Surg* 2005;190(6):941–6.
49. Gunnerson KJ, Kellum JA. Acid-base and electrolyte analysis in critically ill patients: are we ready for the new millennium? *Curr Opin Crit Care* 2003;9(6):468–73.
50. Holmdahl MH, Wiklund L, Wetterberg T, Streat S, Wahlander S, Sutin K, Nahas G. The place of THAM in the management of acidemia in clinical practice. *Acta Anaesthesiol Scand* 2000;44(5):524–7.
51. Nahas GG, Sutin KM, Fermon C, Streat S, Wiklund L. Guidelines for the treatment of acidaemia with THAM. *Drugs* 1998;55(2):191–224.
52. Gentilello LM, Jurkovich GJ, Stark MS, Hassantash SA, O'Keefe GE. Is hypothermia in the victim of major trauma protective or harmful? A randomized, prospective study. *Ann Surg* 1997;226(4):439–47.
53. Arthurs Z, Cuadrado D, Beekley A, Grathwohl K, Perkins J, Rush R, Sebesta J. The impact of hypothermia on trauma care at the 31st combat support hospital. *Am J Surg* 2006;191(5):610–4.
54. Ferrara A, MacArthur JD, Wright HK, Modlin IM, McMillen MA. Hypothermia and acidosis worsen coagulopathy in the patient requiring massive transfusion. *Am J Surg* 1990;160(5):515–8.
55. Hildebrand F, van GM, Giannoudis P, Schreiber T, Frink M, Probst C, Grotz M, Krettek C, Pape HC. Impact of hypothermia on the immunologic response after trauma and elective surgery. *Surg Technol Int* 2005;14:41–50.
56. Gentilello LM, Moujaes S. Treatment of hypothermia in trauma victims: thermodynamic considerations. *J Intensive Care Med* 1995;10(1):5–14.
57. Patel N, Smith CE, Pinchak AC. Comparison of fluid warmer performance during simulated clinical conditions. *Can J Anaesth* 1995;42(7):636–42.
58. Patel N, Knapke DM, Smith CE, Napora TE, Pinchak AC, Hagen JF. Simulated clinical evaluation of conventional and newer fluid-warming devices. *Anesth Analg* 1996;82(3):517–24.
59. Smith CE, Desai R, Glorioso V, Cooper A, Pinchak AC, Hagen KF. Preventing hypothermia: convective and intravenous fluid warming versus convective warming alone. *J Clin Anesth* 1998;10(5):380–5.
60. Smith CE, Parand A, Pinchak AC, Hagen JF, Hancock DE. The failure of negative pressure rewarming (Thermostat) to accelerate recovery from mild hypothermia in postoperative surgical patients. *Anesth Analg* 1999;89(6):1541–5.
61. Danzl D. Hypothermia. *Semin Respir Crit Care Med* 2002;23(1):57–68.
62. Garraway N, Brown DR, Nash D, Kirkpatrick A, Schneidereit N, Van Heest R, Hwang H, Simons R. Active internal re-warming using a centrifugal pump and heat exchanger following haemorrhagic shock, surgical trauma and hypothermia in a porcine model. *Injury* 2007;38(9):1039–46.

63. Gentilello LM, Rifley WJ. Continuous arteriovenous rewarming: report of a new technique for treating hypothermia. *J Trauma* 1991;31(8):1151–4.
64. Gentilello LM. Advances in the management of hypothermia. *Surg Clin North Am* 1995;75(2):243–56.
65. Jurkovich GJ, Greiser WB, Luterman A, Curreri PW. Hypothermia in trauma victims: an ominous predictor of survival. *J Trauma* 1987;27(9):1019–24.
66. Jacobi J, Fraser GL, Coursin DB, Riker RR, Fontaine D, Wittbrodt ET, Chalfin DB, Masica MR, Bjerke HS, Coplin WM, Crippen DW, Fuchs BD, Kelleher RM, Marik PE, Nasraway Jr SA, Murray MJ, Peruzzi WT, Lumb PD. Clinical practice guidelines for the sustained use of sedatives and analgesics in the critically ill adult. *Crit Care Med* 2002;30(1):119–41.
67. Payen JF, Bru O, Bosson JL, Lagrasta A, Novel E, Deschaux I, Lavagne P, Jacquot C. Assessing pain in critically ill sedated patients by using a behavioral pain scale. *Crit Care Med* 2001;29(12):2258–63.
68. Ely EW, Truman B, Shintani A, Thomason JWW, Wheeler AP, Gordon S, Francis J, Speroff T, Gautam S, Margolin R, Sessler CN, Dittus RS, Bernard GR. Monitoring sedation status over time in ICU patients: reliability and validity of the Richmond Agitation-Sedation Scale (RASS). *JAMA* 2003;289(22):2983–91.
69. Chisholm CJ, Zurica J, Mironov D, Sciacca RR, Ornstein E, Heyer EJ. Comparison of electrophysiologic monitors with clinical assessment of level of sedation. *Mayo Clin Proc* 2006;81(1):46–52.
70. Sackey PV, Radell PJ, Granath F, Martling CR. Bispectral index as a predictor of sedation depth during isoflurane or midazolam sedation in ICU patients. *Anaesth Intensive Care* 2007;35(3):348–56.
71. Hall RI, Sandham D, Cardinal P, Tweeddale M, Moher D, Wang X, Anis AS, for the Study Investigators. Propofol vs midazolam for ICU sedation: a Canadian multicenter randomized trial. *Chest* 2001;119(4):1151–9.
72. Maze M, Scarfini C, Cavaliere F. New agents for sedation in the intensive care unit. *Crit Care Clin* 2001;17(4):881–97.
73. Venn RM, Grounds RM. Comparison between dexmedetomidine and propofol for sedation in the intensive care unit: patient and clinician perceptions. *Br J Anaesth* 2001;87(5):684–90.
74. Venn RM, Karol MD, Grounds RM. Pharmacokinetics of dexmedetomidine infusions for sedation of postoperative patients requiring intensive caret. *Br J Anaesth* 2002;88(5):669–75.
75. Duff JF, Moffat J. Abdominal sepsis managed by leaving the abdomen open. *Surgery* 1981;90:774–778.
76. De Waele JJ, De Iaet I, Malbrain ML. Intraabdominal hypertension and abdominal compartment syndrome: we have paid attention, now it is time to understand! *Acta Clin Belg Suppl* 2007;(1):6–8.
77. De Iaet I, Hoste E, Verholen E, De Waele JJ. The effect of neuromuscular blockers in patients with intra-abdominal hypertension. *Intensive Care Med* 2007;33(10):1811–4.
78. Malbrain ML, De Iaet I, Cheatham M. Consensus conference definitions and recommendations on intra-abdominal hypertension (IAH) and the abdominal compartment syndrome (ACS) – the long road to the final publications, how did we get there? *Acta Clin Belg Suppl* 2007;(1):44–59.
79. Cereda M, Weiss YG, Deutschman CS. The critically ill injured patient. Anesthesiol Clin 2007;25(1):13–21, vii.
80. Spinella PC, Priestley MA. Damage control mechanical ventilation: ventilator induced lung injury and lung protective strategies in children. *J Trauma* 2007;62(6 Suppl):S82–3.
81. Plurad D, Martin M, Green D, Salim A, Inaba K, Belzberg H, Demetriades D, Rhee P. The decreasing incidence of late posttraumatic acute respiratory distress syndrome: the potential role of lung protective ventilation and conservative transfusion practice. *J Trauma* 2007;63(1):1–7.
82. Martin GS, Mangialardi RJ, Wheeler AP, Dupont WD, Morris JA, Bernard GR. Albumin and furosemide therapy in hypoproteinemic patients with acute lung injury. Crit Care Med 2002;30(10):2175–82.

83. Putensen C. Volume-controlled versus biphasic positive airway pressure. Crit Care Med 1997;25(1):203–5.
84. Putensen C, Mutz NJ, Putensen-Himmer G, Zinserling J. Spontaneous breathing during ventilatory support improves ventilation-perfusion distributions in patients with acute respiratory distress syndrome. Am J Respir Crit Care Med 1999;159(4 Pt 1):1241–8.
85. The Acute Respiratory Distress Syndrome Network. Ventilation with lower tidal volumes as compared with traditional tidal volumes for acute lung injury and the acute respiratory distress syndrome. The Acute Respiratory Distress Syndrome Network. N Engl J Med 2000;342(18):1301–8.
86. Calfee CS, Eisner MD, Ware LB, Thompson BT, Parsons PE, Wheeler AP, Korpak A, Matthay MA, National Heart, Lung, and Blood Institute Acute Respiratory Distress Syndrome Network. Trauma-associated lung injury differs clinically and biologically from acute lung injury due to other clinical disorders. Crit Care Med 2007;35(10):2243–50.
87. Eisner MD, Thompson T, Hudson LD, Luce JM, Hayden D, Schoenfeld D, Matthay MA, the Acute Respiratory Distress Syndrome Network. Efficacy of low tidal volume ventilation in patients with different clinical risk factors for acute lung injury and the acute respiratory distress syndrome. Am J Respir Crit Care Med 2001;164(2):231–6.
88. Eisner MD, Thompson BT, Schoenfeld D, Anzueto A, Matthay MA. Airway pressures and early barotrauma in patients with acute lung injury and acute respiratory distress syndrome. Am J Respir Crit Care Med 2002;165(7):978–82.
89. Gajic O, Dara SI, Mendez JL, Adesanya AO, Festic E, Caples SM, Rana R, St. Sauver JL, Lymp JF, Afessa B, Hubmayr RD. Ventilator-associated lung injury in patients without acute lung injury at the onset of mechanical ventilation. Crit Care Med 2004;32(9):1817–24.
90. Wolthuis EK, Choi G, Dessing MC, Bresser PM, Lutter R, Dzoljic M, van der Poll T, Vroom MB, Hollmann M, Schultz MJ. Mechanical ventilation with lower tidal volumes and positive end-expiratory pressure prevents pulmonary inflammation in patients without preexisting lung injury. Anesthesiology 2008;108(1):46–54.
91. Chu EK, Whitehead T, Slutsky AS. Effects of cyclic opening and closing at low- and high-volume ventilation on bronchoalveolar lavage cytokines. Crit Care Med 2004;32(1):168–74.
92. Grasso S, Mascia L, Del TM, Del Turco M, Malacarne P, Giunta F, Brochard L, Slutsky AS, Marco Ranieri, V. Effects of recruiting maneuvers in patients with acute respiratory distress syndrome ventilated with protective ventilatory strategy. Anesthesiology 2002;96(4):795–802.
93. Friese RS, Shafi S, Gentilello LM. Pulmonary artery catheter use is associated with reduced mortality in severely injured patients: a National Trauma Data Bank analysis of 53,312 patients. Crit Care Med 2006;34(6):1597–601.
94. Chang MC, Black CS, Meredith JW. Volumetric assessment of preload in trauma patients: addressing the problem of mathematical coupling. Shock 1996;6(5):326–9.
95. Friese RS, Dineen S, Jennings A, Pruitt J, McBride D, Shafi S, Frankel H, Gentilello LM. Serum B-type natriuretic peptide: a marker of fluid resuscitation after injury? J Trauma 2007;62(6):1346–50.
96. Hannemann L, Reinhart K, Grenzer O, Meier-Hellmann A, Bredle DL. Comparison of dopamine to dobutamine and norepinephrine for oxygen delivery and uptake in septic shock. Crit Care Med 1995;23(12):1962–70.
97. Hsu TC, Su CF, Leu SC, Huang PC, Wang TE, Chu CH. Omeprazole is more effective than a histamine H2-receptor blocker for maintaining a persistent elevation of gastric pH after colon resection for cancer. Am J Surg 2004;187(1):20–3.
98. Lasky MR, Metzler MH, Phillips JO. A prospective study of omeprazole suspension to prevent clinically significant gastrointestinal bleeding from stress ulcers in mechanically ventilated trauma patients. J Trauma 1998;44(3):527–33.
99. Phillips JO, Metzler MH, Palmieri MT, Huckfeldt RE, Dahl NG. A prospective study of simplified omeprazole suspension for the prophylaxis of stress-related mucosal damage. *Crit Care Med* 1996;24(11):1793–800.

100. Cook D, Guyatt G, Marshall J, Leasa D, Fuller H, Hall R, Peters S, Rutledge F, Griffith L, McLellan A, Wood G, Kirby A, Tweeddale M, Pagliarello Johnston J, The Canadian Critical Care Trials Group. A comparison of sucralfate and ranitidine for the prevention of upper gastrointestinal bleeding in patients requiring mechanical ventilation. Canadian Critical Care Trials Group. *N Engl J Med* 1998;338(12):791–7.

101. Cook DJ, Fuller HD, Guyatt GH, Marshall JC, Leasa D, Hall R, Winton TL, Rutledge F, Todd T, Roy P, Lacroix J, Griffith L, Willan A, The Canadian Critical Care Trials Group. Risk factors for gastrointestinal bleeding in critically ill patients. Canadian Critical Care Trials Group. *N Engl J Med* 1994;330(6):377–81.

102. Kudsk KA, Croce MA, Fabian TC, Minard G, Tolley EA, Poret HA, Kuhl MR, Brown RO. Enteral versus parenteral feeding. Effects on septic morbidity after blunt and penetrating abdominal trauma. *Ann Surg* 1992;215(5):503–11.

103. Marik PE, Zaloga GP. Early enteral nutrition in acutely ill patients: a systematic review. *Crit Care Med* 2001;29(12):2264–70.

104. Moore EE, Dunn EL, Jones TN. Immediate jejunostomy feeding. Its use after major abdominal trauma. *Arch Surg* 1981;116(5):681–4.

105. Moore EE, Jones TN. Benefits of immediate jejunostomy feeding after major abdominal trauma – a prospective, randomized study. *J Trauma* 1986;26(10):874–81.

106. Moore FA, Feliciano DV, Andrassy RJ et al. Early enteral feeding, compared with parenteral, reduces postoperative septic complications. The results of a meta-analysis. *Ann Surg* 1992;216(2):172–83.

107. Scaife CL, Saffle JR, Morris SE. Intestinal obstruction secondary to enteral feedings in burn trauma patients. *J Trauma* 1999;47(5):859–63.

108. Schunn CD, Daly JM. Small bowel necrosis associated with postoperative jejunal tube feeding. *J Am Coll Surg* 1995;180(4):410–6.

109. Revelly JP, Tappy L, Berger MM, Gersbach P, Cayeux C, Chiolero R. Early metabolic and splanchnic responses to enteral nutrition in postoperative cardiac surgery patients with circulatory compromise. *Intensive Care Med* 2001;27(3):540–7.

110. Zaloga GP, Black KW, Prielipp R. Effect of rate of enteral nutrient supply on gut mass. *JPEN J Parenter Enteral Nutr* 1992;16(1):39–42.

111. Zaloga GP, Roberts P. Permissive underfeeding. *New Horiz* 1994;2(2):257–63.

112. Krishnan JA, Parce PB, Martinez A, Diette GB, Brower RG. Caloric intake in medical ICU patients: consistency of care with guidelines and relationship to clinical outcomes. *Chest* 2003;124(1):297–305.

113. Rubinson L, Diette GB, Song X, Brower RG, Krishnan JA. Low caloric intake is associated with nosocomial bloodstream infections in patients in the medical intensive care unit. *Crit Care Med* 2004;32(2):350–7.

114. Collier B, Guillamondegui O, Cotton B, Donahue R, Conrad A, Groh K, Richman J, Vogel T, Miller R, Diaz Jr J. Feeding the open abdomen. *JPEN J Parenter Enteral Nutr* 2007;31(5):410–5.

115. Cheatham ML, Safcsak K, Brzezinski SJ, Lube MW. Nitrogen balance, protein loss, and the open abdomen. *Crit Care Med* 2007;35(1):127–31.

116. Radhakrishnan RS, Xue H, Moore-Olufemi SD, Weisbrodt NW, Moore FA, Allen SJ, Laine GA, Cox Jr CS. Hypertonic saline resuscitation prevents hydrostatically induced intestinal edema and ileus. *Crit Care Med* 2006;34(6):1713–8.

117. Vassar MJ, Fischer RP, O'Brien PE, Bachulis BL, Chambers JA, Hoyt DB, Holcroft JW. A multicenter trial for resuscitation of injured patients with 7.5% sodium chloride. The effect of added dextran 70. The Multicenter Group for the Study of Hypertonic Saline in Trauma Patients. *Arch Surg* 1993;128(9):1003–11.

118. Hess JR, Holcomb JB, Hoyt DB. Damage control resuscitation: the need for specific blood products to treat the coagulopathy of trauma. *Transfusion* 2006;46(5):685–6.

119. Madigan MC, Kemp CD, Johnson JC, Cotton BA. Secondary abdominal compartment syndrome after severe extremity injury: are early, aggressive fluid resuscitation strategies to blame? *J Trauma* 2008;64(2):280–5.

120. Merten GJ, Burgess WP, Gray LV, Holleman JH, Roush TS,. Kowalchuk GJ, Bersin RM, Van Moore A, Simonton III CA, Rittase RA, Norton HJ, Kennedy TP. Prevention of contrast-induced nephropathy with sodium bicarbonate: a randomized controlled trial. *JAMA* 2004;291(19):2328–34.
121. Ligtenberg JJ, Girbes AR, Beentjes JA, Tulleken JE, van der Werf TS, Zijlstra JG. Hormones in the critically ill patient: to intervene or not to intervene? *Intensive Care Med* 2001;27(10):1567–77.
122. Annane D, Sebille V, Charpentier C, Bollaert P-E, François B, Korach J-M, Capellier M, Cohen Y, Azoulay E, Troché G, Chaumet-Riffaut P, Bellissant E. Effect of treatment with low doses of hydrocortisone and fludrocortisone on mortality in patients with septic shock. *JAMA* 2002;288(7):862–71.
123. Van den BG, Wouters P, Weekers F, Verwaest C, Bruyninckx F, Schetz M, Vlasselaers D, Ferdinande P, Lauwers P, Bouillon R. Intensive insulin therapy in the critically ill patients. *N Engl J Med* 2001;345(19):1359–67.
124. Bochicchio GV, Sung J, Joshi M, Bochicchio K, Johnson SB, Meyer W, Scalea TM. Persistent hyperglycemia is predictive of outcome in critically ill trauma patients. *J Trauma* 2005;58(5):921–4.
125. Laird AM, Miller PR, Kilgo PD, Meredith JW, Chang MC. Relationship of early hyperglycemia to mortality in trauma patients. *J Trauma* 2004;56(5):1058–62.
126. Marik PE, Varon J. Intensive insulin therapy in the ICU: is it now time to jump off the bandwagon? *Resuscitation* 2007;74(1):191–3.
127. Cotton BA, Guillamondegui OD, Fleming SB, Carpenter RO, Patel SH, Morris Jr JA, Arbogast PG. Increased risk of adrenal insufficiency following etomidate exposure in critically injured patients. *Arch Surg* 2008;143(1):62–7.
128. Gannon TA, Britt RC, Weireter LJ, Cole FJ, Collins JN, Britt LD. Adrenal insufficiency in the critically III trauma population. *Am Surg* 2006;72(5):373–6.
129. Fabian TC, Croce MA, Payne LW, Minard G, Pritchard FE, Kudsk KA. Duration of antibiotic therapy for penetrating abdominal trauma: a prospective trial. *Surgery* 1992;112(4):788–94.
130. Luchette FA, Borzotta AP, Croce MA, O'Neill PA, Whittmann DH, Mullins CD, Palumbo F, Pasquale MD. Practice management guidelines for prophylactic antibiotic use in penetrating abdominal trauma: the EAST Practice Management Guidelines Work Group. *J Trauma* 2000;48(3):508–18.
131. Shatz DV, Romero-Steiner S, Elie CM, Holder PF, Carlone GM. Antibody responses in postsplenectomy trauma patients receiving the 23-valent pneumococcal polysaccharide vaccine at 14 versus 28 days postoperatively. *J Trauma* 2002;53(6):1037–42.
132. Suliburk JW, Ware DN, Balogh Z, McKinley BA, Cocanour CS, Kozar RA, Moore FA. Vacuum-assisted wound closure achieves early fascial closure of open abdomens after severe trauma. *J Trauma* 2003;55(6):1155–60.
133. Gracias VH, Braslow B, Johnson J, Pryor J, Gupta R, Reilly P, Schwab CW. Abdominal compartment syndrome in the open abdomen. *Arch Surg* 2002;137(11):1298–300.
134. Cheatham ML, Malbrain ML, Kirkpatrick A, Sugrue M, Parr M, De Waele J, Balogh Z, Leppäniemi A, Olvera C, Ivatury R, D'Amours S, Wendon J, Hillman K, Johansson K, Kolkman K, Wilmer A. Results from the International Conference of Experts on Intra-abdominal Hypertension and Abdominal Compartment Syndrome. II. Recommendations. *Intensive Care Med* 2007;33(6):951–62.
135. Malbrain ML, Cheatham ML, Kirkpatrick A, Sugrue M, Parr M, De Waele J, Balogh Z, Leppäniemi A, Olvera C, Ivatury R, D'Amours S, Wendon J, Hillman K, Johansson K, Kolkman K, Wilmer A. Results from the International Conference of Experts on Intra-abdominal Hypertension and Abdominal Compartment Syndrome. I. Definitions. *Intensive Care Med* 2006;32(11):1722–32.
136. Martin RR, Byrne M. Postoperative care and complications of damage control surgery. *Surg Clin North Am* 1997;77(4):929–42.
137. Hirshberg A, Mattox KL. Planned reoperation for severe trauma. *Ann Surg* 1995;222(1):3–8.

138. Grossman MD, Born C. Tertiary survey of the trauma patient in the intensive care unit. *Surg Clin North Am* 2000;80(3):805–24.
139. Vargo DJ, Battistella FD. Abbreviated thoracotomy and temporary chest closure: an application of damage control after thoracic trauma. *Arch Surg* 2001;136(1):21–4.
140. Phelan HA, Patterson SG, Hassan MO, Gonzalez RP, Rodning CB. Thoracic damage-control operation: principles, techniques, and definitive repair. *J Am Coll Surg* 2006;203(6):933–41.
141. McArthur BJ. Damage control surgery for the patient who has experienced multiple traumatic injuries. *AORN J* 2006;84(6):992–1000.
142. Kaplan LJ, Trooskin SZ, Santora TA. Thoracic compartment syndrome. *J Trauma* 1996;40(2):291–3.
143. Chambers LW, Green DJ, Sample K, Gillingham BL, Rhee P, Brown C, Narine N, Uecker JM, Bohman HR. Tactical surgical intervention with temporary shunting of peripheral vascular trauma sustained during Operation Iraqi Freedom: one unit's experience. *J Trauma* 2006;61(4):824–30.
144. Sriussadaporn S, Pak-art R. Temporary intravascular shunt in complex extremity vascular injuries. *J Trauma* 2002;52(6):1129–33.

Chapter 11
Phase III: Second Operation Repair of All Injuries General and Orthopedics

General

Benjamin Braslow and C. William Schwab

11.1 Timing of Damage Control Phase III

The primary objectives of Damage Control Phase III (DC III) are definitive organ repair and fascial closure. Timing for this stage is critical to successful outcomes. The decision to proceed is predicated upon all physiological and biochemical deficits being corrected. The patient should be normothermic, have normal coagulation studies, have a normal pH, and have normal lactate. This state usually takes 24–36 h to achieve following aggressive ICU management. During this time, a complete tertiary survey of potential missed injuries, particularly extremity soft tissue and orthopedic injuries, is performed. An incidence of missed injuries of 10–20% has been reported in similar patient populations [1]. Additional necessary radiographic and ancillary studies must be completed. Planning by surgical specialty consultants for definitive management of associated injuries is initiated during this time. Occasionally, the timing of definitive repair is influenced by other clinical circumstances. One pressing concern that often leads to early planned reoperation is salvage of an ischemic limb due to shunt occlusion or suboptimal vascular repair following restoration of a normal coagulation profile. Other situations in which early planned reoperation is advisable include: (1) bowel that has been interrupted at several sites, resulting in a closed loop obstruction mechanism that threatens bowel viability and (2) suboptimal control of spillage at the initial laparotomy from packed or drained duodenal, pancreas, kidney, or bladder disruption.

11.2 Damage Control Phase III Techniques

Once in the operating room, the patient is prepped and draped appropriately for the definitive repairs ahead. The temporary abdominal dressing is prepped into the field prior to removal and subsequent exposure of the abdominal contents. All packs are

B. Braslow (✉) and C.W. Schwab
Department of Surgery, University of Pennsylvania School of Medicine, Philadelphia, PA, 19104, USA
e-mail: benjamin.braslow@uphs.upenn.edu

H.-C. Pape et al. (eds.), *Damage Control Management in the Polytrauma Patient*,
DOI 10.1007/978-0-387-89508-6_11, © Springer Science+Business Media, LLC 2010

copiously irrigated and carefully removed, teasing them slowly away from all surfaces to avoid clot disruption. A key aspect in unpacking is that the surgeon must be prepared to stop abruptly and minimize losses if the patient decompensates hemodynamically. On pack removal, if bleeding is encountered that does not originate from an accessible vascular injury and when repeated attempts to control it using local hemostatic measures fail, immediate repacking is the safest course of action to prevent massive blood loss and recurrent physiological deterioration.

11.3 Vascular Repairs

Following successful pack removal, a complete reexamination of the abdominal contents should occur, with particular attention paid to any previous repairs made during Damage Control Phase I (DC I). Significant injuries are often overlooked or only partially defined during the rapidly performed initial laparotomy in an exsanguinating unstable patient. Additional sites of bleeding are controlled, and vascular repairs are performed. If a temporary vascular shunt is in place, the shunt is removed and a Fogarty balloon catheter is passed distally to retrieve any distal clots. Proximal clots are passed by allowing brief spurts of forward flow from the severed vessel. The arterial or venous wall is then trimmed so that the sites of the ligatures or Rummel tourniquets that secured the shunt are not incorporated into the suture line, as these areas usually have sustained full thickness injury [2]. The injury zone is carefully assessed and debrided to exclude any compromised intima or muscular wall. This is especially important when wounds were a result of high velocity or military weaponry. Here the zone of injury can extend in a delayed fashion well beyond the actual missile trajectory secondary to shock wave dissemination [3]. The choice of conduit for interposition grafts depends on the "location" of the injury and the "extent of contamination." In general, reversed autologous vein interposition grafts are best for abdominal vascular repairs, especially in the setting of concomitant bowel or solid organ injury [4]. Cryopreserved artery and vein conduits offer a infection-resistant alternative to autologous vein, but they are very expensive and often not readily available at most hospitals. Polytetrafluoroethylene (PTFE) and Dacron grafts serve well in uncontaminated or only minimally contaminated fields (i.e., proximal extremity injuries from low-velocity missiles), which is rarely the case in laparotomy for damage control.

11.4 Gastrointestinal Repairs

In the majority of patients, delayed primary small bowel and colon anastomosis following destructive injury has been proven to be a safe alternative to stoma creation within the damage control sequence [5, 6]. If fascial closure is not possible, percutaneous feeding tubes and stomas should be avoided, as they are associated with a high complication (leak) rate and make subsequent mobilization and separation of abdominal wall components difficult when closure is eventually performed. Instead, primary anastamoses should be created for gastrointestinal continuity, and both nasogastric tubes and nasoduodenal tubes should be placed and directed into position intraoperatively for proximal decompression and feeding, respectively. Intestinal continuity is restored using standard anastomatic techniques. No study to date has definitively answered the debate over which anastomotic technique is best, especially in this patient population. Some argue that because the damage control sequence often produces edematous bowel secondary to large volume resuscitations with or without concomitant reperfusion injury, handsewn anastomoses are best [7]. The authors note that standard gastrointestinal anastomotic stapling devices are designed for bowel of normal thickness and that edematous bowel makes full closure of the individual staples dubious. This in turn leads to a breakdown of the anastomosis, manifested by either dehiscence when edema is considerable or abscess development when the swelling is not severe enough to completely disrupt the mechanical anastomosis. Stapling proponents claim that stapling is the more efficient anastomotic technique and has not been definitively shown to increase the incidence of abdominal complications in the trauma patient [8, 9]. Regardless of the technique used, any bowel anastomoses should be covered with omentum and/or tucked under mesentery to provide the greatest degree of protection and promote sealing [10]. Some authors believe that if creation of a stoma becomes necessary, it should be placed laterally (lateral to the rectus abdominus muscles) through the obliques. Ideally, an ostomy should lie between the anterior and midaxillary line of the abdominal wall.

11.5   Abdominal Closure

11.5.1   Primary and Delayed Primary Closures

Once all of the repairs are completed, formal abdominal closure without tension is the final step in the planned reoperation sequence. Primary fascial closure is the most preferable closure technique. Maneuvers to temporarily approximate the fascial edges should be performed with clamps. If gentle abduction allows the fascial edges to approximate, a standard fascial closure should be possible. The risk of enterocutaneous fistula (ECF) and recurrent wound problems appears to be lower when primary fascial closure is achieved early. In fact, delayed primary fascial closure before 8 days has been associated with the best outcomes and the fewest complications [11]. However, formal closure may be delayed days to weeks as physiology improves and edema lessens.

Persistent edema within the retroperitoneum, bowel wall, and abdominal wall often renders primary fascial closure impossible at the time of the original take back operation following DC I and DC II. Attempting to close too large a defect can lead to abdominal hypertension and subsequent abdominal compartment syndrome with its associated multisystem physiological demise. Patients who develop this syndrome will require emergent reoperation to release pressure by reopening the abdomen.

A determination will need to be made at the time of closure as to the tension that will be placed on the abdomen and whether it can be closed primarily. The surgeon's judgment is most important here. In general, if the bowels can be seen above the level of the skin when the abdomen is viewed from across the operating room table, then a low-tension primary closure is unlikely. Generally, a gap >10 cm between fascial edges cannot be successfully closed primarily [12] (Fig. 11.1). Another good rule to follow is that if the peak airway pressure rises >10 cmH$_2$O during temporary fascial approximation, then the fascia should be left open and a vacuum dressing is reapplied. The patient is then returned to the ICU, and aggressive diuresis is implemented over the next several days if hemodynamically tolerated. This helps to decrease bowel and body wall edema. During this period, the patient undergoes a daily abdominal washout, reinspection, and meticulous replacement of the vacuum dressing so as not to promote fistula formation. Preventing lateral retraction of the myofascial unit and gradual fascial reapproximation are also essential during this time. These subsequent washouts and vacuum dressing changes can occur at the bedside if personnel and resources are readily available. The majority of damage controlled open abdomens can be primarily closed within 7–10 days, especially if there is no sign of intra-abdominal infection [13].

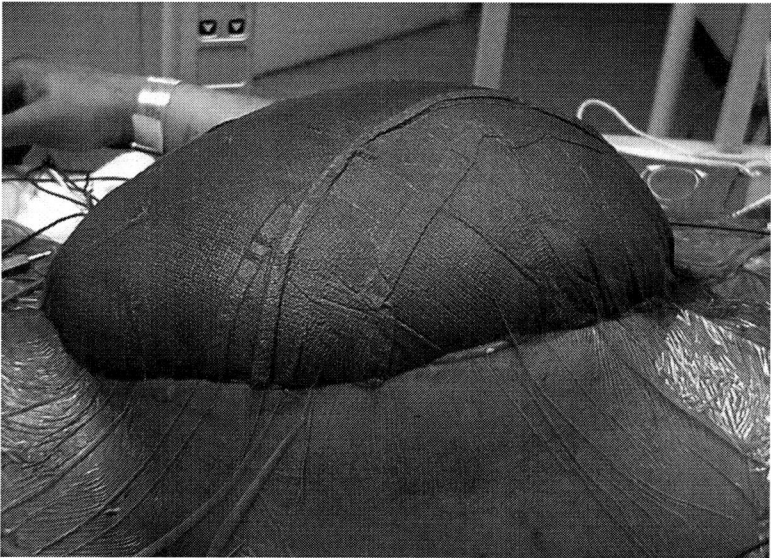

Fig. 11.1 Lateral view of damage control abdomen depicting bowel contents above level of skin

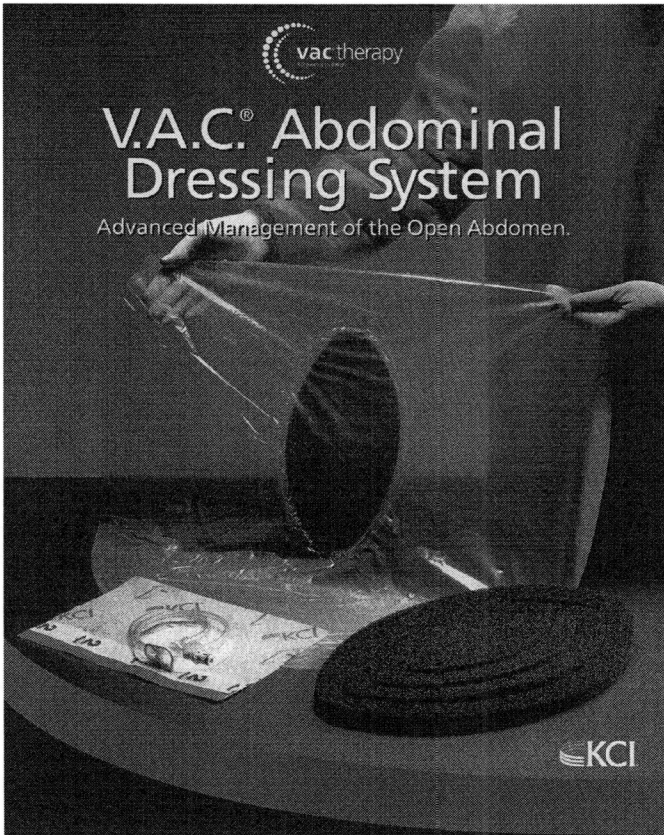

Fig. 11.2   KCI V.A.C.® Abdominal Dressing System (Courtesy of KCI Licensing, Inc., 2008)

Following DC I, the authors have adopted the use of the KCI V.A.C®Abdominal Dressing System (KCI, San Antonio, Texas) (Figs. 11.2–11.4) as our primary damage control dressing. The oval-shaped sponge within the fenestrated nonadherent layer is centered over the wound. The edges of this sheet are trimmed if needed and packed down to the gutters, pelvis, and over the liver. This prevents adherence of the abdominal contents to the underside of the abdominal wall, thus allowing the abdominal wall to slide back toward the midline under negative pressure. Next, the unencapsulated foam ovals are trimmed to the appropriate width to fill the gap between the fascial edges without impeding movement of the fascia toward the midline once suction is applied. The depth of the additional foam sponges should be adequate to apply suction to all layers of the abdominal wall from skin to peritoneum. Several full-thickness subcutaneous sutures are then placed to seal the sponges in place, and gentle tension is further applied on the abdominal wall toward the midline. Excessive tension must be avoided to prevent fascial necrosis. Finally,

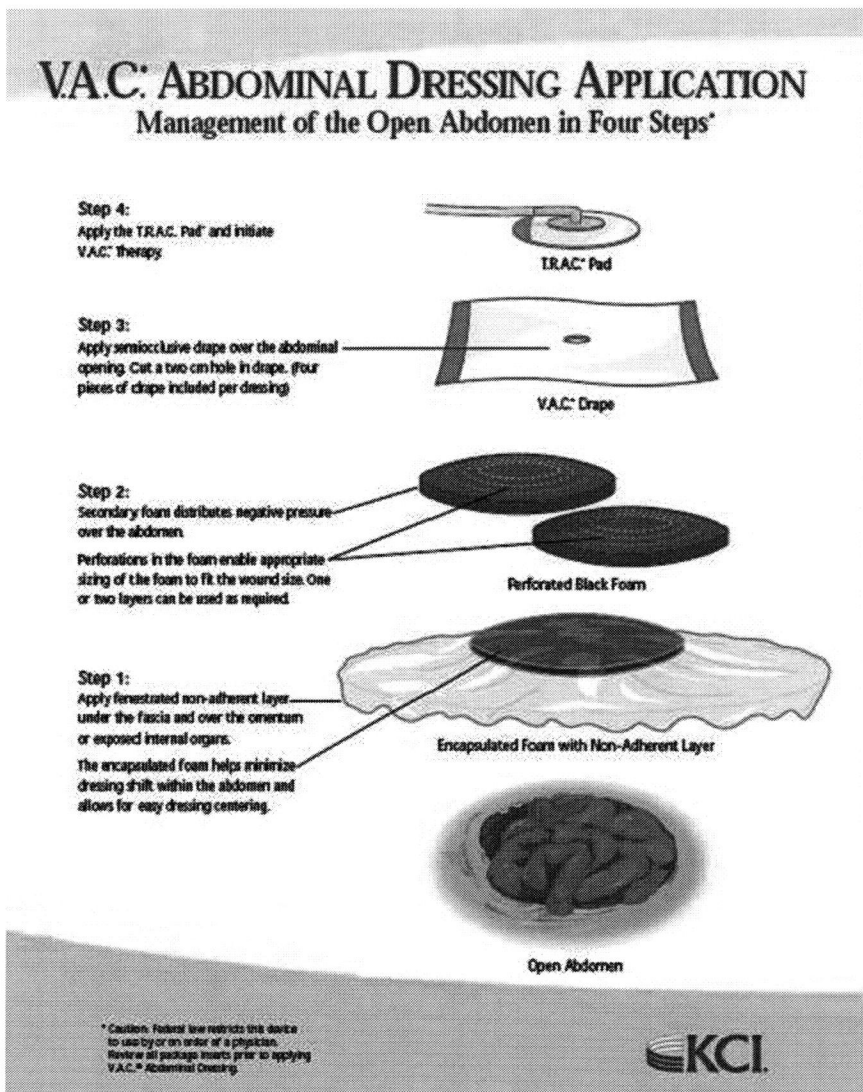

V.A.C. ABDOMINAL DRESSING APPLICATION
Management of the Open Abdomen in Four Steps*

Step 4:
Apply the T.R.A.C. Pad* and initiate
V.A.C.* therapy.

T.R.A.C.* Pad

Step 3:
Apply semiocclusive drape over the abdominal
opening. Cut a two cm hole in drape. (Four
pieces of drape included per dressing)

V.A.C.* Drape

Step 2:
Secondary foam distributes negative pressure
over the abdomen.

Perforations in the foam enable appropriate
sizing of the foam to fit the wound size. One
or two layers can be used as required.

Perforated Black Foam

Step 1:
Apply fenestrated non-adherent layer
under the fascia and over the omentum
or exposed internal organs.

The encapsulated foam helps minimize
dressing shift within the abdomen and
allows for easy dressing centering.

Encapsulated Foam with Non-Adherent Layer

Open Abdomen

*Caution: Federal law restricts this device
to use by or on order of a physician.
Review all package inserts prior to applying
V.A.C.* Abdominal Dressing.

KCI

Fig. 11.3 KCI V.A.C.® Abdominal Dressing Application (Courtesy of KCI Licensing Inc., 2008)

the outer adherent occlusive drape is applied over the entire wound, and the appropriate tubing is applied to allow for connection to the suction device. Suction should be applied within the 100–125 mmHg range. The patient is returned to the OR every 48 h subsequently for abdominal washout and attempted fascial closure.

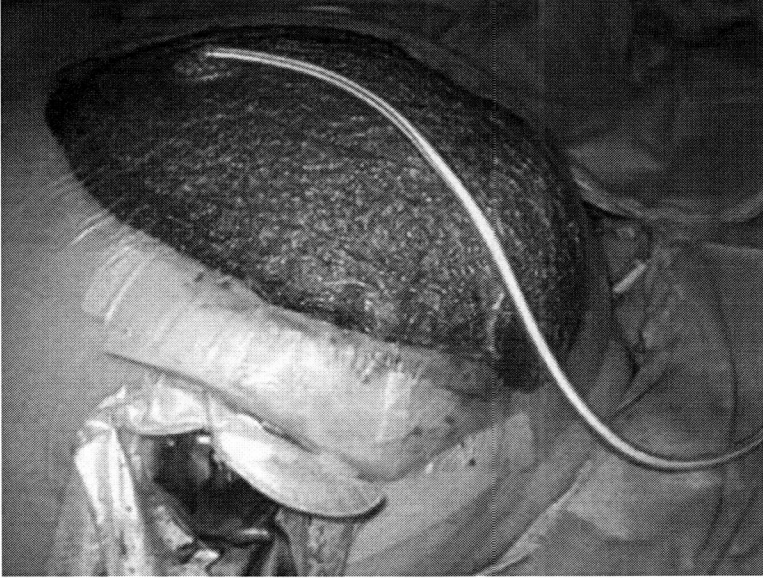

Fig. 11.4 In situ placement of KCI V.A.C.® Abdominal Dressing System (KCI, San Antonio, TX)

If closure is not possible at that time, the system is replaced and the overlying sponges are tailored to the changing dimensions of the abdominal wall.

The authors have occasionally utilized a device known as the Wittmann Patch™ (Star Surgical, Inc., Burlington, Wisconsin) in the past to assist in stepwise fascial closure during the period of diuresis. This device consists of two thin sheets of semirigid material composed of a nonadherent undersurface with a Velcro-like material on the outer surface. Tiny perforations are present over the sheets to allow for the egress of third spaced fluids. These sheets are sutured to the fascia on both sides of the abdominal wound, and when overlapped with slight tension, they allow for partial fascial approximation without threat of loss of domain (Fig. 11.5). The fascia is in effect trained under minimal tension, and the gap between its edges can be slowly obliterated as the patch is trimmed and the defect more closely approximated with each subsequent daily abdominal washout. The nonadherent smooth undersurface prevents fistula formation as the bowel wall is not irritated by contact. The patch is removed prior to definitive fascial closure. A limiting factor in the decision to use this device is its relatively high cost.

Alternatively, a stepwise silo-type closure can be performed utilizing some form of durable nonadherent material (i.e., an opened 3-liter intravenous bag sewn to the fascial edges) in a manner similar to that described in the pediatric surgical literature for neonates with an omphalocele or gastroschisis [14]. Gradual reduction in the size of the silo, and hence the wound, is achieved as the bag is incised, trimmed, and sutured closed during subsequent abdominal washout procedures.

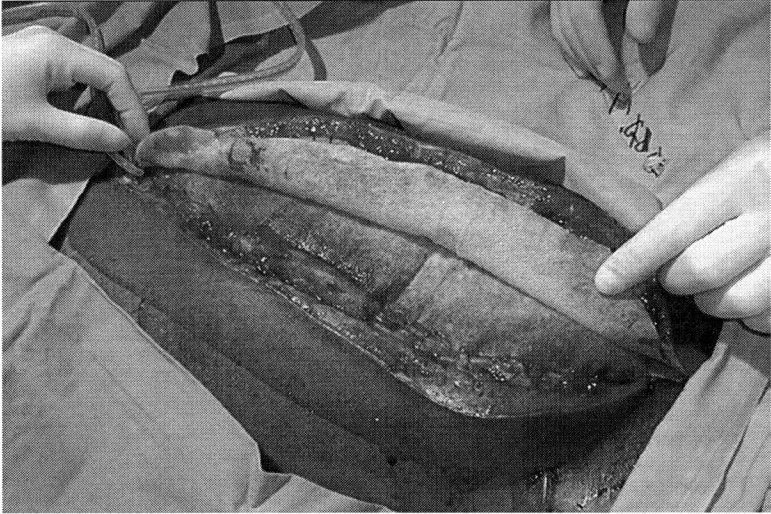

Fig. 11.5 Wittmann Patch™ (Star Surgical, Inc., Burlington, WI) in situ

11.6 Retained Foreign Bodies

The emergent nature of the trauma damage control laparotomy increases the likelihood of retained foreign body [15]. Multiple sponges used for packing as well as certain instruments (vascular clamps, Rumell tourniquets, etc.) are initially intentionally left in the abdomen. These may be unrecognized and left behind after definitive closure, ultimately requiring reexploration and removal.

Do not rely on sponge counts at the time of definitive closure. Obtain an intraoperative abdominal radiograph to ensure no that retained foreign bodies are present prior to proceeding with closure. Be sure that the radiograph displays the entire abdominal cavity. For obese patients, multiple radiographs might be necessary to properly view all four abdominal quadrants.

11.7 Planned Ventral Hernias

Approximately 20% of DC patients fail primary fascial closure and are managed as open abdominal wounds or large ventral hernias. If fascial closure is still not achieved after 7–10 days, the surgeon faces a number of alternatives that will cover the abdominal defect but leave the patient with a large ventral hernia. The first of these involves closing the skin with no attempt at fascial reapproximation. The patient would then undergo repair of the abdominal wall defect several months later. Often, this is not possible as the gap is too wide and, despite skin flap mobilization, the edges cannot be approximated [16].

In a second option, a vicryl (polyglycolic acid) mesh is placed over the entire abdominal wall defect and sutured to the fascial edges or the skin. The vicryl mesh is then covered with saline-soaked wet-to-dry dressings. It is always advisable to drape the greater omentum, if still available, over the bowel so that frequent dressing changes do not promote formation of enteric fistulae. Careful daily dressing changes are performed over this mesh, and the wound is allowed to granulate through the material. Do not allow the intestine to become desiccated. Once a smooth bed of granulation tissue is established (2–3 weeks), a sponge vacuum dressing can then be applied to promote faster granulation.

11.8   Fistula Management in Planned Ventral Hernias

During this process, exposed suture lines, anastomoses, or bowel wall exposed to the mesh or fascial edges may result in the formation of an enteroatmospheric fistulae (Fig. 11.6). Desiccation along with frequent manipulation (i.e., dressing or VAC changes) of the granulating wound compound this risk. An enteroatmospheric fistula is inherently problematic because it lacks a formal fistula tract and overlying well-vascularized soft tissue; therefore, there is no chance that the fistula will close spontaneously, even in the absence of distal obstruction or malnutrition [17]. These can be even more challenging to manage than classic ECF due to the lack of skin on which to apply an ostomy appliance to control drainage. The same principles apply here as to ECF, with the addition of the necessity to provide skin coverage around the fistula site. The anatomy of the fistula (what segment of small bowel or colon is involved) needs to be determined by some kind of contrast radiological study. Likewise, output should be classified as high or low, with the knowledge that high-output fistulae (>300 cc/day) often mandate total parenteral nutritional support and are less likely to close spontaneously without operative repair. It is most important not to attempt split thickness skin grafts until the fistula drainage is controlled, so as to not jeopardize the chance for a successful take. Goverman et al. described the use of a "fistula VAC" technique for the management of enteroatmospheric fistulae arising within the open abdomen (Fig. 11.7) [18]. This technique incorporates standard vacuum dressing supplies and an ostomy appliance. Here, the VAC is not used to close the fistulae but rather to control the "perifistula" environment. The wound surrounding the fistula is treated with the vacuum-assisted device, whereas the enteric contents are completely diverted into an ostomy appliance placed over the fistula, which is segregated from the granulation tissue by a bioocclusive dressing. It may be necessary to stage the split thickness skin grafts. By allowing the fistula output to drain opposite the side of grafting, half of the wound area can be covered before proceeding with grafting the remainder of the wound and allowing the output to drain out the grafted side. This can be accomplished by temporarily positioning the patient in ways to allow gravity to determine the direction of drainage.

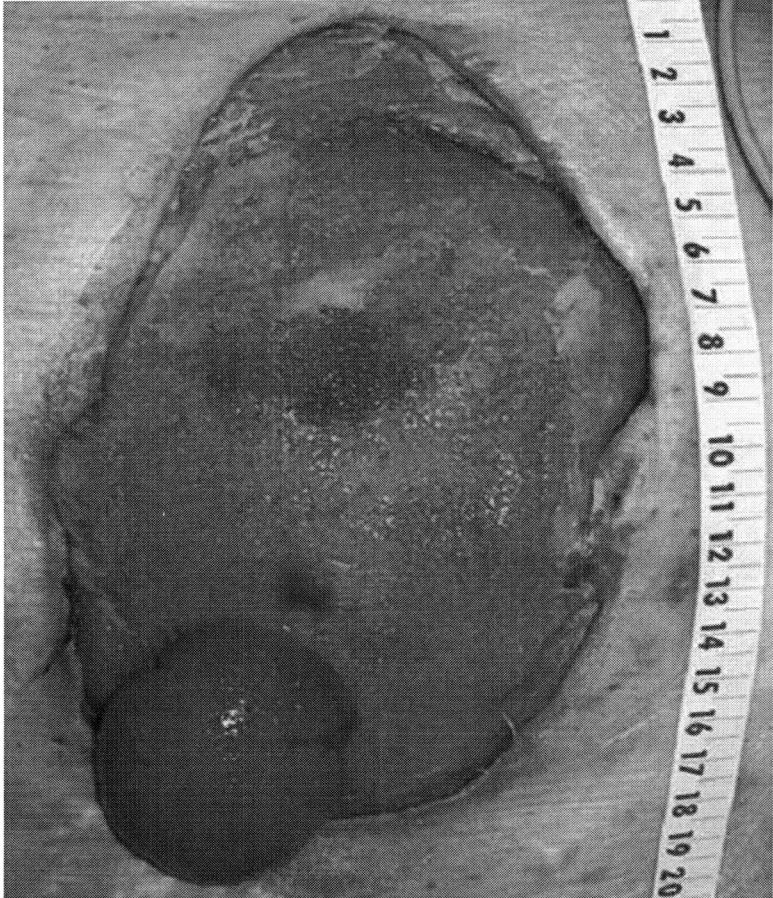

Fig. 11.6 Enteroatmospheric fistulae in open granulating abdominal wound

Another novel approach to the management of enteroatmospheric fistulae is the use of biological dressings. Several groups have described the application of human acellular dermal matrix and fibrin glue to small enteroatmospheric fistulae. Meshed cadaveric skin was also applied to the surrounding abdominal contents to prevent desiccation and contact with dressings. A near 50% closure rate was achieved with this technique [19, 20].

11.9 Definitive Abdominal Wall Reconstruction

The next phase of the planned ventral hernia sequence involves the placement of an autologous split thickness skin graft to the wound once the granulation bed matures. As stated earlier, even the presence of an enteroatmospheric fistula does

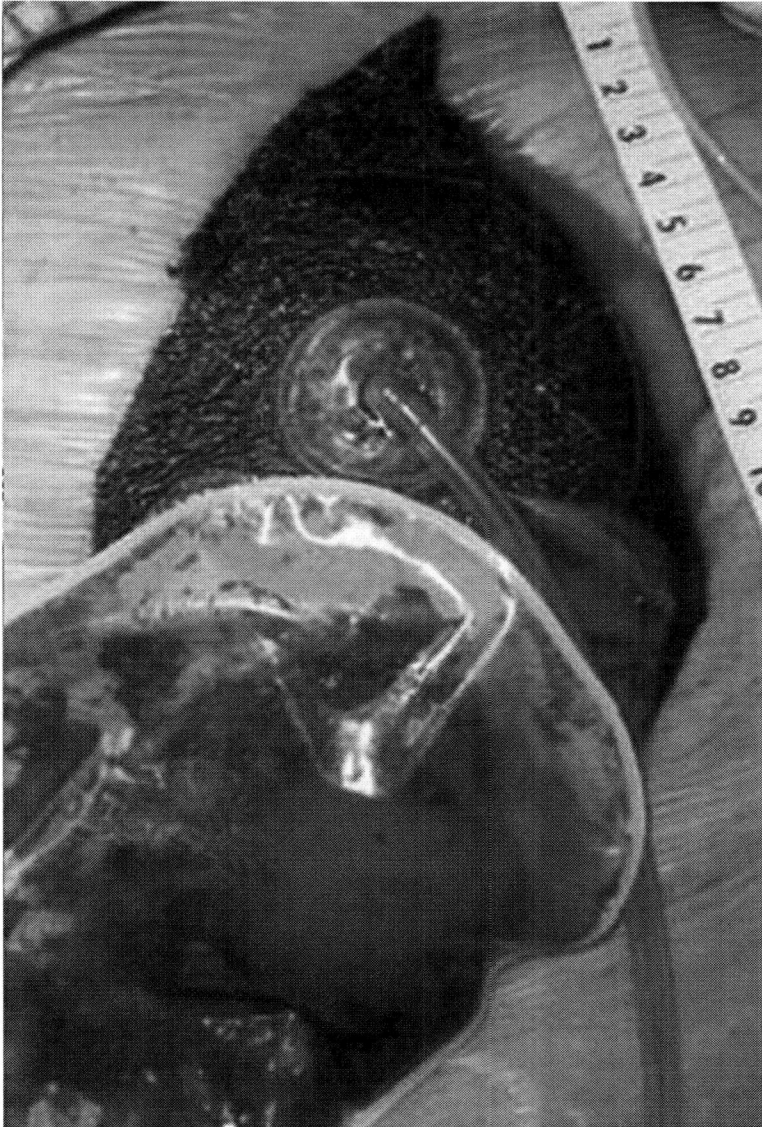

Fig. 11.7 Fistula VAC in situ. Combination of KCI V.A.C® System (KCI, San Antonio, TX) and ostomy appliance

not preclude this step, it just complicates it technically. Over the next 6–12 months, this skin graft will mature, separate, and develop a thin layer of connective tissue or fat between the underlying viscera (Fig. 11.8). At this point, the patient is ready for excision of the skin graft and definitive reconstruction. Many reconstructive techniques have been described in the literature, including the use of preoperative

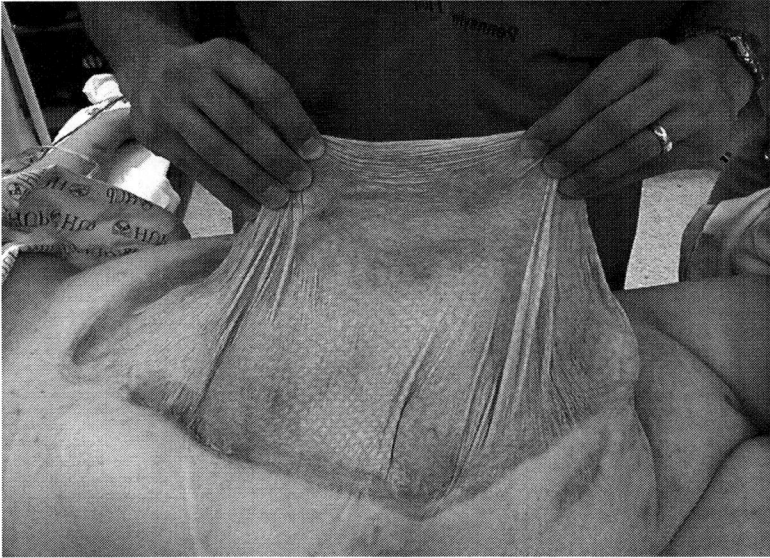

Fig. 11.8 Skin graft separation assessment (the "pinch test")

tissue expanders [21] and abdominal wall component separation with bilateral rectus release to achieve primary component closure with extrafascial mesh support [22]. Here, the external oblique aponeurosis is incised approximately 2 cm lateral to the rectus sheath and separated from the internal oblique (Figs. 11.9 and 11.10). This allows the rectus muscle to be approximated medially and sutured. Various modifications of this technique have been described [23]. The involvement of a plastic surgeon at this step is advisable to lend additional expertise at this delayed setting. Dense abdominal adhesions will make the dissection of the skin graft off of the intestines very difficult. This may lead to prolonged operative times and increase the likelihood of enterotomy, thus contaminating the operative field.

To avoid this scenario, wait at least 6–12 months before scheduling a patient for reconstruction. All acute processes of the original pathology must be resolved, nutritional status must be satisfactory, and the abdomen must pass the "pinch test": The skin graft is pinched and is able to be elevated off of the abdominal contents without palpable adhesions.

There are many alternatives to complex abdominal wall reconstructions. Nonabsorbable mesh is often used to bridge the gap between fascial edges. Unfortunately, this is associated with high recurrence and fistula rates [24, 25]. The main advantage of permanent mesh closure is avoidance of complex abdominal wall reconstruction. Options for permanent prosthesis include polypropylene, expanded polytetrafluoroethylene (ePTFE), composite material, and biological material.

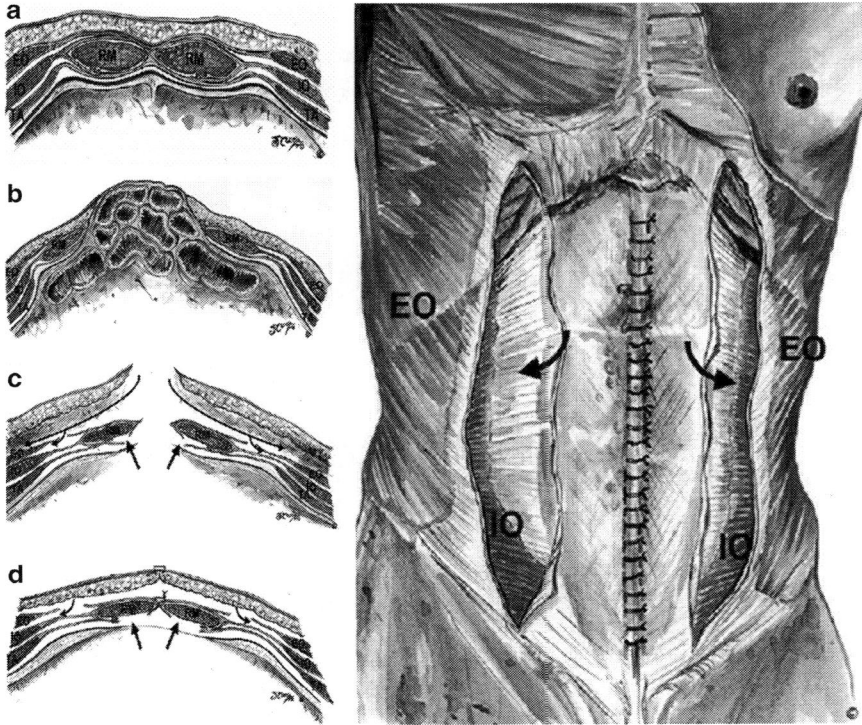

Fig. 11.9 ABCD. Stages of component separation, abdominal wall reconstruction: Schematic rendition. (Reprinted from Rutherford et al. [25]; with permission from Elsevier)

Polypropylene mesh incorporates well (usually within 2 weeks) secondary to fibroblastic reaction, but it can have problems with shrinkage, adhesion formation, seroma and infection (5%), and late recurrence. The ECF rate is approximately 3%. ePTFE has less fibroblastic reaction and adhesions than polypropylene and so has an increased recurrence rate. Although ePTFE can be placed adjacent to bowel, ECF remains a problem. This material is also more expensive than polypropylene. A composite material is available, made up as a "sandwich" of ePTFE placed down on the bowel and polypropylene facing up. This allows an intraperitoneal placement and combines the advantages of both materials while minimizing complications.

There are also many biological materials available for complex abdominal wall closures. Derived from the extracellular matrix (ECM) of animal or human tissue or cadaveric fascia, these materials have a decreased incidence of infection and ECF. Their use is preferred in contaminated wounds. Surgisis® (CBI, West Lafayette, Indiana) is derived from porcine small intestinal submucosa. It is composed mostly of type I collagen from the ECM and is acellular. It has been used

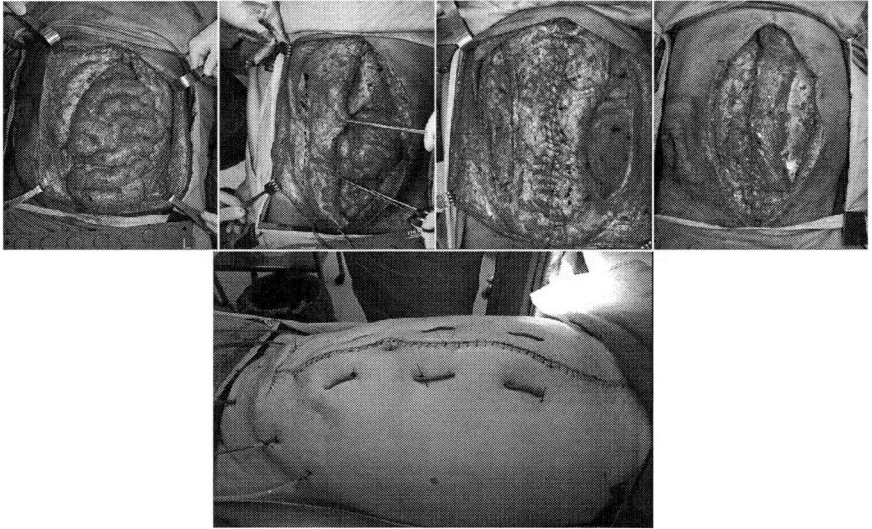

Fig. 11.10 Stages of component separation, abdominal wall reconstruction: Actual human images

successfully in contaminated wounds [26, 27]. Alloderm® (LifeCell Corporation, Branchburg, New Jersey) is human acellular dermis from processed cadaveric skin (Figs. 11.11 and 11.12). It consists of the basement membrane and a dermal collagen matrix. There is no antigenic response, and alloderm has been shown to be effective in abdominal wall reconstruction in patients at increased risk for mesh-related complications [28]. One drawback is its significant expense. Permacol® (Covidien, Mansfield, Massachusetts), a porcine dermal collagen, is another biological material that has been on the market since 2001. These materials work best when placed under tension as an underlay patch with interrupted U-type stitches through a 2–4 cm fascial border. This technique promotes more tensile strength and prolonged integrity while ingrowth of fibroblasts and collagen deposition proceeds.

11.10   Summary and Conclusion

Phase III of the damage control sequence requires meticulous planning and execution. During this phase, the abdomen is reinspected and all definitive vascular and visceral repairs are performed if possible. A "bailout" plan must be in place if the patient decompensates at any point physiologically or if nonsurgical bleeding develops. Attempts at primary fascial closure should be performed to limit subsequent morbidity from the open abdomen; However, if anatomic or physiological

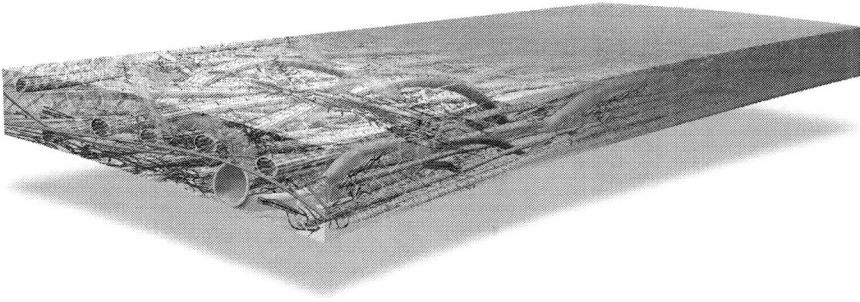

Fig. 11.11 Alloderm® structural schematic (Image courtesy of LifeCell Corporation, Branchburg, New Jersey)

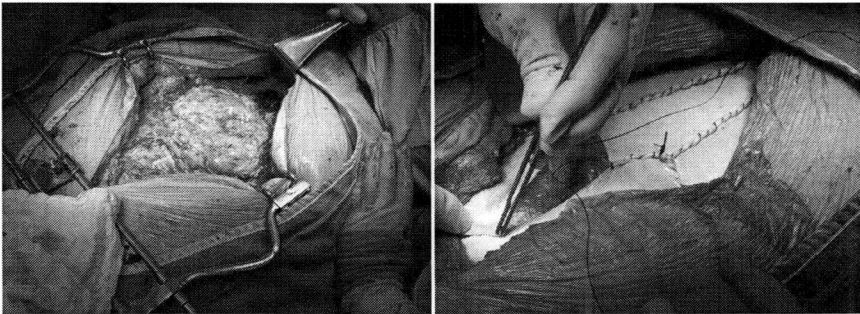

Fig. 11.12 Alloderm® (LifeCell Corporation, Branchburg, New Jersey) placement for abdominal wall reconstruction (in situ)

parameters do not allow this, VAC replacement should be performed with sequential washouts and fascial training toward the midline. Meticulous care of the open abdomen must be taken to limit morbidity, specifically the formation of an enteroatmospheric fistula. Eventual skin coverage is achieved followed by delayed planned complex ventral hernia repair within 8–12 months.

References

1. Hirshberg A, Wall MJ Jr., Mattox KL. Planned reoperation for trauma: A two year experience with 124 consecutive patients. J Trauma 1994;37:365–369.
2. Hirshberg A, Scott BG. Damage control for vascular trauma. In Rich NM, Mattox KL, Hirshberg A (eds) Vascular trauma 2nd ed. Philadelphia: WB Saunders, 2004, 165–176.
3. Braslow B, Schwab CW, Brooks AJ. Damage control. In Mahoney PF, Ryan JM, Brooks AJ, Schwab CW (eds) Ballistic trauma: A practical guide. London: Springer, 2005, 180–208.

4. Fox CJ, Starnes BW. Vascular Surgery on the modern battlefield. Surg Clin N Am 2007;87:1193–1211.
5. Chavarria-Aguilar M, Cockerham WT, Barker DE, Ciraulo DL, Richart CM, Maxwell RA. Management of destructive bowel injury in the open abdomen. J Trauma 2004; 56:560–564.
6. Miller PR, Chang MC, Jason Hoth J, Holmes JH, Meredith JW. Colonic resection in the setting of damage control laparotomy: Is delayed anastomosis safe? Am Surgeon 2007;76:606–610.
7. Brundage SI, Jurkovich GJ, Hoyt DB, Patel NY, Ross SE, Marburger R, Stoner M, Ivatury RR, Ku J, Rutherford EJ, Maier RV, for the WTA Multi-institutional Study Group. Stapled versus sutured gastrointestinal anastomosis in the trauma patient: A multicenter trial. J Trauma 2001;51:1054–1061.
8. Witzke JD, Kraatz JJ, Morken JM, Ney AL, West MA, Van Camp JM, Zera RT, Rodriguez JL. Stapled versus hand sewn anastomosis in patients with small bowel injury: A changing perspective. J Trauma 2000;49:660–666.
9. Demetriades D, Murray JA, Chan LS. Handsewn versus stapled anastomosis in penetrating colon injuries requiring resection: A multicenter study. J Trauma 2002;52:117–121.
10. Behrman SW, Bertken KA, Stefanacci HA, Parks SN. Breakdown of intestinal repair after laparotomy for trauma: Incidence, risk factors, and strategies for prevention. J Trauma 1998;45:227–233.
11. Miller RS, Morris JA, Diaz JJ, Herring MB, May AK. Complications after 344 damage-control open celiotomies. J Trauma 2005; 59:1365–1374.
12. Cioffi WG (Moderator), Biffl WL, Croce MA, Feliciano DV (Panelists). Component separation for the open abdomen (Symposium). Contemp Surg 2006; 62(5):216–220.
13. Miller PR, Meredith JW, Johnson JC, Chang MC. Prospective evaluation of vacuum-assisted fascial closure after open abdomen: Planned ventral hernia rate is substantially reduced. Ann Surg 2004;239:608–616.
14. Rowlands BJ, Flynn TC, Fischer RP. Temporary abdominal wound closure with a silastic "chimney". Contemp Surg 1984;24:17.
15. Gawande AA, Studert DM, Orav EJ, Brennan TA, Zinner MJ. Risk factors for retained instruments and sponges after surgery. N Engl J Med 2003;348(3):229–235.
16. Tremblay LN, Feliciano DV, Schmidt J, Cava RA, Tchorz KM, Ingram WL, Salomone JP, Nicholas JM, Rozycki GS. Skin only or silo closure in the critically ill patient with an open abdomen. Am J Surg 2001 Dec;182(6):670–675.
17. Mastboom WJ, Kuypers HH, Schoots FJ, Wobbes T. Small-bowel perforation complicating the open treatment of generalized peritonitis. Arch Surg 1989;124:689–692.
18. Goverman J, Yelon JA, Platz JJ, Singson RC, Turcinovic M. The "fistula VAC," a technique for the management of enterocutaneous fistulae arising within the open abdomen: Report of 5 cases. J Trauma 2006;60:428–431.
19. Jamshidi R, Schecter WP. Biological dressings for the management of enteric fistulas in the open abdomen: A preliminary report. Arch Surg 2007 Aug;142(8):793–796.
20. Girard S, Siderman M, Spain DA. A novel approach to the problem of intestinal fistulization arising in patients managed with open peritoneal cavities. Am J Surg 2003;184:166–167.
21. Livingston DH, Sharma PK, Glantz AI. Tissue expanders for abdominal wall reconstruction following severe trauma: Technical note and case reports. J Trauma 1992;32:82.
22. Ramirez OM, Raus E, Dellon AL. "Components separation" method for closure of abdominal-wall defects: An anatomic and clinical study. Plast Reconstr Surg 1990;86:519–526.
23. Jernigan TW, Fabian TC, Croce MA, Moore N, Pritchard FE, Minard G, Bee TK. Staged management of giant abdominal wall defects: Acute and long-term results. Ann Surg 2003;238:349–357.
24. Fabian TC, Croce MA, Pritchard FE, Minard G, Hickerson WL, Howell RL, Schurr MJ, Kudsk KA. Planned ventral hernia. Staged management for acute abdominal wall defects. Ann Surg 1994;219:643–650.
25. Rutherford EJ, Skeete DA, Brasel KJ. Management of the patient with an open abdomen: Techniques in temporary and definitive closure. Curr Probl Surg 2004;41(10):821–876.

26. Franklin ME Jr, Gonzalez JJ Jr, Glass JL. Use of porcine small intestinal mucosa as a pros-
    thetic device for laparoscopic repair of hernias in contaminated fields: 2-year follow-up.
    Hernia 2004;8:186–189.
27. Helton WS, Fisichella PM, Berger R, Horgan A, Espat NJ, Abcarian H. Short-term outcomes
    with small intestinal submucosa for ventral abdominal hernia. Arch Surg 2005;140:549–562.
28. Butler CE, Langstein HN, Kronowitz SJ. Pelvic, abdominal, and chest wall reconstruction
    with AlloDerm in patients at increased risk for mesh related complications. Plast Reconstr
    Surg 2005;116:1263–1277.

Orthopedics

Hans-Christoph Pape and Peter V. Giannoudis

11.1 Introduction

The first description of postsurgical dynamics dates back approximately 70 years to a description of the metabolic response (e.g., body temperature, kidney function, intestinal compromise) in patients after major abdominal injuries and femoral fracture fixations [1]. Since then, many pathogenetic pathways have been discovered. In the 1990s, decision making about the timing of surgical intervention in polytrauma patients was based on clinical observations and divided into four stages:

- Stage 1: The initial lifesaving procedures;
- Stage 2: Temporary stabilization of fractures;
- Stage 3: A later surgical phase to perform definitive fixation of major fractures;
- Stage 4: The late reconstruction phase.

Today, the importance of timing to minimize the degree of the second hit stimulus is well described. (*See* Chaps. 5 and 7 for further details.) The term "window of opportunity" has been coined to describe the optimal time interval for performing major reconstructive surgery in the multiply injured patient [2, 3].

Among the factors to consider in planning the timing of operations are the magnitude of the planned operation and the patient's physiological response. Regarding the latter, local tissue and wound factors such as edema, skin condition, or lesions located close to the planned surgical incisions must be considered. In addition, the ability of the patient to withstand the impact of a major operation at a certain time after injury should be considered.

When major operations, such as secondary fixations of periarticular fractures, pelvis, or spinal column procedures, are performed at unfavorable times, almost half of patients demonstrate a new onset of organ failure or deterioration [4]. In contrast, this decline was observed in only 32% of cases after minor operations. Moreover, patients who experienced worsening of their organ functions postoperatively were found to have been in a hyperinflammatory status prior to the procedure.

H.-C. Pape (✉) and P.V. Giannoudis
Department of Orthopaedic Surgery, University of Pittsburgh, Pittsburgh, PA, 15213, USA
e-mail: papeHC@aol.com

As described in the chapter about the parameters for decision making (Chap. 4), a moderate-to-severe hyperinflammatory phase occurs in every polytrauma patient. Subsequently, depending on the general condition and the severity of the injury, a compensatory phase (CARS, the Counterinflammatory Response Syndrome) may occur and is characterized by a period of anergy. Whether the anergic phase will develop is difficult to foresee. The determining factors and the ensuing optimal timing of major secondary operations are discussed next.

11.2 Secondary Orthopedic Stabilization: Pathogenetic Aspects

11.2.1 Clinical Studies of the Effects of Secondary Surgery

It is difficult to separate the inflammatory and immunologic effects of operations from other factors in polytrauma patients. This may be achieved only in well-defined patient populations of adequate numbers. In a review of 4,314 polytrauma patients, those who had blunt trauma and underwent multiple operations were isolated for analysis. Of the long-term surviving patients with an ISS > 18 points, those who were submitted to major secondary operation at days two to four after the initial injury demonstrated a higher incidence of organ dysfunction than those who underwent surgery between days five to eight [3]. Similar observations were made in a prospectively documented cohort study [5] that showed that the clinical course in those patients correlated with parameters of hemostasis, tissue perfusion, and the response of the nonspecific immune system. The authors investigated a well-defined cohort of 133 multiply injured patients with high Injury Severity Scores (ISS). Among these patients, the authors describe a rate of deterioration in the clinical status as high as 38%. One of the major common denominators in this group of patients was that the deterioration of organ function parameters began within 48 h after surgery, a time when inflammatory parameters were already abnormal.

11.3 Clinical Studies of the Relevance of Biochemical Markers

Over the last decade, inflammatory markers have become clinically applicable and were shown as relatively reliable indicators for the assessment of the clinical course [6, 7]. The use of cytokines in determining the magnitude of the surgical impact has been described [8–10]. The acute perioperative inflammatory changes may therefore be more meaningful than the association between the day of surgery and the development of an adverse outcome. Among these parameters, proinflammatory cytokines appear to be particularly relevant. Comparison by Roumen et al. between several inflammatory mediators highlighted that IL-6 is most specific for trauma patients, while TNF-α and IL-1-β demonstrated a greater accuracy in patients with hemorrhage and in nonsurvivors after acute respiratory distress syndrome (ARDS) and multi-organ failure (MOF) [11]. For example. Smith et al. [12] described an IL-10 increase after major surgery, whereas Hensler et al. depicted a noticeable decrease in its secretion [13]. Other authors have demonstrated enhanced IL-10 levels after the surgical insult of a cardiopulmonary bypass operation [14]. Therefore, IL-10 may not be an adequate parameter to monitor the severity of trauma. Likewise, tumor necrosis factor-α is unable to quantify the burden of blunt trauma [15, 16] or of surgical procedures [13]. Furthermore, priming of leukocytes in trauma patients was associated with an increase in IL-8 and TNF, but not in IL-10 concentrations [17].

In contrast, early elevation in IL-6 levels could be used to discriminate trauma patients who would later develop MOF [18]. In patients undergoing orthopedic operations,IL-6 serum levels have been shown to closely relate with the magnitude of the injury (burden of trauma) and the operative procedure (second hit) [19]. Recent clinical findings support these results in that IL-6 concentrations vary according to the type of orthopedic operation. Specifically, the inflammatory response induced by femoral nailing was biochemically comparable to that induced by uncemented total hip arthroplasty. Moreover, in polytrauma patients, primary surgery was determined to further impact the inflammatory response already induced by the initial trauma [19].

There is also a close association between the timing of operation, the complications, and the induced inflammatory response. Indeed, the inflammatory response is different for early (performed days 2–4 after injury) versus late (performed after day 4 following injury) major extremity fixation. In 128 polytraumatized patients, secondary operation on days 2–4 was associated with a higher incidence of postoperative organ dysfunction (46.5%) compared to secondary operation on days 5–8. An association between the initial IL-6 values >500 pg/dl and operation on days 2–4 and the development of MOF ($r = 0.96$, $p< 0.001$) was also observed. In contrast, no discernable correlation was found between the initial IL-6-values >500 pg/dl and operation on days 5–8 ($r = 0.57$, $p< 0.07$). Therefore, no distinct clinical advantage to carrying out early (days 2–4) secondary definitive fracture fixation could be determined [18].

In conclusion, for patients who demonstrate initial IL-6 values above 500 pg/dl, it may be advantageous to delay the interval between primary temporary fracture stabilization and secondary definitive fracture fixation for more than 4 days [20].

Superoxide production stimulated by neutrophils (PMNLs) (concanavalin A, cytochrome d) was elevated in trauma patients at day 3 after trauma and returned to normal by day 7 [21]. Botha et al. [22] found an earlier window of PMNL-priming. The in vitro oxygen radical release by unstimulated PMNLs was resolved by 72 h. The authors concluded that avoidable second hits should be postponed in trauma patients [22]. In burn patients, sustained hyperinflammatory reactions were demonstrated to last until 2 weeks after the initial injury [23]. Others demonstrated a significant priming of PMNLs in trauma patients between days 2 and 13. This reaction was most sustained at days 2 to 5 after the injury and was thought to be related to the length of the inflammatory response. The authors also investigated the effect of a second hit on inflammatory parameters in trauma patients. A 2.5-fold elevation in IL-6 levels and a significant increase in the FMLP response in PMNLs were demonstrated after a second hit [24]. The manifold interactions between different inflammatory cells and their secreted mediators are well described. Johnson et al. reported that IL-6 augments the cytotoxic potential of neutrophils via selective enhancement of elastase release [25]. The plasma of patients at risk for MOF caused an increase in elastase levels and a parallel delay in the apoptosis rate of PMNLs [26]. Apoptosis is known to be an important factor in minimizing the release of proinflammatory cytokines during the deletion of dysfunctional cells in response to trauma. IL-6 has been shown to hamper this potentially beneficial effect by exerting a reduction in the apoptosis rate of neutrophils [27], macrophages [28], and lymphocytes [29]. These studies clearly demonstrate the time dependency of inflammatory changes after trauma and the second hit that interacts with these changes.

In summary, the numerous clinical and experimental investigations regarding the inflammatory response support the theory that the timing of major secondary operation may affect the clinical course in patients with blunt trauma.

11.4   Clinical Parameters that may Act as Aids for Decision Making

The classical surgical risk indicators such as old age and previous cardiac or chronic respiratory illnesses [30] are less important in deciding the operability for secondary surgery in polytrauma patients, since the prevalence of such risk factors is low within the generally young population of the polytraumatized. The classification of the American Society of Anesthesiologists [31] is equally unsuitable for this purpose, since its variability is too high to be used to judge the surgical risk on a daily basis. There are no investigations into the reliability of the clinical prognosis by an experienced surgeon. However, the elevated postsurgical organ dysfunction rate of 38% appears to prove the weakness of such estimates [4]. The Prognostic Index of Shoemaker et al. [32] seemingly predicts outcome in surgical high-risk patients (94%). However, since they use parameters that are assessed postoperatively, the index may not be suitable for planning. Easily accessible parameters such as blood pressure, heart rate, central venous pressure, or pH-value showed little predictive value[33, 34].

The inflammatory changes described in the here can be determined on the basis of clinical parameters. Likewise, Goris described them as rubor, calor, dolor, and tumor of all organs [35].

When the clinical course is uneventful, the clinical signs of posttraumatic inflammation usually diminish within 48–72 h. In patients at high risk for organ failure, the hyperinflammatory state can last longer and is clinically determined by three major factors:

- An ongoing permeability disturbance, as determined by a prolonged positive I/O ratio, signs of fluid overload on the chest X-ray, and associated ventilator settings;
- A failure to normalize hemostatic alterations, which can first be determined by a low factor V and the inability to develop a platelet count >95,000 U/μl;
- A prolonged cardiovascular compromise that often results in a requirement for vasopressors.

According to clinical observations, these patients are at high risk for secondary organ failure, and, therefore, major surgical interventions should be avoided.

Other authors focused mainly on the aspect of pulmonary dysfunction. This seems reasonable because ARDS was once a major cause of death before multiple organ failure syndrome had been described. Certainly, lung function (often assessed via the paO_2/FiO_2 ratio) does play an important role. Patients with close to normal lung function (paO_2/FiO_2-quotient >280) withstood a standard procedure in 89% of the cases, while those with a worse respiratory function developed a postorgan failure in 70% [5].

Fortunately, most patients recover from their injuries and develop a negative fluid balance, normal chest X-rays, and normal cardiovascular status. In these patients, the clinical observation has been made that the fourth postinjury day appears to be the earliest, at which a prolonged nonlifesaving surgery can safely be performed.

In another clinical study, specific parameters were investigated that might have clinical significance [4]. Here, a paO_2/FiO_2-ratio of <280, a C-reactive protein of >11, and a platelet count of <180,000/μl were accompanied by a clearly increased incidence of postoperational organ failure. As a further indicator, there was an increased level in the preoperative inflammatory response, as shown by an increased elastase concentration in the serum (>85 ng/ml). A synopsis of parameters shown to be useful according to empirical observations is listed in Table 11.1 [4, 36, 37].

11.5   Secondary Orthopedic Stabilization: Technical Aspects

One of the major questions that orthopedic surgeons must address after polytrauma is whether the techniques of fracture fixation should be the same as those used for isolated fractures. Fortunately, these aspects appear to be similar regardless of the

Table 11.1 Possible markers for the determination of the sustainability of major secondary surgery

PaO_2/FiO_2 ratio >250
PEEP <8 cm H_2O, each time for at least 24 h preoperatively
No additional infiltration in chest plain radiographs
Platelet count >95,000/μl
Leukocyte count >2,000/μl or <12,000/μl
Balanced or negative fluid ratio for 24 h minimum before surgery
Intra-cranial pressure <15 cm H_2O, no signs of raised ICP in head CT
Serum creatinin <2 mg/dl
Serum bilirubin <3 mg/dl

Reproduced with permission of Wolters Kluwer from [4]; Reproduced with permission of Springer from [36, 37]

severity of injury, provided that the state of the soft tissue and the patient's general condition are taken into account.

However, some aspects of treatment may be different. These are related to the principles of early patient mobilization. To achieve this, some authors have recommended that in cases of polytrauma, humerus shaft fractures should be stabilized by an intramedullary nail. The rationale for this is that mobilization with crutches is achieved earlier when surgical fixation is performed. Usually, many orthopedic fixation techniques remain the same, provided that the soft tissue issues have been addressed (Table 11.2).

As regards the time between conversion from external fixation to the definite stabilization of major fractures, infection is a concern. Conversion should be performed within a 14-day time interval in order to minimize the infection-related

Table 11.2 Fixation principles for orthopedic injuries in polytrauma patients

Anatomic area	Technical aspects	Similar to isolated trauma condition	Different to isolated trauma condition
Proximal humerus	Plate osteosynthesis avoid hemiarthroplasty	+	
Humerus shaft	Intramedullary nail		+
Distal humerus	Locked plate (as in isolated fractures)	+	
Elbow	Cautious timing, beware of formation of heterotopic ossifications	+	
Forearm	May be delayed	+	
Wrist/hand	May be delayed	+	
Proximal femur	Maybe delayed, avoid THA or hemiarthroplasty (patients usually young)		+
Femur shaft	As early as patient condition permits, consider undreamed, plating or ex fix		+
Distal femur	Delayed, technically comparable with isolated trauma	+	
Proximal tibia/ tibial plateau	Delayed, technically comparable with isolated trauma	+	
Tibia shaft	Early, technically comparable with isolated trauma	+	
Distal tibia	Delayed, technically comparable with isolated trauma	+	
Ankle/foot	Delayed, technically comparable	+	
Pelvis	Pelvic binder/C-clamp, consider least amount of blood loss		+
Acetabulum	Delayed, high infectious risk in ICU patients		+
C-Spine	Early if neurodeficit	+	
Thoracic spine	Delayed unless neurodeficit		+
Lumbar spine	Early if neuro deficit		+
Sacrum	Delayed, high infection risk for ICU patients	+	

Table 11.3 Surgical principles for conversion of an external fixateur to an intramedullary nail

Preoperative
Preoperative holding area/OR: Thorough cleaning with alcohol/antiseptic solution
Removal of external fixateur
Prepping/draping
Excision of pin sites, curettage or overdrilling of pin holes
Thorough irrigation of pin sites
Intraoperative
Change of gloves and equipment used for excision (drapes included)
Definitive fixation of major extremity fracture

complications [38], since hospital-acquired infections can be severe. Therefore, conversion should be managed cautiously as summarized in Table 11.3.

11.6   Summary and Conclusion

The pathophysiological sequences after accidental trauma show a biphasic process of the immunomodulatory response. Surgical trauma induced by a secondary operation is shown to represent an additional burden.

Both the magnitude of inflammatory response and the timing of major secondary surgery may affect the further clinical course in patients with blunt trauma.

Studies have shown no clinical advantage to performing earlier secondary definitive surgery in a population of patients with multiple injuries who were initially stabilized by external fixation. The most favorable time for performing major operations appears to be the days after the hyperinflammatory phase is over, i.e., after postinjury day 4 (Table 11.4) [39].

In patients with blunt multiple injuries who have undergone primary temporary fixation of major fractures, the timing of the secondary definitive surgery should be carefully selected, or it may result in a second-hit phenomenon and cause deterioration in the patient's clinical status.

Table 11.4 The type and the timing of fracture treatment in a polytrauma patient in correlation with immunologic markers during the first postinjury week<COMP: PLEASE SET LAST THREE ROWS BORDER IN TABLE 11.4 AS PER ORIGINAL MANUSCRIPT>

Injury	Day 1	Day 3	Day 7	Day 15	Day 20	Day 34
Blunt chest trauma	Vent	Vent	Vent	Vent	Vent	
Pelvic hemorrhage	Laparotomy, packing	Second look		ORIF		
L dist hum frx (open)	Guillotine amp	Closure				
L forearm amp						
Pelvic Frx, Type C	Pelvic Clamp			ORIF		
L fem neck frx	2 K wires				DHS	Reosteosynth
L fem shaft frx (open)	Ex fix, vac	Vac	Vac	Vac	Vac	Retrograde femoral nail, Vac
R fem shaft frx	EX fix					
L patella frx (open)	Partial resection					Reconstruction of patellar tendon
L prox tibia Frx (open)	Ex fix, Vac	Vac	Vac	Vac	Vac	Tibial nail, flap
Duration of surgery	2 h	2 h	45 min	4 h	2 h	9 h
Immunologic markers						
IL-1 beta (ng/liter)	<5	<5	<5	>5	Normal range < 5	
IL-6 (ng/liter)	3,210	1,507	60.4	22.3	Normal range < 5.4	
IL-8 (ng/liter)	2,900	64.4	22.4	<5	Normal range < 62	

Amp amputation; *DFN* distal femoral nail; *DHS* dynamic hip screw; *dist* distal; *ex fix* external fixation; *extub* extubation; *fem* femoral; *flap* myocutaneous skin flap; *fx* fracture; *hum* humerus; *ORIF* open reduction and internal fixation; *prox* proximal; *reconstr* reconstruction; *reosteosynth* reosteosynthesis; *tib* tibial; *vac* wound vac; *vent* ventilation; *UTN* unreamed tibial nail; *IL-1 beta* interleukin-1 beta; *IL-6* interleukin-6; *IL-8* interleukin-8
Reproduced with permission of Wolters Kluwer from [39]

References

1. Cuthbertson D. Post-shock metabolic response. Lancet 1942;1:433–437.
2. Krettek C, Simon RG, Tscherne H. Management priorities in patients with polytrauma. Langenbecks Arch Surg 1998;383:220–227.
3. Pape H-C, Stalp M, van Griensven M, Weinberg A, Dahlweit M, Tscherne H. Optimal timing for secondary surgery in polytrauma patients: An evaluation of 4,314 serious-injury cases. Chirurg 1999;70–11:1287–1293.
4. Waydhas C, Nast-Kolb D, Trupka A et al. Posttraumatic inflammatory response, secondary operations, and late multiple organ failure. J Trauma 1996;40:624–631.
5. Waydhas C, Nast-Kolb D, Kick M, Zettl R, Wiesholler J, Trupka A, Jochum M, Schweiberer L. Operation planning of secondary interventions after polytrauma. Unfallchirurg 1994;97:244–249.
6. Pape HC, Giannoudis PV, Krettek C, Trentz O. Timing of fixation of major fractures in blunt polytrauma: Role of conventional indicators in clinical decision making. J Orthop Trauma 2005;19:551–562.
7. Harwood PJ, Giannoudis PV, van Griensven M, Krettek C, Pape HC. Alterations in the systemic inflammatory response after early total care and damage control procedures for femoral shaft fracture in severely injured patients. J Trauma 2005;58:446–452.
8. Roberts CS, Pape HC, Jones AL, Malkani AL, Rodriguez JL, Giannoudis PV. Damage control orthopaedics: Evolving concepts in the treatment of patients who have sustained orthopaedic trauma. Instr Course Lect 2005;54:447–462.
9. Giannoudis PV, Hildebrand F, Pape HC. Inflammatory serum markers in patients with multiple trauma. Can they predict outcome? J Bone Joint Surg Br 2004;86:313–323.
10. Pape HC, Grimme K, Van Griensven M, Sott AH, Giannoudis P, Morley J, Roise O, Ellingsen E, Hildebrand F, Wiese B, Krettek C; EPOFF Study Group. Impact of intramedullary instrumentation versus damage control for femoral fractures on immunoinflammatory parameters: Prospective randomized analysis by the EPOFF Study Group. J Trauma 2003; 55:7–13.
11. Roumen RM, Redl H, Schlag G, Zilow G, Sandtner W, Koller W, Hendriks T, Goris RJ. Inflammatory mediators in relation to the development of multiple organ failure in patients after severe blunt trauma. Crit Care Med 1995;23:474–480.
12. Smith RM, Giannoudis PV, Bellamy MC, Perry SL, Dickson RA, Guillou PJ. Interleukin-10 release and monocyte human leukocyte antigen-DR expression during femoral nailing. Clin Orthop Relat Res 2000;373:233–240.
13. Hensler T, Hecker H, Heeg K, Heidecke CD, Bartels H, Barthlen W, Wagner H, Siewert JR, Holzmann B. Distinct mechanisms of immunosuppression as a consequence of major surgery. Infect Immun 1997;65:2283–2291.
14. Naldini A, Borrelli E, Carraro F, Giomarelli P, Toscano M. Interleukin 10 production in patients undergoing cardiopulmonary bypass: Evidence of inhibition of Th-1-type responses. Cytokine 1999;11:74–79.
15. Pape HC, Remmers D, Grotz M, Schedel I, von Glinski S, Oberbeck R, Dahlweit M, Tscherne H. Levels of antibodies to endotoxin and cytokine release in patients with severe trauma: Does posttraumatic dysergy contribute to organ failure? J Trauma 1999;46:907–913.
16. Rabinovici R, John R, Esser KM, Vernick J, Feuerstein G. Serum tumor necrosis factor-alpha profile in trauma patients. J Trauma 1993;35:698–702.
17 Zallen G, Moore EE, Johnson JL, Tamura DY, Aiboshi J, Biffl WL, Silliman CC. Circulating postinjury neutrophils are primed for the release of proinflammatory cytokines. J Trauma 1999;46:42–48.
18. Pape HC, van Griensven M, Rice J, Gansslen A, Hildebrand F, Zech S, Winny M, Lichtinghagen R, Krettek C. Major secondary surgery in blunt trauma patients and perioperative cytokine liberation: Determination of the clinical relevance of biochemical markers. J Trauma 2001;50:989–1000.

19. Giannoudis PV, Smith RM, Bellamy MC, Morrison JF, Dickson RA, Guillou PJ. Stimulation of the inflammatory system by reamed and unreamed nailing of femoral fractures. An analysis of the second hit. J Bone Joint Surg Br 1999;81:356–361.
20. Pape HC, Remmers D, Grotz M, Kotzerke J, von Glinski S, van Griensven M, Dahlweid M, Sznidar S, Tscherne H. Reticuloendothelial system activity and organ failure in patients with multiple injuries. Arch Surg 1999;134:421–427.
21. Tanaka H, Ogura H, Yokota J, Sugimoto H, Yoshioka T, Sugimoto T. Acceleration of super-oxide production from leukocytes in trauma patients. Ann Surg 1991;21:187–192.
22. Botha AJ, Moore FA, Moore EE, Kim FJ, Banerjee A, Peterson VM. Postinjury neutrophil priming and activation: An early vulnerable window. Surgery 1995;118:358–365.
23. Nijsten MWN, Hack CE, Helle M, ten Duis HJ, Klasen HJ, Aarden LA. Interleukin-6 and its relation to the humoral immune response and clinical parameters in burned patients. Surgery 1991;109:761–767.
24. Ogura H, Tanaka H, Koh T, Hashiguchi *N, Kuwagata Y, Hosotsubo H, Shimazu T, Sugimoto H*. Priming, second hit priming, and apoptosis in leukocytes from trauma patients. J Trauma 1999;46:774–783.
25. Johnson JL, Moore EE, Tamura DY, Zallen G, Biffl WL, Silliman CC. Il-6 augments neutrophil cytotoxic potential via selective enhancement of elastase release. J Surg Res 1998;76:91–94.
26. Biffl WL, Moore EE, Zallen G, Johnson JL, Gabriel J, Offner PJ, Silliman CC. Neutrophils are primed for cytotoxicity and resist apoptosis in injured patients at risk of MOF. Surgery 1999;126:198–202.
27. Kettritz R, Gaido M, Haller H, Luft FC, Jennette CJ, Falk RJ. Interleukin 6 delays spontaneous and TNF alpha–mediated apoptosis of human neutrophils. Kidney Int 1998;53:84–91.
28. Afford S, Pongracz J, Stockley R, Croker J, Burnett D. The induction of human Il-6 of apoptosis in the promonocytic cell line U937 and human neutrophils. J Biol Chem 1992;267:21612–21616.
29. Teague T, Marrack P, Kappler J, Vella AT. Il-6 rescues resting mouse T cells from apoptosis. J Immunol 199;158:5791–5796.
30. Goldman L, Caldera DL, Nussbaum SR, Southwick FS, Krogstad D, Murray B, Burke DS, O'Malley TA, Goroll AH, Caplan Ch, Nolan J, Carabello B, Slater EE. Multifactorial index of cardiac risk in noncardiac surgical procedures. N Engl J Med 1977;297:845–850.
31. Vacanti CJ, VanHouten RJ, Hill RC. A statistical analysis of the relationship of physical status to postoperative mortality in 68,388 cases. Anesth Analg 1970;49:564–566.
32. Shoemaker WC, Appel PL, Bland R, Hopkins JA, Chang P. Clinical trial of an algorithm for outcome prediction in acute circulatory failure. Crit Care Med 1982;10:390–397.
33. Goris RJA, Boekhorst TPA, Nuytinck JKS, Gimbrere JSF. Multiple organ failure: Generalized autodestructive inflammation? Arch Surg 1985;120:1109–1115.
34. Baker SP, O'Neill B, Haddon W, Long WB. The injury severity score: A method for describing patients with multiple injuries and evaluating emergency care. J Trauma 1974;14:187–196.
35. Goris RJ. Multiple organ failure: Whole body inflammation? Schweiz Med Wochenschr 1989;119:347–353.
36. Regel G, Pohlemann T, Krettek C, Tscherne H. Frakturversorgung beim Polytrauma. Zeitpunkt und Taktik. Unfallchirurg 1997;100:234–248.
37. Waydhas C, Flohe S. Intensive medicine criteria for operability. Unfallchirurg 2005;108:866–871.
38. Harwood PJ, Giannoudis PV, Probst C, Krettek C, Pape HC.The risk of local infective complications after damage control procedures for femoral shaft fracture. J Orthop Trauma 2006;20:181–189.
39. Przkora R, Bosch U, Zelle B, Panzica M, Garapati R, Krettek C, Pape HC. Damage control orthopedics: A case report. J Trauma 2002;53:765–769.

Chapter 12
Phase IV: Late Reconstruction Abdominal Wall Closure: Staged Management Technique

Timothy C. Fabian

12.1 Damage Control: Background for Laparotomy

There has been an evolution in managing the laparotomy wound associated with devastating abdominal injuries over the past 25 years. The pathophysiology of the scenario resulting in intra-abdominal hypertension has been fairly well worked out in both laboratory models as well as in clinical observational studies. It has been observed that closure of the laparotomy incision under such circumstances results in a compartment syndrome. As an alternative to closure under tension, the development of multiple methods of open abdominal wound management has evolved. However, while this progress has positively influenced some of these problems, a new dilemma has emerged: the giant ventral hernia [1–6].

A clinical study by Ivatury and colleagues looked at different ways to close the abdomen [7]. Those investigators reported a group of 45 patients who had sustained major abdominal trauma and had primary abdominal closure with interposition mesh; they compared them to an historical group ($n=25$) who had fascial closure. The two groups were matched for injury severity, worst based deficit, and transfusion requirements over the first 24 h. They found that 22% of the mesh-closed group developed abdominal hypertension versus 52% of the fascial closure patients ($P=0.012$). More importantly, they noted a mortality of 10.6% in the mesh-closure group versus 36% in those with fascial closure ($P=0.003$). While other clinicians had synchronously begun similar prophylactic approaches for prevention of intra-abdominal hypertension and compartment syndrome, those investigators were among the first to clearly demonstrate an outcome efficacy.

Those observations threw open the era of open abdomen techniques. It became clear that such approaches not only lessened the occurrence of intra-abdominal hypertension and abdominal compartment syndrome, but they also resulted in a

T.C. Fabian (✉)
Department of Surgery, University of Tennessee Health Science Center,
910 Madison Avenue, #203, Memphis, TN, 38163, USA
e-mail: tfabian@utmem.edu

H.-C. Pape et al. (eds.), *Damage Control Management in the Polytrauma Patient*,
DOI 10.1007/978-0-387-89508-6_12, © Springer Science+Business Media, LLC 2010

marked diminution in necrotizing fasciitis and intestinal fistulae, which invariably accompanied abdominal closure under extreme tension. Many different techniques have been utilized for coverage of the open abdomen including use of absorbable mesh, permanent mesh, silastic and polyvinyl chloride sheets, and biosynthetic devices [8–11]. The era of open abdominal wound management also introduced the era of giant abdominal wall defects, the reconstruction of which is the focus of this chapter.

12.2 Staged Management of Abdominal Wall Defects

The author and colleagues have developed a staged approach to managing the open abdominal wound in Memphis. Management is divided into three stages (Fig. 12.1): Stage One involves the insertion of a biosynthetic replacement in the open abdominal wall; Stage Two consists of the creation of a "planned ventral hernia"; and Stage Three is the definitive reconstruction of the hernia. The staged approach will be detailed, and complications encountered with the various stages of management will be discussed. Complications include the incidences of mortality, fistula formation, and hernia recurrences.

At the Presley Regional Trauma Center, the author and colleagues currently treat approximately 50 patients each year with open abdomen techniques. Recent results reported with the staged method include outcomes of 274 patients managed in this fashion [12]. Over the period of study, there were about 2,600 trauma laparotomies performed. Approximately 10–15% of the trauma patients requiring laparotomy are managed with open abdomen techniques. Nearly all of these incisions are large, and the open wounds measure approximately 25×35 cm. The overall mortality rate of 40% underscores the severity of the traumatic insult the patients selected for open abdomen have sustained.

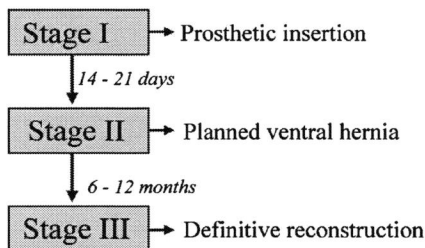

Fig. 12.1 Abdominal wall reconstruction: Staged management technique (Reproduced with permission of Wolters Kluwer from Fabian et al [17].)

12.3   Stage One: Initial Techniques for Temporary Coverage of the Open Abdominal Wound

A variety of approaches has been utilized for temporary coverage or staged fascial closure of the open abdominal wound. Most of the experiences of the author and his colleagues' have been with the use of prosthetic materials to maintain the intestines within the peritoneal cavity. Permanent prostheses including Polytetrafluorethylene (PTFE) sheets as well as polypropylene sheets have been used, but these are currently not in favor. There are two major problems with the utilization of those materials. PTFE is expensive when used as a temporary fascial closure device. While polypropylene mesh has been one of the more commonly used prosthetic materials for maintenance of the viscera within the peritoneal cavity, the author and colleagues have avoided it due to the propensity for development of intestinal fistulae. Indeed, a summary of 14 studies involving 128 patients who had polypropylene mesh used in the emergency setting demonstrated a fistula rate of 23% [13].

Based on those considerations, approach at the author's institution has gravitated to the use of *absorbable mesh* as a means for maintenance of the abdominal viscera in the peritoneal cavity. Polyglactin 910 woven mesh has been used throughout this experience. An attempt is made to tighten up this absorbable mesh over the first week following the initial laparotomy in order to achieve secondary fascial closure. This is accomplished by incising and suturing the prosthesis. However, a substantial portion of patients cannot have the mesh adequately placed to permit fascial closure due to ongoing edema. Therefore, these open wounds are allowed to granulate and are covered with split-thickness skin grafts. While it would seem that absorbable mesh might be completely absorbed, the author and colleagues have found that this is *not* the case with the woven product utilized in this experience. Within 2.5–3.5 weeks, the wounds granulate enough so that the mesh is removed without difficulty. There is generally a suppurative interface that develops between the granulation tissue and the graft that allows it to be removed without danger to the bowel. In cases in which the mesh is left for a prolonged period of time, the author and his colleagues have found a significant incidence of intestinal fistulae. As a consequence, split-thickness skin grafts are placed on these wounds as soon as the granulation tissue is mature and the abdominal contents are stuck to the native peritoneal cavity preventing evisceration.

An alternative approach to utilization of a mesh prosthesis in Stage One is application of the vacuum pack technique. Brock and colleagues were among the first to report this procedure [14]. Their original description utilized a surgical towel covering the omentum and intestines with sump drains placed on top of the drape. An adhesive-backed plastic drape was placed on top of the drains. Subsequently, this concept has been commercialized (Vacuum Assisted Closure, VAC®, KCI Inc., San Antonio, TX) and has been widely adopted in North America. Theoretically, the vacuum approach mobilizes intraperitoneal fluids and may prevent fascial retraction and loss of abdominal domain. A welcome feature of this strategy is that a high percentage of abdominal wounds might be closed without formation of a planned ventral hernia. Indeed, success rates with secondary fascial closure have been reported to be as high as 80% with this vacuum technique [15]. However, it is not clear as yet that all investigators are comparing similar populations with the various acute open abdomen techniques.

12.4 Stage Two: Formation of Planned Ventral Hernia

While the author and colleagues make an attempt to pleat the absorbable mesh during Stage One to achieve secondary fascial closure, this is successful in only 25% of patients, leaving the remaining population to undergo granulation of the wound with split-thickness skin grafting. One of the greatest banes of open abdomen management is the development of intestinal fistulae. There are three factors that can minimize the propensity for fistula development. These include choice of fascial substitute, secondary fascial approximation, and early coverage of the granulating open wound. As discussed earlier, avoidance of polypropylene mesh will indeed decrease the incidence of fistula development. The ability to attain secondary closure of the fascia is preferable in order to both avoid a large defect and minimize fistula formation. Unfortunately, a large percentage of patients having damage control laparotomy will be unable to have secondary closure of their fascia. For those patients who are left with a large open wound, the data from the author's institution would suggest that the earlier the granulating wound is covered with split-thickness skin graft, the less likely it is for intestinal fistulae to develop. Additionally, the large wounds function as a catabolic drain.

The author and colleagues' experience with utilization of absorbable mesh followed by split-thickness skin grafting has resulted in an 8% fistula rate in those patients who have survived the acute trauma. Analysis of those data allowed for the addressing of issues of management techniques that might reduce the fistula rate [12]. Approximately, three quarters of intestinal fistulae occur in the small bowel with most of the remainder being colonic. These fistulae are occasionally the result of failed suture lines, but they are most often associated with either mesh erosion or breakdown of granulation tissue with bowel erosion. An analysis of the timing of wound closure and the development of intestinal fistulae revealed that the patients who developed fistulae had their mesh in place for an average of nearly 4 weeks compared to approximately 2½ weeks for those patients who were successfully managed without fistula development. Thus, the author and colleagues believe that this is an important component of management of those open wounds that cannot be tightened and closed by secondary fascial closure. Split-thickness grafting should be done as soon as the bowel is stuck to the edges of the wound. The complication of intestinal fistula formation cannot be completely eliminated in the face of open abdomen management, but it is likely that, with judicious application of wound care principles, the fistula rate can be kept below 5%.

12.5   Stage Three: Definitive Reconstruction

Appropriate *timing* is of major importance to obtain optimal results for definitive abdominal wall reconstruction. It takes six to 12 months for the intra-abdominal inflammation and adhesions to adequately resolve to allow safe, definitive reconstruction. Patients are followed, and the time of resolution of adhesions is ascertained by examination of the skin graft over the abdominal viscera. In the initial months, adhesions of the graft to the viscera are dense, and the two cannot be separated on physical examination. If the reconstruction is attempted too early, the dissection of the graft from the underlying viscera is extremely difficult. This results in inadvertent enterotomy and the potential for serious wound infection and reconstruction failure. As time passes and the healing process progresses, the dense adhesions resolve. On examination, the skin graft can be pinched away from the underlying viscera with the fingers. Once this degree of adhesion resolution has occurred, it is time to reconstruct the abdominal wall. Waiting too long to perform reconstruction is associated with loss of abdominal domain and high hernia recurrence rates.

There are two general approaches to abdominal wall reconstruction. While the largest percentage of these giant ventral hernias are probably repaired with permanent prosthetic materials worldwide, the preferred method of the author and colleagues is to use autologous tissue transfer for reconstruction. Important considerations related to outcomes of reconstruction include the development of recurrent hernias and infection. The advantage of prosthetic materials is simplicity of repair. The use of an autologous tissue transfer technique has the appeal of avoiding foreign materials and consequent reduction of infection rates. Infections of large prostheses are quite morbid, and nearly always require prosthetic removal, which can be a formidable procedure. Subsequent management involves months and often years of care, entailing multiple operative procedures and significant morbidity. However, a concern for adequacy of coverage of these large defects with tissue transfer is a significant hernia recurrence rate.

The component separation technique was described by Ramirez and colleagues in 1990 [16]. This technique was devised to repair large abdominal hernias by tissue transfer. That description involved medial mobilization of the musculofascial units of the rectus abdominus muscles. This allows for autologous continuity combined with dynamic support. That approach permits approximately five to eight centimeters of mobilization on each musculofascial unit. Patients must be monitored for development of a further ACS for 24–48 h following repair. A problem may occur with the very large ventral hernias that result from open abdomen techniques utilized today. A standard component separation operation may not allow for closure of a high percentage of those wounds and results in the need for adjunctive prosthetic mesh. Consequently, the author and colleagues developed a modified components separation technique [17]. That approach is graphically demonstrated in Fig. 12.2.

The modified component separation technique has now been performed on approximately 150 patients in Memphis with a mean follow-up of around 3 years.

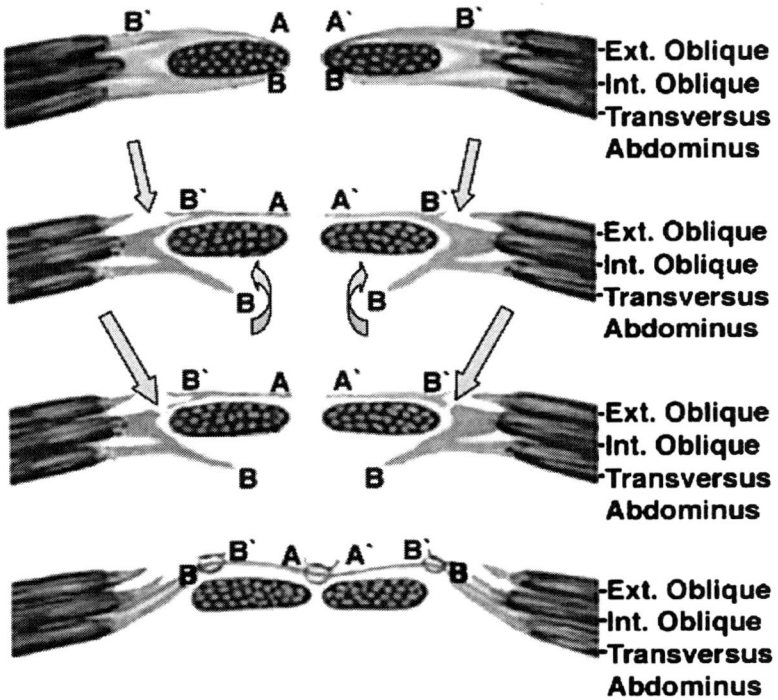

Fig. 12.2 Modified components separation technique (Reproduced with permission of Wolters Kluwer from Jernigan et al [12].; and from Fabian et al [17].)

The rate of recurrent herniation is around 5%. It has been found that recurrent hernias are associated with prolongation of definitive time to reconstruction. If reconstruction is delayed beyond a year, the hernia rate is much higher. This is due to progressive loss of domain with resultant need for closure under a higher degree of tension. Using a similar single stage components repair, Van Geffen and colleagues have reported 26 patients with a mean follow-up of 27 months and a recurrence rate of 8% – results comparable to those of the author and his colleagues [18]. The author and colleagues have also noted that 10% of patients have required adjunctive mesh to avoid closure under tension and, similar to recurrent hernias, the required adjunctive mesh has been in those patients who were definitively reconstructed beyond a year with a mean interval of 20 months from injury to reconstruction in those needing adjunctive mesh. Van Geffen and colleagues reported that 15% of their patients required adjunctive mesh. Considering complications compared with time of reconstruction from the author and his colleagues' population, the percent of complication (hernia or adjunctive mesh) when reconstruction was done under 1 year was 7.6% compared to 25% complication rate in those who were reconstructed 12 months or later.

12.5.1   Operative Approach

In the operating room, the skin graft is pinched away from the underlying viscera somewhere near the midportion of the wound. The graft is sharply incised, and, with a combination of sharp and blunt dissection, it is dissected from the underlying viscera. This excision generally takes approximately 1 h. The most dense adhesions are usually over the liver as well as at the native myofascial edge of the wound. It is imperative to gently dissect the adhesions from the liver, with attention to avoiding dissection beneath Glissen's capsule, which results in significant troublesome oozing. The myofascial edge is virtually always more densely adherent than the adhesions to the omentum or intestines. However, occasionally, small areas of dense adhesions to small bowel are encountered. Injury to the intestine may require short areas of resection. Avoidance of permanent mesh for reconstruction is desirable due to the risk of infection of the foreign body.

The anatomy of the abdominal wall must be considered in understanding the mobilization and tissue transfer involved with modified components separation. Both the anterior rectus fascia and the posterior rectus fascia comprise two lamellae. The anterior rectus fascia is composed of an extension of the external oblique fascia combined with a component of the internal oblique fascia. Thus, a fusion of the external oblique and a lamellum of the internal oblique fascia produces the anterior rectus sheath. The posterior rectus fascia comprises the medial fascia of the trans versus abdominus muscle and the posterior lamella of the internal oblique fascia. Thus, the internal oblique fascia splits to form a component of both anterior rectus fascia and posterior rectus fascia above the accurate line.

Performance of the modified components separation technique begins with a division of the external oblique component of the anterior rectus sheath. The lateral plane where this division occurs is located by grasping the rectus abdominus muscle between the thumb anteriorly and the fingers posteriorly and squeezing this tissue; this allows for identification of the lateral portion of the anterior rectus fascia. This is approximately 1 cm lateral to the lateral board of the rectus and is where the incision of the external oblique fascia is begun. This incision is extended 6 to 8 cm above the costal margin superiorly and down to the pubis inferiorly. Following division of the external oblique component of the anterior rectus sheath, blunt dissection is carried out between the external oblique fascia and the internal oblique fascia, bilaterally out to the area of the anterior axillary line to allow for mobilization of the rectus musculofascial component. Following division of the external oblique fascia, the posterior rectus fascia is sharply dissected from the rectus abdominus muscles bilaterally. Care is taken to avoid injury to the inferior epigastric vessels, which provide blood supply to the rectus abdominus muscles. For moderate-size defects, that may be all of the mobilization required to allow for fascial closure. However, most of the large abdominal wall defects will require further separation of abdominal wall components. The modification of the components' separation description of Ramirez and colleagues that the author and colleagues have added is to next divide the internal oblique component of the anterior rectus sheath.

The location of the internal oblique component is readily seen after the external oblique component of the anterior sheath has been divided. The internal oblique component is divided superiorly up over the lower costal margin, but it is very important to not divide it inferiorly below the linea semilunaris, because there is no posterior rectus sheath below that point. If the internal oblique component of the anterior rectus sheath were divided lower than the semilunar line, then a large hernia defect would be produced. The complete mobilization of these abdominal wall components provides approximately 10 cm of medial advancement in the epigastium, 20 cm in the midabdomen, and 8 cm in the lower abdomen. The epigastric region is always the tightest and is the most common location for the occasional need for adjunctive mesh. Following these steps, the abdominal wall reconstruction is completed by approximating the medial edge of the posterior rectus sheath to the lateral portion of the anterior rectus sheath with polypropylene suture. The repair is completed by reapproximating the medial edges of the anterior rectus sheaths in the midline.

Analysis of 73 patients who had definitive abdominal wall reconstruction using the modified components separation technique found that recurrent hernia developed in four patients (5%). The mean follow-up of patients undergoing reconstruction was 24 months [12]. The author and colleagues have discovered that waiting too long for abdominal wall reconstruction produces inferior results. When need for adjunctive mesh was grouped with hernia recurrence and they were considered as complications, the complication rate was 7.6%. Patients with those complications were reconstructed at 20 months following discharge compared with 10 months in those without complications. This is probably secondary to progressive loss of abdominal domain and consequent closure under tension. Ideally, reconstruction should take place when the skin graft can be pinched from the intestines; this is usually the case within 6–12 months from initial hospital discharge.

12.6   Summary and Conclusion

The *staged management* of patients with giant abdominal wall defects without the use of permanent mesh provides for a safe and effective approach for both initial and definitive reconstruction. The staged approach produces low morbidity, and there was no technique-related mortality in our study. Absorbable mesh provides effective temporary abdominal wall coverage with a low fistula rate. Granulating wounds should be covered early. From the experience of the author and his colleagues, the component separation technique is the procedure of choice for definitive abdominal wall reconstruction, though other techniques too have been described and continue to be studied. Definitive reconstruction should not be delayed beyond the time at which adhesion resolution indicates a nonhostile abdomen.

References

1. Stone HH, Strom PR, Mullins RJ. Management of the major coagulopathy with onset during laparotomy. *Ann Surg* 1983; 197:532–5.
2. Kron IL, Harman PK, Nolan SP. The measurement of intra-abdominal pressure as a criterion for abdominal re-exploration. *Ann Surg* 1984; 199(1):28–30.
3. Fietsam R, Villalba M, Glover JL, Clark K. Intra-abdominal compartment syndrome as a complication of ruptured abdominal aortic aneurysm repair. *Am Surg* 1989; 55:396–402.
4. Richardson JD, Trinkle JK. Hemodynamic and respiratory alterations with increased intra-abdominal pressure. *J Surg Res* 1976; 20:401–404.
5. Diebel LN, Dulchavsky SA, Wilson RF. Effect of increased intra-abdominal pressure on mesenteric arterial and intestinal mucosal blood flow. *J Trauma* 1992; 33:45–49.
6. Maxwell RA, Fabian TC, Croce MA, Davis KA. Secondary abdominal compartment syndrome: An underappreciated manifestation of severe hemorrhagic shock. *J Trauma* 1999; 47:995–999.
7. Ivatury RR, Porter JM, Simon RJ, Islam S, John R, Stahl WM. Intra-abdominal hypertension after life-threatening penetrating abdominal trauma: Prophylaxis, incidence, and clinical relevance to gastric mucosal pH and abdominal compartment syndrome. *J Trauma* 1998; 44:1016–1023.
8. Silverman RP, Li EN, Holton LH III, Sawan KT, Goldberg NH. Ventral hernia repair using allogenic acellular dermal matrix in a swine model. *Hernia*. 2004; 8:336–342.
9. Menon NG, Rodriguez ED, Byrnes CK, Girotto JA, Goldberg NH, Silverman RP. Revascularization of human acellular dermis in full-thickness abdominal wall reconstruction in the rabbit model. *Ann Plast Surg* 2003; 50:523–527. Erratum in: *Ann Plast Surg* 2003; 51:228.
10. An G, Walter RJ, Nagy K. Closure of abdominal wall defects using acelluar dermal matrix. *J Trauma* 2004; 56:1266–1275.
11. Scott BG, Welsh FJ, Pham HQ, Carrick MM, Liscum KR, Granchi TS, Wall Jr MJ, Mattox KL, Hirshberg A. Asher Early Aggressive Closure of the Open Abdomen. *J Trauma* 2006; 60:17–22.
12. Jernigan TW, Fabian TC, Croce MA, Moore N, Pritchard FE, Minard G, Bee TK. Staged management of giant abdominal wall defects: Acute and long term results. *Ann Surg* 2003; 238:349–357.
13. Jones JW, Jurkovich GJ. Polypropylene mesh closure of infected abdominal wounds. *Am Surg* 1989; 55(1):73–76.
14. Brock WB, Barker DE, Burns RP. Temporary closure of open abdominal wounds: The vacuum pack. *Am Surg* 1995; 61:30–35.
15. Miller Pr, Meredith JW, Johnson JC, Chang MC. Prospective evaluation of vacuum-assisted fascial closure after open abdomen: Planned ventral hernia rate is substantially reduced. *Ann Surg* 2004; 239:608–616.
16. Ramirez OM, Ruas E, Dellon AL. "Components separation" method for closure of abdominal-wall defects: An anatomic and clinical study. *Plast Reconstr Surg* 1990; 86:519–526.
17. Fabian TC, Croce MA, Pritchard FE, Minard G, Hickerson WL, Howell RL, Schurr MJ, Kudsk KA. Planned ventral hernia. Staged management for acute abdominal wall defects. *Ann Surg* 1994; 219:643–653.
18. Van Geffen JH, Simmermacher RK, van Vroohoven TJ, van der Werken C. Surgical treatment of large contaminated abdominal wall defects. *J Am Coil Surg* 2005; 201(2):206–212.

Chapter 13
Phase IV: Late Reconstruction: Reconstruction of Posttraumatic Soft Tissue Defects

Jörn Redeker and Peter M. Vogt

13.1 Introduction

The surgical care of wounds for patients with complex extremity trauma follows the principles of polytrauma care. The primary focus is to stabilize the patient. This may lead to the decision that a prompt amputation of the severely injured limb is necessary. The "life before limb" principle must be respected.

It is first essential to properly evaluate the wound condition. Therefore, it is important to understand the mechanism of injury. A high velocity injury or an injury with an extended crush zone may lead to secondary necrosis of the soft tissue.

Prior to wound closure the following questions should be addressed:

1. How big the defect will be after a serial debridement?
2. What are the requirements of the region to be covered?
3. Does the area of defect require sensation or is it an area that needs to sustain severe pressure load (e.g., heel) or great flexibility (e.g., elbow or knee joint)?
4. Is it necessary to maintain the integrity of the dominant vessels or subdermal plexus?
5. Is there a relevant comorbidity, such as diabetes mellitus or arteriosclerosis?
6. Is the patient compliant?

Success of wound treatment is no longer measured simply on the basis of closure, but also on the functional outcome. The advantage of a lower leg amputation with a rapid resumption of daily life activity must be weighed against the complex, lengthy reconstruction of a limb.

J. Redeker (✉)

Department of Plastic, Hand, and Reconstructive Surgery, Hannover Medical School,
Carl Neuberg Str. 1, Hannover, 30625, Germany
e-mail: redeker.joern@mh-hannover.de

H.-C. Pape et al. (eds.), *Damage Control Management in the Polytrauma Patient*,
DOI 10.1007/978-0-387-89508-6_13, © Springer Science+Business Media, LLC 2010

13.2 Radical Debridement

The initial débridement should be performed by using a tourniquet. All dead and devitalized tissue should be removed. At the end of the first débridement, the tourniquet is released and all questionable necrosed or compromised tissue is resected. The wound is washed out several times. Jet lavage may be used for further wound cleaning. Neither the prospect of developing a wound surface of great depth and size nor the utilization of second look surgery or the application of antibiotic will relieve the surgeon from performing the initial radical first débridement.

While small bone fragments are removed, large bone fragments are cleaned, handled with care to make sure that the periosteum will not be stripped, and then reinserted into the defect as a free graft. Major neurovascular structures should be preserved if possible, even if initially they have no soft tissue protection. The exposed vessels may be covered using surrounding muscle or, in exceptional cases, with a primary free or pedicaled flap. Unprotected bone, nerve, and tendon undoubtedly require proper vascularized soft tissue for protection as quickly as possible, but, with the use of vacuum-assisted closure for temporary wound dressing, which was established in the late 1990s, one has the opportunity to delay further surgery. Other considerations regarding the timing of reconstruction are further described in the following sections.

13.3 Stabilization of Fractures

The fracture management depends mainly on whether the patient is stable enough to tolerate a definitive osteosynthesis or not. While in the 1980s the concept of early total care (ETC) was advocated in all patient groups regardless of the injury severity and distribution, in the 1990s the concept of damage control orthopedics (DCO) was established. The reason for leaving the general concept of ETC was that several studies showed that extended operative procedures during the early phase of polytrauma were associated with adverse outcome [1]. The principles of DCO contain the advantages of immediate temporary fracture stabilization and secondary definitive management [2]. For this reason, the fixateur extern is the preferred treatment in the beginning. For the definitive osteosynthesis, intramedullary unreamed nails are favorable because they are weight-bearing systems and need only a small incision. Plates do have the disadvantages of postoperative disturbed wound healing because of decreased skin perfusion around contused regions and incision lines.

13.4 Methods of Soft Tissue Closure

Soft tissue closure techniques are selected according to the wound ground, the exposed structures, and the local region of the defect. A stepwise algorithm is used to determine the closure technique, beginning with the simplest and least complex closure options to the more complex techniques. The flaw of this simplified metaphor is that its aim is to achieve the simplest wound closure solution rather than the method that will produce the best functional outcome. This principle misleads inexperienced surgeons to choose the allegedly "simple" wound closure option.

Using the vacuum-assisted wound closure for as long as required to generate sufficient granulation and reduce the size of the wound might be attractive upon first glance. However, in the long term, this will likely create problems such as unstable scars or fistulae due to prolonged treatment and infection. The lack of well-vascularized tissue may also delay bone healing. If there is an option of closing the defect with a local or free flap, one must take into account the donor-site morbidity and the time factor for uncomplicated healing. An open lower extremity fracture with exposed tendon and bone distal to the middle third of the tibia may be closed with a combination of a pedicled gastrocnemius flap and an additional hemisoleus flap. Predicting whether the combined muscle flaps will sufficiently cover the defect is more difficult than if one chooses a free flap large enough to cover the entire defect (Fig. 13.1a,b). Also, the donor-site morbidity of a hemisoleus muscle flap is considerable. The fourth compartment of the calf is crucial for venous drainage. This is even more important when impaired drainage is present in an open lower limb fracture.

In conclusion, an apparently complex microvascular free tissue transfer [e.g., ALT-perforator flap (Fig. 13.2a,b), parascapular flap] may entail less chance of donor-site morbidity and a safer predictable functional outcome than would a local flap. Again, the challenge is not solely the technical implementation of the defect coverage, but also determining the method that offers the best long-term functional outcome.

The semantic discussion of the metaphor "reconstructive ladder" has spawned other metaphors such as the "reconstructive elevator" [3] or the "reconstructive triangle," [4] all of which attempt to express that the decision-making process for selecting a reconstructive procedure is not linear [5]. A more realistic conceptualization of defect reconstruction is a chess game in which the different methods are represented by chess pieces with specific characteristics rather than a ladder or elevator, which implies steps and levels.

13.4.1 Chess Game of Reconstruction

This is how this chess game analogy works:

- The queen is the free flap because both possess the greatest freedom of movement. However, like the queen, the free flap is very valuable because it presents only once.
- The castle symbolizes a pedicle flap with great power but with limited versatility.
- The knight compares with the local flap, an important figure with limited range of motion.

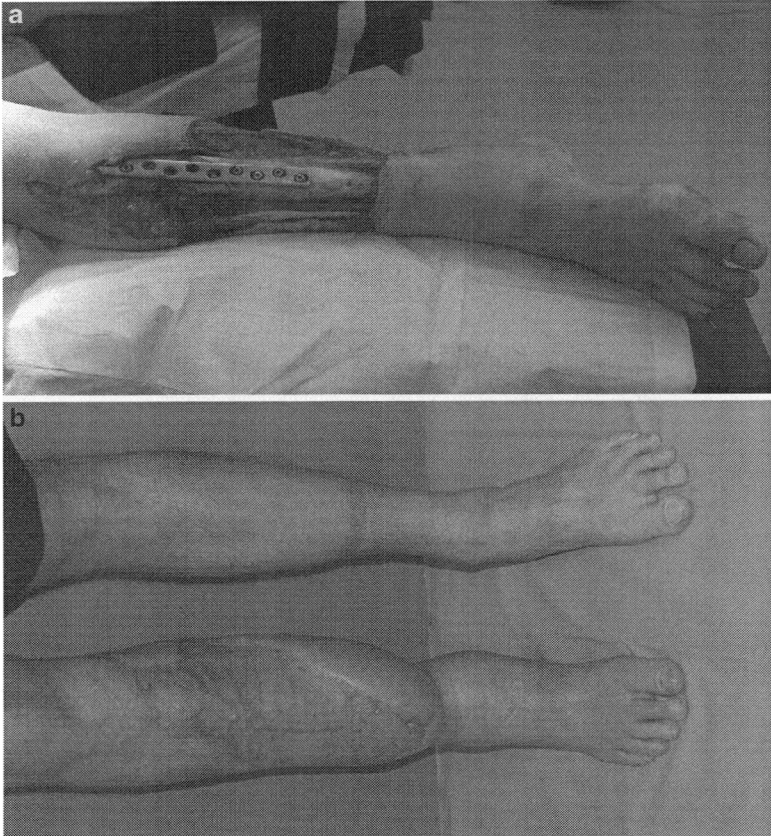

Fig. 13.1 Fifty-four-year old man with an open tibial fracture Gustilo 3 b with a great soft tissue loss of the anterior calf and exposed osteosynthesis material. (**a**) Preoperative; (**b**) Six months after reconstruction with a free myocutaneus latissimus dorsi flap

- The bishop resembles the vacuum-assisted wound closure, which may flank many procedures in modern reconstructive surgery.
- As a bishop can never move to a different colored square, the second bishop compares to a skin graft, which can be used widely but requires sufficient vascularized wound ground.
- The pawn is the most basic chess piece, and it is comparable to the fundamental techniques of stepwise wound closure.

Although the "chess game of reconstruction" is a simplification, it better reflects the time-dependent decisions inherent in plastic surgery. The concepts and figures of chess compare to the daily practice of the plastic surgeon, who not only understands the capabilities of the techniques but also the tactical meaning of the procedures.

This game is deceptively easy to learn, but takes a lifetime to master.

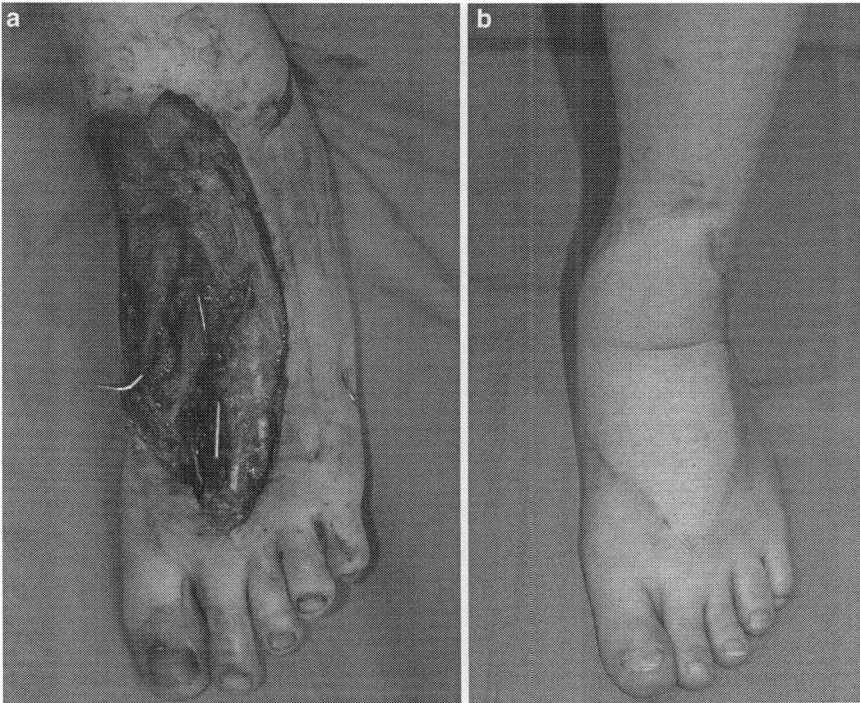

Fig. 13.2 Twenty-eight-year old woman with open luxated fractures of the metatarsal bones 2–4 and soft tissue defect of the dorsum of the foot. (**a**) Preoperative; (**b**) Eight months after reconstruction with a ALT-perforator flap

13.4.2   Techniques

These are the different techniques:

- Primary wound closure: Edges can be approximated directly.
- Dynamic skin suture: Consists of a technique that diminishes local pressure on skin and permits progressive tightening of the sutures for stepwise incisional closure. Indications are restricted to minimal excision wounds or after release of compartment syndromes [6].
- Secondary wound closure: Primary closure cannot be achieved. The inflammation and fibroplasia leads to wound-contracture. The wound will be reepithelialized from the margin of an intact epithelium on the wound ground. If tertiary closure (using skin graft or flaps for bridging the defect) is impossible because of morbidity (e.g., tumor), sometimes secondary wound closure is the only treatment left. It can be supported by the techniques of vacuum-assisted closure.

- Split-thickness skin graft: Includes only a portion of the dermis and so has the advantage of being able to tolerate less vascularity. Its disadvantages include shrinkage, reduced sensory recovery, and susceptibility to pressure and shear force. It is used at the trunk and the genitalia.
- Full-thickness skin graft: Contains epidermis and the entire dermis. Therefore, it requires a better vascularized wound ground. It resists contraction, and its texture and pigmentation make it more suitable for use in the regions of the face and hand.

For both types of skin graft, the survival rate may be increased if small incisions are made in the skin to prevent graft loss from seroma and hematoma. Additional shearing forces may be reduced by using a tie-over-dressing. This can be made with fluffed gauze and sutures or foam material and staples. This dressing is left for 5 days and is then carefully removed.

13.4.3   Flaps

13.4.3.1   Local Flaps

These include transposition, advancement, and rotation-flaps. To safely employ these local flaps, a detailed knowledge about the cutaneous vessel-perforators is mandatory. All too often, when applying these local flaps partial necrosis can be observed due to damaged perforators in posttraumatic skin after crush injuries. This is one of the reasons why these flaps are rarely applied in lower leg injuries.

13.4.3.2   Distant Flaps

These are used to cover nonadjacent defects. They may be transferred directly, tubed, or transferred by microvascular technique. For the upper extremity, the groin flap and interosseus posterior flaps are suitable to cover defects on the hand. For the lower leg muscle, flaps like the gastronemius or suralis flap are often used for coverage. Preoperatively, it is necessary to assure that the dominant vessels are not compromised by the injury or from atherosclerosis. This can be done with Doppler ultrasound or conventional angiography.

13.4.3.3   Free-Flaps

When local or distant flaps are not available and a simple skin graft is not suitable for a soft tissue defect, a free flap is required, and its use is well accepted. The main advantage of free flap surgery is the possibility of designing a custom-made flap that matches size, form, and tissue components of the wound. The intrinsic blood perfusion of free muscle flaps not only guarantees reduced partial necrosis as compared to local flaps, but it may also help to heal infection or support bone fusion [7]. The combination of different tissues – such as skin, muscle, and bone – perfused by one arterial axis as in the subscapularis and thoracodorsalis system presents the opportunity to reconstruct even complex tissue defects. This is performed in a single operation using the so-called chimeric flap [8]. Another innovation in microsurgery is the perforator flap. Based on a musculocutaneous perforating vessel, these flaps have the significant advantage of decreasing donor-site morbidity. They also comprise a refinement of the functional and esthetic design. For better planning, the preoperative assessment should trace the perforator by a Doppler probe. Anatomic variations and the intramuscular local-ization of the perforator are often of interest. CT angiography for the preoperative mapping is used to reduce complication rate [9]. The risk of total flap necrosis is about 2–5% [10].

13.4.4   Acute Bone-Shortening/Bone Transport

High energy injuries usually cause complex wounds with soft tissue defects and open fractures of the upper and lower limb. In cases of temporary shortening of the bone with or without angulation, the soft tissue defect can be closed. Later, a dis-traction osteogenesis is performed with an Ilizarov external fixation. A free flap can be interposed to add the missing soft tissue before starting with the distraction. Distraction osteogenesis underneath the flap is possible when the dominant vessels are preserved. Delayed gradual limb lengthening can be performed without a free flap if there are no recipient vessels available [11]. The disadvantage of this proce-dure is the time-consuming therapy extending over months. Without adequate tissue coverage, the bone might be easily exposed to an instable scar tissue. A better alternative is to use an arteriovenous loop with the advantage of attaining tension-free anastomoses outside the zone of injury. This can be done in a single-stage or multistage procedure [12].

13.4.5   Vacuum-Assisted Closure

Since its introduction in the 1990s, the vacuum-assisted wound closure has become more and more popular. A layer of foam under an occlusive dressing with continu-ous negative pressure decreases edema. It supports building of granulation tissue, which, in selected cases, helps to close a wound by a skin graft. However, unstable scars may result, requiring flaps in the long term. Recent data suggest that the out-come for vacuum-assisted closure is improved when it is applied in the critical phase between 5 days and 3 months.

13.5   Timing of Soft Tissue Closure

Both the timing of wound treatment and possible defect closure are the subject of controversial debates. For the polytrauma patient, the concept of DCO is established. For this group of patients, early wound closure with time-consuming reconstructive plastic surgery is not recommended. Even if the necessity of a free flap is obvious, surgery for the potentially unstable patient must be delayed. Temporary external fixation for open fractures is essential and should be done first after the radical débridement. Then, in most cases, temporary wound closure can be attained by using vacuum-assisted therapy. Ideally, the orthopedic trauma surgeon will involve the plastic surgeon early on in the process management to discuss the indication for early soft tissue reconstruction. This approach also facilitates aggressive débridement, which helps to reduce bacterial contamination.

For patients who have sustained a severe mono-trauma injury and who are clinically stable, for example an isolated Gustilo III lower leg crush injury, there is a consensus on the benefit of early reconstruction with free microsurgical tissue transfer within 1 week [13–16].

Justification of early definitive wound closure is the minimization of the risk of infection, better fracture healing, decreased flap failure, the length of hospital stay, and, finally, a shorter convalescence [14, 17]. Godina retrospectively evaluated patients with lower leg crush injuries who were treated with free tissue transfer. Patients treated with a flap within 72 h were labeled the early group and showed a decreased incidence of osteomyelitis or nonunion as compared with the delayed treatment group, which was comprised of patients who received a free flap up to 3 months after the accident [14]. These data were obtained when open wound coverage with vacuum-assisted closure was not available and superinfected granulation tissue was detrimental to microsurgery. But the scientific evidence regarding the impact of timing is still unclear [18]. Other authors have acknowledged that early wound closure diminishes the risk of infection. Godina found that early wound coverage is superior when performed within 72 h, Byrd within 5 days [13]. New data show that free flap can be performed safely in conjunction with vacuum therapy.

13.5.1   Classification

The nomenclature for time categories in the literature has caused confusion with regard to overlapping terms. For example, the term "emergency flap" suggests a procedure comparable to a replantation, which is mandatory in the first hours after trauma at the end of primary debridement. The definition indicates the first surgical procedure within 24 h after the accident [14, 19].

Other terminologies used are:

- Emergency (within 24 h) [17, 19–24]
- Immediate (within 24 h) [20]
- Early (less then 72 h), delayed (within 3 months), late (greater than 3 months) [14]
- Early (1–7 days), late (8–30 days) [25]
- Acute (within 5 days), subacute (1–6 weeks), chronic (>6 weeks) [13]

Ninkovic and colleagues tried to establish a more standardized classification: [26]

1. Primary free flap closure (12–24 h)
   a. With primary repair
   b. With primary reconstruction
   c. With late reconstruction
2. Delayed primary free flap closure (2–7 days)
   a. With primary repair
   b. With primary reconstruction
3. Secondary free flap closure (>7 days)
   a. With late reconstruction

The authors would suggest the following classification according to practical applications:

1. Immediate: During primary operation (<12–24 h)
2. Delayed: After stabilization of the patient (<7 days)
3. Secondary: After secondary referral to plastic surgery (>7 days)

Immediate reconstruction of injured blood vessels may preserve tissues and limbs (replantation/revascularation). This includes rare cases in which an amputated limb is the source of tissue parts (so-called banked tissue) required for the salvage of the contralateral injured limb [27], or the salvage of valuable functional tissue parts in the same limb. Saving additional limb length with sensation may result in better fitting prosthesis or preserve the function of a joint [28]. Another indication for immediate wound closure with vital tissue is the exposure of dominant blood vessels, which cannot be safely covered with vacuum-assisted closure because of the danger of erosive-bleeding.

Therefore the decision-making between amputation and salvage sometimes cannot be delayed.

All other wound closures can be done safely when delayed, keeping in mind that the delay should be as short as possible. This delay enables the surgeon to consider the treatment plan and gives him/her the opportunity to discuss the plan with the patient. There is no need for a possibly exhausted or inexperienced team to take on this challenging operation in the middle of the night. Misjudging the situation and preserving a limb with a nonfunctioning free flap represents the worst case scenario. Since plastic surgery may not be available in some institutions, secondary referral to a center may be discussed as soon as possible.

13.6   The Importance of the Interdisciplinarity

As soon as possible , after the patient has been stabilized, radical débridement and sufficient external fixation will be performed by the trauma surgeon. The early involvement of an experienced plastic surgeon is of great value for the outcome of the patients with severe complex soft tissue defects. Multidisciplinarity is cost effective.

Benefits of involving plastic surgery include:

- Skillful reconstruction of injured blood vessels and nerves with the potential salvage of the injured limb;
- Primary wound closure with the entire spectrum of plastic reconstructive techniques available;
- Incision lines during the first débridement or for necessary osteosynthesis could be modified to preserve axial or perforator vessels;
- Arrangements for the exact position of possible fixation-pins;
- Preserving vessels necessary for further microsurgical tissue transfer;
- Early evaluation of the wound situation and direct communication with the orthopedic trauma surgeon;

13.7   Regions of Trauma-Associated Defects: Wound Closure

13.7.1   Upper Limb

Most severe accidents involving the upper extremity are crush or avulsion injuries. Because of the good muscle envelope, the defects in most cases are sufficiently grafted with split-thickness skin grafts.

For more expansive wounds, there is range of available local and distant flaps, so that free flaps are not used as often as in the lower limb. Exposed osteosynthesis material, tendon, vessels, or open elbow joint and bone defects are possible indications for a free flap.

13.7.1.1   Upper Arm

Local and distant flaps:

- Pedicled latissimus dorsi flap
- Pectoralis muscle flap
- Lateral upper arm flap
- Forearm Flap

13.7.1.2   Elbow/Forearm

Local and distant flaps:

- Distally pedicled lateral upper arm flap
- Proximally pedicled radial forearm flap

Frequently used free flaps:

- Parascapular/scapular flap
- Latissimus dorsi flap
- Lateral upper arm flap
- Antero lateral thigh perforator flap
- Free osteocutaneous fibula flap

13.7.1.3   Back of the Hand

Local and distant flaps:

- Radial forearm flap
- Interosseus posterior flap
- Groin flap

Free flaps:

- Serratus anterior fascial flap
- Parascapular/scapular flap
- Latissimus dorsi flap
- Lateral upper arm flap
- Antero lateral thigh perforator flap

13.7.2   Lower Limb

Soft tissue damage often results from direct high energy trauma or due to secondary soft tissue loss on the basis of postischemic necrosis. Due to its thin skin envelope, the distal third of the lower leg is the most at risk. In the thigh region, most of the defects requiring tissue reconstruction are secondary, such as after osteomyelitis or soft tissue loss following total endoprosthesis of the hip and knee.

13.7.2.1   Thigh

In general, the rich muscle coverage of the femur provides protection and is typically eligible for a split thickness skin graft. Only defects over the bony prominence of the trochantor major region require local or distant flaps.

Local and distant flaps include:

• Tensor fascia lata flap
• Vastus lateralis flap
• Rectus femoris flap
• Biceps femoris flap

13.7.2.2 Knee

The muscle flap of first choice is the gastrocnemius flap. The medial and lateral head of the gastrocnemius can be used. The muscle is dissected up to the insertion at the femur condyle and then rotated into the defect. The lateral head of the gastronemius muscle is smaller than medial head. The peroneus must be preserved during the operation. The muscle can be denervated to avoid disturbing contractures during walking. The muscle will be covered with split-thickness skin graft. If the muscle is used with a turnover technique, it is useful to carefully resect the tendon aponeurosis because the skin graft will adhere in a better manner to the muscle. The flap may be raised as a myocutaneous-flap.

Local and distant flaps about the knee region are:

• Gastrocnemius flap
• Distal pedicled anterolateral thigh flap

13.7.2.3 Calf

The tibia is very vulnerable to direct trauma because of its thin soft tissue layer. Soft tissue defects of the upper two-thirds can be closed with one or both heads of the M. gastrocnemius. More distal defects are sometimes treated with an additional M. hemisoleus flap. The donor site morbidity of the hemisoleus has been discussed earlier.

Defects of the distal third of the tibia usually require free flap closure. Pedicled fasciocutaneus or muscle flaps are possible alternative treatment options in selected cases.

The distal pedicaled M. peroneus brevis flap or the suralis flap are limited in size and mobility.

Preoperative angiography of the injured leg is mandatory. Sometimes the angiography shows a posttraumatic lesion, but more often it shows atherosclerotic narrowing at several locations. This examination should be done under standby condition for an interventional angiography, which can be used to guide balloon angioplasty catheters and stents to stretch the walls of a narrowed blood vessel, restoring normal blood flow.

If the distal vessels of the leg are not sufficient for primary anastomosis, arteriovenous loops provide adequate perfusion out of the zone of injury or far from scar or irradiated tissue [29].

Local and distant flaps:

- Gastrocnemius flap
- Hemisoleus flap
- Peroneus flap
- Suralis flap

Free flaps:

- Latissimus dorsi flap
- Serratus anterior flap
- Parascapula/scapular flap
- Anterolateral thigh flap
- Radial forearm flap
- Lateral arm flap

13.7.2.4   Foot

For small defects, a variety of local flaps is available, such as the lateral calcaneal artery flap for reconstruction of the calcaneal and malleolar regions. For large defects, free fasciocutaneus muscle or pure fascial flaps are applied. Tissue defects of the heel region are a challenging problem, so that in some cases a lower leg amputation must be considered. After traumatic amputation or mutilating injuries of the forefoot, the technique of tibiocalcanear arthrodesis may be regarded as a limb salvage procedure for selected patients and may yield satisfactory long-term results. The advantage compared to below-knee amputation is that the patient is able to walk short distances without any prosthesis.

Local and distant flaps:

- Suralis flap
- Instep flap
- Lateral calcanear artery flap

Free flaps:

- Latissimus dorsi flap
- Serratus anterior flap
- Parascapula/scapular flap
- Anterolateral thigh flap
- Radial forearm flap
- Lateral arm flap

13.8   Summary and Conclusion

There are many ways in which to deal with soft tissue defects. To reach the best restoration of function and the best esthetic outcome, it is not only necessary to be familiar with the complete spectrum of plastic surgery techniques, it is also essential to operate in the ideal time slot. Therefore, close involvement in interdisciplinary cooperation is mandatory. In cases with severe soft tissue injuries, consulting a plastic surgeon in the very beginning will allow concerted treatment for complex wound closure.

In the authors' opinion, there is no need to follow the so-called sequential reconstructive ladder. Instead, find an ideal strategy using the whole armamentarium of plastic surgery. This can mean immediate salvage operation or delayed wound closure with a free flap in the first line, as well as vacuum therapy and secondary wound closure with split skin graft. Choosing the right treatment for the individual soft tissue reconstruction is the real challenge for the medical team.

References

1. Hildebrand F, Giannoudis P, Kretteck C, Pape HC. Damage control: Extremities. *Injury* 2004;35:678–89.
2. Pape HC, Giannoudis P, Krettek C. The timing of fracture treatment in polytrauma patients: Relevance of damage control orthopedic surgery. *Am J Surg* 2002;183:622–9.
3. Gottlieb LJ, Krieger LM. From the reconstructive ladder to the reconstructive elevator. *Plast Reconstr Surg* 1994;93:1503–4.
4. Mathes SJ, Nahai F. *Reconstructive Surgery: Principles, Anatomy, and Technique.* London: Churchill Livingstone, 1997.
5. Lineaweaver WC. Microsurgery and the reconstructive ladder. *Microsurgery* 2005;25:185–6.
6. Strich R, Bohm HJ. [Dynamic skin suture for secondary skin closure and treatment of skin defects]. *Swiss Surg* 1995:236–40.
7. Mathes SJ. The muscle flap for management of osteomyelitis. *N Engl J Med* 1982;306:294–5.
8. Huang WC, Chen HC, Wei FC, Cheng MH, Schnur DP. Chimeric flap in clinical use. *Clin Plast Surg* 2003;30:457–67.
9. Rosson GD, Williams CG, Fishman EK, Singh NK. 3D CT angiography of abdominal wall vascular perforators to plan DIEAP flaps. *Microsurgery* 2007;27:641–6.
10. Nakatsuka T, Harii K, Asato H, Takushima A, Ebihara S, Kimata Y, Yamada A, Ueda K, Ichioka S. Analytic review of 2372 free flap transfers for head and neck reconstruction following cancer resection. *J Reconstr Microsurg* 2003;19:363–8; discussion 9.
11. Ullmann Y, Fodor L, Ramon Y, Soudry M, Lerner A. The revised "reconstructive ladder" and its applications for high-energy injuries to the extremities. *Ann Plast Surg* 2006;56:401–5.
12. Freedman AM, Meland NB. Arteriovenous shunts in free vascularized tissue transfer for extremity reconstruction. *Ann Plast Surg* 1989;23:123–8.
13. Byrd HS, Cierny G III, Tebbetts JB. The management of open tibial fractures with associated soft-tissue loss: External pin fixation with early flap coverage. *Plast Reconstr Surg* 1981;68:73–82.
14. Godina M. Early microsurgical reconstruction of complex trauma of the extremities. *Plast Reconstr Surg* 1986;78:285–92.
15. Gopal S, Majumder S, Batchelor AG, Knight SL, De Boer P, Smith RM. Fix and flap: The radical orthopaedic and plastic treatment of severe open fractures of the tibia. *J Bone Joint Surg Br* 2000;82:959–66.
16. Machens HG, Kaun M, Lange T, Egbers HJ, Wenzl M, Paech A, Reichert B, Mailänder P. [Clinical impact of operative multidisciplinarity for severe defect injuries of the lower extremity]. *Handchir Mikrochir Plast Chir* 2006;38:403–16.

17. Breidenbach WC III. Emergency free tissue transfer for reconstruction of acute upper extremity wounds. *Clin Plast Surg* 1989;16:505–14.
18. Levin LS. Early versus delayed closure of open fractures. *Injury* 2007;38:896–9.
19. Chen SH, Wei FC, Chen HC, Chuang CC, Noordhoff MS. Emergency free-flap transfer for reconstruction of acute complex extremity wounds. *Plast Reconstr Surg* 1992;89:882–8; discussion 9–90.
20. Arnez ZM. Immediate reconstruction of the lower extremity--an update. *Clin Plast Surg* 1991;18:449–57.
21. Brenner P, Lassner F, Becker M, Berger A. Timing of free microsurgical tissue transfer for the acute phase of hand injuries. *Scand J Plast Reconstr Surg Hand Surg* 1997;31:165–70.
22. Georgescu AV, Ivan O. Emergency free flaps. *Microsurgery* 2003;23:206–16.
23. Lister G, Scheker L. Emergency free flaps to the upper extremity. *J Hand Surg [Am]* 1988;13:22–8.
24. Ninkovic M, Schoeller T, Benedetto KP, Anderl H. Emergency free flap cover in complex injuries of the lower extremities. *Scand J Plast Reconstr Surg Hand Surg* 1996;30:37–47.
25. Cierny G III, Byrd HS, Jones RE. Primary versus delayed soft tissue coverage for severe open tibial fractures. A comparison of results. *Clin Orthop Relat Res* 1983:54–63.
26. Ninkovic M, Mooney EK, Kleistil T, Anderl H. A new classification for the standardization of nomenclature in free flap wound closure. *Plast Reconstr Surg* 1999;103:903–14; discussion 15–7.
27. Weinberg A, Mosheiff R, Liebergall M, Berlatzky Y, Aner H, Neuman RA. Amputated lower limbs as a bank of organs for other organ salvage. *Injury* 1999;30(Suppl 2):B34–8.
28. Dubert T, Oberlin C, Alnot JY. Partial replantation after traumatic proximal lower limb amputation: A one-stage reconstruction with free osteocutaneous transfer from the amputated limb. *Plast Reconstr Surg* 1993;91:537–40.
29. Vogt PM, Steinau HU, Spies M, Kall S, Steiert A, Boorboor P, Vaske B, Jokuszies A. Outcome of simultaneous and staged microvascular free tissue transfer connected to arteriovenous loops in areas lacking recipient vessels. *Plast Reconstr Surg* 2007;120:1568–75.

Chapter 14
The Role of Interventional Radiology

Thomas M. Scalea and Patrick C. Malloy

14.1 Introduction

Damage control is a philosophy of care that involves addressing only the most life-threatening injuries during the initial phases. Nonurgent injuries are temporized and discussed later, when the patient's physiology allows. While damage control was first described for use in patients with penetrating abdominal injury, the principles have been generalized to injuries in the thorax, pelvis, and the remainder of the body.

Clearly, the foremost principle in the use of damage control is rapid hemorrhage control. While this often involves direct surgical approaches, interventional radiologic techniques can also be quite helpful. Diagnostic angiography can precisely identify sites of bleeding that may not be obvious to the surgeon, such as deep in the substance of the liver, in the retroperitoneum, or in deep pelvis. Transcatheter embolization can be life saving in helping to achieve hemostasis. Stent grafting can provide definitive therapy for vascular injuries. Endovascular management may enhance the possibility of success or possibly even eliminate the need for traditional surgery, in some cases allowing for retention of solid organ function in situations when traditional surgical techniques may have mandated organ resection.

The decision to employ interventional techniques is obviously not made in isolation. These techniques must be part of a well-thought-out total patient-care scheme. In patients physiologically unstable enough to require damage control, diagnostics, surgical therapeutics, and interventional procedures may happen simultaneously or in close sequence. Communication among all services providing care is critical to facilitate rapid and efficient care and to optimize outcomes.

T.M. Scalea (✉)
R. Adams Cowley Shock Trauma Center, 22 S. Greene Street, Baltimore, MD, 21201, USA
e-mail: tscalea@umm.edu

H.-C. Pape et al. (eds.), *Damage Control Management in the Polytrauma Patient*,
DOI 10.1007/978-0-387-89508-6_14, © Springer Science+Business Media, LLC 2010

14.2 Factors Affecting Decision Making

A trauma patient who is a candidate for damage control often presents with partially compensated or uncompensated shock due to acute hemorrhage. Rapid assessment (physical examination and limited radiographs) and triage to identify those patients who will benefit from emergency surgical exploration are essential. Adjunct bedside techniques such as diagnostic peritoneal lavage or Focused Abdominal Ultrasound (FAST) help guide decision making. A plain radiograph such as a chest or pelvis x-ray can rapidly identify cavitary threatening hemorrhage or bony injury associated with arterial disruption and hemorrhage.

This evaluation will identify most patients needing emergency surgical procedures; however, there is also a subgroup that will benefit from additional evaluation and intervention outside of the trauma resuscitation unit. In the past, diagnostic angiography was used more commonly to identify sites of bleeding [1]. Currently, imaging with multidetector Computerized Tomography (CT) is most often the next appropriate step in the assessment of stable or meta-stable patients. Due to the short scan times, multidetector CT offers the ability to image the patient in multiple phases of perfusion from early arterial to late venous phases. Scans now take only seconds to perform and minutes to review. Multidetector CT can provide an accurate assessment of the location and extent of solid organ injury and can often detect sites of vascular disruption, including frank arterial extravasation, pseudoaneurysm formation, dissection, or occlusion. Properly performed CT is often able to specifically guide the interventional radiologist to the vascular bed that is injured or, in some instances, to specific vessels that will benefit from a transcatheter intervention [2–4].

Several technical factors will impact the quality of the CT evaluation. Multidetector CT units may range from 4 slices per rotation to the currently available 64 slices per rotation. Due to marked increases in temporal and special resolution, new generation scanners can more effectively suppress motion and delineate anatomic detail. In the acute trauma patients who often cannot cooperate with breathing or motion restrictions, these newer more rapid units can optimize the examination. Properly timed contrast enhancement is essential for anatomic detail and vascular evaluation. Ideally, patients should be evaluated in the early and late arterial phases, as well as in the venous and delayed phases. Although the majority of solid organ injuries are well delineated on axial reconstructions, 3D reconstructions are often useful in vascular injury and disruption, particularly in solid viscera and muscle beds. CT evaluation is often the most important factor in triaging a meta-stable patient. However, CT provides only a snapshot in time in a patient who often has injuries in a state of rapid evolution. Therefore, CT scans with minimal findings can give false assurances in patients who are yet to manifest the findings of their injuries. For instance, a patient with blunt solid organ injury who, at the time of CT, is seen to have a devascularized segment without hemorrhage can evolve to have a pseudoaneurysm with extravasation and active hemorrhage. Finally, the patient who is going to be treated via interventional radiologic techniques must be able to undergo a procedure that lasts a minimum of 30–35 min and to a maximum of 3–4 h from vascular access to completion. These procedures take place in an interventional suite separate and sometimes remote from the trauma resuscitation unit. The patient's injuries continue to evolve, and support in the interventional radiology suite is critical. Though the procedure time may be kept to a minimal, ongoing resuscitation monitoring and evaluation must continue throughout the angiography. This requires interdisciplinary critical care support, including nursing, respiratory therapy, and the active participation of all clinical specialties. Clearly, local expertise, logistics, and the layout of the hospital will impact the decision on when and how to use interventional radiologic techniques safely and efficiently.

14.3   Interventional Radiology as Part of Damage Control

14.3.1   Extremity Injuries

Interventional radiologic techniques are an important part of damage control in the extremity. This is most often used in patients with a mangled extremity. These patients present with massive soft tissue, bony, and vascular injury. Operative exploration is almost always the initial intervention, with intraluminal shunting of damaged blood vessels and on-table angiography. These angiograms are not always of the highest quality, and unless performed using fluoroscopy, they are static and may not accurately characterize blood flow or more distal vascular injury. Temporary bony stability is usually gained with external fixation. Restoring blood flow often activates bleeding that may have been quiescent during hypovolemia and hypotension, for example, bleeding from the deep muscular branches off the profunda femoral circulation. These can be extremely difficult to control with standard surgical techniques.

If the trauma operating room is equipped with biplanar angiographic capability, this is a perfect role for interventional techniques as part of damage control. The angiogram can be performed with better technique than an on-table study, and selective coil embolization for small branch vessel can be employed rather than direct surgical therapy [5]. In addition, injuries below the popliteal arteries and involving the trifurcation can be treated with endovascular techniques. An expendable vessel, such as the peroneal artery, in many cases, can be far more rapidly treated by coil embolization than surgical bypass.

Central larger vessel injury in the extremity can be treated with stent grafts [6]. Stent grafts should be avoided in peripheral vessels in regions of motion or bending such as the femoral and popliteal region. The long term outcome of stent grafts in the extremity is not known, but in certain cases, they obviate the need for surgical exploration, saving time to address more pressing injuries in the thorax and abdomen. If extremity pseudoaneurysms are identified, these can sometimes be managed expectantly and then treated at a later date with direct thrombin injection.

14.3.2 Thoracic Injury

Traditionally, blunt aortic injuries were diagnosed with angiography, followed by surgical exploration and interposition grafting. This required left thoracotomy, time, and, even in the most experienced surgeon's hands, had the physiologic consequences of aortic cross clamping. In some cases, cardiopulmonary bypass plus heparinization was required, and patients with injuries elsewhere were at risk for hemorrhage. More recently, aortic injury has been treated with beta-blockade and delayed surgical repair [7]. This has the advantages of delaying the repair until the patient is more physiologically stable and until all injuries have been addressed. The disadvantages include the hemodynamic consequences of beta-blockade, especially in patients with Central Nervous System (CNS) injuries. In addition, some patients are resistant to conventional beta blockade, requiring very large doses, and a few never achieve adequate beta-blockade and blood pressure management. Clearly, these patients remain at risk for rupture of their aorta.

Endovascular stent grafting of the injured aorta has been described recently with encouraging results [8, 9] (Fig. 14.1a–c). Advantages of stent grafting include rapid and definitive repair using minimally invasive techniques. The technique avoids aortic cross clamping and the risks of paraplegia. Short-term outcome from stent grafts has been quite encouraging. In a recent review, Bansal et al. found many case series reporting success with Endovascular Stenting (EVS) for traumatic aortic injury, with minimal morbidity and mortality. In addition, they cited multiple series comparing open repair with EVS, which all showed a decreased mortality and a decreased incidence of paraplegia [10]. While long-term outcome needs to be determined, this technique should be strongly considered in patients with critical CNS and thoracic injury or in patients requiring damage control. This approach can be especially helpful in patients requiring angioembolization for any other reason, such as pelvic fracture bleeding or solid visceral bleeding. Aortic injuries can be stented after damage control surgical therapy for abdominal or extremity injuries.

Interventional techniques in other areas of the thorax include coil embolization of intercostal arterial injuries. These may be symptomatic and require surgical exploration and ligation for the therapy; however, coil embolization provides definitive therapy.

14.3.3 Intraabdominal Injuries

The use of surgical exploration and packing for hemorrhage control for abdominal injuries are well known and an efficacious part of abdominal damage control. While complete resection of an injured spleen is both straightforward and curative, nephrectomy can have significant consequences, and total hepatectomy is almost always fatal. Transcatheter embolization has a far ranging role for adjunctive hemostasis for solid organ injury. Virtually, any solid organ is amenable to selective embolization.

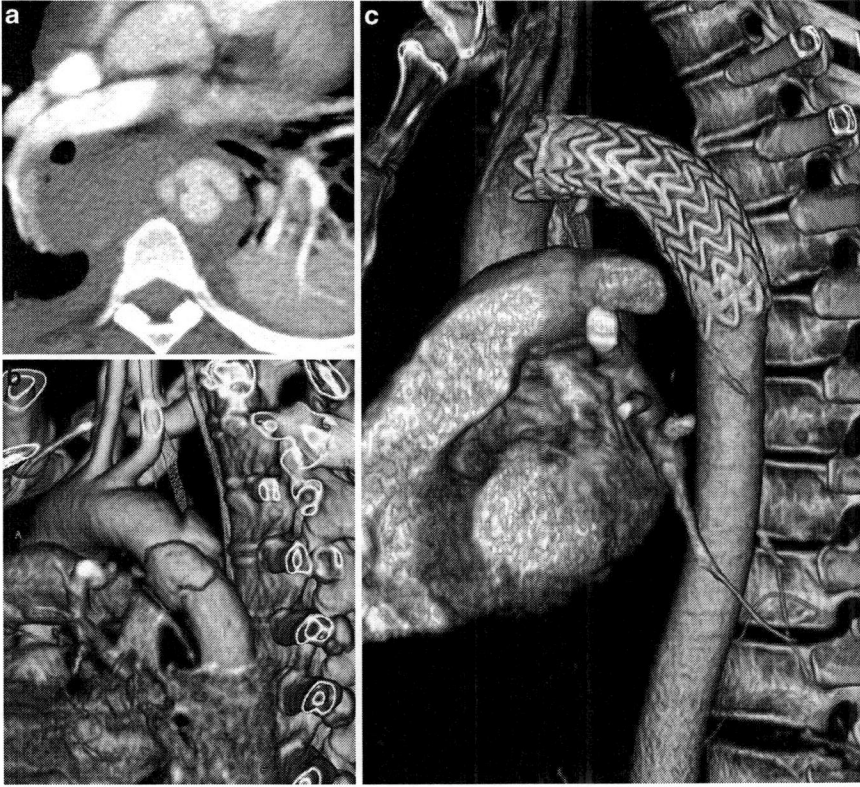

Fig. 14.1 High speed vehicular crash with significant thoracoabdominal injures: (**a**) CT scan demonstrates traumatic aortic injury with associated mediastinal hemorrhage; (**b**) this is confirmed on coronal images; (**c**) the patient was successfully treated with an endovascular stent graft. Postoperative CT scan shows the stent in good place

In patients requiring damage control, blunt hepatic injury often requires operative exploration and packing. However, bleeding from the deep substance of the liver can be difficult to control, and small segmental and subsegmental arterial injuries can cause significant hemorrhage. Pre-op CT scan, if obtained, can identify the site of liver injury and the sites of hepatic vascular disruption and extravasation. Selective embolization, either preoperatively or postoperatively, is a necessary part of the control of bleeding [11, 12] (Fig. 14.2a–d).

Angiography is highly successful for the diagnosis and treatment of intrahepatic vascular injury. Hepatic disruption, contrast extravasation, and pseudoaneurysms are commonly seen on nonselective angiography, including nonselective aortic flush imaging. Actively bleeding vessels often respond with severe vasoconstriction and require a more selective diagnostic approach. Superselective embolization with coils is the preferred method of hemostasis. Gel foam should be avoided if possible to avoid the possible consequences of hepatic infarction and/or biliary ischemia.

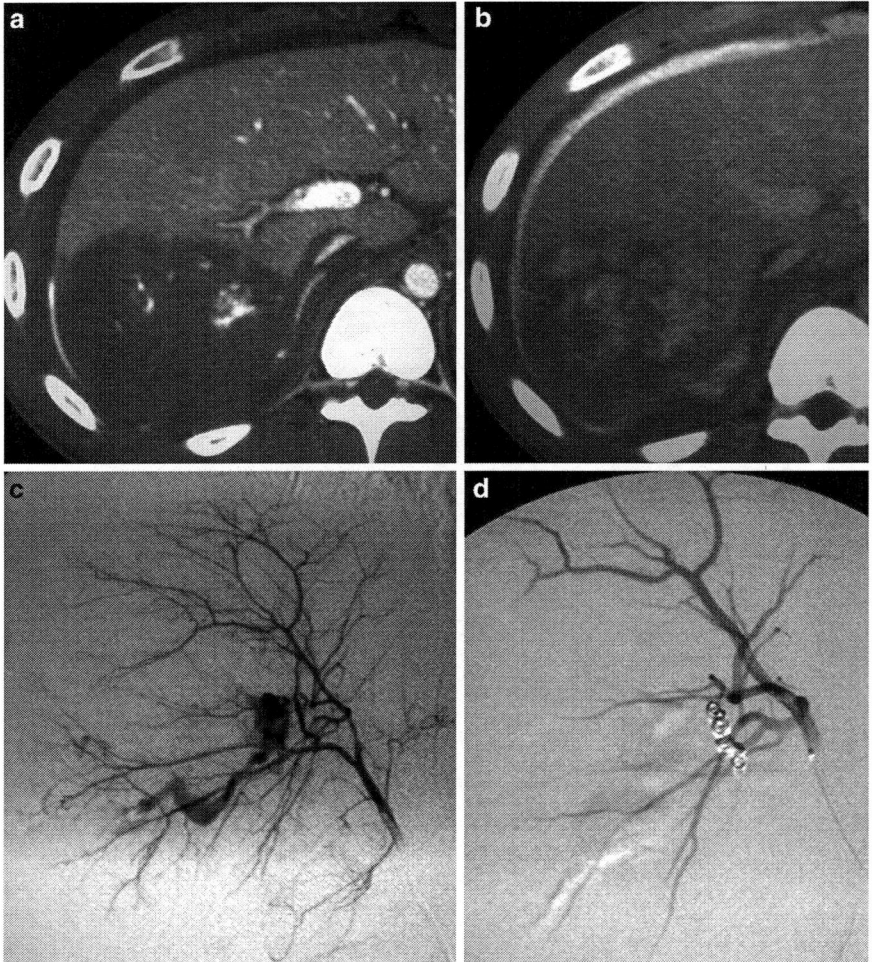

Fig. 14.2 Multitrauma high speed vehicular crash with obvious injury to the right upper quadrant: (**a**) CT scan demonstrates a Grade IV liver injury with contrast extravasation. There is a suggestion of extravasation outside the capsule of the liver; (**b**) delayed images clearly demonstrate active contrast extravasation outside the liver; (**c**) hepatic artery angiography demonstrates a large vascular injury with active bleeding; (**d**): this was successfully treated with selective coil embolization

Portal venous injury is a particularly difficult injury to treat. Direct surgical exploration and repair require significant expertise and experience [13]. The diagnosis of extra hepatic portal venous injury can be made on CT scan. These can be treated with stent graft deployment via a transhepatic "TIPS" approach.

Similar techniques can be used for hemostasis in the kidney. High grade renal lacerations may produce significant retroperitoneal hemorrhage. However, only retroperitoneal hemotoma that are pulsatile or rapidly expanding are generally explored at the time of laparotomy. Again, CT scanning can be very helpful in both diagnosing and classifying the extent of renal injury, including identifying active extravasation or pseudoaneurysm formation. Subselective and superselective coil embolization can often save the majority of functioning renal parenchyma and are preferable, since operative exploration often results in nephrectomy. Large vessel pseudoaneurysms can be treated with small stent grafts; transected or occlusive dissected vessels should be embolized with coil even in the absence of active extravasation in order to prevent bleeding later [14, 15].

In patients requiring damage control, splenic injuries identified at the time of laparotomy are almost always treated with splenectomy. Splenectomy is rapid, safe, and provides definitive hemostasis. However, some patients with significant intraparenchymal splenic injury may have relatively normal appearing spleens at the time of laparotomy. In addition, patients undergoing imaging later as part of damage control may have splenic injuries identified. Proximal coil embolization is very attractive as an alternative to immediate relaparotomy for splenectomy, thus allowing the patient time to stabilize in the ICU. Blunt trauma to the spleen produces regional vascular injury that may manifest as devascularization, pseudo-aneurysm, or active extravasation. Proximal coil embolization is the preferred technique and occludes the main splenic artery at a point between the origin to just proximal to the last collateral near the hilum (Fig. 14.3a–c). This reduces splenic perfusion pressure while the spleen remains viable via collateral circulation. In the finding of active extravasation, superselective embolization may be beneficial if it can be accomplished expeditiously. Depending on individual anatomy, however, this may be a time-consuming procedure, and patients unstable enough to require damage control are usually better served by proximal embolization or splenectomy. Particulate and gel foam embolization should be avoided in the trauma patient, as it leads to a high rate of splenic infarct and abscess [16].

14.3.4   Treatment of Blunt Pelvic Fracture Bleeding

Care of the hemodynamically unstable patient with hemorrhage due to blunt pelvic fracture may be the best example of multidisciplinary trauma care. The therapies available to treat pelvic fracture bleeding are many and must occur simultaneously or in tight sequence in order to control significant pelvic hemorrhage. The most important initial steps are to rule out free cavitary bleeding in the chest and abdomen and to characterize the pelvic fracture. Those with widely displaced pelvis fractures should have a pelvic binder or sheet applied and tightened for reduction. Patients who continue to be hypotensive are best served by rapid angiography and coil embolization. Finally, patients who are too unstable to undergo angiography should undergo operative exploration and extraperitoneal pelvic packing, which can be used as a bridge to angiography [17].

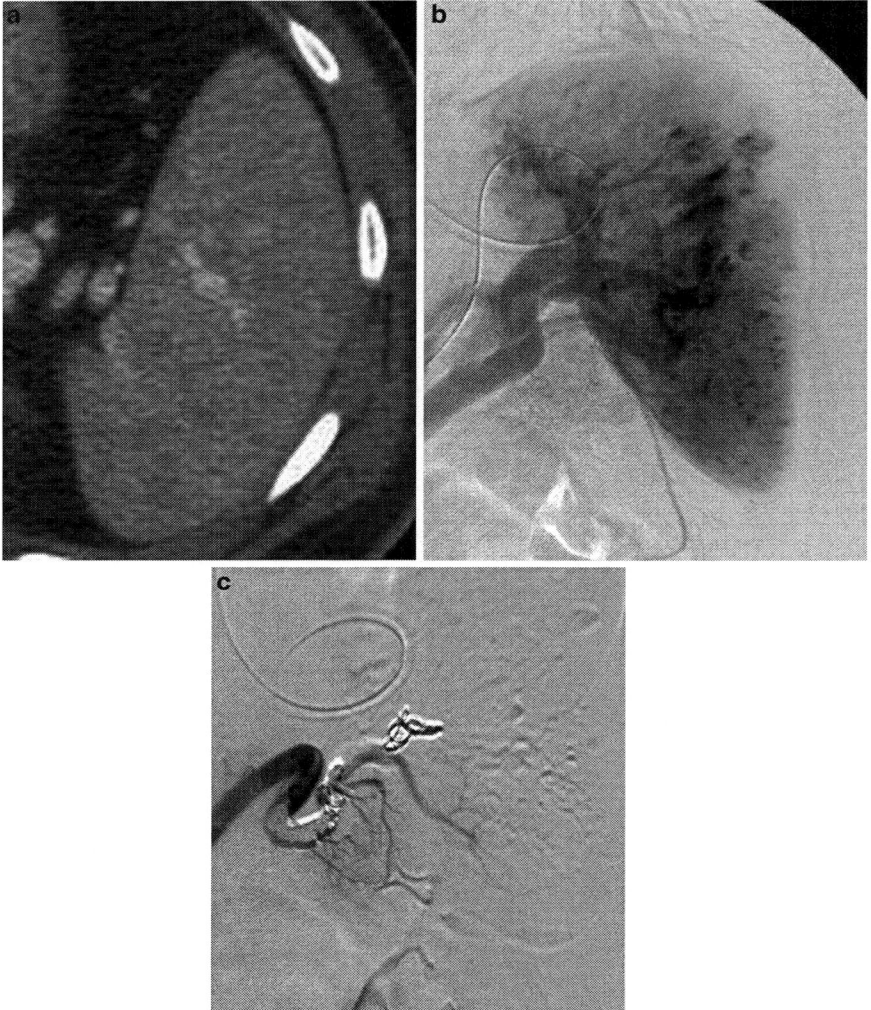

Fig. 14.3 Polytrauma to the abdomen: (**a**) CT scan demonstrates high grade splenic injury with multiple areas of pseudoaneurysm formation; (**b**) coronal sections confirmed contrast extravasation; (**c**) selective splenic artery angiography demonstrates a large number of pseudoaneurysms that was treated with proximal coil embolization

Patients who continue to bleed after external compression or patients whose fracture pattern is not amenable to external compression, such as those following lateral compression pelvic fractures, are often best served by angiographic embolization (Fig. 14.4a–d). Table 14.1 depicts our indications for angiography. Major vascular injuries can sometimes be identified on a flush distal aortography.

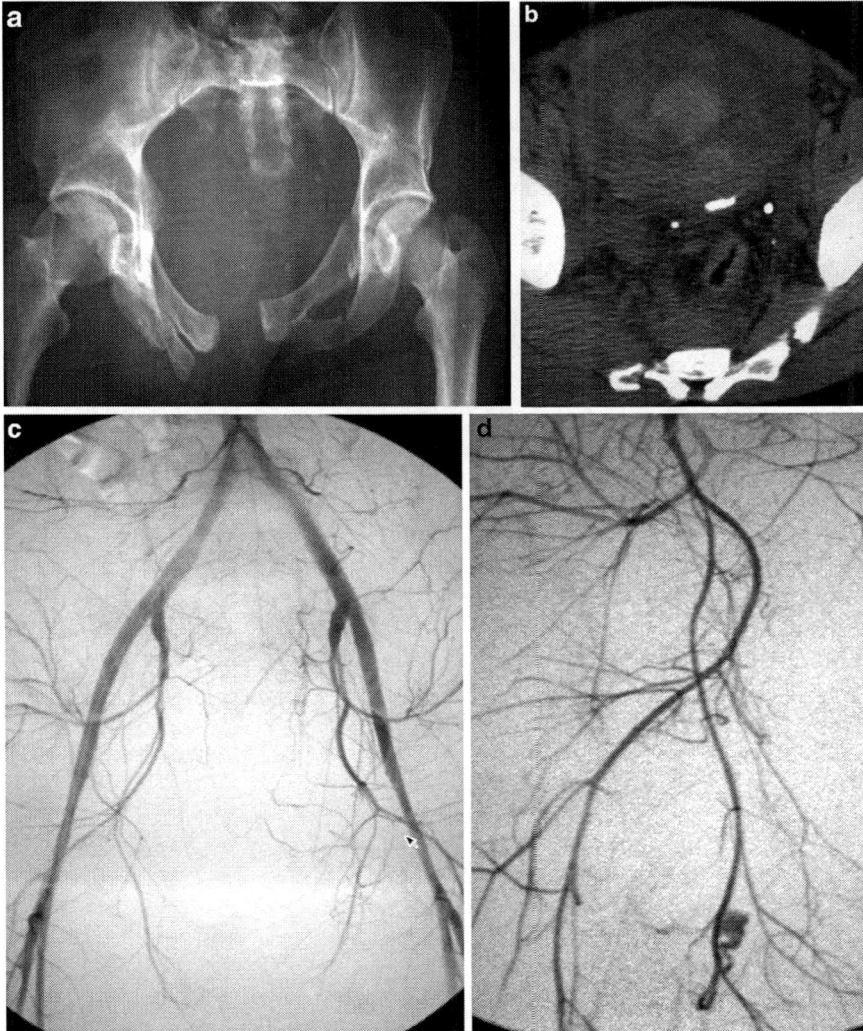

Fig. 14.4 High speed motorcycle crash with polytrauma. Multitrauma to abdomen with multiple solid organ injuries: (**a**) plain films of the pelvis demonstrate AP III injury; (**b**) CT scan demonstrates significant retroperitoneal hemorrhage with contrast blush; (**c**) aortography suggests an injury within the left hypogastric arterial distribution; (**d**) selective hypogastric injection demonstrates significant contrast extravasation. This was treated with selective coil embolization

Identifying more subtle vascular injuries requires selective iliac and hypogastric cannulation and diagnostic angiography. The entire pelvic vasculature must be studied, including bilateral iliac systems, before the angiogram is considered complete. Approximately 50% of patients with one vascular injury will have a second concomitant injury identified [18].

Table 14.1 Indications for angiography after blunt pelvic trauma

1. Large pelvic hematoma on CT
2. Uncontrollable pelvic bleeding at exploratory laparotomy
3. Major pelvic fracture and hemodynamic instability
4. Pelvic pseudo aneurysm on helical CT
5. Greater than 4 units transfused for pelvic bleeding in under 24 h
6. Greater than 6 units transfused for pelvic bleeding in under 48 h

Ideally, embolization should be performed as selectively as possible. This limits the possibility of pelvic ischemia and may limit complications. Hemodynamically unstable patients, particularly those with more than one vascular injury, may not be candidates for selective embolization, which can be quite time consuming. In these patients, particulate or gel foam embolization may be the wisest course. Proximal hypogastric coil embolization is also an option. This will drop perfusion pressure to the pelvis, allowing spontaneous thrombosis of small vascular injuries. It eliminates the possibility of using repeat embolization, however, if bleeding persists [19–21]. Bilateral hypogastric artery embolization is associated with a high incidence of gluteal necrosis and should be employed with caution.

Some patients may be bleeding from the pelvis too rapidly to allow safe transport to the angiography suite. Alternatively, patients may be found to have expanding pelvic hematomas at the time of laparotomy. Both of these subsets of patients are good candidates for extraperitoneal pelvic packing as part of damage control. Extraperitoneal pelvic packing is a technique that has been used in Europe for some time, but it has only recently gained some popularity in the United States. This involves making either a lower midline incision or a pfanansteil incision. The extraperitoneal space is entered below the peritoneal reflection. The pelvic hematoma can then be evacuated. The pelvis is packed utilizing the pelvic peritoneum in order to increase pressure in the pelvic space, helping to tamponade the bleeding. The fascia can be closed to increase the tamponade, or it can simply be packed open with a vacuum dressing, in a technique similar to that used for damage control in the abdomen.

There are two recent series that support the use of extraperitoneal packing. The group from Denver General uses pelvic packing more liberally than many, packing patients who remained hypotensive after two units of blood. Perhaps not surprisingly, angiography was often not necessary in their series [22]. The group from Oslo used pelvic packing more as a component of damage control [23]. In this series, patients underwent pelvic packing only if they were too unstable to undergo angiography. Pelvic packing was used as a bridge to angiography, and the subsequent angiograms were positive approximately 90% of the time. The authors' own experience with pelvic packing is similar to the Oslo group's experience. The authors have used this technique 13 times in the last several years and used it only in patients who are too unstable to be taken to the angiography suite. Virtually, every patient in the authors' institution then undergoes angiography following pelvic packing. Unpublished data from the authors' institution have also shown angiography to be positive approximately 90% of the time.

14.4 Summary and Conclusion

Endovascular management of both blunt and penetrating injury has the potential to be lifesaving, while resulting in retained organ function and decreased morbidity as compared to traditional surgical techniques when used with the same injuries. When utilizing these techniques as part of damage control, they can be used both as an alternative and in conjunction with surgical techniques. The use of endovascular therapy rarely precludes future surgical intervention. Percutaneous techniques are minimally invasive, and in those with critical injuries, they may be the preferred to multiple operations. Endovascular embolization does carry the risk of organ dysfunction and delayed fracture healing. These procedures are dependent on institutional and individual interest and expertise. Institutional support is necessary at a high level in order to be able to safely use these techniques as part of the damage control strategy.

References

1. Sclafani SJ, Cooper R, Shaftan GW, Goldstein AS, Glanz S, Gordon DH. Arterial trauma: diagnostic and therapeutic angiography. Radiology 1986;161:165–172.
2. Shanmuganathan K, Mirvis SE, Boyd-Kranis R, Takada T, Scalea TM. Nonsurgical management of blunt splenic injury: use of ct criteria to select patients for splenic arteriography and potential endovascular therapy. Radiology 2000;217:75–82.
3. Poletti PA, Mirvis SE, Shanmuganathan K, Killeen KL, Coldwell D. CT criteria for management of blunt liver trauma: correlation with angiographic and surgical findings. Radiology 2000;216:418–427.
4. Busquets AR, Acosta JA, Colon E, Alejandro KV, Rodriguez P. Computed tomographic angiography for the diagnosis of traumatic arterial injuries of the extremities. J Trauma 2004;56(3):625–628.
5. Mavili E, Donmez H, Ozcan N, Akcali Y. Endovascular treatment of lower limb penetrating arterial traumas. Cardiovasc Intervent Radiol 2007;30(6):1124–1129 .
6. Stecco K, Meier A, Seiver A, Dake M, Zarins C. Endovascular stent-graft placement for treatment of traumatic penetrating subclavian artery injury. J Trauma 2000;48(5):948–950.
7. Symbas P, Sherman AJ, Silver JM, Symbas JD, Lackey JJ. Traumatic rupture of the aorta: immediate or delayed repair? Annals of Surgery 2002;235(6):796–802.
8. Semba CP, Kato N, Kee ST, Lee GK, Mitchell RS, Miller DC, Dake MD. Acute rupture of the descending thoracic aorta: repair with use of endovascular stent-grafts. J Vasc Interv Radiol 1997;8:337–342.
9. Neschis D, Moaine S, Gutta R, Charles K, Scalea T, Flinn W, Griffith G. Twenty consecutive cases of endograft repair of traumatic aortic disruption: Lessons learned. J Vascu Surg 2007;45(3):487–492.
10. Bansal V, Lee J, Coimbra R. Current diagnosis and management of blunt traumatic rupture of the thoracic aorta. J Vasc Bras 2007;6(1):64–73.
11. Carrillo EH, Platz A, Miller FB, Richardson JD, Polk Jr HC. Non-operative management of blunt hepatic trauma. Br J Surg 1998;85:461–468.
12. Wahl WL, Ahrns KS, Brandt MM, Franklin GA, Taheri PA. The need for early angiographic embolization in blunt liver injuries. J Trauma 2002;52(6):1097–1101.
13. Stone HH, Fabian TC, Turkleson ML. Wounds of the portal venous system. World J Surg 1982;6:335–341.

14. Dinkel H-P, Danuser H, Triller J. Blunt renal trauma: minimally invasive management with microcatheter embolization – experience in nine patients. Radiology 2002;223:723–730.
15. Pappas P, Leonardou P, Papadoukakis S, Zavos G, Michail S, Boletis J, Tzortzis G. Urgent superselective segmental renal artery embolization in the treatment of life-threatening Renal Hemorrhage Department of Radiology, Laiko General Hospital, Athens, Greece. Urol Int 2006;77:34–41.
16. Haan JM, Bochicchio GV, Kramer N, Scalea TM. Nonoperative management of blunt splenic injury: a 5-year experience. J Trauma 2005;58(3):492–498.
17. Ertel W, Oberholzer A, Platz A, Stocker R, Trentz O. Incidence and clinical pattern of the abdominal compartment syndrome after "damage-control" laparotomy in 311 patients with severe abdominal and/or pelvic trauma. Crit Care Med 2000;28(6):1747–1753.
18. O'Neill PA, Riina J, Sclafani S, Tornetta III P. Angiographic findings in pelvic fractures. Techniques and outcome in pelvic fractures. Clin Orthop Relat Res 1996;329:60–67.
19. Velmahos GC, Toutouzas K, Vassiliu P, Sarkisyan G, Chan LS, Hanks SH, Berne TV, Demetriades D. A prospective study on the safety and efficacy of angiographic embolization for pelvic and visceral injuries. J Trauma 2002;53(2):303–308.
20. Ramirez JI, Velmahos GC, Best CR, Chan S, Demetriades D. Male sexual function after bilateral internal iliac artery embolization for pelvic fracture. J Trauma 2004;56(4):734–741.
21. Obaro RO, Sniderman KW. Case report: avascular necrosis of the femoral head as a complication of complex embolization for severe pelvic haemorrhage. Br J Radiol 1995;68:920–922.
22. Cothren CC, Osborn PM, Moore EE, Morgan SJ, Johnson JL, Smith WR. Preperitonal pelvic packing for hemodynamically unstable pelvic fractures: a paradigm shift. J Trauma 2007;62:834–842.
23. Totterman A, Madsen JE, Skaga NO, Roise O. Extraperitoneal pelvic packing: a salvage procedure to control massive traumatic pelvic hemorrhage. J Trauma 2007;62:843–852.

Part III
Special Aspects of Damage Control

Chapter 15
Head Injuries in Polytrauma Patients

James M. Schuster

The management of a head injured patient with multiple other injuries presents one of the most challenging and difficult clinical scenarios in trauma critical care. This is, in part, due to the fact that the treatment of other injuries, such as orthopedic, spine, and craniofacial fractures, has the potential for worsening the neurologic outcome. This potential worsening is not necessarily directly related to the primary repair or the timing of surgery, but more to the fact that additional surgery with potential blood loss and possible resultant hypotension or hypoxia can adversely affect an injured brain. A single episode of hypotension or hypoxia can adversely affect the outcome of all severities of head injury [1–6].

Management of polytrauma patients with head injury requires strict adherence to Advanced Trauma Life Support (ATLS®) principles and close coordination and communication between all involved surgical specialties, including simultaneous procedures when appropriate. Decision-making is all about assessing relative risk, with priority initially given to life-threatening and neurologic injuries, but with a simultaneous evaluation and possible management of orthopedic, spine, and craniofacial injuries. This often requires flexibility on the part of the involved services, as surgical decisions should not be based on convenience of the physicians. This approach provides an opportunity for imaginative and innovative surgical management. Definitive repair procedures are not always possible or appropriate because of the length of the case, the inability to appropriately provide neurologic monitoring, and the potential for significant blood loss and fluid administration. Other options include placement of external fixation, choosing a surgical approach based on reduced operative time and reduced blood loss, or staged procedures.

The trauma surgery team often serves as the coordinator of care for multiply injured patients, as each involved service can be somewhat myopic in its approach to the patient. However, once the patient has stabilized and once life-threatening injuries are addressed immediately, the neurosurgery consultant feels the obligation

J.M. Schuster (✉)
Department of Neurosurgery, University of Pennsylvania, 3400 Spruce Street, Silverstein, 3rd Floor, Philadelphia, PA, 19104, USA
e-mail: schustej@uphs.upenn.edu

H.-C. Pape et al. (eds.), *Damage Control Management in the Polytrauma Patient*,
DOI 10.1007/978-0-387-89508-6_15, © Springer Science+Business Media, LLC 2010

to protect the brain and spinal cord at all costs. While the neurosurgeons are usually very involved with the simultaneous management of spine injuries, they must be well informed about the effects of delayed treatment of orthopedic or craniofacial injuries. Again, this decision-making often comes down to an assessment of relative risk. Ultimately, while patients with lost or suboptimally functioning limbs or craniofacial defects can return to independent functioning; this is less often the case in patients with significant brain injuries. Again, avoidance of secondary injury must be paramount. The intent of this chapter is to provide a template for rapid management of head injury in polytrauma patients, including an initial assessment paradigm (Fig. 15.1) to aid in making decisions about the need for emergent neurosurgical intervention, as well as to provide a system for prioritizing and coordinating the treatment of other injuries.

15.1 Initial Assessment

The overall approach to a head injured patient should be aggressive and timely treatment of the primary injury and avoidance of secondary injury. The basic underlying questions that need to be addressed early in the assessment are as follows:

- Does this problem need immediate surgical intervention?
- Is the injury likely to require intervention in the near future?
- Or is this an injury not likely to need surgical intervention?

These decisions are based on a clinical and radiographic assessment of the patient. Injuries such as Epidural Hematomas (EDH), Subdural Dematomas (SDH), intraparenchymal hemorrhage, contusions, or penetrating injuries with altered neurologic status (especially pupillary abnormalities and lateralizing motor finding) often require immediate surgical intervention. The question of salvageability of the patient often arises, especially in patients with fixed, dilated pupils and Glascow Coma Score of 3 [7, 8]. While the decision should be individualized, the survivability of such injuries is debatable. However, it is imperative that the clinical assessment is not altered by pharmacologic muscle paralysis or injuries/medications that can alter pupillary function. There is also a danger of being too reassured by a patient's initial clinical assessment such as in patients with the "talk and die syndrome." This is generally seen in a young patient with bifrontal or subfrontal injuries (often contusions) who initially may be awake and talking (Fig. 15.2a–c). Because of basal-frontal swelling near the brainstem, any perturbation, such as a seizure or hypoxemia, can set in motion a rapidly progressive clinical spiral, leading to fixed dilated pupils, which then requires emergent surgery to avoid poor outcome [9].

Once the decision is made that a patient needs an operation, the question then arises: What operation? The operative plan must take into account the presence of intracranial hematomas, overall brain swelling, intracranial foreign bodies, involvement of major vascular structures, and the involvement of air sinuses that need to

Polytrauma patient with head injury

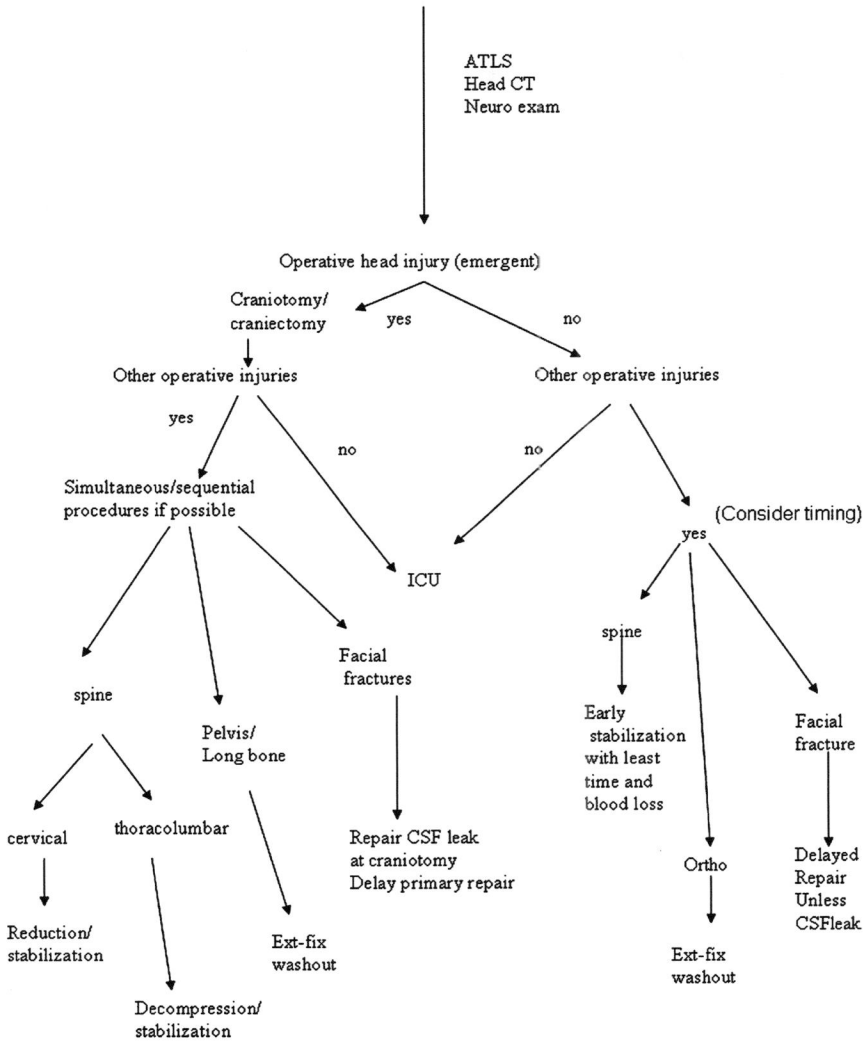

ATLS
Head CT
Neuro exam

Operative head injury (emergent)

Craniotomy/
craniectomy   yes   no

Other operative injuries   Other operative injuries

yes

Simultaneous/sequential
procedures if possible   (Consider timing)
                                                          yes
                              no   no

                              ICU

                                        spine

                          Facial
                          fractures

spine   Early
                                        stabilization   Facial
                                        with least   fracture
              Pelvis/   time and
              Long bone   blood loss

cervical   thoracolumbar   Repair CSF leak
                                 at craniotomy   Ortho   Delayed
                                 Delay primary repair   Repair
                                                                       Unless
Reduction/   CSFleak
stabilization   Ext-fix
                           washout
                                                         Ext-fix
            Decompression/   washout
            stabilization

Fig. 15.1 Decision-making flow sheet for polytrauma patient with associated head injury

be addressed to avoid CSF leak. The general approach is to evacuate hematomas, debride devitalized tissue, remove accessible foreign bodies, and repair CSF leaks. The likelihood of the patient developing significant problems with raised intracranial pressure postoperatively must also be addressed. Concerns for postoperative management often drive the decision to perform a craniectomy, with storage of the bone subcutaneously in the abdomen or in the freezer until the brain swelling has

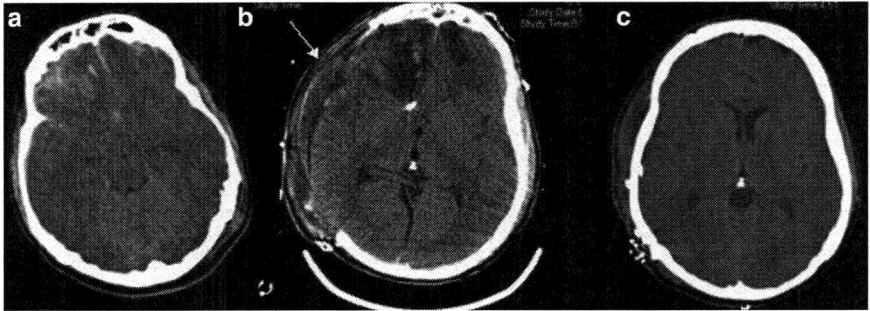

Fig. 15.2 Patient at risk for "Talk and Die" Syndrome. (**a**) CT scan showing frontal contusions. (**b**) CT scan showing right hemicraniectomy (*arrow*) after progressive neurologic decline. (**c**) CT showing replacement of bone at 8 weeks after patient made excellent neurologic recovery

subsided and the bone can be replaced. This procedure also requires dural augmentation with pericranium or a dural substitute to allow swelling of the brain out of the bone defect, thus decompressing the brain. The procedure can be performed unilaterally, bifrontally, or bihemispherically, depending on the pattern of injury [10–14] (Fig. 15.2b, c). The removal of bone must be adequate to insure that, as the brain swells out of the defect, it is not lacerated or contused against a bone edge. Craniectomy, if performed adequately, is the most effective and durable way to reduce intracranial pressure. While ultimate outcome is still heavily tied to the severity of the initial injury and neurologic status, there is evidence that hemicraniectomy can reduce intracranial pressure and improve brain oxygenation as measured by invasive monitoring in head injured patients [15, 16]. The other advantage of hemicraniectomy and the subsequent improvement in ICP and brain oxygenation is that it often makes postoperative management less physiologically stressful to the patients as they are less likely to require osmotic diuretics, blood pressure support, and heavy sedation. In patients with less severe injuries but labile intracranial pressure, the placement of a ventriculostomy for CSF diversion can be an extremely effective and less physiologically stressful treatment of raised intracranial pressure.

After aggressive surgical treatment of the primary intracranial injury, the introduction of aggressive neurocritical care has been shown to positively impact brain injured patients [17–19]. Using monitoring to measure brain oxygenation and intracranial pressure, the use of continuous EEG to detect seizures and ischemia and the use of protocol-driven approaches to glycemic control and hyperthermia are routinely implemented [20–22]. Early tracheostomy and enteral access are initiated to facilitate patient care [23, 24].

Finally, consulting services such as orthopedics often inquire regarding when a patient is stable enough to allow further surgery. This decision needs to be individualized based on injury severity, clinical exam, neurophysiologic stability based on monitoring, the perceived urgency of the proposed surgery, and the potential physiologic stress of the surgery, including length and risk of large blood loss or large fluid volume administration. Physiologic monitoring is also recommended during the case (ICP, brain oxygenation), which may affect positioning and the potential to abort the procedure if a problem arises. Essentially, management in the OR must be an extension of the management in the ICU, with the same vigilance with regard to monitoring and proactive intervention [25].

As can be seen from the above discussion, there is an apparent paradox in the treatment approach to a patient with a head injury and associated injuries. We aggressively and definitively treat the primary CNS injury in order to avoid secondary injury, while treating other associated injuries in a damage control fashion. This is, in part, due to the fragile nature of CNS structures, characterized by little reparative capability, little functional reserve, and a narrow window of time with regard to salvageability after injury. The authors will discuss this approach in the subsequent sections. Finally, surgical decision making involves relative risk assessment, and, therefore, it is imperative that patients and families understand the complexity of these interactions and have realistic expectations for outcome and recovery.

15.2 Head Injury Associated with Major Chest/Abdominal Injury

Stabilizing a patient's cardiopulmonary status must always be the highest priority in dealing with a trauma patient. However, there are clinical scenarios in which a patient is taken emergently to the operating room to deal with life-threatening thoracoabdominal trauma with a suspected brain injury, but without confirmatory neuroimaging. There is traditional support for placing burr holes on the side of a "blown" pupil in the ED or in the OR during thoracoabdominal surgery. While, if performed correctly, there is the potential to relieve pressure from an evolving EDH or SDH, this may not be the definitive procedure, and a craniotomy may also be required [26, 27]. This in theory could follow after cardiopulmonary stabilization. In the case of bilateral "blown" pupils, practitioners must keep in mind that hypoxia/hypotension can cause pupillary abnormalities that do not indicate an intracranial space occupying mass [28]. As neurosurgeons, we are sometimes asked to place intracranial monitors in patients undergoing "crash" thoracotomies or exploratory laporotomies with suspected intracranial pathology. However, elevated ICP is difficult to interpret in a patient lying flat or head down and receiving massive fluid resuscitation. Additionally, therapeutic interventions such as mannitol would not be indicated in a hypotensive patient. The key in the management of the patient with brain injury in this setting is early cranial imaging. A rapid helical CT scan, preoperatively if possible, or utilization of a portable CT scanner intraoperatively would obviate this problem.

15.3   Head Injury Associated with Cranial Facial Injury

Head injury from blunt force trauma or penetrating wounds has the potential for involvement of the air sinuses, such as the frontal sinus, as well as cranial facial structures [29, 30]. Although not absolute indications for surgical intervention, the presence of pneumocephalus or a CSF leak must be closely monitored. Increasing pneumocephalus or rhinorrhea/otorrhea that does not resolve spontaneously may require surgical intervention. The goal of an operation in a patient with significant intracranial pathology (hematoma, contusion) associated with pneumocephalus/CSF leak (i.e., from an anterior skull base fracture/frontal sinus fracture) is to adequately deal with the intracranial pathology and stop the CSF leak, essentially isolating the brain from the nose [31, 32]. There is often input from multiple services, including neurosurgery and ENT, OMFS, or plastics, but it is generally in the patient's interest to delay the definitive repair of facial fractures because of the overall extension of the operative time [33]. If CSF diversion is required to protect the repair, a ventriculostomy is preferred to a lumbar drain in a patient with suspected intracranial swelling. Compression of the optic nerve could also be addressed by this approach if indicated [34].

Skull base fractures can also cause damage to carotid arteries. There should be a high index of suspicion with these types of fractures. Treatment options include medical management or more invasive surgical or endovascular therapy. Therapy depends on the risk-benefit ratio of each option, considering the natural history of each injury type: mild intimal irregularities, intimal flaps, pseudoaneurysms, fistulas, and occlusions. The need for treatment is determined in part by the collateral circulation to the brain and the degree to which the lesion is thrombogenic [35]. It is beyond the scope of this chapter to discuss the management of traumatic carotid injury, but the risk of anticoagulation must be considered in a patient with significant intracranial injury [36].

15.4   Head Injury with Spine Injury

There is a high incidence of associated spine fracture with head injury, especially with falls and motor vehicle accidents [37]. It is often difficult to clinically clear the cervical spine in a patient with a significant head injury, even without obvious radiographic abnormalities. But the more pressing difficulty occurs with the combination of an operative head injury and an operative spine injury. In the case of spine fracture/dislocation with a spinal cord injury such as with bilateral jumped facets and burst fractures, early decompression and stabilization are optimal [38, 39]. While these injuries can be decompressed in traction, this delays mobilization, which has been shown to negatively impact outcome secondary to pulmonary issues [40–43]. With simultaneous operative injuries, the cranial portion could be completed and the cervical spine be reduced and stabilized through an anterior approach if possible. In critically ill patients with unstable thoracolumbar fractures, a posterior approach can be utilized in a time efficient and less physiologically stressful manner for decompression/stabilization, even if an anterior approach will subsequently be required. This staged stabilization/decompression allows mobilization and thus helps avoid life threatening pulmonary complications [42, 43]. These stabilization procedures can sometimes be performed in a percutaneous/minimally invasive method, significantly reducing blood loss and physiologic stress [44].

Blunt vertebral artery injury is associated with complex cervical spine fractures involving subluxation, extension into the foramen transversarium, or upper C1 to C3 fractures [45]. The posterior circulation stroke rate has been reported as high as 12–24% after traumatic vertebral artery injury [46, 47]. Treatment of vertebral artery injuries, such as dissections, pseudoaneurysms, fistulas, and occlusions, must be individualized with regard to the use of anticoagulation and/or endovascular treatment based on the patient's clinical status, risk of ischemic/thrombotic potential for the individual lesions, and the suitability of the patient for anticoagulation based on intracranial pathology and other injuries [46–48].

15.5 Head Injury with Orthopedic Injury

The combination of head injuries and significant orthopedic injuries is relatively common with motor vehicle accidents and falls. Major orthopedic trauma can be both life-threatening (pelvic fractures with vascular injuries) as well as limb-threatening, especially with open and potentially contaminated extremity injuries. Ideally, head injuries and orthopedic injuries can be assessed and, if possible, treated simultaneously. If the patient is going to the OR for an operative head injury, every effort should be made to treat orthopedic injuries in a damage control fashion. Any injury that can realistically be splinted or casted and treated definitively in a delayed fashion. Any injury that can be treated with external fixation or washed out and closed when the patient initially goes to the OR for a head injury should be treated simultaneously. This damage control method has been shown to be both safe and effective [49–55]. The problem often arises when these injuries are not treated simultaneously and early. Once the patient is in the ICU, there is generally resistance to allow the patient to go to the OR if they have labile vital signs, especially brain oxygenation and intracranial pressure difficulties. In this case, these decisions need to be made in a coordinated fashion between the involved services. This often results in a compromise in which the patient is allowed to go to the OR for a less time-consuming and less physiologically-stressful procedure. While this is an area of discussion, there is growing evidence to support this approach [51–53, 56].

15.6 Summary and Conclusion

The management of a polytrauma patient with a significant head injury represents one of the most complicated clinical scenarios encountered by the trauma team. However, it provides an opportunity to implement innovative and imaginative management strategies that require communication, coordination, and flexibility among the involved subspecialties. Primary intracranial pathologies need to be treated aggressively, and secondary injuries need to be avoided. Head injuries, spine injuries, orthopedic injuries, and craniofacial injuries with CSF leaks need to be assessed and treated simultaneously if possible. The definitive treatment of the extra-cranial injuries can often be delayed, with the initial therapy designed to stabilize spine, pelvis, and long bone injuries as well as to repair CSF leaks associated with cranial facial injuries. This facilitates management in the ICU and helps prevent pulmonary complications, which are a major source of morbidity and mortality. Additionally, neurocritical care, provided in the ICU, needs to be extended to the OR to avoid secondary brain injury. Subsequently, with stabilization and improvement of the head injury, the extra-cranial injuries can be readdressed.

References

1. Chesnut RM. Secondary brain insults after head injury: clinical perspectives. *New Horiz* 1995;3(3):366–75.
2. Chesnut RM, Marshall LF, Klauber MR, Blunt BA, Baldwin N, Eisenberg HM, Jane JA, Marmarou A, Foulkes MA. The role of secondary brain injury in determining outcome from severe head injury. *J Trauma* 1993;34(2):216–22.
3. Chesnut RM, Marshall SB, Piek J, Blunt BA, Klauber MR, Marshall LF. Early and late systemic hypotension as a frequent and fundamental source of cerebral ischemia following severe brain injury in the Traumatic Coma Data Bank. *Acta Neurochir Suppl (Wien)* 1993;59:121–5.
4. Chi JH, Knudson MM, Vassar MJ, McCarthy MC, Shapiro MB, Mallet S, Holcroft JJ, Moncrief H, Noble J, Wisner D, Kaups KL, Bennick LD, Manley GT. Prehospital hypoxia affects outcome in patients with traumatic brain injury: a prospective multicenter study. *J Trauma* 2006; 61(5):1134–41.
5. Jeremitsky E, Omert L, Dunham CM, Protetch J, Rodriguez A. Harbingers of poor outcome the day after severe brain injury: hypothermia, hypoxia, and hypoperfusion. *J Trauma* 2003;54(2):312–9.
6. Manley G, Knudson MM, Morabito D, Damron S, Erickson V, Pitts L. Hypotension, hypoxia, and head injury: frequency, duration, and consequences. *Arch Surg* 2001;136(10):1118–23.
7. Tien HC, Cunha JR, Wu SN, Chughtai T, Tremblay LN, Brenneman FD, Rizoli SB. Do trauma patients with a Glasgow Coma Scale score of 3 and bilateral fixed and dilated pupils have any chance of survival? *J Trauma* 2006;60(2):274–8.
8. Udekwu P, Kromhout-Schiro S, Vaslef S, Baker C, Oller D. Glasgow coma scale score, mortality, and functional outcome in head-injured patients. *J Trauma* 2004;56(5):1084–9.
9. Reilly PL. Brain injury: the pathophysiology of the first hours. 'Talk and Die revisited'. *J Clin Neurosci* 2001;8(5):398–403.
10. Hutchinson PJ, Corteen E, Czosnyka M, Mendelow AD, Menon DK, Mitchell P, Murray G, Pickard JD, Rickels E, Sahuquillo J, Servadei F, Teasdale GM, Timofeev I, Unterberg A, Kirkpatrick PJ. Decompressive craniectomy in traumatic brain injury: the randomized multicenter RESCUEicp study (www.RESCUEicp.com). *Acta Neurochir Suppl* 2006;96:17–20.
11. Jagannathan J, Okonkwo DO, Dumont AS, Ahmed H, Bahari A, Prevedello DM, Jane JA Sr, Jane JA Jr. Outcome following decompressive craniectomy in children with severe traumatic brain injury: a 10-year single-center experience with long-term follow up. *J Neurosurg* 2007;106(4 Suppl):268–75.

12. Munch E, Horn P, Schurer L, Piepgras A, Paul T, Schmiedek P. Management of severe traumatic brain injury by decompressive craniectomy. *Neurosurgery* 2000;47(2):315–22; discussion 322–3.

13. Polin RS, Shaffrey ME, Bogaev CA, Tisdale N, Germanson T, Bocchicchio B, Jane JA. Decompressive bifrontal craniectomy in the treatment of severe refractory posttraumatic cerebral edema. *Neurosurgery* 1997;41(1):84–92; discussion 92–4.

14. Shaffrey M, Farace E. Decompressive craniectomy. *Crit Care Med* 2003;31(10):2560–1.

15. Stiefel MF, Heuer GG, Smith MJ, Bloom S, Maloney-Wilensky E, Gracias VH, Grady MS, LeRoux PD. Cerebral oxygenation following decompressive hemicraniectomy for the treatment of refractory intracranial hypertension. *J Neurosurg* 2004;101(2):241–7.

16. Timofeev I, Kirkpatrick PJ, Corteen E, Hiler M, Czosnyka M, Menon DK, Pickard JD, Hutchinson PJ. Decompressive craniectomy in traumatic brain injury: outcome following protocol-driven therapy. *Acta Neurochir Suppl* 2006;96:11–6.

17. Diringer MN, Edwards DF. Admission to a neurologic/neurosurgical intensive care unit is associated with reduced mortality rate after intracerebral hemorrhage. *Crit Care Med* 2001;29(3):635–40.

18. Fakhry SM, Trask AL, Waller MA, Watts DD. Management of brain-injured patients by an evidence-based medicine protocol improves outcomes and decreases hospital charges. *J Trauma* 2004; 56(3):492–9; discussion 499–500.

19. Hyman SA, Williams V, Maciunas RJ. Neurosurgical intensive care unit organization and function: an American experience. *J Neurosurg Anesthesiol* 1993;5(2):71–80.

20. Jordan KG. Continuous EEG monitoring in the neuroscience intensive care unit and emergency department. *J Clin Neurophysiol* 1999;16(1):14–39.

21. Kilpatrick MM, Lowry DW, Firlik AD, Yonas H, Marion DW. Hyperthermia in the neurosurgical intensive care unit. *Neurosurgery* 2000; 47(4):850–5; discussion 855–6.

22. Van den Berghe G, Wouters PJ, Bouillon R, Weekers F, Verwaest C, Schetz M, Vlasselaers D, Ferdinande P, Lauwers P. Outcome benefit of intensive insulin therapy in the critically ill: Insulin dose versus glycemic control. *Crit Care Med* 2003;31(2):359–66.

23. Bouderka MA, Fakhir B, Bouaggad A, Hmamouchi B, Hamoudi D, Harti A. Early tracheostomy versus prolonged endotracheal intubation in severe head injury. *J Trauma* 2004;57(2):251–4.

24. Perel P, Yanagawa T, Bunn F, Roberts IG, Wentz R. Nutritional support for head-injured patients. *Cochrane Database Syst Rev* 2006;(4):CD001530.

25. Grotz MR, Giannoudis PV, Pape HC, Allami MK, Dinopoulos H, Krettek C. Traumatic brain injury and stabilisation of long bone fractures: an update. *Injury* 2004;35(11):1077–86.

26. Liu JT, Tyan YS, Lee YK, Wang JT. Emergency management of epidural haematoma through burr hole evacuation and drainage. A preliminary report. Acta *Neurochir (Wien)* 2006;148(3):313–7; discussion 317.

27. Springer MF, Baker FJ. Cranial burr hole decompression in the emergency department. *Am J Emerg Med* 1988;6(6):640–6.

28. Andrews BT, Levy ML, Pitts LH. Implications of systemic hypotension for the neurological examination in patients with severe head injury. *Surg Neurol* 1987;28(6):419–22.

29. Alvi A, Doherty T, Lewen G. Facial fractures and concomitant injuries in trauma patients. *Laryngoscope* 2003;113(1):102–6.

30. Martin RC, 2nd, Spain DA, Richardson JD. Do facial fractures protect the brain or are they a marker for severe head injury? *Am Surg* 2002;68(5):477–81.

31. Rocchi G, Caroli E, Belli E, Salvati M, Cimatti M, Delfini R. Severe craniofacial fractures with frontobasal involvement and cerebrospinal fluid fistula: indications for surgical repair. *Surg Neurol* 2005; 63(6):559–63; discussion 563–4.

32. Bell RB, Dierks EJ, Homer L, Potter BE. Management of cerebrospinal fluid leak associated with craniomaxillofacial trauma. *J Oral Maxillofac Surg* 2004;62(6):676–84.

33. Weider L, Hughes K, Ciarochi J, Dunn E. Early versus delayed repair of facial fractures in the multiply injured patient. *Am Surg* 1999;65(8):790–3.

34. Levin LA, Beck RW, Joseph MP, Seiff S, Kraker R. The treatment of traumatic optic neuropathy: the International Optic Nerve Trauma Study. *Ophthalmology* 1999;106(7):1268–77.
35. Larsen DW. Traumatic vascular injuries and their management. *Neuroimaging Clin N Am* 2002;12(2):249–69.
36. Cothren CC, Moore EE, Biffl WL, Ciesla DJ, Ray CE, Jr, Johnson JL, Moore JB, Burch JM. Anticoagulation is the gold standard therapy for blunt carotid injuries to reduce stroke rate. *Arch Surg* 2004;139(5):540–5; discussion 545–6.
37. Holly LT, Kelly DF, Counelis GJ, Blinman T, McArthur DL, Cryer HG. Cervical spine trauma associated with moderate and severe head injury: incidence, risk factors, and injury characteristics. *J Neurosurg* 2002;96(3 Suppl):285–91.
38. Fehlings MG, Perrin RG. The timing of surgical intervention in the treatment of spinal cord injury: a systematic review of recent clinical evidence. *Spine* 2006;31(11 Suppl):S28–35; discussion S36.
39. Fehlings MG, Perrin RG. The role and timing of early decompression for cervical spinal cord injury: update with a review of recent clinical evidence. *Injury* 2005;36(Suppl 2):B13–26.
40. Chipman JG, Deuser WE, Beilman GJ. Early surgery for thoracolumbar spine injuries decreases complications. *J Trauma* 2004;56(1):52–7.
41. Holland MC, Mackersie RC, Morabito D, Campbell AR, Kivett VA, Patel R, Erickson VR, Pittet JF. The development of acute lung injury is associated with worse neurologic outcome in patients with severe traumatic brain injury. *J Trauma* 2003;55(1):106–11.
42. McHenry TP, Mirza SK, Wang J, Wade CE, O'Keefe GE, Dailey AT, Schreiber MA, Chapman JR. Risk factors for respiratory failure following operative stabilization of thoracic and lumbar spine fractures. *J Bone Joint Surg Am* 2006;88(5):997–1005.
43. McLain RF, Benson DR. Urgent surgical stabilization of spinal fractures in polytrauma patients. *Spine* 1999;24(16):646–54.
44. Rampersaud YR, Annand N, Dekutoski MB. Use of minimally invasive surgical techniques in the management of thoracolumbar trauma: current concepts. *Spine* 2006;31(11 Suppl):S96–102; discussion S104.
45. Cothren CC, Moore EE, Biffl WL, Ciesla DJ, Ray CE Jr., Johnson JL, Moore JB, Burch JM. Cervical spine fracture patterns predictive of blunt vertebral artery injury. *J Trauma* 2003; 55(5):811–3.
46. Biffl WL, Moore EE, Elliott JP, Ray C, Offner PJ, Franciose RJ, Brega KE, Burch JM. The devastating potential of blunt vertebral arterial injuries. *Ann Surg* 2000;231(5):672–81.
47. Miller PR, Fabian TC, Bee TK, Timmons S, Chamsuddin A, Finkle R, Croce MA. Blunt cerebrovascular injuries: diagnosis and treatment. *J Trauma* 2001; 51(2):279–85; discussion 285–6.
48. Lee YJ, Ahn JY, Han IB, Chung YS, Hong CK, Joo JY. Therapeutic endovascular treatments for traumatic vertebral artery injuries. *J Trauma* 2007;62(4):886–91.
49. Giannoudis PV, Pape HC. Damage control orthopaedics in unstable pelvic ring injuries. *Injury* 2004;35(7):671–7.
50. Harwood PJ, Giannoudis PV, Probst C, Krettek C, Pape HC. The risk of local infective complications after damage control procedures for femoral shaft fracture. *J Orthop Trauma* 2006;20(3):181–9.
51. Pape HC, Giannoudis P, Krettek C. The timing of fracture treatment in polytrauma patients: relevance of damage control orthopedic surgery. *Am J Surg* 2002;183(6):622–9.
52. Pape HC, Grimme K, Van Griensven M, Sott AH, Giannoudis P, Morley J, Roise O, Ellingsen E, Hildebrand F, Wiese B, Krettek C. Impact of intramedullary instrumentation versus damage control for femoral fractures on immunoinflammatory parameters: prospective randomized analysis by the EPOFF Study Group. *J Trauma* 2003;55(1):7–13.
53. Pape HC, Hildebrand F, Pertschy S, Zelle B, Garapati R, Grimme K, Krettek C, Reed RL 2nd. Changes in the management of femoral shaft fractures in polytrauma patients: from early total care to damage control orthopedic surgery. *J Trauma* 2002;53(3):452–61; discussion 461–2.
54. Renaldo N, Egol, K. Damage-control orthopedics: evolution and practical applications. *Am J Orthop* 2006;35(6):285–91; discussion 291.

55. Taeger G, Ruchholtz S, Waydhas C, Lewan U, Schmidt B, Nast-Kolb D. Damage control orthopedics in patients with multiple injuries is effective, time saving, and safe. *J Trauma* 2005;59(2):409–16; discussion 417.
56. Brundage SI, McGhan R, Jurkovich GJ, Mack CD, Maier RV. Timing of femur fracture fixation: effect on outcome in patients with thoracic and head injuries. *J Trauma* 2002;52(2):299–307.

Chapter 16
Spinal Injuries in Polytrauma Patients

Clinton James Devin, Gbolahan O. Okubadejo, and Joon Y. Lee

16.1   Epidemiology

In the United States, there are nearly 11,000 acute spinal cord injuries annually. Most injuries occur during motor vehicle collisions, with approximately 2–4% of blunt trauma patients presenting with a spinal column injury [1]. Groups that are at an increased risk for cervical spine injury include males, patients over 65 years old, and those of white or "other" ethnicity [2].

16.2   Transport and Clinical Evaluation

In the polytraumatized patient, it should be assumed that a spine injury exists until it is proven otherwise. Therefore, appropriate precautions and immobilization must be undertaken to protect the spinal column. It is estimated that between 3% and 25% of spinal cord injuries occur during transport from the scene to the emergency room [3–5]. Toscano determined that 32 of 123 trauma patients suffered neurological deterioration during transport from the scene of the accident to the hospital [6]. Prior to the standardized immobilization techniques in the 1970s, nearly 55% of spinal cord injury victims had complete injuries; but once immobilization protocols were implemented in the 1980s, only 39% complete spinal cord injuries were seen.[7].

Once the patient is brought to the emergency room, the process of "clearing the spine" should begin as soon as possible to prevent morbidity caused by prolonged immobilization. A common complication is the development of decubitus ulceration about the face secondary to cervical spine collars pressing around the chin and the neck. Similarly, length of time on a rigid spinal board has been shown to correlate with an increased risk of developing pressure ulcers, especially in patients

C.J. Devin (✉)
Fondren Orthopedics at Texas Orthopedic Hospital, 7401 South Main Street, Houston, TX, 77003, USA
e-mail: clintondevin@gmail.com

H.-C. Pape et al. (eds.), *Damage Control Management in the Polytrauma Patient*,
DOI 10.1007/978-0-387-89508-6_16, © Springer Science+Business Media, LLC 2010

who have lost protective sensation due to a spinal cord injury [8]. This can occur even in as few as 2 h in patients who are not frequently turned [9]. In addition, cervical collars can act as a tourniquet, resulting in elevated jugular venous pressure leading to an increased Intracranial Pressure (ICP). This may be significant in 3.5–6% of blunt trauma patients who have both a cervical spine injury as well as a severe head injury [10, 11]. Patients with a severe head injury may have little reserve to tolerate even a slightly elevated ICP from a rigid collar. Therefore, many advocate controlled release of the collar if the ICP remains elevated or using an alternative means of cervical immobilization, such as a halo, or sand bags and tape in this subset of patients [12]. Cervical spine immobilization has also been shown to potentially increase the risk of aspiration and limit respiratory function [13]. Therefore, once a patient arrives in the emergency room, every effort should be made to move him/her to a semi-rigid cushion from the spine board and to remove the cervical collar whenever possible.

16.3   Imaging and Cervical Spine Clearance

Unfortunately, a rate of missed spinal fractures of up to 33% has been reported [14, 15] in high energy trauma patients. Therefore, it is imperative that a complete and thorough examination observing strict spine precautions, is undertaken when evaluating a polytraumatized patient. Cervical spine clearance protocol has been evaluated through two large clinical studies: National Emergency X-Radiography Utilization Study (NEXUS) and the Canadian C-Spine Rule (CCR).

The NEXUS and CCR clearance criteria have helped to do away with unnecessary radiographs, particularly in low-energy trauma patients. However, with the advanced imaging modalities such as helical CT scans, plain radiographs are rapidly becoming obsolete. It has been shown that helical CTs can be more time efficient, cost effective, and, most importantly, much more sensitive than the standard three views (AP, Lateral, and odontoid views) in detecting cervical spine injuries [16–19]. CT scans may not detect subtle ligamentous injuries, and MRI should be used in cases in which subtle ligamentous injury is suspected [20].

16.4   Specific Injury Types

Injuries to the atlanto-occipital articulation are usually fatal. However, those patients who survive these injuries require immediate immobilization with a halo vest. Excessive transfers should be avoided, and surgical fixation of the injury must be performed as soon as physiologically possible [21].

Atlas fractures comprise 10% of all cervical spine injuries (Jefferson's fracture). It is rare to have neurological injury with atlas fractures because usually there is ample space available for the spinal cord at this level. The patient can be immobilized with a rigid collar until the polytrauma algorithm is complete. Most patients can be definitively treated with a collar or a halo vest. Rarely, patients with progressive displacement may require occiput-C2 arthrodesis [22].

Odontoid fractures constitute about 8–18% of all cervical fractures, with neurological deficits occurring in 10–20% of cases. Initial collar immobilization is recommended during the polytrauma evaluation; however, more rigid fixation is recommended for most odontoid fractures. Type III odontoid fractures (fractures within the C2 body) can usually be treated in a collar. However, treatment of type II (base of the odontoid) fractures is more controversial. Halo vests are recommended for nondisplaced type II fractures in younger patients. Relative indications for surgery for type II odontoid fractures include multiple injuries, associated closed head injury, initial displacement of 4 mm or more, angulation greater than 10°, delayed presentation (>2 weeks), multiple risk factors for nonunion, the inability to treat with a halo due to advanced age, and presence of associated upper cervical fractures. No interference with the polytrauma algorithm is to be expected [22, 23].

Traumatic spondylolisthesis of the axis (Hangman's fractures) is usually placed in a rigid collar and treated as such definitively. Rarely will these fractures require surgical fixation, and no interference to the polytrauma protocol is to be expected.

Subaxial fractures/subluxations/dislocations require initial rigid collar immobilization, followed by a careful evaluation of the stability of the spinal column and the injury assessment of the spinal cord. Assessment of the stability of the subaxial spinal column will often require analysis of the CT scan for osseous injuries and, often, MRI evaluation for the soft tissue trauma. Subluxations and dislocations will require urgent reduction followed by an urgent surgical fixation. Unilateral facet and bilateral facet dislocations are common injuries that require either closed reduction with graduated weights and manipulation or open surgical reduction. The status of the spinal cord is assessed with a careful neurological examination in awake and alert patients or with an MRI in obtunded patients. The use of steroids in patients with neurological injuries remains highly controversial [24–26].

Thoracolumbar spine fractures often result from both low and high-energy mechanisms. Four general types of thoracolumbar fractures are described: compression, burst, flexion-distraction (chance), or fracture-dislocation.

Compression fractures occur because of anterior spinal column failure caused by an axial load mechanism. The majority of these fractures are stable and can be treated with a rigid thoracolumbar orthosis. Burst fractures are also due to axial loading forces. This pattern commonly involves at least two columns of the spine, most often the anterior and middle columns. Neurologic status ,along with overall alignment, determines whether or not surgical intervention may be necessary [27].

Flexion-distraction injuries, also called Chance fractures, occur secondary to the primary anterior force vector acting along an axis of rotation located anterior to the spinal column. As such, the posterior and middle structures fail in tension, while the anterior column may fail in either tension or compression. This pattern of fracture can be too subtle to detect on plain radiographs, and CT has been helpful in diagnosis of these injuries. A "bony" Chance fracture will have a fracture line that extends through the vertebral body, whereas a "soft-tissue" Chance fracture will fail through the posterior facets and the disc space. High-speed motor vehicle accidents in which the lap belt is used without a shoulder belt are common causes of this injury pattern. There is also a high rate of concomitant intra-abdominal injury, (of about 45%), with a risk of neurologic injury (around 10–15%). These fractures are potentially unstable and require urgent surgical fixation [27, 28].

Fracture-dislocations in the thoracolumbar spine represent the most extreme presentation of trauma to that region. This is an extremely unstable injury that involves all three columns of the spine. Definitive management should occur without delay and involves reduction and surgical stabilization [27].

16.5 Timing of Fixation in Patients with Proven Spinal Cord Injury

Difficulty arises with those patients from whom an accurate exam cannot be obtained because of their altered mental status; this is often the case in those suffering a spinal cord injury. Fairly objective cursory findings that may indicate a spinal cord injury in the acute period include flaccidity, diaphragmatic breathing without the assistance of accessory muscles, priapism, and the presence of greater than three beats of clonus in the unconscious patient without decerebrate rigidity [29]. The timing of surgical decompression is somewhat controversial. Initial reports advocated delaying surgery for more than 4 days to allow for medical and neurological stabilization. This was based on data demonstrating an increased rate of medical complications in those undergoing surgery within 5 days [30]. Implementation of more aggressive medical management and improved spine techniques has allowed patients to undergo surgery within 5 days without increased complication rates when compared to their nonoperative counterparts [31, 32]. Vaccaro and others performed the only prospective randomized trial evaluating the effect of surgical timing on neurological outcome for patients with spinal cord injury. They found no difference in the neurological outcome, the length of acute postoperative intensive care stay, or the length of inpatient rehabilitation noted [33]. La Rosa and colleagues performed a systematic review of the literature between 1966 and 2000, comparing neurological outcomes in patients undergoing decompression within 24 h of injury with those in patients undergoing decompression after this time point. They concluded that improved neurological outcomes were demonstrated in earlier decompression; however, there were no randomized prospective studies included within this review [34]. Currently, there is a multicenter, prospective study evaluating neurological outcomes in acute cervical spinal cord injuries that undergo urgent (<24 h) vs. delayed decompression. Aside from potential neurological improvement from early decompression, it may also decrease the incidence of nonspine related complications. This has been shown to be particularly important in patients with thoracic spinal trauma and associated spinal cord injury. These injuries require a high-energy mechanism; therefore, it is not unusual for patients to have associated rib fractures, pulmonary contusions, or hemothorax.

Keeping a patient with thoracic trauma in a supine position for a prolonged period of time prior to surgical stabilization can lead to multiple complications. There have been a number of studies demonstrating decreased incidence of pneumonia and deep venous thrombosis as well as shorter ICU and overall hospital length of stay with earlier stabilization of those with thoracic spine injuries [35, 36]. Therefore, the optimal timing for surgical intervention has not been conclusively demonstrated. However, there is likely some neurological benefit to early decompression for patients with incomplete injuries or for those with neurological deterioration. It also assists in mobilizing patients, thereby preventing medical complications.

16.6   Summary and Conclusion

Rapid diagnosis followed by prompt implementation of definitive treatment for spinal injuries is crucial in successfully managing polytrauma patients. In polytrauma patients who are alert, awake, and cooperative, every effort should be made to rapidly clear the cervical/thoracic/lumbar spine for rapid mobilization. Many factors favor early stabilization of spinal injuries. In general, patients who are critically ill from visceral or head trauma will require temporary spinal stabilization with either traction, rigid collar, or careful thoraco/lumbar precautions prior to definitive surgical fixation when safe. For patients who are in borderline or unstable condition, consideration should be given to the presence or absence of any neurological deficit. If the neurological deficit is progressive, urgent surgical stabilization/fixation should be considered.

References

1. Levi AD, Hurlburt RJ, Anderson P, Fehlings M, Rampersaud R, Massicotte EM, France JC, Le Huec JC, Hedlund R, Arnold P. Neurologic deterioration secondary to unrecognized spinal instability following trauma: a multicenter study. *Spine* 2006;31:451–8.
2. Lowery DW, Wald MM, Browne BJ, Tigges S, Hoffman JR, Mower WR. Epidemiology of cervical spine victims. *Annals of Emergency Medicine* 2001;38:12–6.
3. Burney RE, Waggoner R, Maynard FM. Stabilization of spinal injury for early transfer. *Journal of Trauma* 1989;29:1497–9.
4. Hachen HJ. Emergency transportation in the event of acute spinal cord lesion. *Paraplegia* 1974;12:33–7.
5. Prasad VS, Schwartz A, Bhutani R, Sharkey PW, Schwartz ML. Characteristics of injuries to the cervical spine and spinal cord in polytrauma patient population: experience from a regional trauma unite. *Spinal Cord* 1999;37:560–8.
6. Toscano J. Prevention of neurological deterioration before admission to a spinal cord injury unit. *Paraplegia* 1988;26:43–150.
7. Garfin SR, Shakford SR, Marshall LF, Drummond JC. Care of the multiply injured patient with cervical spine injury. *Clinical Orthopaedics and Related Research* 1989;239:19–29.
8. Mawson AR, Biundo Jr JJ, Neville P, Linares HA, Winchester Y, Lopez A. Risk factors for early occurring pressure ulcers following spinal cord injury. *American Journal of Physical Medicine and Rehabilitation* 1988;67:123–7.

9. Linares HA, Mawson AR, Suarez E, Biundo JJ. Association between pressure sores and immobilization in the immediate postinjury period. *Orthopedics* 1987;10:571–3.

10. Soicher E, Demetriades D. Cervical spine injuries in patients with head injuries. *British Journal of Surgery* 1991;78:1013–4.

11. Michael DB, Guyot DR, Darmody WR. Coincidence of head and cervical spine injury. *Journal of Neurotrauma* 1989;6:177–89.

12. Ho AM, Fung KY, Joynt GM, Karmakar MK, Peng Z. Rigid cervical collar and intracranial pressure of patients with severe head injury. *Journal of Trauma, Injury, Infection, and Critical Care* 2002;53:1185–8.

13. Totten VY, Sugarman DB. Respiratory effects of spinal immobilization. *Prehospital Emergency Care* 1999;3:347–52.

14. Bohlman HH. Acute fractures and dislocations of the cervical spine. *Journal of Bone and Joint Surgery* 1979;61A:1119–40.

15. Davis JW, Phreaner DL, Hoyt DB, Machersie RC. The etiology of missed cervical spine injuries. *Journal of Trauma* 1993;34:342–6.

16. Grogan EL, Morris Jr J, MJ, Dittus RS, Moore DE, Poulose BK, Diaz JJ, Speroff T. Cervical spine evaluation in urban trauma centers: lowering institutional costs and complications through helical CT scan. *Journal of American College of Surgeons* 2005;200:160–5.

17. Nunez D, Zuluaga A, Fuentes-Bernardo D, Rivas L, Becerra J. Cervical spine trauma: how much more do we learn by routinely using helical CT?. *Radiographics* 1996;16:1307–18.

18. Mathen R, Inaba K, Munera F, Teixeira PGR, Rivas L, McKenney M, Lopez P, Ledezma CJ. Prospective evaluation of multislice computed tomography versus plain radiographic cervical spine clearance in trauma patients. *Journal of Trauma, Injury, Infection, and Critical Care* 2006;62:1427–31.

19. McCulloch PT, France J, Jones DL, Krantz W, Nguyen TP, Chambers C, Dorchak J, Mucha P. Helical computed tomography alone compared with plain radiographs with adjunct computed tomography to evaluate the cervical spine after high-energy trauma. *Journal of Bone and Joint Surgery* 2005;87A:2388–94.

20. Stassen NA, Williams VA, Grestring ML, Cheng JD, Bankey PE. Magnetic resonance imaging in combination with helical computed tomography provides safe and efficient method of cervical spine clearance in the obtunded patient. *Journal of Trauma, Injury, Infection, and Critical Care* 2006;2006:171–7.

21. Bucholz RW, Heckman JD, Court-Brown C. *Rockwood and Green's Fractures in Adults*. 6th Edition. Philadelphia, PA: Lippincott Williams & Wilkins, 2006, pp. 1402–500.

22. Jackson RS, Banit DM, Rhyne AL, Darden BV. Upper cervical spine injuries. *Journal of American Academy of Orthopaedic Surgeons* 2002;10:271–80.

23. Anderson LD, D'Alonzo RT. Fractures of the odontoid process of the axis. *Journal of Bone and Joint Surgery* 1974;56A:1663–74.

24. Effendi B, Roy D, Cornish B, Dussault RG, Laurin CA. Fractures of the ring of the axis – a classification based on the analysis of 131 cases. *Journal of Bone and Joint Surgery* 1981;63:319–27.

25. Levine AM, Edwards CC. The management of traumatic spondylolisthesis of the axis. *Journal of Bone and Joint Surgery* 1985;67:217–26.

26. Levine AM, Edwards CC. Treatment of injuries in the C1-C2 complex. *Orthopaedic Clinics of North America* 1986;17:31–44.

27. Vaccaro AR, Kim KH, Brodke DS, Harris M, Chapman J, Schildhauer T, Routt MLC, Sasso RC. Diagnosis and management of thoracolumbar spine fractures. *Journal of Bone and Joint Surgery* 2003;85A:2456–70.

28. Denis F. The three column spine and its significance in the classification of acute thoracolumbar spinal injuries. *Spine* 1983;8:817–31.

29. Sneed RC, Stover SL. Undiagnosed spinal cord injuries in brain-injured children. *American Journal of Diseases of Children* 1988;142:965–67.

30. Marshall LF, Knowlton S, Garfin SR, Klauber MR, Eisenberg HM, Kopaniky D, Miner ME, Tabbador K, Clifton GL. Deterioration following spinal cord injury. A multicenter study. *Journal of Neurosurgery* 1987;66:400–4.

31. Vale FL, Burns J, Jackson AB, Hadley MN. Combined medical and surgical treatment after acute spinal cord injury: results of a prospective pilot study to assess the merits of aggressive medical resuscitation and blood pressure management. *Journal of Neurosurgery* 1997;87:239–46.
32. Levi L, Wolf A, Belzerg H. Hemodynamic parameters in patients with acute cervical cord trauma: Description, intervention, and prediction of outcome. *Neurosurgery* 1993;33:1007–17.
33. Vaccaro AR, Daugherty RJ, Sheehan TP, Dante SJ, Cotler JM, Balderston RA, Herbison GJ, Northrup BE. Neurologic outcome of early versus late surgery for cervical spinal cord injury. *Spine* 1997;22:2609–13.
34. La Rosa G, Conti A, Cardali S, Cacciola F, Tomasello F. Does early decompression improve neurological outcome of spinal cord injured patients? Appraisal of the literature using a meta-analytical approach. *Spinal Cord* 2004;42:503–12.
35. Kerwin AJ, Frykberg ER, Schinco MA, Griffen MM, Murphy T, Tepas JJ. The effect of early spine fixation on non-neurologic, outcome. *Journal of Trauma, Injury, Infection, and Critical Care* 2005;58:15–21.
36. Croce MA, Bee TK, Pritchard E, Miller PR, Fabian TC. Does optimal timing for spine fracture fixation exist? *Annals of Surgery* 2001;233:851–8.

Chapter 17
Pelvic Fractures in Polytrauma Patients

Peter V. Giannoudis, Christopher C. Tzioupis, and Hans-Christoph Pape

17.1   Introduction

In recent years, the surgical insult has been described, measured, and quantified with inflammatory mediators such as interleukins and other chemokines [1–3]. The "two-hit" theory for trauma patients indicates that the likelihood of developing post-traumatic complications is increased if several adverse impacts such as hemorrhage, infection, or surgery occur sequentially.

Despite the introduction of organized trauma systems, pelvic ring disruptions continue to be a significant source of morbidity and mortality [4–7]. Indeed, in closed pelvic fractures with hemodynamic instability, a mortality rate of up to 42% has been reported [8]. Other factors that have been found to correlate with increased mortality rates include age injury severity score, bony pelvic instability, size and status of the wound in open injuries, presence of rectal injury, number of blood units transfused, and presence of associated injuries [9–11]. Furthermore, mortality following pelvic fractures has been shown to have a trimodal distribution: early at the scene (within minutes), delayed (within 48 h), and late (days to weeks later) [12]. Late mortality is due to multiple organ dysfunction syndrome and sepsis, whereas early mortality is due to uncontrollable hemorrhage (shock), clotting disturbances, and an exaggerated systemic inflammatory response syndrome.

Patients with pelvic fractures can be divided into two subgroups:

- The first group comprises patients who sustain stable pelvic fractures, with most of the injury confined to the ligamentous tissues. Management in these circumstances is confined to reconstruction of the osteoligamentous structures on a more semielective basis. Different stabilization procedures have been established and are associated with good long-term outcomes [13–16].

P.V. Giannoudis (✉)
Trauma and Orthopaedic Surgery, University of Leeds, Leeds General Infirmary,
University Hospital, Clarendon Wing, Floor A, Great George Street, Leeds, Yorkshire,
LS1 3EX, UK
e-mail: pgiannoudi@aol.com

H.-C. Pape et al. (eds.), *Damage Control Management in the Polytrauma Patient*,
DOI 10.1007/978-0-387-89508-6_17, © Springer Science+Business Media, LLC 2010

- The second group has patients who sustain displaced pelvic ring fractures and who require emergency hemorrhage control and a multidisciplinary team approach for the associated injuries. The prevalence of pelvic fractures presenting with hemodynamic instability ranges from 2% to 20% [17–22]. The major causes of death in these patients are early exsanguination and late sequelae of prolonged shock and massive transfusion. Hemodynamic instability compounds the necessity for prompt, effective triage, and swift implementation of definitive therapies. One of the most difficult decisions for a trauma surgeon is whether to proceed to the operating room for laparotomy or whether to transfer the patient to the interventional suite for pelvic arterial embolization. In North America, immediate recognition of instability caused by pelvic trauma is typically followed with resuscitation using blood products, external mechanical stabilization, and emergent pelvic angioembolization [23–27]. In severely multiply injured patients who are "unstable" or "in extremis," damage control orthopedics is the current treatment of choice. By performing limited surgical interventions, the subsequent reduction in blood loss and transfusion requirements can only be beneficial in these critically ill patients, reducing the risk of developing systemic complications and early mortality.

Over the years, the overall improvement of the mortality in pelvic fractures can be attributed to the progress made in modern critical care medicine, the implementation of ATLS® (Advanced Trauma Life Support), and multidisciplinary protocols, the early aggressive fracture stabilization, and the selective fecal diversion in cases of open fractures.

17.2   Control of Pelvic Hemorrhage

Upon arrival in the emergency department, patients should be resuscitated according to the guidelines of the Advanced Trauma Life Support Course (ATLS®) of the American College of Surgeons' Committee on Trauma [28]. The primary survey emphasizes immediate assessment of the airway and breathing while maintaining spinal precautions. In patients who have sustained high-energy injuries, pelvic fracture should always be suspected. Quickly identifying the site of hemorrhage in the hemodynamically unstable patient is both critical and time-dependent.

Arterial bleeding (iliac vessels and their branches to the inferior abdominal viscera and pelvic organs) is a major contributor to hemorrhagic shock in pelvic fractures. Other sources of bleeding include the low-pressure venous plexus and fractured cancellous bone surfaces. The retroperitoneum can contain up to 4 L of blood, and bleeding will continue until intravascular pressure is overcome and physiological tamponade has occurred. However, where extensive disruption of the retroperitoneal muscle compartments has taken place, this can lead to uncontrolled hemorrhage with the risk of exsanguination. This is because the retroperitoneum is not a closed space, and pressure-induced tamponade cannot be expected [29].

The first step in restoring hemodynamic stability includes the administration of intravenous crystalloid fluids and whole blood. However, it is important to note that volume resuscitation without hemorrhage control is ineffective and may lead to secondary iatrogenic complications such as hypothermia and coagulopathy. Hemorrhage control consists of stopping external bleeding by direct pressure and expeditiously determining whether surgery or other interventions are required for internal control of bleeding. If the patient shows signs of hypovolemia, a thorough and systematic search must be initiated to identify the source of bleeding. Depending on the hemodynamic status, patients with pelvic fractures are divided into four categories:

1. Stable: Patients without clinical signs of shock
2. Borderline: Patients with a systolic blood pressure between 80 and 100 mmHg, AIS 2 or more, blood transfusion 2–8/2 h
3. Unstable: Patients unable to maintain a systolic blood pressure of >90 mmHg, pulse of <100 beats/min, CVP >5 cmH$_2$O, or Urine Output of >30 ml/h despite adequate fluid resuscitation and blood transfusion over a period of 2 h
4. In extremis: Patients with either absent vital signs or presence of severe shock due to uncontrollable hemorrhage needing mechanical resuscitation or repeated catecholamine infusion, despite complete blood volume replacement within 120 min (>12 blood transfusions/2 h) [30]

In most patients with stable pelvic ring injuries and stable vital signs, bleeding into the closed pelvic space will be self-limiting [31]. By contrast, unstable pelvic fractures will frequently be associated with disruption of retroperitoneal muscle compartments [29]. This can lead to uncontrolled hemorrhage creeping cranially above the psoas muscle or along the gluteal muscles, with the risk of exsanguination or pelvic and abdominal compartment syndromes. This phenomenon has been named the chimney effect [32]. According to Heetveld and colleagues [8], every 3 min of hemodynamic instability without hemorrhage control increases the mortality by 1%.

Complex reconstructive work is delayed until the patient is hemodynamically stable and in a better physiological condition to withstand the additional surgical burden. Avoidance of coagulation disturbances, the systemic inflammatory response, adult respiratory distress syndrome, and multiple organ dysfunction syndrome is of paramount importance for reduced mortality rates [33–35]. Treatment options that should be considered for the emergency hemostasis of patients with pelvic fractures at risk of exsanguination include the pelvic sling, arterial inflow arrest, external fixation devices, internal fixation, direct surgical hemostasis, pelvic packing, pelvic angiography, and embolization.

17.3 Radiographic Assessment and Fracture Classification

The basic radiographic "trauma series" includes lateral cervical spine, anterior posterior chest, and pelvis films [36]. If the patient is hemodynamically stable, inlet (beam directed caudad at 60(), outlet (beam directed cephalad at 45() [37], and

Judet (Iliac and Obturator oblique) pelvic radiographs yields more information regarding the fracture pattern. If the pelvic X-ray shows a pelvic fracture, there is 32% probability of intra-abdominal bleeding and a 52% probability of retroperitoneal bleeding [8].

After the initial clinical assessment and the ATLS® radiographs (cervical spine, chest, and pelvis) and in cases in which patients respond transiently to the fluid resuscitation, an intra-abdominal/intra-pelvic hemorrhage should be suspected, and a Focused Abdominal Sonogram in Trauma (FAST) or diagnostic peritoneal lavage is recommended. FAST is 83–95% accurate in identification of free fluid in the abdominal cavity. If performed soon after the injury, there is a risk of nondetection of the hemorrhage because it may not be significant enough [38]. FAST should be repeated within 1 h to increase sensitivity to 95%: false negatives have been reported in 19–29% of the cases.

Computed Tomography scan (CT scan) is used for the assessment of the pelvis in the hemodynamically stable patients; osseous and soft tissue windows are used as well as 3D reconstruction [39]. Extraluminal gas, hemorrhage, or bowel wall thickening will help in the assessment of the intestinal injuries. Vaginal lacerations or previous diagnostic peritoneal lavage can provide false-positive results and should be taken into account [40–43].

The utility of the Pelvic X-Ray (PXR) has recently come into question with stable patients. Compared to CT scan, PXRs detect only 66–87% of pelvic fractures and miss nonbony pelvic injuries [44, 45]. However, for the unstable blunt trauma patient, the pelvic radiograph is necessary because these patients can neither provide a reliable physical examination nor undergo immediate CT scan. As a result, PXR provides a useful gross estimate of pelvic injury. As would be expected, in unstable pelvic fracture patterns, the sensitivity of the plain film is improved over minor pelvic fractures, 75–91% [44].

The fracture pattern on the initial anterior-posterior pelvic X-ray is the best initial guide to determine the probability of pelvic arterial bleeding. The Young and Burgess classification system is an expansion of the original classification developed by Pennal and Sutherland in which the fractures were classified based on the direction of three possible injury forces: Anterior Posterior Compression (APC), Lateral Compression (LC), and Vertical Shear (VS) [46, 47]. Young and Burgess developed subsets on the LC and APC injuries to quantify the forces applied. They also added a fourth injury force category of combined mechanical injury [48]. The Young and Burgess classification system has been utilized more frequently than the Tile system [24] when comparing the potential association between pelvic fracture type and retroperitoneal hemorrhage [36, 49].

A significant correlation has been reported between greater blood product requirement and unstable fracture patterns [50, 51]. However, a limitation of predicting hemorrhage based on classifying the initial pelvic X-ray is that major posterior element disruption may not be detected in 9–22% of fractures when compared with CT [52–54].

17.4   Pelvic Fracture Treatment

In hemodynamically unstable patients with no obvious site of hemorrhage, careful clinical examination of the pelvis is mandatory even when radiographs look normal or a pelvic image demonstrates a stable fracture configuration. Physical examination of the pelvis should include thorough inspection of the flanks, lower abdomen, groin, perineum, and buttocks to detect any wounds or bruises. Remember that as often as 60% of the time, the chest or the abdomen may be the source of active blood loss in the hemodynamically unstable patient with a pelvic fracture.

Injuries to cervix, uterus, and ovaries are rare [55]. Inspection of the external genitalia is the first action to take, and then a more meticulous digital examination can reveal lacerations, blood at the external urethral meatus, a high-riding prostate, perineal hematoma, hematuria, or vaginal bleeding. Any of these findings or the inability to urinate in association to an anterior pelvic ring fracture should be an indication for retrograde urethrogram [56, 57]. If a urethral injury has been diagnosed, a cystogram should follow through a suprapubic catheter. In this way, both the urethral and the bladder integrity can be assessed. The nature of the pelvic fracture, whether it is closed or open, and the hemodynamic status of the patient will determine the treatment plan. In unstable patients, apart from the fluid resuscitation, there is a need to enhance the tamponade effect in the pelvis to increase the intrapelvic pressure and to facilitate hemostasis. This can be achieved by either invasive or noninvasive measures.

17.4.1   Noninvasive Measures

The noninvasive techniques include application of a circumferential sheet, pelvic binder, internal rotation of both legs, traction of the lower limbs, and application of Military AntiShock Trousers (MAST). Military antishock trousers achieve direct compression and immobilization of the pelvic ring and the lower extremities via pneumatic pressure [58]. However, access to the traumatized region is limited, and assessment and treatment of concomitant injuries is impaired. Major complications, including compartment syndromes and impaired peripheral perfusion necessitating amputation, are reported, particularly after long-term application [32, 59]. A recent Cochrane review of 1,075 patients in two randomized trials of MAST found no evidence for reduction in mortality, length of hospitalization, or length of ICU stay [60]. During the past decade, direct pelvic compression using a bed sheet, pelvic sling, or pelvic belt has been introduced for emergency stabilization of pelvic fractures. It achieves satisfactory pelvic compression without seriously limiting access to the patient [61, 62].

Vermeulen and colleagues [63] first illustrated the prehospital use of an external pelvic compression belt (Geneva belt) in a series of 19 patients in 1999. Their device was applied by paramedics at the accident scene within 3 s on clinical suspicion of unstable pelvic fractures. Since then, a variety of commercial material compression splints have been manufactured. Examples include the Stuart splint, the London splint, the Dallas pelvic binder, and the Trauma Pelvic Orthotic Device, TPOD™ (Cybertech Medical, California). They are generally applied at the level of greater trochanters/symphysis pubis directly on to the patient's skin. One study determined the mean (SD) force required to reduce unstable open book pelvic fractures (180 (50) N) on cadaveric models. This led to the development of new commercial splints (SAM Sling™, SAM Medical Products, Oregon), which use controlled and consistent stabilization with an autostop buckle to reduce the risk of overcompression in case of internal rotation injuries of the pelvic ring [61, 64]. It has been shown that simple application of this sling increases pelvic stability by 61% in response to rotational stress and 55%, flexion–extension [64].

Clinical judgment and reassessment are important in using these techniques. Potential complications include skin necrosis if left in place too long or applied too tightly. In LC injuries with transforaminal sacral fractures, possible visceral or neural injury may occur if applied too vigorously [60].

17.4.2 Invasive Measures

17.4.2.1 External Fixation

The anterior fixator is thought to contribute to hemostasis by maintaining a reduced pelvic volume, allowing tamponade, and by decreasing bony motion at the fracture site, allowing clots to stabilize [65]. External fixation-stabilization is a widely accepted emergency measure for the resuscitation's outcome, as this has already been demonstrated [66, 67]. In patients who are both hemodynamically and mechanically unstable and in whom the major bleeding is thought to be related to the pelvic fracture, external stabilization of the pelvis indeed becomes the first priority.

The best results of external pelvic stabilization are achieved in rotationally unstable LC fracture types II and III and APC types II and III. Stabilization can be achieved in 64–83% of these fractures [14]. With additional vertical instability (VS or CM type injury), stabilization can be achieved in only 27% of cases, and supplementary ipsilateral skeletal traction is needed [68]. Anterior external fixation has been shown to be effective in the acute phase of resuscitation. However, definitive fixation of unstable type C or open book fractures with external fixator constructs has shown a high rate of secondary displacement [69]. Percutaneous methods are favored posteriorly [70].

17.4.2.2 Pelvic C-Clamp

To deal with posteriorly unstable fractures, Ganz and colleagues [71] developed a pelvic C-clamp, now available in most trauma units. These clamps have been applied in hemodynamically unstable patients and prophylactically in stable patients with unstable pelvic-ring disruptions. Their use is, however, limited to a specific set of indications. For example, they are not applicable in fractures of the ilium and transiliac fracture dislocations. Complications include injury to gluteal neurovascular structures and overcompression with the risk of secondary nerve injury in sacral fractures [71]. Although potentially life-saving, these devices should be applied by an experienced surgeon and considered only in cases of posteriorly unstable pelvic fractures accompanied by hemodynamic instability.

17.4.2.3   Acute Fracture Fixation

Provisional fixation of unstable pelvic-ring disruptions with a pelvic clamp or an external frame with a supracondylar pin has proved markedly beneficial in the resuscitative phase of management [72]. If, however, the patient undergoes a laparotomy to deal with visceral injuries, symphyseal disruption and medial ramus fractures should be plated at the same time. Because neither blood loss nor operative time is greatly increased, combining these repairs decreases the risk of complications in a patient who is already compromised [73].

A role has also been suggested for percutaneous fixation; however, only surgeons appropriately trained should use this technique. Percutaneous pelvic fixation techniques allow for acute and definitive treatment of anterior and posterior pelvic ring injuries without extensive dissection.

Fixation can be performed acutely, even as a component of the patient's resuscitation. Operative blood loss is minimal and wound complications are unusual. Minimally invasive anterior ring fixation includes fixation with retrograde or anterograde screws in the medulla of the superior ramus. Closed reduction and fixation with percutaneous sacroiliac screws offers definitive stable fixation for many posterior pelvic ring injuries, such as fracture/dislocation of the sacroiliac joint or sacral fractures, with the advantage of minimal dissection and a reduction in wound complications [29, 43, 74]. Nevertheless, in the acute setting and especially in the "extremis" clinical condition of the patient, such an approach is not advocated as it is time consuming, and, often, extensile approaches are necessary, predisposing the patient to uncontrollable hemorrhage, coagulation disturbances, and early mortality.

17.4.2.4   Arterial Inflow Arrest

In cases in which exsanguination of the patient is imminent, occlusion of the aorta can be used as a temporary measure to control the hemorrhage. This can be performed directly by open crossclamping or via percutaneous or open balloon catheter techniques [75]. Other authors have reported satisfactory control of arterial bleeding with ligation of the hypogastric artery, attributing this to the remarkable collateral supply within the pelvis [76, 77].

17.4.2.5   Pelvic Angiography and Embolization

Information about the rate of arterial injury in pelvic trauma has primarily been derived from angiographic studies, with reported rates ranging from 0.01% to 2.3% [12, 34, 35] for all pelvic trauma and from 9% to 80% in unstable pelvic injuries [26, 49, 78–81].

Timely identification and control of pelvic hemorrhage is pivotal to decrease pelvic fracture-related mortality [6, 82, 83]. The main controversy regarding the treatment of patients with profuse, exsanguinating hemorrhage relates to the role of angiography and embolization.

This technique is time consuming and can be performed in only approximately 10% of the cases [24, 26, 84]. Simultaneous treatment of other injuries cannot be performed during this procedure, and mortality of up to 50% has already been reported, despite effective bleeding control. Angiography requires a skilled radiologist and technical staff as well as transportation of a critically ill patient to the angiography suite knowing that there have been series in which 20% of these patients had cardiorespiratory arrest during the procedure. However, in a hospital where interventional radiology is available, angiography is both diagnostic and therapeutic for pelvic hemorrhage [24, 26, 80, 81, 85–88].

Indeed, early angiography and embolization have proven to be one of the most important interventions to control arterial pelvic hemorrhage [26, 88]. Extravasation of contrast, false aneuryms, and occlusion due to thrombus or vasospasm are all signs of arterial injury, which may require embolization [24]. Embolization is safe and effective and achieves up to 90% success rates [69].

Nevertheless, there are several aspects of the current management strategy of early angioembolization for hemodynamically unstable patients with pelvic fractures that are concerning.

Predicting the patient who does or does not require embolization remains a challenge [89]. Furthermore, although angioembolization may be effective in controlling pelvic arterial bleeding [86], it has not been shown to decrease the necessity for blood product resuscitation. Third, there are a number of institutions that do not have angiographic capabilities, hence necessitating transfer of any such patient – not an ideal option in the already hemodynamically unstable patient.

Current consensus is that, before angiography, aggressive resuscitation needs to be initiated, other sources of bleeding (chest/abdominal) need to be ruled out, and provisional pelvic stabilization with either a sheet or external fixator should be performed. If the patient remains hypotensive, angiography is indicated [17, 90].

17.4.2.6   Pelvic Packing

Where ongoing hemodynamic instability is encountered, pelvic packing can complement the external fixation. It is effectuated through a lower abdominal laparotomy, adjusted to the pelvic wound. Packs have to be inserted in the prevesical and presacral spaces and must be removed or changed within 48 h [69]. Abdominal injuries are simultaneously assessed and treated.

In some European centers, external fixation of the pelvic fracture and surgical packing of the retroperitoneum is performed in favor of angiography [23, 91–93].

Pelvic Packing (PP) eliminates the often arduous decision by the trauma surgeon: OR vs. IR? All patients can be rapidly transported to the operating room, and PP can be accomplished in less than 30 min. It may be also ideally suited for austere conditions and in settings in which angiography is unavailable or unable to be done expeditiously. Emergent retroperitoneal packing appears to be a safe procedure that has a role in damage control of critically injured patients. It can be done immediately and with ease in conjunction with external fixation of the pelvis and other surgical procedures to stabilize the patient.

17.5 Damage Control Orthopedics for Pelvic Fractures with Hemodynamic Instability

In patients with pelvic fractures in an "unstable" or "extremis" clinical condition, prolonged operative interventions could initiate a series of reactions at the molecular level, predisposing the patient to an adverse outcome. Any surgical intervention must be considered immediately life saving and should therefore be simple, quick, and well performed. Rigid rules relating to timing should be avoided to prevent unnecessary delay: time is usually critical to survival of the patient [34]. Protocols designed to reduce mortality should stop bleeding, detect and control associated injuries, and restore hemodynamics. A staged diagnostic and therapeutic approach is required. The severity of bleeding is a crucial hallmark for survival during the early period after injury.

Numerous clinical pathways were developed and published during the last 20 years for management of hemodynamically unstable patients. All of them consist of abdominal diagnostic procedures, pelvic binding and/or external fixation, pelvic retroperitoneal packing, angioembolization, and orthopedic fixation of the pelvis.

Trauma care providers in different trauma care systems (i.e., German vs. Anglo-American systems) have varied levels of interest and expertise in the management of the injured pelvis. In Germany and in countries following the German system in which comprehensive trauma surgeons (traumatologists) are responsible for orthopedic trauma, pelvic fractures tend to be fixed earlier and large expanding retroperitoneal hematomas are managed with packing against the restored pelvic ring [82, 92]. In the United States, where general surgical trauma surgeons are responsible for the resuscitation, arterial bleeding in hemodynamically unstable patients is embolized or excluded in the angiography suite before definitive pelvic fixation is performed by the consulting orthopedic trauma specialists [26, 82, 92].

Because of the disastrous sequelae of uncontrolled hemorrhage in young patients, only external devices that are easy to apply can be used effectively. These devices, by external compression, reduce the intrapelvic volume and create a tamponade effect against ongoing bleeding. Pelvic packing should be considered in cases in which, despite the application of the external fixator, ongoing bleeding is encountered. Angiographic embolization is not usually indicated in this patient population.

However, in cases in which hemodynamic stability with volume replacement can be achieved but ongoing pelvic hemorrhage is suspected (expanding hematoma), then angiography could be considered as an adjunct to the treatment protocol.

17.6 Ongoing Treatment

If definitive stabilization is needed, it should be effectuated according to the principles of damage control orthopedics [30, 33–35]. Definitive stabilization in closed pelvic fractures with internal fixation is recommended between the third and seventh day postinjury. In open fractures, the timing is not adequately delineated, and fixation techniques are controversial. Traditionally, only external fixation has been used [94], but there are authors publishing good results after internal fixation [95] or suggesting internal fixation when there is no gross contamination of the fracture site [94]. In comminuted iliac wing fractures, early open internal fixation is preferred since external fixation cannot be applied [96]. Combination of internal and external fixation has been described by Leenen and colleagues [97], and percutaneous internal fixation has been used for open fractures with fewer complications [95].

When wounds are associated with the pelvic fractures, their treatment includes extensive irrigation, debridement (up to healthy tissue with capillary bleeding), and removal of foreign bodies and bony fragments. For the washout, either free flow or pulsed lavage techniques can be used. The wounds can either be left open, or vacuum-sealed dressings can be used to drain them. A second look, with or without closure, should be effectuated after 48–72 h [98, 99].

The possibility of a compartment syndrome associated to the above-mentioned injuries should not be neglected. The major pelvic compartments are the iliopsoas, the gluteus maximus, and the gluteus medius/minimus. Measurement of the compartment pressure is mandatory.

Plastic surgical techniques can be undertaken to treat these wounds and eliminate dead spaces. Split or full thickness skin grafts are used as well as suction drains, vacuum-sealed drainage, or free flaps.

The management of the open pelvic fracture should follow the same guidelines and principles as for any open fracture of the extremities. The perineal wounds must be judged (because of their location) for a potential contamination of the fracture site and/or of the retroperitoneal hematoma. Perineal wounds involving the rectum require fecal diversion, early sphincter repair (when injured), and local wound management [100]. When placing the stoma, bear in mind the eventual location of any orthopedic incision, suprapubic catheter, and external fixator pins [101]. The restoration of the continuity has an important rate of complications, and therefore awareness of the patient with regard to this issue is of paramount importance [102, 103].

In "complex" pelvic and acetabular fractures, perineal soft tissue swelling and "butterfly" hematoma are frequently present. This is the result of the extravasation of the retroperitoneal hematoma through the superficial perineal fascia of Colles. It can be managed with a scrotal sling for 5–7 days and then with a triangular sponge wedge (usually after surgical management of the lesions) [104]. Surgical insult to the perineum, local venous thrombosis, the pudendal post during skeletal traction [105], transient hypoalbuminemic state, and scrotal skin breakdown with sloughing and local infection can contribute to the expansion of the swelling.

17.7   Hemipelvectomy

A particular type of pelvic injury is the hemipelvectomy. This can be defined as an unstable ligamentous or osseous hemipelvic injury with rupture of the pelvic neurovascular bundle. Usually, it is characterized by wide separation of the pubic symphysis and the Sacro-Iliac Joint, with various degrees of soft tissue and neurovascular disruption and stretching. The nonviable limb may still be attached to the trunk. Simultaneous and not sequential care is mandatory. Only in stable patients can one proceed to pelvic X-ray, USS, DPL, and Retrograde Urethro-Cystogram. Direct pressure or obvious arterial clamping should be immediate. It must be noted that a partial hemipelvectomy should be preferably completed. This is a life-saving procedure as bleeding cannot be controlled when the limb remains partially attached. Partial vessel injuries do not allow closure of the vessel lumen by muscular contraction. The remaining pelvis can be fixed internally, and the hemipelvectomy can be converted to a hip disarticulation if there is no massive wound contamination. Ultimate closure requires a spectrum of plastic surgical techniques [106]. Some complications seen with this type of injury include problems with wound healing, soft tissue and skin flap necrosis, iliopsoas necrosis from avulsion of its blood supply, local infection leading to lethal systemic sepsis, and meningitis probably secondary to ascending infection along the avulsed lumbar and sacral roots [105].

17.8   Summary and Conclusions

Pelvic fractures can be one of the most devastating orthopedic injuries, mainly because of their association to high-energy trauma. Hemodynamic stabilization is of capital importance and should be taken into account starting from the prehospital care of the injured. Patients need to be managed in a synchronous fashion by a multidisciplinary team upon their admission to the trauma center. When a pelvic fracture is suspected, temporarily stabilization should be attempted before admission. The hemodynamic and pelvic stability, primarily, and the associated injuries will determine the sequence of management. The early adequate treatment of the pelvic fractures, starting from the hemodynamic parameters, decreases the mortality and improves the outcome.

References

1. Probst C, Probst T, Gaensslen A, Krettek C, Pape HC. The timing and duration of the initial pelvic stabilization after multiple trauma in patients from the German trauma registry: is there an influence on outcome. J Trauma 2007;62:370–377.
2. Pape HC, Van GM, Rice J, Gansslen A, Hildebrand F, Zech S, Winny M, Lichtinghagen R, Krettek C. Major secondary surgery in blunt trauma patients and perioperative cytokine liberation: determination of the clinical relevance of biochemical markers. J Trauma 2001;50:989–1000.
3. Seekamp A, Jochum M, Ziegler M, van Griensven M, Martin M, Regel G. Cytokines and adhesion molecules in elective and accidental trauma-related ischemia/reperfusion. J Trauma 1998;44:874–882.
4. Giannoudis PV, Hildebrand F, Pape HC. Inflammatory serum markers in patients with multiple trauma Can they predict outcome? J Bone Joint Surg Br 2004;86:313–323.
5. Eastridge BJ, Burgess AR. Pedestrian pelvic fractures: 5 year experience of a major urban trauma center. J Trauma 1997;42:695–700.
6. Flint L, Babikian G, Anders M, Rodriguez J, Steinberg S. Definitive control of mortality from severe pelvic fracture. Ann Surg 1990;211:703–707.
7. Rommens PM. Pelvic ring injuries: a challenge for the trauma surgeon. Acta Chir Belg 1996;96:78–84.
8. Heetveld MJ, Harris I, Schlaphoff G, Sugrue M. Guidelines for the management of haemodynamically unstable pelvic fracture patients. ANZ J Surg 2004;74:520–29.
9. Jones AL, Powell JN, Kellam JF, McCormack RG, Dust W, Wimmer P. Open pelvic fractures: A multicenter retrospective analysis. Orthop Clin North Am 1997;28:345–350.
10. Rieger H, Joosten U, Probst A, Joist A. Significance of score systems in open complex trauma of the pelvis. Zentralbl Chir 1999;124:1004–1010.
11. Baker SP, O'Neil B, Haddon W, Long WB. The injury severity score: A method for describing patients with multiple injuries and evaluating emergency care. J Trauma 1974;14:187–196.
12. Ertel WK. General assessment and management of the polytrauma patient. In Tile M, Helfet DL, Kellam JF (eds), Fractures of the pelvis and acetabulum. 3rd Edition. Philadelphia, PA: Lippincott Williams & Wilkins, 2003, pp 61–79.
13. Borelli J, Koval K, Helfet D. The crescent fracture: A posterior fracture dislocation of the sacroiliac joint. J Orthop Trauma 1996;10:165–170.
14. Kellam J. The role of external fixation in pelvic disruptions. Clin Orthop 1989;241:66–82.
15. Pohlemann T, Gänsslen A. Separation of the symphysis pubis. Orthop Traumatol 1999;7:144–154.
16. Routt M, Simonian P. Closed reduction and percutaneous skeletal fixation of sacral fractures. Clin Orthop 1996;329:121–128.
17. Mirza A, Ellis T. Initial management of pelvic and femoral fractures in the multiply injured patient. Crit Care Clin 2004;20:159–170.
18. Pohlemann T, Bosch U, Gansslen A, Tschern H. The Hannover experience in management of pelvic fractures. Clin Orthop 1994;305:69–80.
19. Failinger MS, McGanity PL. Unstable fractures of the pelvic ring. J Bone Joint Surg Am 1992;74:781–791.
20. Buckle R, Browner B, Morandi M. Emergency reduction for pelvic ring disruptions and control of associated hemorrhage using the pelvic stabilizer. Tech Orthop 1995;9:258–266.
21. Gaensslen A, Pehlemann T, Paul C, Lobenhoffer P, Tscherne H. Epidemiology of pelvic ring injuries. Injury 1996;27:S-A13–S-A19.
22. Poka A, Libby E. Indications and techniques for external fixation of the pelvis. Clin Orthop 1996;329:54–59.
23. Cothren CC, Osborn PM, Moore EE, Morgan SJ, Johnson JL, Smith WR. Preperitonal pelvic packing for hemodynamically unstable pelvic fractures: A paradigm shift. J Trauma 2007;62:834–839.

24. Velmahos GC, Toutouzas KG, Vassiliu P, Sarkisyan G, Chan L, Hanks S, Berne TV, Demetriades D. A prospective study on the safety and efficacy of angiographic embolization for pelvic and visceral injuries. J Trauma 2002;53:303–308.

25. Kimbrell BJ, Velmahos GC, Chan LS, Demetriades D. Angiographic embolization for pelvic fractures in older patients. Arch Surg 2004;139:728–733.

26. Agolini SF, Shah K, Jaffe J, Newcomb J, Rhodes M, Reed JF. Arterial embolization is a rapid and effective technique for controlling pelvic fracture hemorrhage. J Trauma 1997;43:395–399.

27. Durkin A, Sagi HC, Durham R, Flint L. Contemporary management of pelvic fractures. Am J Surg 2006;192:211–223.

28. American College of Surgeons. *Advanced trauma life support, 7th edition*. Chicago: American College of Surgeons, 2004.

29. Grimm M, Vrahas M, Thomas K. Pressure-volume characteristics of the intact and disrupted pelvic retroperitoneum. J Trauma 1998;44:454–459.

30. Pape HC, Giannoudis PV, Krettek C. The timing of fracture treatment in polytrauma patients: Relevance of damage control orthopaedic surgery. Am J Surg 2002;183:622–629.

31. Downs AR, Dhalla S. Hemorrhage and pelvic fractures. Can J Surg 1988;31:89–90.

32. Vahedi M, Ayuyao A, Parsa M, Freeman HP. Pneumatic antishock garment-associated compartment syndrome in injured lower extremities. J Trauma 1995;38:616–618.

33. Giannoudis PV. Current concepts of the inflammatory response after major trauma: An update. Injury 2003;34:397–404.

34. Giannoudis PV. Surgical priorities in damage control in polytrauma. Joint Bone Joint Surg 2003;85-B:478–484.

35. Pape HC, Giannoudis PV, Krettek C, Trentz O. Timing of fixation of major fractures in blunt polytrauma: Role of conventional indicators in clinical decision making. J Orthop Trauma 2005;19:551–562.

36. Cryer HM, Miller FB, Evers BM, Rouben LR, Seligson DL. Pelvic fracture classification: Correlation with haemorrhage. J Trauma 1988;28:973–980.

37. Pennal GB, Tile M, Waddell JP. Pelvic disruption: Assessment and classification. Clin Orthop 1980;151:12–22.

38. Boulanger BR, Kearney PA, Brenneman FD, Tsuei B, Ochoa J. FAST utilization 1999: Results of a survey of North American trauma centers. Am Surg 2000;66:1049–1055.

39. Theumann NH, Verdon JP, Mouhsine E, Denys A, Schnyder P, Portier F. Traumatic injuries: Imaging of pelvic fractures. Eur Radiol 2002;12:1312–1330.

40. Ebraheim NA, Savolaine ER, Rusin JR, Jackson WT, Asensio JA. Occult rectal perforation in a major pelvic fracture. J Orthop Trauma 1988;2:340–343.

41. Kumar BA, Chojnowski AJ. Open pelvic fractures with vaginal laceration: An unusual clinical feature. Injury 2000;31:68–70.

42. Magen AB, Moser RP, Woomert CA, Guidici MA. Septic arthritis of the hip: a complication of a rectal tear associated with pelvic fractures. Am J Roentgenol 1991;156: 817–818.

43. Ross GL, Dodd O, Lipham JC, Campbell JK. Rectal perforation in unstable pelvic fractures: The use of flexible sigmoidoscopy. Injury 2001;32:67–68.

44. Berg EE, Chebuhar C, Bell RM. Pelvic trauma imaging: a blinded comparison of computed tomography and roentgenograms. J Trauma 1996;41:994–998.

45. Guillamondegui OD, Pryor JP, Gracias VH, Gupta R, Reilly PM, Schwab CW. Pelvic radiography in blunt trauma resuscitation: A diminishing role. J Trauma 2002;53:1043–1047.

46. Dalal SA, Burgess AR, Siegel JH, Young JW, Brumback RJ, Poka A, Dunham CM, Gens D, Bathon H. Pelvic fracture in multiple trauma: Classification by mechanism is key to pattern of organ injury, resuscitative requirements and outcome. J Trauma 1989;29:981–1002.

47. Young JWR, Burgess AR, Brumback RJ, Poka A. Pelvic fractures: Value of plain radiography in early assessment and management. Radiology 1986;160:445–451.

48. Burgess AR, Eastridge BJ, Young JWR, Ellison TS, Ellison Jr PS, Poka A, Bathon GH, Brumback RJ. Pelvic ring disruptions: Effective classification system and treatment protocols. J Trauma 1990;30:848–856.

49. Poole GV, Ward EF, Muakkassa FS, Hsu HSH, Griswold JA, Rhodes RS. Pelvic fracture from major blunt trauma. Ann Surg 1991;213:532–539.
50. Gruen GS, Leit ME, Gruen RJ, Peitzman AB. The acute management of hemodynamically unstable multiple trauma patients with pelvic ring fractures. J Trauma 1994;36:706–713.
51. Eastridge BJ, Starr A, Minei JP, O'Keefe GE. The importance of fracture pattern in guiding therapeutic decision-making in patients with hemorrhagic shock and pelvic ring disruptions. J Trauma 2002;53:446–451.
52. Moreno C, Moore EE, Rosenberger A, Cleveland HC. Haemorrhage associated with major pelvic fracture. J Trauma 1986;26:987–989.
53. Resnik CS, Stackhouse DJ, Shanmuganathan K, Young JW. Diagnosis of pelvic fractures in patients with acute pelvic trauma: efficacy of plain radiographs. Am J Roentgenol 1992;158:109–112.
54. Robertson DD, Sutherland CJ, Chan BW, Hodge JC, Scott WW, Fishman EK. Depiction of pelvic fractures using 3D volume tric holography: Comparison of plain X-ray and CT. J Comput Assist Tomogr 1995;19:967–974.
55. Govender S, Sham A, Singh B. Open pelvic fractures. Injury 1990;21:373–376.
56. Koraitin MM. Pelvic fracture urethral injuries: The unresolved controversy. J Urol 1999;161:1433–1441.
57. Morehouse DD. Injuries to the urethra and urinary bladder associated with fractures of the pelvis. Can J Surg 1988;31:85–88.
58. Frank LR. Is MAST in the past? The pros and cons of MAST usage in the field. J Emerg Med Serv 2000;25:38–41.
59. Clarke G, Mardel S. Use of MAST to control massive bleeding from pelvic injuries. Injury 1993;24:628–629.
60. Dickinson K, Roberts I. Medical anti-shock trousers (pneumatic anti-shock garments) for circulatory support in patients with trauma (Cochrane Review). *The Cochrane Library, Issue 2.* Oxford: Update Software, 2003.
61. Bottlang M, Krieg JC, Mohr M, Simpson TS, Madey SM. Emergent management of pelvic ring fractures with use of circumferential compression. J Bone Joint Surg 2002;84-A(Suppl 2):43–47.
62. Routt M, Falicov A, Woodhouse E, Schildhauer TA. Circumferential pelvic antishock sheeting: A temporary resuscitation aid. J Orthop Trauma 2002;16:45–48.
63. Vermeulen B, Peter R, Hoffmeyer P, Unger P-F. Prehospital stabilization of pelvic dislocations: A new strap belt to provide temporary hemodynamic stabilization. Swiss Surg 1999;5:43–46.
64. Bottlang M, Simpson T, Sigg J, Krieg JC, Madey SM, Long WB. Noninvasive reduction of open-book pelvic fractures by circumferential compression. J Orthop Trauma 2002;16:367–373.
65. Mears DC. Clinical techniques in the pelvis. In Mears DC (ed), *External skeletal fixation.* Baltimore, MD: Williams and Wilkins, 1983, p 342.
66. Connor GS, McGwin G Jr PA, Alonso JE, Rue 3rd LW. Early versus delayed fixation of pelvic ring fractures. Am Surg 2003;69:1019–1023.
67. Tile M. Pelvic fractures: should they be fixed? J Bone Joint Surg 1988;70-B:1–12.
68. Garcia JM, Doblare M, Seral B, Seral F, Palanca D. Three dimensional finite element analysis of several internal and external pelvis fixations. J Biomech Engin 2000;122:516–522.
69. Gänsslen A, Giannoudis P, Pape HC. Haemorrhage in pelvic fracture: Who needs angiography? Curr Opin Crit Care 2003;9:515–523.
70. Giannoudis PV, Tzioupis CC, Pape HC, Roberts CS. Percutaneous fixation of the pelvic ring: An update. J Bone Joint Surg Br 2007;89-B:145–154.
71. Ganz R, Krushell AJ, Jakob RP, Kuffer J. The antishock pelvic clamp. Clin Orthop 1991;267:71–78.
72. Mohanty K, Musso D, Powell JN, Kortbeek JB, Kirkpatrick AW. Emergent management of pelvic ring injuries: An update. Can J Surg 2005;48:49–56.
73. Tile M. Acute pelvic fractures: II. Principles of management. J Am Acad Orthop Surg 1996;4:152–161.

74. Barei DP, Bellabarba C, Mills WJ, Routt ML Jr. Percutaneous management of unstable pelvic ring disruptions. Injury 2001;32(Suppl 1):S-A33–S-A44.
75. Buhren V, Trentz O. Intraluminare ballonblockade der aorta bei traumatischer massivblutung. Unfallchirurg 1989;92:309–313.
76. Platz A, Friedl H, Kohler A, Trentz O. Chirurgisches management bei schweren becken-quetschverletzungen. Helv Chir Acta 1992;58:925–929.
77. Saueracker AJ, McCroskey BL, Moore EE, Moore FA. Intraoperative hypogastric artery embolization for life-threatening pelvic hemorrhage: A preliminary report. J Trauma 1987;27:1127–1129.
78. Tötterman A, Madsen JE, Skaga NO, Røise O. Extraperitoneal pelvic packing: A salvage procedure to control massive traumatic pelvic hemorrhage. J Trauma 2007;62:843–852.
79. Huittinen V-M, Slatis P. Postmortem angiography and dissection of the hypogastric artery in pelvic fractures. Surgery 1973;73:454–462.
80. Biffl WL, Smith WR, Moore EE, Gonzalez RJ, Morgan SJ, Hennessey T, Offner P, Ray Jr CE, Franciose RJ, Burch JM. Evolution of a multidisciplinary clinical pathway for the management of unstable patients with pelvic fractures. Ann Surg 2001;233:843–850.
81. Perez JV, Hughes TM, Bowers K. Angiographic embolisation in pelvic fracture. Injury 1998;29:187–191.
82. Balogh Z, Caldwell E, Heetveld M, D'Amours S, Schlaphoff G, Harris I, Sugrue M. Institutional practice guidelines on management of pelvic fracture-related hemodynamic instability: Do they make a difference? J Trauma 2005;58:778–782.
83. The Eastern Association for the Surgery of Trauma website. Available at: http://www.east.org/tpg/pelvis.pdf. Accessed July 7th, 2007.
84. Hagiwara A, Minakawa K, Fukushima H, Murata A, Masuda H, Shimazaki S. Predictors of death in patients with life-threatening pelvic haemorrhage after successful transcatheter arterial embolisation. J Trauma 2003;55:696–703.
85. Panetta T, Sclafani SGA, Goldstein AS, Phillips TF, Shaftan GW. Percutaneous transcatheter embolisation for massive bleeding from pelvic fractures. J Trauma 1985;25:1021–1029.
86. Hamill J, Holden A, Paice R, Civil I. Pelvic fracture pattern predicts arterial hemorrhage. ANZ J Surg 2000;70:338–343.
87. Miller PR, Moore PS, Mansell E, Meredith JW, Chang MC. External fixation or arteriogram in bleeding pelvic fracture: initial therapy guided by markers of arterial hemorrhage. J Trauma 2003;54:437–443.
88. Velmahos GC, Chahwan S, Falabella A, Hanks SE, Demetriades D, Moore EE. Angiographic embolisation for intraperitoneal and retroperitoneal injuries. World J Surg 2000;24:539–545.
89. Gourlay D, Hoffer E, Routt M, Bulger E. Pelvic angiography for recurrent traumatic pelvic arterial hemorrhage. J Trauma 2005;59:1168–1174.
90. Wolinsky PR. Assessment and management of pelvic fracture in the hemodynamically unstable patient. Orthop Clin North Am 1997;28:321–329.
91. Ertel W, Karim E, Keel M, Trentz O. Therapeutic strategies and outcome of polytraumatized patients with pelvic injuries. Eur J Trauma 2000;6:278–286.
92. Ertel W, Keel M, Eid K, Platz A, Trentz O. Control of severe hemorrhage using c-clamp and pelvic packing in multiply injured patients with pelvic ring disruption. J Orthop Trauma 2001;15:468–474.
93. Giannoudis PV, Pape HC. Damage control orthopaedics in unstable pelvic ring injuries. Injury 2004;35:671–677.
94. Rout ML Jr, Nork SE, Mills WJ. High energy pelvic ring disruptions. Orthop Clin North Am 2002;33:59–72.
95. Routt Jr ML, Nork SE, Mills WJ. Percutaneous fixation of pelvic ring disruptions. Clin Orthop 2000;375:15–29.
96. Switzer JA, Nork SE, Routt Jr ML. Comminuted fracture of the iliac wing. J Orthop Trauma 2000;14:270–276.
97. Leenen LP, van der Werken C, Schoots F, Goris RJ. Internal fixation of open pelvic fractures. J Trauma 1993;35:220–225.

98. Parker MJ, Roberts C. Closed suction surgical wound drainage after orthopaedic surgery. Cochrane Database Syst Rev 2001;4:CD001825
99. Kudsk KA, Hanna MK. Management of complex perineal injuries. World J Surg 2003;27:895–900.
100. Kudsk KA, Sheldon GF, Walton RL. Degloving injuries of the extremity and the torso. J Trauma 1981;21:835–839.
101. Faringer PD, Mullins RJ, Feliciano PD, Duwelius PJ, Trunkey DD. Selective faecal diversion in complex open pelvic fractures from blunt trauma. Arch Surg 1994;129:958–963.
102. Wong RW, Rappaport WD, Witzke D, Putnam CW, Hunter GC. Factors influencing the safety of colostomy closure in the elderly. J Surg Res 1994;57:289–292.
103. Bulger EM, McMahon K, Jurkovich GJ. The morbidity of penetrating colon injury. Injury 2003;34:41–46.
104. Raman R, Senior C, Segura P, Giannoudis PV. Management of scrotal swelling after pelvic and acetabular fractures. Br J Nurs 2004;13:458–461.
105. Klingman R, Smith P, Stromberg B, Valentine J, Goebel M. Traumatic hemipelvectomy. Ann Plast Surg 1991;27:156–163.
106. Rieger H, Dietl KH. Traumatic hemipelvectomy: An update. J Trauma 1998;45:422–426.

Chapter 18
Vascular Injuries in Polytrauma Patients

Luke P. H. Leenen and Frans L. Moll

The highest goal in damage-control surgery is to stop the bleeding. Major injuries to the vessels, therefore, pose one of the greatest challenges in the damage-control approach. Vascular injuries of the torso are an immediate threat to the life of the victim, whereas vascular injuries to the extremities threaten the preservation of the limb.

18.1 General Techniques

During damage control, simple techniques have to be employed in order to gain control as quickly as possible. Time-consuming complex repairs are not indicated in most instances as they result in the loss of the patient, most often on the operating table.

Draping, in case of suspicion of major vessel injury, should be done from sternal notch to the knees, since it might be possible to regain control of inflow and outflow in adjacent compartments.

In damage-control situations, only a limited number of preoperative measures and diagnostic procedures are possible. Airway and breathing management should precede further management.

18.1.1 Temporary Occlusion

In the prehospital or preoperative situation with extensive external blood loss, temporary occlusion with simple manual or digital pressure provides a simple, effective measure for reducing further blood loss. Alternatively, in extremity injury, a tourniquet can be applied.

L.P.H. Leenen (✉)
Department of Surgery, Department of Vascular Surgery, University Medical
Center Utrecht, Utrecht University Hospital, G 04 129, Heidelberglaan 100,
Utrecht, 3584 CX, The Netherlands
e-mail: lleenen@umcutrecht.nl

H.-C. Pape et al. (eds.), *Damage Control Management in the Polytrauma Patient*,
DOI 10.1007/978-0-387-89508-6_18, © Springer Science+Business Media, LLC 2010

After being banned from clinical practice because of the danger of venous congestion and the imminent danger of further damage by injudicious application, the tourniquet is back as a result of the Iraqi conflict, in which it found renewed interest [1–3].

Another adjunct measure to temporary tamponade is the extraluminal balloon tamponade, which can be utilized in a wide variety of situations and anatomic localizations. A Foley catheter is placed through the trajectory of the injury, and the balloon is inflated. Slight traction may bolster the effect. If the opening in the skin is too wide, it can be sewn together to minimize the opening. This technique can also be used during operation, for example, in the case of penetrating liver injury. For longer trajectories, a drain placed in a glove can be used as a temporary occlusion device.

Intraoperative bleeding can be stopped or diminished by manual compression or swabs on the in- and outflow trajectory. In low pressure systems, for example, veins, which are easily damaged by clamping or attempts to dissect, this provides a quick and effective approach to bleeding control. For immediate control of abdominal aorta, an aortic occluder can be used, which is placed in the diaphragmatic aperture. Intraluminal balloon occlusion can be used intraoperatively if the vascular structure can be readily identified. In- and outflow control can also be obtained with rubber tourniquets, without further damaging vulnerable vascular structures.

18.1.2   Flow Restoration

18.1.2.1   Shunts

In recent years, intraluminal shunts are used more and more as a temporary vascular conduit for almost any anatomic location. Basic research shows that even under low pressure circumstances the shunt remains patent for a considerable amount of time [4]. Recent experiences in Iraq showed a huge success for introduction of shunts even in the field. In a series of 54 shunts placed in the field, 43 in the proximal limb 37 (85%) remained patent until arrival in the definitive care area [5]. Even shunts placed in the venous system remained patent [6]. Commercially available shunts, for example, those used for carotid surgery, can be utilized; however, they also can be constructed from simple IV lines or endotracheal suctioning tubing. The shunt is secured from dislodging with a simple tie of any kind, but sophisticated clamps can also be used when available.

Shunts can be left in place for a considerable amount of time without major drawbacks. The use of anticoagulants is *not* advised since most patients are coagulopatic and have other, potentially bleeding, injuries. The patency of the shunts depends on the physiological situation, local circumstances, and time of the distal ischemia. Shunts allow for quick revascularization of the organ or limb, minimizing the acidotic load to the patient and minimizing the reperfusion reaction. The skin can be closed over the shunt temporarily, after which other injuries can be addressed and/or the patient can be further resuscitated in the ICU. Repair of the vessel can be attempted when the patient is in a more favorable condition, and an optimal plan for repair with the optimal operation team can be worked out. In the case of a concomitant orthopedic injury, vascular repair can follow the repair of the fracture [7].

Problems encountered with shunts are dislodgement, usually due to inadequate fixation, rebleeding, and obstruction of the shunt. Reintervention with refixation should be done as soon as possible. This is even possible in the ICU. Occlusion of the shunt can be diagnosed when the extremity is becoming pale and pulseless. With the use of T-shaped, so-called irrigation catheters, patency can be checked, and, in cases of repeated occlusion, even local heparin on a pump can be given as a local adjunct.

18.1.2.2 Lateral Repair

Simple lateral repair, in suitable cases, is preferable as a quick and effective measure. Lesions of larger truncal or extremity vessels can benefit from this technique. The lesion has to be clean, and no devitalization of the vessel wall should be present. Frayed ends or complete transaction are a contraindication for lateral repair. A major disadvantage is the high probability of creating a stenosis, even with larger vessels such as the aorta or vena cava. If possible, the repair should be transverse, even in the case of a lengthy tear. Revision of the repair at another opportunity is advised, and, where needed, revision before thrombosis is recommended.

18.1.2.3 Stents

With the increased availability of intraluminal stents, their use in selected cases has increased. For numerous indications, stents can be used, with the major advantage of obviating the operative trauma. Of course, in the case of bleeding, covered stents should be used. The main indication for stenting is the thoracic aorta, which will be discussed in the thoracic section in this chapter, but this has become the method of choice for vascular repair in other regions as well. Upper thoracic aperture vessel injuries, auxiliary injuries, and also iliac vessel injuries can be treated in this manner in a damage-control fashion. There is considerable debate whether these stent procedures should be regarded as bridge procedures, with removal of the stent and direct repair at a later phase. As most patients are young and the natural course of these stents is still unknown, this is the tendency.

18.1.2.4 Complex Repairs and Grafts

In the context of damage-control surgery, complex repairs and extended repairs with the use of grafts are not wise choices. The lengthy operations needed are ill-advised in a cold coagulopathic patient, and the quality of the repair in many cases is not optimal because of the time pressure with which the surgeon is confronted.

18.1.3 Definitive Occlusion

18.1.3.1 Ligation

The simplest method for regaining bleeding control is clamping and ligation of the bleeder. In a large range of bleeding problems, this remains a very attractive measure; however, every named artery has its own rules as to whether a simple tie will be tolerated. Care has to be taken in the procedure of clamping. Wild undirected clamping in a pool of blood results in more damage, and vulnerable structures such as veins are the first to be severed. Moreover, the venous structures are the most difficult ones to repair. Controlling inflow and outflow at some distance in an untouched area can be of great help in order to gain overview. To accomplish this, a vessel loop passed twice around a vessel and held in place with a clip, clamp, or tubing can be used.

18.1.3.2 Coiling

A modern method for occluding the bleeding vessel is coiling through the intravascular route. Although a hemodynamically unstable patient in the angio suite is a bad combination, the disadvantages of additional operative trauma may lead to this approach. Moreover, in a modern combined operation-angio suite, which should be part of a state-of-the-art level 1 trauma center, the best of these two worlds can be combined, and a versatile approach to vascular trauma can be utilized. Of course, the nature of the bleeding must be arterial.

18.1.3.3 Hemostatic Agents and Glues

In the case of severe bleeding and devastating wounds, sorting out the exact location of the bleeding can be very demanding. As these patients are usually already coagulopathic, everything bleeds, and discriminating between the structures is usually not possible. The hospital hemostatic agents have been developed mainly for use outside of the hospital, and these stop the bleeding immediately. These mineral hemostatic agents mainly draw water from the surroundings in an exothermic process, developing temperatures of up to 55°C. In a comparative analysis in an animal model of lethal groin injury, the efficacy of zeolith was compared to classic dressings and other commercially available hemostatic agents. The results were astonishing: zeolite reduced blood loss 4–180 min after application to 10 ml/kg body weight, and no deaths occurred. However, this was at the cost of high exothermic reaction, with temperatures of up to 55°C [8]. This could be attenuated by modification of the zeolite hemostatic dressing [9].

Another adjunct to damage control in vascular lesions is the use of fibrin sealant. Kheirabadi and colleagues [10] evaluated the use of fibrin sealant dressing in a high pressure vascular lesion animal model and concluded that fibrin sealant can seal an arterial bleed and prevent rebleeding for at least 7 days. It can therefore be used as a bridging procedure for subsequent stenting or open repair procedures.

18.1.3.4 Amputation

A very definitive way of dealing with a major bleeding problem can be amputation. In the case of a mangled extremity with multiple injuries and severe hemorrhage, it can be wise to use amputation in order to save the patient. This team decision should be made early and expeditiously in order to gain time and prevent needless blood loss and additional shedding of waste products into circulation. The preferred technique is a guillotine amputation, with compressive dressing afterward in order to prevent a lengthy procedure of modeling and flap creation. The guillotine amputation also offers the opportunity to have a second look and to judge whether the remaining tissues are viable and suitable for the creation of an adequate amputation stump.

18.2 Specific Lesions

18.2.1 Maxillofacial

Maxillofacial hemorrhage as a reason for hypotension is fairly uncommon; however, it is overlooked in some cases as the focus of important bleeding because much of the blood is either aspirated, swallowed, or on the floor. Nevertheless, if it is revealed as the site of important hemorrhage, two techniques are available. For acute management, double balloon tamponade can be used. By introducing two Foley catheters through the nose and into the epipharynx and filling these with up to 10 ml of water or saline, an adequate tamponade usually is achieved. Providing some traction on it frequently will add to the effect [11].

The second method is the transcatheter embolization of the maxillofacial artery. Bynoe and colleagues [12] reported this method in 11 out of 912 patients with maxillofacial injuries, with good success in all cases. Complications seen were partial necrosis of the tongue in one case and a facial nerve palsy in another case. In two other patients, minor groin hematomas were seen. Two patients died secondary to concomitant brain injury.

18.2.2 Neck

Every zone in the neck has its own peculiarities, both from initial and definitive treatment. Generally, in penetrating injury with ongoing hemorrhage, the hemorrhage can be treated with direct focal pressure or with a Foley catheter passed through the trajectory and then inflating the balloon. Current diagnostics are duplex sonography and CT angiography; however, in the damage-control situations with profuse external bleeding, the patients are taken immediately to the operating room. Other indications for immediate operative intervention are air bubbles evacuating from the wound (in the absence of a pneumothorax), stridor, hemoptysis, and expanding pulsatile hematomas. If the bleeding is controlled with the previously mentioned methods, nonoperative options should be considered. Lesions in zone I and zone III, because of the anatomically inconvenient localization, can be treated with transcatheter embolization or stenting.

18.2.2.1   Carotid Injuries

Carotid injuries go along with high mortality and morbidity. In a classic series, Demitriades and colleagues reported 56% dead prehospital, whereas those operated upon died in another 22% [13]. An aggressive approach is advocated. Depending on clinical signs alone is dangerous, as many of these victims are drugged, have high blood alcohollevels, or are hypovolemic, making interpretation of level of consciousness and neurological signs difficult. Clear-cut coma, however, makes it very debatable to revascularize the carotid artery because of the often devastating reperfusion reaction intracranially. If there is time for evaluation, infrequently encountered in damage-control situations, a CT scan can be performed to rule out cerebral infarction, which is regarded as a contraindication for revascularization [14]. In case of a high carotid injury, a mandible joint dislocation procedure or even a mandible osteotomy can be performed.

In a recent series from Capetown [15] involving 22 urgently operated patients, ligation in three patients resulted in one death; however, an improved level of consciousness was reached in two. The remaining patients underwent repair with improved results. External carotid injuries can be ligated without any drawbacks [16].

18.2.2.2   Cervical Venous Injuries

In a damage-control situation, virtually all venous lesions in the neck can be treated with ligation. Even the internal jugular vein, as is known from cancer surgery and a few small trauma series [17], can be ligated without further detrimental effects. Some engorgement can result; however, it will subside several days after initial surgery.

18.2.2.3   Vertebral Arteries

Because of the hidden position of the vertebral artery, lesions to this structure pose a real management challenge. In these days of intravascular embolization and because of the very challenging anatomic position of the vertebral artery, these lesions are almost always dealt with by endovascular treatment. Bowley and colleagues

[18] advise tight packing and closure of the neck with the endotracheal tube *in situ* for ventilation. At reoperation, rebleeding is rarely seen. Higher lesions of the vertebral artery, after leaving the vertebral canal, usually are the terrain of the neurosurgeon; however, because of the time needed to open up the skull at this location, endovascular treatment *also* remains the treatment of choice in these cases.

18.2.2.4   Subclavian Arteries

Injuries to the subclavian vessels have remained a challenge over the years. Because of the anatomic circumstances, it is not easy to reach and control them. The change in weapons used, as reported from South Africa, affected the outcome of these lesions dramatically, doubling the mortality from 20% to 47% for gunshot wounds as compared to stab wounds [19].

At presentation, the Fogarty balloon is an excellent device used to control the bleeding in zone I of the neck. In case of a concomitant hemothorax, a second balloon can sometimes be used as a counterfit [18].

The approach is fiercely discussed over the years, but sternotomy provides an excellent possibility for proximal control, after which a supraclavicular incision can be used. On the left side, an anterolateral thoracotomy provides adequate possibilities for proximal control, after which further exposure is dictated by the lesion found. The long promoted trap-door incisions are not advocated any longer because of difficulties with this approach.

18.2.3   Thorax

18.2.3.1   Aorta

Most patients with penetrating lesions to the thoracic aorta do not reach the hospital. Mediastinal traversing injuries are a special case. Degiannis and colleagues [20] evaluated these lesions and found 47% hemodynamically unstable, requiring immediate surgery. Of these 51 patients, 8 had an aortic injury, and only one survived. Repair can be done by lateral repair, patch, or graft; however, patients with lesions large enough to require graft repair do not reach the emergency department alive.

Blunt aortic injury is more commonly found as part of the multiply injured patient. However, these patients are usually not hemodynamically unstable, and, therefore, in the strictest sense, they do not fall into the category of needing damage-control procedures. Nevertheless, controlling this and further damage with a bridging procedure of endovascular stenting deserves mention in this chapter. The main objective in the treatment of these patients is to minimize the operative risks that undoubtedly go along with open repair of aortic tears in the thorax. Selective hypotension in the preoperative phase is wise and is even suggested as the only treatment in these cases. The rule of thumb, however, is 1% mortality per hour warrants treatment for these injuries.

As hypotension generally is not due to the aortic lesion, treatment of other lesions causing hypotension should prevail. After control is regained, the patient should remain in the operating room. With adequate fluoroscopic facilities, preferably a combined angio/operating suite, entry through the femoral vessels should be sought, and a guidewire with length gauge should be inserted. The exact placement of the stent depends on the exact location of the lesion. In some cases, overstenting of the left subclavian artery is mandated; however, in most cases, this is well tolerated.

First results reported in the literature are good; however, some problems must still be addressed [21, 22]. The devices clearly are *not* specifically designed for this anatomic region. Most stents are designed for straight application, whereas, in the aortic arch, because of the differences in inner and outer radii, a more curvilinear design would be preferable. Moreover, since these patients are young, the diameter of the aorta is usually too small for the stent to fit conveniently. Both problems mentioned above can culminate in a wrinkling of the stent in the aortic arch.

Because these patients generally are young and the long-term effects of aortic stenting in this area are still unknown, it is questionable as to whether this should be regarded as a bridging procedure, after which, in due course after recovery of most injuries, a second, more definitive operation in an elective setting should be considered.

18.2.3.2   Pulmonary Vessels

Since most injuries to the pulmonary hilum have concomitant pulmonary injuries, these are dealt with elsewhere in this book. In the rare case in which there is a lesion of the pulmonary vessels in the small distance between the lung and the heart, clamping of the hilum is a problem, and pulmonary twist also is not possible. Opening of the pericardium and intrapericardial clamping are the options available.

18.2.3.3   Thoracic Vena Cava

The superior vena cava is very rarely severed. But, even in those rare cases, lateral venorrhaphy is usually possible. Intrathoracic injury to the inferior vena cava gives rise to intrapericardial hematoma and tamponade. It is highly lethal [23], up to 60%, and very difficult to approach. At times, a shunt is needed, or a cardiopulmonary bypass is performed. Again, balloon tamponade can be of help.

18.2.3.4   Azygos Vein

Although rare, lesions of the azygos vein can occur as result of blunt [24] or penetrating trauma, but also as a result of operative trauma during blind transhiatal esophagectomy. Because of the high flow, considerable blood loss can occur, and this lesion is potentially fatal. Usually there are combined injuries to the bronchus or other structures in the thoracic aperture, resulting in severe problems for adequate repair. The azygos vein itself can be best ligated without further consequences [24].

18.2.4   Abdomen

In presumed vascular injuries of the abdomen, it is essential to follow the principles of wide draping, sternal notch to knees, in order to obtain inflow and outflow control when needed in adjacent compartments. Large amounts of abdominal towels and preferably two suction devices should be available, when possible connected to an autotransfusion device.

The number of severed vascular structures is directly related to mortality [25]: 33% in one lesion to 100% in four or more vascular structures damaged. An early decision to convert to the damage-control mode is essential for survival.

Frank intraperitoneal bleeding leads the way to the source of bleeding; however, in some instances, a large retroperitoneal hematoma is encountered. This can be central or lateral in the pelvic area. Access to the upper aorta, celiac axis, superior mesenteric artery, splenic and left renal vessels can be gained by a left medial reflection of the organs (Mattox maneuver). This will reflect spleen, colon, pancreas, and, if needed, the kidney medially, so that the dorsal side of the aorta also can be approached. Lateral abdominal hematomas usually originate in the kidneys and can be left alone, provided they are not expanding or pulsatile. Of course, the colon must be intact. A pelvic hematoma should be explored only if there is a definitive need, for example, expanding or pulsatile. In the case of a pelvic fracture, stabilization of the pelvis with a pelvic clamp should be considered; thereafter, the pelvis can be packed with abdominal towels. (See Chap. 17 on Pelvic Ring Injuries). Embolization is an option in sustaining arterial bleeding. In other cases, inflow control should be gained by cross-clamping the aorta. Veins are very fragile in this area, and hence adequate packing is the method of choice.

18.2.4.1   Abdominal Aorta

Lesions to the truncal abdominal vessels go along with a high mortality rate. Injury of the abdominal aorta is only manageable with prompt surgical intervention. Prehospital or preoperative fluid resuscitation before managing the hole in the vessel is counterproductive [26]. Access to the aorta is gained by medial rotation of the abdominal viscera to the right. It is a point of discussion as to whether clamping of the aorta should be done in the hilum or through a left anterolateral thoracotomy. The authors prefer to use an aortic occluder placed in the hilum to compress the aorta against the vertebral column. This needs no extensive dissection and is placed in an instance. Another possibility is the use of a large Prewitt balloon that can be advanced through the lesion up into the aorta. After inflating the balloon, good control is achieved.

Repair in damage-control situations, when possible, is done by lateral aortoraphy. Care should be taken not to narrow the vessel too much, but, in the damage-control situation, this is usually the only option. Upon second look, these repairs should be revised, and, in most cases, a graft repair is necessary and can be done at this time. The use of artificial conduits usually leads to thrombosis and is not a good option for extended duration. Ligation of the aorta, distal to the renal vessels, is a possibility, but this is usually associated with severe distal ischemia, which calls for an extraanatomic bypass.

Mortality for free intraperitoneal bleeding from the aorta is high. Degiannis and coworkers [27] and Velmahos and colleagues [28] found an 85% lethality for gunshot wounds to the abdominal aorta. Factors contributing to mortality were lack of response to resuscitation, the need for emergency room thoracotomy, and free intraperitoneal bleeding.

18.2.4.2 Celiac Axis

Injuries to the celiac axis are mostly hidden in a central hematoma. Inflow control is essential. This can be done by a left anterior thoracotomy [29] or locally. By dividing the crus of the diaphragm, more room is achieved. Exposure is done by the medial reflection procedure. Repair is extremely difficult, and, when staying proximal to the main branches, ligation is well tolerated, in case of an intact superior mesenteric artery. Splenic and left gastric arteries can be ligated without consequences. The hepatic artery can be safely ligated proximal to the gastroduodenal artery [30].

18.2.4.3 Superior Mesenteric Artery and Vein

Lesions to the superior mesenteric artery can be hidden by the pancreas and are sometimes not very accessible via the medial rotation. In selected cases, transection of the pancreas along the mesenteric artery axis is needed to gain access. Shunting is a good option. Definitive repair can be done at a later stage. Ligation of the superior mesenteric artery is an option in desperate cases; however, this necessitates subtotal small bowel resection and lifelong Total Parenteral Nutrition (TPN).

A lesion of the mesenteric vein also remains a challenge. In these devastating cases, which derive mostly from penetrating injury and warrant a damage-control approach [31], ligation is advocated. Survival is seen in 40% of cases. If primary repair is possible, survival rises to 60%. Combined injuries to superior mesenteric vein and artery have a survival rate of 55%. Combined injuries of portal and superior mesenteric veins have a survival rate of 40% [31].

18.2.4.4 Inferior Mesenteric Artery

The inferior mesenteric artery can be ligated without any problem. In other intraabdominal devastating lesions, the viability of the colon should be checked at closure or at the time of the second look.

18.2.4.5   Renal Vessels

The kidney is very sensitive for ischemia and tolerates only a limited time of hampered blood flow. Stenting in selected cases may be an option; however, it is usually not feasible in the damage-control situation. In case of complete transection of the renal artery, removal of the kidney should be considered instead of a tedious repair.

Provided the spermatic vein is intact, the left renal vein can be safely ligated.

18.2.4.6   Iliac Vessels

Proximal and distal control should be gained before entering the hematoma distal from the aortic bifurcation. Proximal control is gained by cross-clamping the aorta, and distal control can be achieved by a separate incision in the groin and clamping the femoral vessels. The sigmoid colon is mobilized; however, it is usually already lifted by the hematoma. On the right side, the coecum is mobilized to the midline. Care should be taken of the ureters crossing the iliac vessels at their bifurcation. The veins are the main problem. They are very adherent to the dorsal pelvic wall and to the dorsal side of the right iliac artery. Mobilizing and trying to clamp them ordinarily is ill-advised, as these veins are very fragile. Such an attempt will usually result in even more bleeding, filling up the pelvic cavity in no time. Adequate remote control or vigorous packing with abdominal towels is the only viable option. Case reports [32, 33] as well as the recent Iraq experience [5, 6] show good results with shunting over a prolonged period of time even under low flow circumstances.

18.2.4.7   Inferior Vena Cava

The suprahepatic vena cava is accessed through a sternotomy, incising the diaphragm and opening the pericardium. The frequently recommended procedure of cava-atrial shunts is written about more than practiced and will not be considered here.

The infrahepatic vena cava is approached by a right medial visceral rotation, also called the Cattel-Braasch maneuver. This is followed by a Kocher maneuver and mobilization of the root of the mesentery of the small bowel to fully expose the cava. Best control is achieved with direct pressure on this low pressure system [34]. This also lessens the chance of extra damage to the vena cava. Two stick swabs are very adequate to provide a dry operating field. In penetrating trauma, care should be taken of the dorsal side of the cava. As the dorsal side is not readily exposed by rotation without endangering the friable lumbar veins, inspection and repair should take place through the ventral entry wound. In devastating cases, the inferior cava, distal of the renal veins, can be ligated [34, 35]. Direct venorrhaphy is the first choice of repair and is associated with low thrombosis and low embolic complication rates [34].

18.2.4.8 Portal Vein

Damage of the portal vein is usually accompanied by damage to the choledochus and the hepatic artery, since they are part of the ligamentum hepatoduodenale. Since the portal vein follows through the pancreas and is dorsal to the duodenum, a Kocher maneuver may be necessary to gain control in more proximal lesions. In more distal lesions, control may be possible by a Pringle maneuver. Clamping the portal vein gives rise to small bowel congestion, and hence a stent should be considered at an early stage. If no other options remain, ligation may be the only choice, at the cost of major morbidity. Nevertheless, an early decision to make this move is essential, since up to 84% of cases with lesions in the porta hepatis region expire because of exsanguination [36].

18.2.4.9 Groin

The groin is a special region with regard to damage control and repair. It is a less protected area in modern body armor, and vascular structures are very superficial and vulnerable. To support these cases in the field, several options have been developed, one of these being hemostatic dressings, which were dealt with in the techniques section earlier in this chapter. In recent years and boosted by the experiences in Iraq, the intravascular shunt has been utilized as part of the damage-control procedure, even in the field [5]. Clouse and colleagues, in their series of 54 severe groin wounds with vascular damage provided with an intravascular shunt, 43 were open at the time the patient arrived in the definitive treatment area [5].

18.2.5 Extremity Vessels

Injuries to the extremity arteries require damage-control procedures only in a limited number of cases; however, in a patient with other severe injuries and concomitant vascular injury, a damage-control procedure can be necessary, as illustrated in Fig. 18.1a–d. Lesions to the femoral vessels lead only rarely to death; common femoral vessel injury is associated with poor outcome [37, 38]. The current approach that uses shunts as a temporary measure minimizes the initial ischemic trauma and reperfusion injury. Valuable time can be spent on other injuries since there is less time pressure to complete the repair.

Perhaps the most important procedure after long-term ischemia of the extremity is the fasciotomy, which should be in the armamentarium of every surgeon dealing with trauma. There should be a low threshold for performing a fasciotomy in a patient after damage-control procedures and involvement of the extremities. There is much discussion about when to perform a fasciotomy, and there is a call for measurements in obtunded patients; however, in the case of a patient in shock, thresholds differ, very often resulting in a delayed fasciotomy with late sequelae [39].

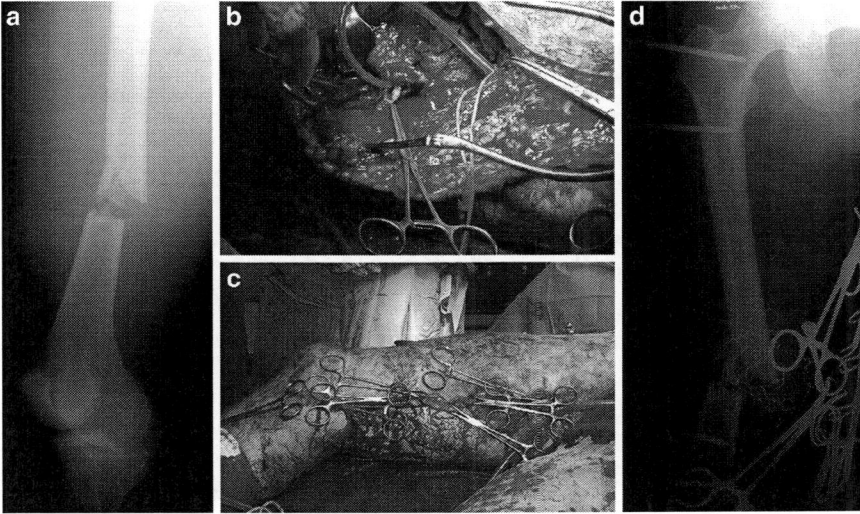

Fig. 18.1 Patient with severe shock after a crane incident with concomitant neurological deficit necessitating CT and craniotomy for drainage of an epidural hematoma: (**a**) femoral fracture; (**b**) femoral artery transection with shunt in place; (**c**) temporary closure before transport to CT; (**d**) temporary external fixation

A separate journey to the OR is not needed for a fasciotomy since it can be performed as a bedside procedure in the ICU itself.

18.3 Summary and Conclusion

The highest goal in damage-control surgery is to *stop the bleeding*. Major injuries to the vessels, therefore, pose the biggest challenge in the damage-control approach. In the acute phase, such as in the field or in the prehospital stage, hemostatic agents such as zeolith are becoming more important additives for first responders. Other general techniques include temporary closure by tourniquets, compression devices, and intra- as well as extravascular balloons. Intra-operative manual compression and stick swabs can be used for temporary control of the bleeding. For more definitive closure, ligation as well as endovascular coiling can be used. For temporary flow restoration, indwelling stents can be used, whereas, for more permanent flow restoration, both anatomic stent grafting as well as extraanatomic stent grafting are used.

Complex repairs and extensive grafting procedures should be avoided since temporary measures in the damage-control situation can be followed up by more definitive procedures as the patient survives the initial phase.

References

1. Kragh JF, Baer DG, Walters TJ. Extended (16 hour) tourniquet application after combat wounds: a case report and review of current literature. J Orthop Trauma 2007;21:274–8.
2. King RB, Filips D, Blitz S, Logsetty S. Evaluation of possible tourniquet systems for use in the Canadian forces. J Trauma 2006;60:1061–71.
3. Welling DR, Burris DG, Hutton JE, Minken SL, Rich NM. A balanced approach to tourniquet use: lessons learned and relearned. J Am Coll Surg 2006;203(1):106–15.
4. Dawson DL, Putnam AT, Light JT, Ihnat DM, Kissinger DP, Rasmussen TE, Bradley DV. Temporary arterial shunts to maintain limb perfusion after arterial injury: an animal study. J Trauma 1999;47:64–76.
5. Clouse WD, Rasmussen TE, Peck MA, Eliason JL, Cox MW, Bowser AN, Jenkins DH, Smith DL, Rich NM. In-theater management of vascular injury: 2 years of balad vascular registry. J Am Coll Surg 2007;204:625–32.
6. Rasmussen TE, Clouse WD, Jenkins DH, Peck MA, Eliason JL, Smith DL. The use of temporary vascular shunts as a damage control adjunct in the management of wartime vascular injury. J Trauma 2006;61:8–15.
7. Reber PU, Patel AG, Sapio NLD, Ris HB, Beck M, Kniemeyer HW. Selective use of temporary intravascular shunts in coincident vascular and orthopedic upper and lower limb trauma. J Trauma 2004;47:72–6.
8. Alam HB, Chen Z, Jaskill A, Querol RILC, Koustov E, Inocencio R, Conran R, Seufert A, Ariaban N, Toruno K, Rhee P. Application of a zeolite hemostatic agent achieves 100% survival in a lethal model of complex groin injury in swine. J Trauma 2004;56:974–83.
9. Ahuja N, Ostomel TA, Rhee P, Stucky GD, Conran R, Chen Z, Al-Mubarak GA, Velmahos G, Demoya M, Alam HB. Testing modified zeolite hemostatic dressings in a large animal model of lethal groin injury. J Trauma 2006;61:1312–20.
10. Kheirabadi BS, Acheson EM, Deguzman R, Crissey JM, Delgado AV, Estep SJ, Holcomb JB. The potential ability of fibrin sealant dressing in repair of vascular injury in swine. J Trauma 2007;62:94–103.
11. Shimoyama, T, Kaneko T, Horie N. Initial management of massive oral bleeding after midfacial fracture. J Trauma 2003;54:332–6.
12. Bynoe RP, Kerwin AJ, Parker HH, Nottingham JM, Bell RM, Yost MJ, Close TC, Hudson ER, Sheridan DJ, Wade MD. Maxillofacial injuries and life-threatening hemorrhage: treatment with transcatheter arterial embolization. J Trauma 2003;55:74–9.
13. Demitriades D, Skalkides J, Sofianos C, Melissas J, Franklin J. Carotid artery injuries: experience with 124 cases. J Trauma 1989;29:91–4.
14. Murray JA, Demetriades D, Asensio JA. Carotid injury: post revascularization hemorrhagic infarction. J Trauma 1996;41:760–2.
15. Navsaria P, Omoshoro-Jones J, Nicol A. An analysis of 32 surgically managed penetrating carotid artery injuries. Eur J Vasc Endovasc Surg 2002;24:349–55.
16. Mittal VK, Paulson TJ, Colaiuta E, Habib FA, Penney DG, Daly B, Young SC. Carotid artery injuries and their management. J Cardiovasc Surg (Torino) 2000;41:423–31.
17. Nair R, Robbs JV, Muckart DJ. Management of penetrating cervicomediastinal venous trauma. Eur J Vasc Endovasc Surg 2000;19:65–9.
18. Bowley DM, Degiannis E, Goosen J, Boffard KD. Penetrating vascular trauma in Johannesburg, South Africa. Surg Clin North Am 2002;82:221–35.
19. Degiannis E, Velmahos G, Krawczykowski D, Levy RD, Souter I, Saadia R. Penetrating injuries of the subclavian vessels. Br J Surg 1994;81:524–26.
20. Degiannis E, Benn CA, Leandros E, Goosen J, Boffard K, Saadia R. Transmediastinal gunshot injuries. Surgery 2000;128(1):54–8.
21. Dinkelman MK, Leenen LPH, Verhagen HJM, Blankensteijn JD. Endovascular treatment of 4 patients with a traumatic rupture of the thoracic aorta. Ned Tijdschr Geneeskd 2003;147:2291–94.

22. Dunham MB, Zygun D, Petrasek P, Kortbeek JB, Karmy-Jones R, Moore RD. Endovascular stent grafts for acute blunt aortic injury. J Trauma 2004;56:1173–8.
23. Mattox KL. Injury to the thoracic great vessels. In: Feliciano DV, Moore EE, Mattox KL (eds), Trauma, 3rd edition. New York: Appleton & Lange, 1995.
24. Nguyen LL, Gates JD. Simultaneous azygos vein and aortic injury from blunt trauma: a case report and review of literature. J Trauma 2006;61(2):444–6.
25. Tyburski JG, Wilson RF, Dente C, Steffes C, Carlin AM. Factors affecting mortality rates in patients with abdominal vascular injuries. J Trauma 2001;50:1020–6.
26. Bickell WH, Wall MJ, Pepe PE, Martin RR, Ginger VF, Allen MK, Mattox KL. Immediate versus delayed fluid resuscitation for hypotensive patients with torso injuries. New Engl J Med 1994;331:1105–9.
27. Degiannis E, Levy RD, Florizoone MG, Badicel TV, Badicel M, Saadia R . Gunshot injuries of the abdominal aorta a continuing challenge. Injury 1997;28:195–7.
28. Velmahos GC, Degiannis E, Souter I, Allwood AC, Saadia R. Outcome of a strict policy on emergency department thoracotomies. Arch Surg 1995;130:774–7.
29. Linuma Y, Yamazaki Y, Hirose Y, Kinoshita H, Kumagai K, Tanaka T, Miyajima M, Katayanagi N, Kuwabara S, Nakazawa S. A case of isolated celiac axis injury by blunt abdominal trauma. J Trauma 2006;61:451–3.
30. Asensio JA, Forno W, Roldan G. Visceral vascular injuries. Surg Clin North Am 2002;82:1–20.
31. Asensio JA, Petrone P, Garcia-Nunez L, Healy M, Martin M, Kuncir E. Superior mesenteric venous injuries: to ligate or to repair remains the question. J Trauma 2007;62:668–75.
32. Nalbandian MM, Maldonado TS, Cushman J, Jacobowitz GJ, Lamparello PJ, Riles TS. Successful limb reperfusion using prolonged intravascular shunting in a case of an unstable trauma patient – a case report. Vasc Endovasc Surg 2004;38:375–9.
33. Kuncir EJ, Demitriados D. Transection of common iliac arteries and veins bilaterally. Eur J Trauma 2004;30:191–4.
34. Carr JA, Kralovich KA, Patton JH, Horst HM. Primary venorrhaphy for traumatic inferior vena cava injuries. Am Surg 2001;67:207–13.
35. Kuehne J, Frankhouse J, Modrall G, Golshani S, Aziz I, Demetriades D, Yellin AE. Determinants of survival after inferior vena cava trauma. Am Surg 1999;65:976–81.
36. Jurkovic GJ, Hoyt DB, Moore FA, Ney AL, Morris JA, Jurkovich GJ, Scalea TM, Pachter HL, Davis JW, Bulger E, Simons RK, Moore EE, McGill JW, Miles WS. Portal triad injuries. J Trauma 1995;39:426–34.
37. Asensio JA, Kuncir EJ, García-Núñez LM, Petrone P. Femoral vessel injuries: analysis of factors predictive of outcomes. J Am Coll Surg 2006;203:512–20.
38. Pearl JP, McNally MP, Perdue PW. Femoral vessel injuries in modern warfare since Vietnam. Mil Med 2003;168:733–5.
39. Brand JHG van den, Sosef NL, Verleisdonk EJMM, Werken Chr van der. Acute compartment syndrome after lower leg fracture. Eur J Trauma 2004;30:93–7.

Chapter 19
Pediatric Trauma and Polytrauma Pediatric Patients

Yigit S. Guner, Henri R. Ford, and Jeffrey S. Upperman

19.1 Epidemiology of Childhood Injuries

The latest version of the pediatric report of the National Trauma Databank (NTDB) contains 221,451 records from U.S. trauma centers from 2000 to 2004 [1]. In this report, blunt mechanisms of injury including motor vehicle crashes (43%) and falls from a height (19.9%) account for the majority of injuries, whereas penetrating injuries comprise only 9% of the total [1]. Trauma is the leading cause of death in children between ages 1 and 14 years in the United States [2]. Injury-related death in childhood is also a global problem as it is the leading cause of death in both industrial and developing countries [3]. Nearly 16,000,000 children visit emergency departments for injuries each year. Of those, 15,000 die and 20,000 are disabled. There are nearly 10 million pediatric injury-related primary care visits in the U.S. annually [4]. In fact, injury is the principal reason for medical spending for children 5–14 years of age [2]. These figures underscore the public health impact of pediatric trauma in contemporary society.

19.2 Differences between Children and Adults

19.2.1 Anatomic Differences

There are some intrinsic differences between children and adults that influence the pattern of injuries seen in children following blunt trauma. In children, energy from an impact is dispersed over a smaller surface area, which means that the force of

Y.S. Guner (✉)
Childrens Hospital Los Angeles/University of Southern California, Department of Pediatric Surgery, University of California Davis Medical Center, 4650 Sunset Boulevard, MS35, Los Angeles, CA, 90027, USA
e-mail: yguner@chla.usc.edu

H.-C. Pape et al. (eds.), *Damage Control Management in the Polytrauma Patient*,
DOI 10.1007/978-0-387-89508-6_19, © Springer Science+Business Media, LLC 2010

impact is greater. Children's connective tissues are weaker and their bones are more pliable. Children also have less fat and muscle tissue to protect their internal organs from injury. The ability of the thoracic cage and pelvis to shield the underlying organs is therefore limited [5]. Indeed, pulmonary contusions and splenic lacerations often occur in children without underlying rib fractures. As children's internal organs are in relatively close proximity, the odds of multiple organ injuries are amplified in comparison to their adult counterparts.

19.2.2 Physiological Differences

The cues needed to recognize early signs of shock are less apparent in pediatric patients. The heart rate is the most important marker of hypovolemia in children since cardiac output is maintained predominantly by increasing heart rate rather than stroke volume as in adults. Children do not develop hypotension until they have lost 45% of their blood volume. It is also important to note that the blood volume changes throughout developmental stages. In the newborn, the blood volume is 90 mL/kg, and, by 1 year of age, it is approximately 80 mL/kg. By adolescence, the circulating blood volume is the same as adults, which is 70 mL/kg. Small children have greater water and thermal losses due to their high body surface area to weight ratio.

19.2.3 Psychological Differences

There are also behavioral and emotional differences between pediatric and adult trauma victims. Following injury, children often regress in maturity due to stress and panic associated with pain and the traumatic event. Such exaggerated behavior can misguide and frustrate physicians performing physical examination.

19.3 Initial Assessment

The basic principles of ATLS® trauma resuscitation apply to children; however, there are specific considerations that are important for timely diagnosis and treatment of injured children. The trauma team must document stability or perform various maneuvers in order to stabilize the patient. Based on the American College of Surgeons Advanced Trauma Life Support (ATLS®) guidelines for adults and children, the trauma team must address the following functions of the patient in an orderly fashion:

- airway (A)
- breathing (B)
- circulation (C)
- disability (D)
- exposure (E)

Clinicians must verify the child's ability to speak, cry, or breathe spontaneously to determine that the airway is patent. Infants and young children have small airways, and edema can rapidly lead to severe airway compromise. Signs that could indicate airway obstruction include stridor, nasal flaring, sternal retractions, or hoarseness. Adequate breathing must be determined by auscultation of both lung fields. In order to reduce respiratory noise from the contralateral lung, axillary auscultation may be helpful. Physicians must also assess symmetric chest rise, respiratory rate, and pulse oximetry. If placement of an endotracheal tube is needed, Cole's formula [size (mm internal diameter)=(age/4)+4] can be used to estimate tube size [6].

The trauma team must assess circulation by determining heart rate, blood pressure, pulses, and capillary refill. Vital signs are age-related, and the physiologic response to shock differs in children. As explained in the previous section, blood pressure alone is not a reliable indicator of volume status because children are able to maintain normal blood pressure in the face of hypovolemia by increasing their heart rate. Therefore, elevated heart rate is the most important early indicator of hypovolemic shock in pediatric trauma patients.

19.4   Secondary Survey and Management

19.4.1   Neurologic Trauma

Traumatic brain injury (TBI) is the most common cause of death and disability in children [7, 8]. Approximately 75% of pediatric deaths from trauma are due to head injury [1, 7]. Nearly half a million children under the age of 14 years sustain TBI yearly [8]. TBI rates are greatest for ages 0–4 years [7]. The most common cause of TBI is motor vehicle collision. A modified version of the Glasow coma scale (GCS) should be used to assess neurologic status in children less than 6 years during the primary survey. The modified GCS is adjusted to accommodate for the differences in the communication skills of young children. All children with GCS of 8 or less should undergo airway control. Ideally, prior to intubation, the trauma team should examine the pupils and note any obvious motor or sensory deficit. Treatment depends on accurate diagnosis, which is best accomplished by a noncontrast computerized tomography (CT) scan of the head. Clinicians should obtain a CT scan on most children who suffer a loss of consciousness or who have an abnormal GCS. Young children with scalp hematomas and a reasonable mechanism should also get head CT scans [9]. If a clinician is not sure whether an injured child has experienced loss of consciousness, he/she should have a low threshold for obtaining a head CT and evaluating the child for possible TBI. For almost all neurological injuries, neurosurgery consultation is necessary. Intracranial pressure monitoring may be needed for children with a GCS of 8 or less. Cerebral perfusion pressure should be kept above 40 mmHg [10]. Elevated intracranial pressure can be managed with a combination of cerebrospinal fluid (CSF) drainage, neuro-muscular blockade, hypertonic saline, or mannitol [10]. Currently, hyperventilation is not recommended because it leads to vasoconstriction and decreased cerebral blood flow. Clinicians may start children with severe head injuries on anticonvulsant prophylaxis with phenytoin in order to prevent seizure-induced increases in intracranial pressure and additional brain injury [10]. However, phenytoin use remains controversial as it is not proven to significantly decrease early seizure rate in children with moderate to severe blunt head trauma [11].

19.4.2 Fractures

The most common skull fractures in children are linear skull fractures. Linear skull fractures are frequently found in children less than 1 year of age who are dropped [10]. Typically, they do not require surgical treatment. Depressed skull fractures are also common fractures. These are repaired when the depression is greater than 1 cm, or when there is open and gross contamination, an underlying large hematoma, a CSF leak, neurological deficits, or poor cosmesis [10]. As a result of a skull fracture, children may develop a leptomeningeal cyst, also known as growing skull fractures. In these cases, children may present with a subacute fluctuant swelling at the fracture site [12]. The treatment of leptomeningeal cysts requires the repair of the underlying tear in the dura [12]. Children often present late with leptomeningeal cysts and, thus, child abuse should be considered.

19.4.3 Diffuse Head Injuries

Rapid acceleration or deceleration forces may generate massive shearing forces that cause diffuse brain injury. Types of brain injury seen after shear forces include concussion and diffuse axonal injury (DAI). Concussions are closed head injuries with reversible neurologic dysfunction, often without any radiographic findings on CT scan [10]. Postconcussive symptoms and signs may include headaches, lethargy, irritability, nausea/vomiting, or a short period of amnesia. The postconcussive period can last up to 6–8 weeks; one may experience ongoing symptoms during this period [10]. Children who sustain head injury with severe rotational forces may develop DAI due to myelin disruption and complete axonal tearing. In severe DAI cases, coma can last longer than 24 h without a focal radiographic neurological lesion. DAI is often associated with immediate unconsciousness and decorticate or decerebrate posturing [10]. Magnetic resonance imaging (MRI) is more sensitive than CT for detecting DAI [13]. DAI treatment is mainly supportive since, in most cases, the patient's intracranial pressures are usually not elevated [10]. In severe DAI, long term disability is certain and mortality is high [14].

19.4.4   Focal Head Injuries

Children may sustain subdural hematomas after motor vehicle crashes, falls, or nonaccidental trauma [10]. Children with small subdural hematomas are usually observed in Level 1 trauma centers. On the other hand, if children have associated neurological deficits or midline shifts, they may require surgical decompression and evacuation of the hematoma. If an infant with a subdural has an open fontanelle, the neurosurgeon may elect to perform a needle aspiration of the hematoma [15]. Epidural hematomas due to an injury of the middle meningeal artery are uncommon in young children [10]. Children may have epidural hematomas without a skull fracture. Epidural hematomas in young children may be due to bleeding bone edges, dura, or venous structures [10]. The indications for surgery for epidural hematoma are similar to those for subdural hematoma, and they include neurological deficits, midline shifts, or brain stem compression [10].

19.4.5   Cervical Spine

The incidence of cervical spine injuries in pediatric patients is fairly low (1–2%) [16]. However, they account for 60–80% of all spinal injuries seen in children [16]. Cervical spine injuries are associated with significant mortality (27%) and neurological deficits (66%) [16]. Compared to adults, children have a large head to body size ratio, and, therefore, children tend to hyper-flex their necks with sudden acceleration or deceleration maneuvers. In addition, children's neck muscles and ligaments are not as strong and thus are unable to stabilize the head with rapid forces. Therefore the head and neck anatomy of children predisposes them to cervical spine injury up to about 8 years of age [16]. Younger children (<8 years of age) are prone to upper cervical spine injuries, and older children have lower cervical spine injuries [16].

Cervical spine immobilization is a key step during the initial workup and evaluation. Clearance of the cervical spine should start with physical examination. Children who exhibit neck pain or focal midline tenderness, head injury, and other high force injuries typically need X-rays to rule out underlying injuries. When cervical spine clearance is not possible based on physical exam, either due to neurologic issues or abnormal findings on physical examination, routine cervical spine imaging in pediatric trauma patients should include anterior-posterior, lateral, and odontoid views. Considerable debate exists on how to adequately clear the cervical spine in conscious children less than 5 years of age. In this age group (<5), physical examination may be limited, and it may be difficult to obtain an open mouth odontoid view.

Some have advocated the routine use of a limited CT scan of C1–C2 in younger children due to inability to obtain an adequate open mouth odontoid radiograph [17]. It should, however, be noted that there is a paucity of data in the literature supporting the routine use of CT or MRI as screening tools in pediatric patients. One major concern regarding the routine use of CT scanning of the cervical spine in children is the potential for cancer due to excess radiation [18]. If the initial imaging studies are deemed to be normal and the child meets National Emergency X-Radiography Utilization Study (NEXUS) criteria (absence of midline tenderness, normal level of alertness, normal neurological exam, absence of distracting injury), the cervical spine can be cleared [19]. Younger children are also more prone to ligamentous injuries, and, therefore, some clinicians suggest the use of flexion-extension views in detecting cervical spine instability [20]. Regardless, flexion/extension X-rays should be the next step in those children who do not meet NEXUS criteria [19]. If the flexion/extension study is normal, then the cervical spine can be cleared. If flexion or extension is limited or other abnormalities are noted, a neurosurgeon should be consulted [19]. Overall, the clearance of the cervical spine should be done in a systematic manner. Lee and colleagues have demonstrated that, by employing a cervical spine clearance pathway, the time required for cervical clearance was significantly decreased [17]. Viccellio and coworkers further estimated that the use of NEXUS guidelines could reduce the use of spine imaging in children by 20% [21]. When injuries are identified leading to neurological deficits, steroid use remains controversial. Most physicians follow the adult guidelines from the national acute spinal cord trauma study in terms of steroid use and doseage [22].

Children may also sustain Spinal Cord Injury Without Radiological Abnormality (SCIWORA). SCIWORA occurs when a traumatic force stresses lax ligaments and joint capsules with excess mobility, resulting in neck injury without actually causing spine subluxation or fractures. MRI detects injury to the ligamentous structures; therefore, the term essentially refers to an era when technology was not as sensitive. Platzer and coworkers showed that the rate of these injuries is more common in children less than 8 years of age [16]. A child suspected of having a cervical spine injury without plain radiograph or CT evidence should undergo the more sensitive MRI study.

19.4.6 Thoracic Trauma

The incidence of thoracic trauma in children is fairly low at about 4–6% [23]. Blunt trauma causes 80–97% of the thoracic injuries in children [24, 25]. Isolated pediatric thoracic trauma mortality is 4–15% [26–28]. When thoracic trauma is combined with extra-thoracic injuries, the mortality rate climbs to 29% [26]; in the presence of heart or great vessels injury, mortality rises to 50% [29]. Anatomic differences in children lead to differences in injury patterns in children as opposed to adults. For instance, the rib cage is more flexible in children; therefore, rib fractures are less likely, but underlying cardiac or pulmonary contusions are more likely.

In young children, the trachea is narrow, and the airway caliber is small, which makes them more prone to obstruction by blood, debris, or saliva that a child may aspirate after significant head and thoracic injury. Moreover, since children have higher oxygen consumption than adults, hypoxia may develop quickly, thus requiring oxygen supplementation and possibly airway control. Controlling the pediatric airway is not a trivial matter, but one may use a bag-valve mask for long periods with a child. During pediatric intubation, right main-stem intubation is a common mishap due to the short length of the trachea; therefore, experienced personnel in airway management should perform this maneuver. Field intubations in the pediatric population do not improve outcomes and lead to an increased rate of complications [30]. DiRusso and colleagues suggested that, except for circumstances in which bag-valve ventilation has failed, field intubation should not be practiced [30]. In rare instances, one should perform emergency department thoracotomy in children with hemodynamically unstable penetrating thoracic injuries with very rapid deterioration despite maximal emergency treatment [31, 32]. However, as in adults, the results of ED thoracotomy is extremely poor for blunt trauma, and it therefore should be avoided [32, 33].

19.4.7 Bony Injuries of the Chest

Most children with rib fractures are involved in motor vehicle crashes [24]. Rib fractures are rare in infants and young children due to the highly compliant chest walls [34]. Young children with rib fractures should be screened for more serious underlying injuries. In addition, kids with rib fractures that are attributed to "minor" mechanisms should be screened for nonaccidental trauma, since significant force is necessary to break young ribs unless there is an underlying medical condition causing fragile bones (e.g., osteogenica imperfecta). In fact, in children less than 3 years of age, nonaccidental trauma is the predominant cause for rib fractures [35]. Although rib fractures are not usually the primary cause of death in injured children, the mortality rate in injured children associated with rib fractures ranges from 40 to 70% [28, 35]. Management of isolated rib fractures is pain management and aggressive pulmonary toilet.

Children who sustain a crush injury to the thorax may quickly develop traumatic asphyxia because the chest is pliable and the jugular and because innonimate veins are valveless, resulting in displacement of the blood cephalad, leading to cyanosis, subconjunctival hemorrhages, and facial edema. Treatment for traumatic asphyxia is supportive, but it requires intensive care monitoring and may require mechanical ventilation. Traumatic asphyxia is commonly associated with pulmonary contusions and hemo- or pneumothorax [25]. Flail chest is extremely rare in injured children, but it happens in 1–2% of children with rib fractures [25]. Patients with flail chest have poor respiratory mechanics due to the paradoxical outward and expanding motion of the flail segment during respiration. Similar to children with rib fractures, flail chest patients require aggressive pain control, possibly including epidural analgesia. Injured children with hemo- or pneumothorax may need a tube thoracostomy. In severe cases, they may need positive pressure ventilation until chest wall mechanics are reestablished.

Thoracic spine injuries are rare, related to motor vehicle crashes and seen more commonly in children greater than 8 years of age [28]. Injured children with focal back tenderness or abnormalities on neurological exam should undergo radiological examination including plain spine X-rays and/or CT scan [28]. Children with SCIWORA of the thoracic spine should have an MRI [36]. Younger children (<8) are more likely to have more profound or even complete spinal injuries [37].

19.4.8 Pulmonary Contusion

Pulmonary contusion is the most common thoracic injury in children due to blunt trauma [24]. Blunt trauma causes damage to the vasculature, causing leakage of blood and plasma, which results in fluid accumulation in the alveoli and hypoventilation. As a consequence, hypoxemia develops, and this leads to further lung consolidation, edema formation, and decreased compliance. The pathophysiology of hypoxemia associated with pulmonary contusion is due to intrapulmonary-shunting. Blunt injured children can develop progressive lung inflammation and edema, which may lead to worsening hypoxemia in the first 24–48 h [38]. The degree of hypoxemia depends on the volume of lung injured. The diagnosis of pulmonary contusion may be made with an initial chest radiograph during resuscitation; however, plain film changes may lag 4–6 h behind the initial injury [25]. Patients with pulmonary contusion should receive supplemental oxygen, and, if they are unstable with poor oxygenation and ventilation, they should be intubated and supported with mechanical ventilation. Patients intubated for pulmonary contusion usually require a short duration of positive pressure ventilation [24, 28]. However, children with pulmonary contusion may develop complications such as respiratory distress syndrome or pneumonia [39, 40]. If patients with severe pulmonary contusions fail mechanical ventilation, then some clinicians suggest using extracorporeal life support [41].

19.4.9 Pneumothorax

Pneumothoraces in children are often due to motor vehicle crashes and falls [27]. A pneumothorax is typically caused by broken ribs puncturing the lung parenchyma and allowing air to escape into the thoracic cavity. Other causes include disruption of the pulmonary parenchyma by a sudden increase in intra-bronchial pressure or injury to the trachea or bronchi. The incidence of pneumothorax associated with blunt injury in children ranges from 34 to 37% [24, 42]. If a clinician obtains the appropriate history and detects diminished breath sounds or chest wall crepitus, these findings usually point to pneumothorax, and the clinician may elect to perform a tube thoracostomy in an unstable patient. If the patient is stable, one may obtain a plain chest radiograph or chest CT scan to confirm the injury (Fig. 19.1). All traumatically injured patients with a significant pneumothorax should undergo tube thoracostomy. Thoracostomy or chest tube placement will evacuate the air in the pleural space and expand the lung. Left untreated, a significant pneumothorax with unmitigated pressure will develop into a tension pneumothorax. Since a child's mediastinum is quite mobile, the physiologic effect of tension pneumothorax is more likely to lead to respiratory and cardiovascular compromise. Initial treatment of a tension pneumothorax can be either the placement of a temporizing angiocatheter or chest tube. An occult or very small pneumothorax, detected on abdominal CT scan and not on the plain chest radiograph, may be observed if the patient is not going to require positive pressure ventilation. If these patients require positive pressure ventilation, then they should undergo chest tube insertion [43, 44].

19.4.10 Hemothorax

Hemothorax occurs in 13% of the children with blunt chest trauma [24]. On initial evaluation, a clinician may obtain a history of penetrating or blunt chest trauma and diminished breath sounds with respiratory compromise. This is sufficient evidence

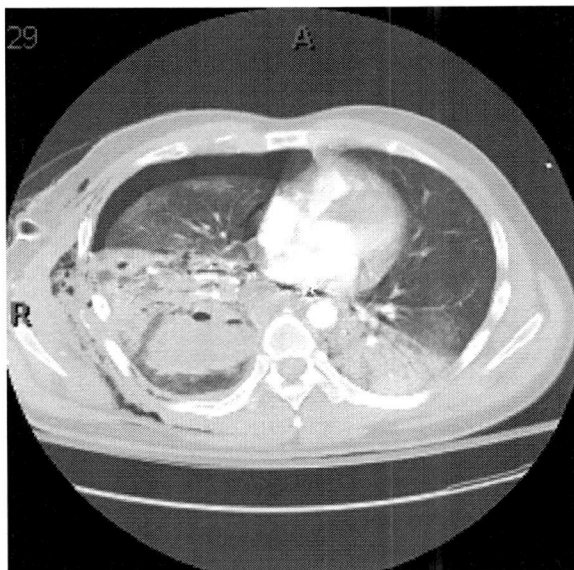

Fig. 19.1 Right pneumothorax and bilateral pulmonary contusions

to perform a tube thoracostomy. In other instances in stable patients, clinicians may confirm a hemothorax on a chest X-ray or chest CT scan and perform a tube thoracostomy. After the blood is drained with a chest tube, the lung will expand, and this should improve respiration and possibly tamponade bleeding from the lung parenchyma. Most thoracic bleeding after chest trauma is due to injury to the lung parenchyma or intercostals vessels. Severe injuries may also include damage to the great vessels, heart, bronchi or trachea, esophagus, and diaphragm, resulting in massive hemorrhage, cardiac tamponade, large pneumothorax, or persistent air leak [33]. After the placement of a chest tube, the trauma team should monitor drainage; if 20–25 mL/kg of blood is drained immediately, they should consider a thoracotomy. If clinicians detect continued bleeding at a rate of 2 cc/kg/h, they may consider a thoracotomy. During such an operation, surgeons can oversew pulmonary lacerations and resect nonviable portions of the lung. If surgeons identify central pulmonary injuries, they should be alert to potential exsanguination or air embolism. Surgeons who detect severe damage involving major blood vessels may need to clamp the pulmonary hilum in order to facilitate complete assessment and repair. If the injuries are irreparable, they may elect to perform a pneumonectomy. Retained blood in the thoracic cavity may develop into a localized infection or empyema. Most advocate draining a hemothorax within 7 days of injury in order to avoid an infectious complication or lung trapping and fibrosis [45].

19.4.11 Tracheobronchial Injuries

Airway injuries are rare in children, but they carry a mortality rate of greater than 30% [25]. Most tracheobronchial injuries are due to blunt trauma [25]. If patients continue to have large persistent air leaks or pneumothoraces, then clinicians should consider a tracheobronchial injury. Following stabilization, the trauma team can evaluate for a potential tracheobronchial injury with bronchoscopy. Treatment consists of thoracotomy to fix the trachea or a bronchus injury. Surgeons may opt for nonoperative treatment if the injury is less than one third the diameter of the bronchus or if a tube thoracostomy controls the pneumothorax [25].

19.4.12 Cardiac Injuries

Blunt injury to the heart is rare in children. Tiao and colleagues found only 0.8% of the children who sustained blunt trauma had injury to the heart [46]. Mortality associated with blunt cardiac injury ranges from 10 to 14% [47, 48]. The disease spectrum ranges from cardiac contusion to rupture of the ventricles or atria. If the injury is severe, these injuries are uniformly fatal [25]. Cardiac contusions are the most common blunt injury to the heart [46, 48]. Cardiac contusions in children have minimal symptoms and require only supportive care [25]. If the cardiac output remains diminished despite adequate fluid resuscitation, cardiac contusion should be suspected. Children with EKG abnormalities or elevation of cardiac isoenzymes need close monitoring for the first 24 h. Common clinical signs of cardiac contusion include tachycardia, arrhythmias, EKG changes, and wall motion abnormalities on echocardiography. The most likely period for arrhythmias is the first 24 h.

Cardiac tamponade is a rare finding in children following thoracic blunt trauma. Clinicians may identify Beck's triad (diminished heart sounds, jugular-venous distention, and hypotension) during initial screening, but this is often difficult to assess in infants. Cardiac tamponade may be treated with pericardiocentesis during the initial resuscitation. If emergency abdominal surgery is performed, a pericardial window can be created during laparotomy to evaluate the possibility of a cardiac tamponade. *Commotio cordis* is a unique condition in the 12–13 years of age group that is a sudden change in heart rhythm after chest wall impact leading to sudden death [25, 28]. The most common projectile associated with *commotio cordis* is a baseball. In *commotio cordis*, unlike in cardiac contusion, there is no structural damage to the heart despite the chest wall impact [49]. Defibrillation in the field may be lifesaving in *commotio cordis* [25]. Youth baseball leagues now require protective chest wall devices to prevent this injury.

19.4.13 Great Vessel Injuries

Aortic or great vessel injuries in the pediatric population are deadly but extremely rare [29]. They are typically caused by blunt trauma [24, 33, 50]. Unlike adults, children with traumatic aortic injuries do not have associated chest wall injuries, but, instead, they undergo a rapid deceleration or severe crush mechanism [50]. When screening for aortic disruption on chest radiograph, one should be aware of the large thymic silhouettes seen in young children that appear as a widened mediastinum. In addition, clinicians may note a widened mediastinum with a superior mediastinal hematoma due to traumatic aortic injury. Some suggest that deviation of the esophagus, as demonstrated by a displaced nasogastric tube, may be a more accurate sign in young children of a mediastinal hematoma [33]. Similar to the adult population, children with first rib fractures may have associated great vessel injuries [51]. In a hemodynamically stable child with an abnormal chest X-ray revealing a widened mediastinum or apical capping, one should consider additional tests such as CT-based angiography or standard angiography [52]. Aortic transection at the level of ligamentum arteriosum is most commonly reported for children greater than 8 years of age [50]. Additional studies for determining an aortic disruption include transthoracic or transesophageal echocardiogram, CT angiogram, or aortogram [50]. Most consider an arch aortogram as the gold standard for diagnosing a disrupted aorta [53]. Bruckner and colleagues showed that chest CT scans have a negative predictive value of 99% of ruling out aortic injury; yet its specificity is fairly low due to artifacts [54]. Aortography is therefore still required for clarification when suspicious findings are present on computed tomography. If an aortic injury is identified, operative repair is usually performed with great success [50]. Surgeons caring for a child with aortic disruption should manage blood pressure with a β-blockade in order to reduce rupture risk.

There are two methods of repairing the aorta: (1) Clamp and sew technique; (2) Aortic bypass with temporary conduit for maintaining distal perfusion. The clamp and sew method does not involve aortic cannulation, and, therefore, anticoagulation is not required. On the other hand, anticoagulation is needed for the aortic bypass approach [25]. Paraplegia is a devastating complication of both operations, and the incidence is reported to be 9–16% in retrospective pediatric series [50, 55, 56]. Recent reports suggest endovascular stent grafting, a new alternative for open aortic repair in injured children [57]. The complications reported with stent grafting technique include perigraft leak, graft migration, infection, and occlusion of the left main stem bronchus [58]. The long-term outcome with this type of a repair is not yet known in adults or children. It is currently recommended as a bridge technique for children who are otherwise too unstable to undergo open operative repair [57, 58].

19.4.14   Diaphragm Injury

Small retrospective reports or case series suggest that diaphragmatic injuries are rare in children [28, 59]. A diaphragmatic injury is usually associated with other injuries after blunt trauma [59, 60]. Most believe that severe blunt forces cause diaphragmatic injury when there is a sudden increase in intra-abdominal pressure. For instance, lap belts malpositioned high on a child's abdomen and not in the correct lap position may rapidly squeeze the abdominal wall on sudden impact, resulting in swift increase in abdominal pressure. The rapid increase in intraabdominal pressure can rupture the diaphragm [28]. The left hemidiaphragm is more likely to rupture compared to the right because the right hemidiaphragm is protected by the liver [25, 61]. The diaphragm typically bursts at the central tendon and the lateral chest wall attachment. Clinicians make the diagnosis of diaphragmatic rupture with a chest radiograph in only 20–30% of the cases [25, 62]. Radiographic findings include hemidiaphragm elevation, mediastinal shift, and abdominal viscera herniation into the chest [60]. CT is also an excellent imaging modality that has a high specificity to demonstrate diaphragmatic injuries [25]. If a ruptured diaphragm is diagnosed late, the herniated abdominal viscera can become strangulated. Clinical signs and symptoms include dyspnea, tachypnea, abdominal pain or tenderness, and diminished breath sounds on the affected side [60]. Diaphragmatic injuries should be repaired via laparatomy so that other intra-abdominal organs can be readily assessed. On occasion, some patients remain asymptomatic after diaphragmatic injury. If suspected, such occult injuries can be detected by laparoscopy with 100% specificity in adult patients; however, similar data are lacking for the pediatric population [63].

19.4.15 Abdominal Trauma

The most common mechanism responsible for abdominal trauma in children are traffic accidents. Children are killed twice as frequently by blunt abdominal trauma than by thoracic trauma [27]. The risk of intraabdominal injury is increased in children because intraabdominal solid organs are in close proximity to each other, which predisposes the patient to multiple injuries. Overall, when the same force applied to an adult is applied to a small-sized child, this leads to greater impact per body surface area for the child. Commonly injured intra-abdominal organs include the spleen, liver, and kidney [27]. Children wearing improperly positioned lap belts may sustain a classic combination of injuries in car crashes including abdominal wall abrasions, intestinal perforation, and lumbar spine fracture, also known as Chance fractures [64]. Children involved in bike crashes may sustain handlebar injuries such as duodenal hematoma or perforation, or pancreatic contusions [64].

Advance trauma life support recommends primary and secondary survey for a child, similar to the adult protocol. Examining an anxious frightened child is challenging and requires patience. Crying children may have misleading abdominal findings. Crying young children swallow large amounts of air and develop gastric distention; in some cases, clinicians may confuse air swallowing associated gastric distention with pathological abdominal distention from other causes. If clinicians suspect abdominal injury, they must perform serial abdominal exams. There is some debate regarding the routine use of ATLS®-recommended digital rectal exams in children. Since digital rectal exams may confuse and scare children, this distraction may thwart the physician's ability to interpret the child's overall exam. Kristinsson and colleagues demonstrated that the sensitivity of physical examination with or without digital rectal exam in children was equivalent [65]. Nevertheless, clinicians should always check for gross blood in the perineum and associated perineal injuries. In children with penetrating trauma, perineal blood close to the rectum requires rectal exams [66, 67].

Many trauma centers send predetermined laboratory panels based on suspected injury severity or trauma level designation. Laboratory tests are typically ordered and obtained during initial intravenous catheter placement for resuscitation. Initial blood samples often include a type and cross-match, hemoglobin or hematocrit, alanine aminotranferase (ALT), aspartate aminotransferase (AST), amylase, and lipase. In addition, clinicians usually obtain urine samples for routine urinalysis. Liver injury in children is implicated by enzyme level elevation, such as AST (>400 IU/L) or ALT (>250 IU/L) [68]. Nadler and colleagues showed that serum amylase greater than 200 IU/L and serum lipase greater than 1,800 IU/L are indicative of major pancreatic ductal injury in a pediatric population [69]. Most moderately injured pediatric blunt trauma victims have minimal laboratory abnormalities [70], but serology studies combined with other diagnostic studies may be useful. For instance, Holmes and colleagues showed that low systolic blood pressure, abdominal tenderness, femur fracture, urine analysis with greater 5 RBC per high powered field, and initial hematocrit less than 30% were all highly associated with intraabdominal injury in children [71]. In summary, serology tests add information when screening for intraabdominal injuries, but they must be used in combination with a thorough physical exam and select radiographic studies. The following section will outline radiographic studies that are key in pediatric trauma evaluations for abdominal injury.

Injured, hypotensive children with no evidence of extremity or neurologic injury and normal chest and pelvis X-rays are believed to have intra-abdominal bleeding until proven otherwise. Some advocate an emergency abdominal ultrasound also known as a Focused Assessment with Sonography for Trauma (FAST) in trauma patients to identify either free fluid or solid organ injuries. The FAST exam in children has 33–92% sensitivity and 95–97% specificity for identifying free fluid or solid organ injury [72–74]. The most important diagnostic test for determining abdominal injury is CT. More details on the utility of this test will follow in the specific organ section.

Children with free intraperitoneal fluid on CT scan without solid organ injury may have an undetected solid organ or bowel injury. Many clinicians observe these children with serial abdominal examinations, and, if the tenderness persists or worsens, they often consider an abdominal exploration. Until recently, the diagnostic peritoneal lavage (DPL) was viewed as the gold-standard procedure for determining evidence of intraabdominal injury. However, the wide scale adoption of nonoperative management for solid intraabdominal organ injury has resulted in a decline in the use of DPL in pediatric trauma because intraperitoneal hemorrhage is not an absolute indication for laparotomy [75]. In hemodynamically unstable children with neurological injuries, DPL may be indicated if the need for rapid neurosurgical intervention precludes adequate radiographic evaluation of intraabdominal injury [64]. An alternative to DPL is diagnostic laparoscopy or minimally invasive surgery. These approaches make it possible to evaluate brain-injured patients without a formal laparotomy. Feliz and coworkers retrospectively analyzed 113 children and found that, by performing laparoscopy, laparotomy was avoided in over half the patients, and no injury was missed [76]. These findings are preliminary and require further study. The following sections will review specific abdominal organ injuries.

19.4.16   Spleen

In children, the spleen is the most commonly injured organ following blunt abdominal trauma. Isolated splenic trauma is associated with a low mortality [77]. Traffic crashes and falls account for the most common blunt mechanisms associated with splenic injury [78]. Some patients may describe left shoulder pain, which is due to diaphragmatic irritation (Kehr's sign). Left lower rib fractures are often associated with splenic injury in adults (20–25%), but this association is less common in children [78]. In hemodynamically stable patients, the diagnosis of splenic laceration or hematoma is made by CT scan with intravenous contrast (Fig. 19.2). Radiologists

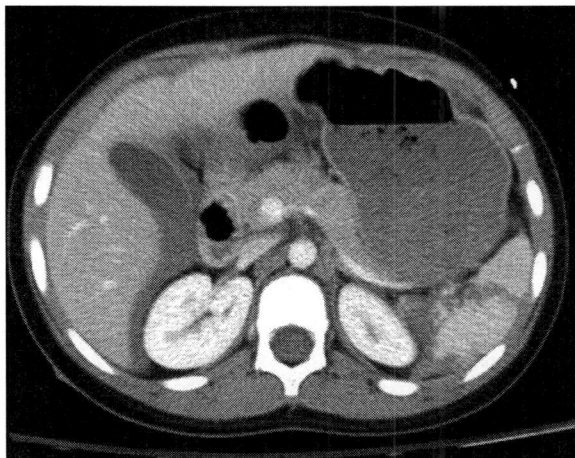

Fig. 19.2 CT scan demonstrates a complex splenic laceration involving the hilum. This patient required a splenectomy due to massive blood loss

and trauma surgeons grade CT scan findings according to the severity of splenic injury. The radiographic grade can also be used to guide the treatment and convalescence algorithm in stable patients [79–82].

Most splenic injuries in hemodynamically stable patients can be managed nonoperatively [77, 78, 82]. Blood transfusions are required in less than 10% of these injured children [83, 84]. Not all children with splenic injuries need intensive care unit admission. For Grade I-III splenic injuries, the incidence of splenectomy is 3% [85]. Grade IV injuries are associated with a 13% laparotomy rate and a 26% transfusion rate; therefore, such patients are typically admitted to the intensive care unit for the first day of admission [85]. The exact length of hospital stay following splenic injury is debated. Gandhi and colleagues showed that hemodynamically stable children with isolated splenic trauma can be safely treated with a 4-day hospital stay [81]. The American Pediatric Surgical Association (APSA) committee on trauma advocates estimating the hospital stay by assessing the splenic injury grade (based on abdominal CT scan) and adding one day to the grade value. In hemodynamically stable patients with isolated spleen or liver injury, estimating the length of stay in this manner is gaining wide support [85]. In addition to the length of stay calculation, APSA recommends estimating the safe interval of rest or limited physical activity by adding 2 weeks to the injury grade [85]. For example, a child with a grade III spleen laceration should be hospitalized for 4 days and should have restricted physical activity for 5 weeks. Routine follow-up imaging to ensure healing is not recommended unless patients are symptomatic [82, 85].

Although nonoperative treatment of splenic trauma is the gold standard of care, it is not successful in every patient. If children fail conservative management, surgeons should consider exploration and possibly splenorrhaphy or splenectomy. The risk of infection after splenectomy is age-dependent, since children who are younger than 5 years of age have infection rates of approximately 10% [78]. If the surgeon is unable to preserve any splenic parenchyma, the patient is at-risk for overwhelming post-splenectomy sepsis (OPSI). Splenorrhaphy and partial splenectomy may be performed successfully in most children who require laparotomy, and these maneuvers often decrease the risk of OPSI [86]. Compared to adults, children are at increased risk for OPSI; in particular, children who undergo elective splenectomy for medical indications have the greatest risk of OPSI [78, 87]. The incidence of OPSI in children following splenectomy for trauma is 2% [87]. Streptococcus pneumonia is the most common pathogen responsible for OPSI. Other encapsulated organisms implicated include *Haemophilus influenza type b* and *Neisseria meningitides* [78].

The optimal timing for immunizing adults or children against encapsulated bacteria following trauma splenectomy is controversial due to lack of sufficient evidenced-based data [78]. Shatz and colleagues measured the levels of serum immunoglobulin G in adult trauma patients who were given pneumococcal vaccine 1–28 days after emergency splenectomy [88, 89]. In these studies, maximal immunoglobulin response was seen 14 days following splenectomy. Administration of the vaccine at 28 days did not improve antibody response [89]. These authors also showed that antibody response was limited in asplenic trauma patients in comparison to healthy adults immunized with pneumococcal vaccine [88]. Current guidelines do not mandate a particular post-operative day for vaccination, but they recommend administering vaccines prior to hospital discharge [78]. The practice of immunizing prior to discharge has the advantage of avoiding patients being lost to follow-up [90]. Due to reports of delayed presentation of OPSI, revaccination is recommended [90, 91]. Pneumococcal vaccine has limited effectiveness in children who are younger than 2 years of age [92]. Therefore, children <2 years old should be on oral penicillin or amoxicillin prophylaxis and should be vaccinated after they reach two years of age [90, 92]. The exact length of oral antibiotic prophylaxis remains controversial as well [90]. Pneumococcal vaccine should be repeated 3–5 years following the initial dose [75, 78]. Trauma personnel should educate all parents about OPSI, and the parents should receive contact numbers and a medical alert card.

Selective percutaneous splenic artery embolization is an alternative and less invasive method in children who fail nonoperative management [93]. This method is used as either a bridge to operative treatment to decrease blood loss or as a definitive treatment. Laparoscopic splenectomy is another minimally invasive method for performing splenectomy in trauma patients. Huscher and colleagues have reported successful laparoscopic splenectomy in 6 adults and laparoscopic splenic salvage in another 5 patients [94]. Minimally invasive approaches are untested in the pediatric population. Both interventional and laparoscopic techniques need additional studies to determine their effectiveness in children.

19.4.17   Liver

The liver is the second most commonly injured intra-abdominal organ, but the most common cause of death in children after blunt intra-abdominal trauma [27, 64, 77]. Traffic crashes and falls are the two most common mechanisms leading to injury [27]. Serious liver injuries are rare, but associated damage may include injuries to the inferior vena cava and hepatic veins. Some falls are associated with avulsion injuries, and such extensive liver injuries can lead to massive uncontrolled hemorrhages [95].

Since the right lobe of the liver is larger than the left side, it is injured more often. In the setting of liver injury, most children complain of abdominal and sometimes right shoulder pain. Elevated transaminases (AST >400, ALT >250) are indicative of liver injury in children [68]. Hemodynamically unstable patients that do not respond to fluid resuscitation are potential candidates for laparotomy. In stable patients, liver injury is typically detected with a CT scan (with intravenous contrast). Surgeons and radiologists grade liver injury similar to splenic injuries from Grades 1 to 6 [79]. Injury grade does not always predict outcome, and, therefore, it should not be used as a sole determinant of clinical decision-making [79]. Historically, indications for operative management for liver injury were deep lacerations involving major vascular structures, lacerations with nonviable liver segments, or injury to vena cava or hepatic veins [95]. In recent times, trauma surgeons treat nearly 60% of children with massive liver injuries (grade 4 or higher) without operative intervention [64, 96].

When an operative intervention is required, current thinking suggests that the liver should be packed and the abdomen closed temporarily (Fig. 19.3) [97]. In the interim period, hypothermia, hypovolemia, and coagulopathy must be corrected, and other injuries must be addressed pending patient stability. After a stabilization period of 24–48 h, patients return to the operating room for packing removal and other maneuvers to control the hemorrhage if necessary. At this time, a major liver resection may be undertaken. Some patients may require multiple trips to the operating room for debridement of necrotic portions of the liver. Complications of management include bleeding, abscess formation, bile leak, and, rarely, hemobilia [95]. If injured children are hemodynamically stable and do not have peritoneal signs, nonoperative treatment can continue at the end of the stabilization period. Even with nonoperative treatment, patients may require bile drainage, bile duct stenting, or arterial embolization for bleeding. Two large studies showed that 90–93% of children can be successfully treated nonoperatively, with an associated mortality rate of 1–5% [96, 98]. Landau and coworkers showed that transfusion requirements and hospital stay were less in the nonoperative group than in the operative group [96]. Most of the deaths in these series were due to associated head injury rather than to the hepatic injury. Reported complications of nonoperative treatment are similar to post-surgical complications such as biloma, abscess, and hepatic artery pseudo-aneurysm with hemobilia [98]. Guidelines for hospital stay and resuming regular activity are the same as for splenic injuries. ICU admission

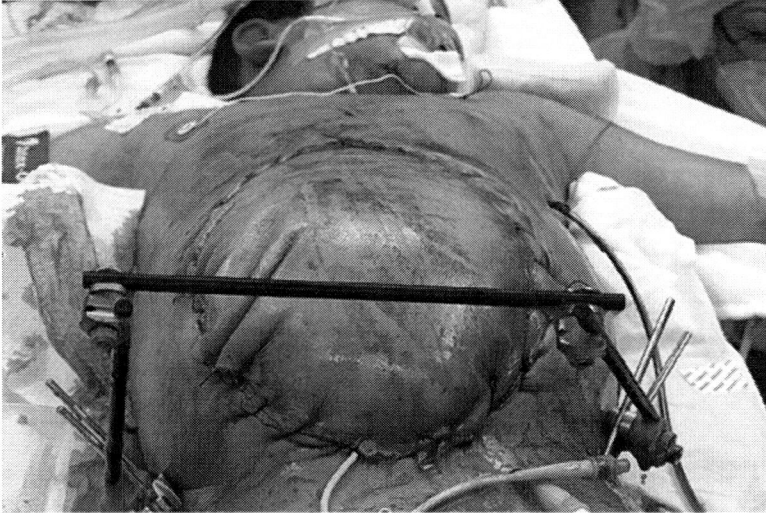

Fig. 19.3 Due to massive intraabdominal injuries and need for aggressive resuscitation, delayed abdominal closure was performed in this child

should be entertained for all grade V injuries; hospital stay should be CT grade plus 1 day, and patients may return to full activity status at CT grade plus 2 weeks [85]. In addition, follow-up CT scan in asymptomatic children is not recommended as it does not affect patient management [82, 85].

19.4.18 Kidney

Injury to the kidney is most commonly caused by blunt trauma and accounts for 10–20% of blunt intra-abdominal injuries in children [99]. Mortality associated with isolated kidney injuries is extremely low [64]. Physicians should bear in mind that young children may have preexisting tumors or hydronephrosis, which may be incidentally discovered as a result of hematuria following mild injury. Anatomic differences, such as the lack of perirenal fat, larger size of kidney relative to rest of the body, and weaker abdominal wall musculature, predispose children to renal injuries [99, 100]. Signs and symptoms in children may include flank or abdominal pain and gross hematuria. However, it should be noted that gross hematuria may be absent, even with severe renal injuries. Hemodynamically stable children who are symptomatic should be worked-up with a CT scan. If children are asymptomatic, a CT scan should be ordered if the urine analysis shows >50 red blood cells per high powered field for blunt trauma, or >5 red blood cells for penetrating trauma [99, 101]. Children who are unstable require urgent operative exploration.

CT staging should be determined for both penetrating and blunt trauma [80, 102]. American Association for the Surgery of Trauma (AAST) organ injury severity score for kidney injuries has been validated to predict management in adult and pediatric patients [80, 102]. Most of the blunt injuries in children are mild (grade I-III) and are almost always successfully managed nonoperatively. Children with grade I-III injuries should be admitted, placed on bed rest, and observed for at least 24 h. Recurrent bleeding and hemodynamic instability are most common in the first 24–48 h. After the resolution of hematuria, children can be discharged home. Follow-up imaging is not recommended for grade I or II injuries, and, if grade III injury was not associated with hemodynamic instability, complications are usually rare [101]. Activity restrictions can be discontinued after the resolution of microscopic hematuria [100].

Severe renal injuries (grade IV-V) are often associated with head injury [99]. Children with such injuries must be admitted to the intensive care unit and kept on strict bed rest. If these patients cannot be stabilized and continue to require blood products, surgical exploration is required. Selective nonoperative treatment of blunt grade IV and V renal injuries is possible, but this may require the use of angiography to embolize bleeding segmental renal arteries [99]. Urinary extravasation can also be treated by placement of uretheral stents or percutaneous drains [99]. Low-grade fevers and a mild ileus can be seen secondary to the retroperitoneal hematoma. Bed rest and urinary drainage with a foley catheter should be continued until the resolution of gross hematuria. Delayed bleeding is more common with severe injuries. Follow-up imaging is only recommended for grade IV and V injuries [101].

19.4.19 Gastrointestinal Injuries

Gastrointestinal injuries are the fourth most common injury following blunt trauma in children [23]. Small intestinal injuries are most common followed by injuries to the duodenum, colon, and stomach [103]. Diagnosing intestinal injury poses a special challenge to both adult and pediatric surgeons. Signs and symptoms related to intestinal injury may be minimal initially. This is further confounded by the fact that CT scan of the abdomen is not reliable in diagnosing intestinal injuries. Perforations as a result of blunt trauma may take several days to manifest, with no evidence of injury on initial physical exam [104]. Tso and colleagues showed that delay in diagnosis can be seen in 10% of children with abdominal injuries [104]. Children suspected of having intestinal injuries should be serially examined, and, if they develop peritoneal signs, they should be taken to the operating room. Focal perforations are most common and can be repaired primarily. Streck and colleagues recently reported their successful series of laparoscopic repair of traumatic bowel injuries in 14 children [105].

The lap portion of the seatbelt is designed to rest at the level of the pelvis in adults. The tightening of the seatbelt against the pelvis protects abdominal organs from compression due to sudden deceleration. However, the lap portion of the seatbelt in children will often ride near the level of the umbilicus. As a result, intestinal blowout can occur from compression of the intestine against the lumbar spine [106]. This mechanism can also cause fractures of the lumbar spine, known as "Chance fractures." Campbell and colleagues showed that up to 46% of children with seatbelt contusion required laparotomy [107]. Seatbelt contusions are also associated with bladder injuries, mesenteric disruptions, and duodenal perforation [75]. Booster seats are available to prevent this type of injury. According to a recent study, toddlers in child seats had 81.8% lower odds of injury than belted toddlers [108].

Child abuse is the second most common blunt mechanism leading to small intestinal perforation [103]. These children can present late, as the person who inflicted the injury will most likely not seek medical care. When the mechanism is not clear, physicians should suspect child abuse and obtain additional work-up. One must be particularly suspicious of parents who give the explanation that their child fell down the stairs. This may seem like a plausible story, as falls from stairs are actually a common mechanism for injury during childhood. Nevertheless, Huntimer and coworkers found no evidence of intestinal perforation after reviewing 677 cases of falls on stairs [109]. Moreover, a sudden blow to the epigastrium can cause duodenal perforation and/or pancreatic injury. Consistent with that hypothesis, Gaines and colleagues showed nonaccidental trauma to be a common cause of duodenal injury in children who are 4 years old or younger [110].

Pancreatic and duodenal injuries are most commonly caused by handle-bar injuries in children [75]. Duodenal injuries are only seen in 3% of all gastrointestinal injuries and in 4% of pancreatic injuries [27]. The diagnosis of both may be made with the use an abdominal CT scan with oral and intravenous contrast [110, 111]. Duodenal injuries include either a wall hematoma or perforation. A duodenal hematoma will cause upper gastrointestinal obstruction and commonly spontaneously resolves after a period of bowel rest, nasogastric decompression, and parenteral nutrition. If duodenal hematoma is encountered as a part of an exploratory laparotomy, the clot within the duodenal wall should be evacuated. Duodenal perforations may lead to retroperitoneal or intraperitoneal air and/or contrast leak. The repair of duodenal injuries depends on the position of the injury. These repairs have a risk of anastomotic dehiscence and fistula formation. The techniques that may be employed include observation, primary serosal patch repair, duodenal diverticularization, pyloric exclusion with gastrojejunostomy, and duoudenostomy tube. Although it was a small series, Ladd and colleagues showed that pyloric exclusion was associated with decreased morbidity in contrast to other methods [112]. If duodenal injuries are accompanied with severe pancreatic injuries, a Whipple procedure may be needed.

Trauma is amongst the top causes of pancreatitis in children [111]. Handle-bar injuries may lead to transection of the pancreas at its mid-section. If this injury is suspected, serum amylase and lipase should be checked. Pancreatic ductal injury is likely if serum amylase is greater than 200 and serum lipase greater than 1,800 [69]. CT imaging is a good initial study, but for accurate diagnosis of ductal injury magnetic resonance cholangiopancre (MRCP) may also be utilized. Ultimately, endoscopic retrograde cholangiopancreatography (ERCP) may be needed to determine the extent of the ductal injury and need for operative intervention. Spleen sparing distal pancreatectomy is a good option in children whose injuries are identified early [111]. Nonoperative treatment is also a feasible option for mild to moderate pancreatic injuries. Pseudocyst formation, however, is a complication of nonoperative treatment, and these may require a drainage procedure if they persist or become symptomatic [75].

19.5   Summary and Conclusion

Injury is the leading cause of death for children aged 1–14. Blunt trauma is responsible for the majority of these injuries. Clinicians must be aware of the anatomic and physiological differences between children and adults as well as differences in injury patterns between these groups. When the mechanism does not fit the injury, nonaccidental trauma must be suspected, and work-up should be extended to look for evidence of prior injuries. Other than size and volume issues, there are no differences in the initial approach to resuscitation of adults and children. Patience and caution are required as children often regress in maturity level as a result of injury, and they may require multiple exams to determine the true extent of their injuries. TBI is the foremost cause of morbidity and mortality in children. Practitioners must also bear in mind the higher incidence of spinal cord injuries without radiological abnormalities. The spleen is the most commonly injured solid organ as a result of blunt trauma in children. Most of these injuries, as well as liver and kidney injuries, can be managed nonoperatively, with minimal need for blood transfusions. Overall, pediatric trauma is a preventable health problem.

References

1. American College of Surgeons. National Trauma Data Bank Pediatric Report. 2005:1–21
2. Dowd MD, Keenan HT, Bratton SL. Epidemiology and prevention of childhood injuries. Crit Care Med 2002;30(11 Suppl):S385–S392
3. Krug EG, Sharma GK, Lozano R. The global burden of injuries. Am J Public Health 2000;90(4):523–526
4. Hambidge SJ, Davidson AJ, Gonzales R, Steiner JF. Epidemiology of pediatric injury-related primary care office visits in the United States. Pediatrics 2002;109(4):559–565
5. DeRoss AL, Vane DW. Early evaluation and resuscitation of the pediatric trauma patient. Semin Pediatr Surg 2004;13(2):74–79
6. Cole F. Pediatric formulas for the anesthesiologist. AMA 1957;94(6):672–673
7. Langlois JA, Rutland-Brown W, Thomas KE. The incidence of traumatic brain injury among children in the United States: Differences by race. J Head Trauma Rehabil 2005;20(3):229–238
8. Keenan HT, Bratton SL. Epidemiology and outcomes of pediatric traumatic brain injury. Dev Neurosci 2006;28(4–5):256–263
9. Listman DA, Bechtel K. Accidental and abusive head injury in young children. Curr Opin Pediatr 2003;15(3):299–303

10. Khoshyomn S, Tranmer BI. Diagnosis and management of pediatric closed head injury. Semin Pediatr Surg 2004;13(2):80–86

11. Young KD, Okada PJ, Sokolove PE, Palchak MJ, Panacek EA, Baren JM, Huff KR, McBride DQ, Inkelis SH, Lewis RJ. A randomized, double-blinded, placebo-controlled trial of phenytoin for the prevention of early posttraumatic seizures in children with moderate to severe blunt head injury. Ann Emerg Med 2004;43(4):435–446

12. Muhonen MG, Piper JG, Menezes AH. Pathogenesis and treatment of growing skull fractures. Surg Neurol 1995;43(4):367–372; discussion 72–73

13. Mittl RL, Grossman RI, Hiehle JF, Hurst RW, Kauder DR, Gennarelli TA, Alburger GW. Prevalence of MR evidence of diffuse axonal injury in patients with mild head injury and normal head CT findings. Am J Neuroradiol 1994;15(8):1583–1589

14. Smith DH, Meaney DF, Shull WH. Diffuse axonal injury in head trauma. J Head Trauma Rehabil 2003;18(4):307–316

15. Macdonald RL, Hoffman HJ, Kestle JR, Rutka JT, Weinstein G. Needle aspiration of acute subdural hematomas in infancy. Pediatr Neurosurg 1994;20(1):73–76; discussion 7

16. Platzer P, Jaindl M, Thalhammer G, Dittrich S, Kutscha-Lissberg F, Vecsei V, Gaebler C. Cervical spine injuries in pediatric patients. J Trauma 2007;62(2):389–396; discussion 94–96

17. Lee SL, Sena M, Greenholz SK, Fledderman M. A multidisciplinary approach to the development of a cervical spine clearance protocol: Process, rationale, and initial results. J Pediatr Surg 2003;38(3):358–362; discussion -62

18. Rice HE, Frush DP, Farmer D, Waldhausen JH. Review of radiation risks from computed tomography: Essentials for the pediatric surgeon. J Pediatr Surg 2007;42(4):603–607

19. Anderson RC, Scaife ER, Fenton SJ, Kan P, Hansen KW, Brockmeyer DL. Cervical spine clearance after trauma in children. J Neurosurg 2006;105(5 Suppl):361–364

20. Mauldin JM, Maxwell RA, King SM, Phlegar RF, Gallagher MR, Barker DE, Burns RP. Prospective evaluation of a critical care pathway for clearance of the cervical spine using the bolster and active range-of-motion flexion/extension techniques. J Trauma 2006;61(3):679–685

21. Viccellio P, Simon H, Pressman BD, Shah MN, Mower WR, Hoffman JR. A prospective multicenter study of cervical spine injury in children. Pediatrics 2001;108(2):E20

22. Bracken MB, Shepard MJ, Collins WF, Holford TR, Young W, Baskin DS, Eisenberg HM, Flamm E, Leo-Summers L, Maroon J, Marshall LF, Perot PL Jr, Piepmeier J, Sonntag VKH, Wagner FC, Wilberger JE, Winn HR. A randomized, controlled trial of methylprednisolone or naloxone in the treatment of acute spinal-cord injury. Results of the Second National Acute Spinal Cord Injury Study. N Engl J Med 1990;322(20):1405–1411

23. Cooper A. Thoracic injuries. Semin Pediatr Surg 1995;4(2):109–115

24. Nakayama DK, Ramenofsky ML, Rowe MI. Chest injuries in childhood. Ann Surg 1989;210(6):770–775

25. Sartorelli KH, Vane DW. The diagnosis and management of children with blunt injury of the chest. Semin Pediatr Surg 2004;13(2):98–105

26. Black TL, Snyder CL, Miller JP, Mann CM, Jr., Copetas AC, Ellis DG. Significance of chest trauma in children. South Med J 1996;89(5):494–496

27. Cooper A, Barlow B, DiScala C, String D. Mortality and truncal injury: The pediatric perspective. J Pediatr Surg 1994;29(1):33–38

28. Bliss D, Silen M. Pediatric thoracic trauma. Crit Care Med 2002;30(11 Suppl):S409–S415

29. Peclet MH, Newman KD, Eichelberger MR, Gotschall CS, Garcia VF, Bowman LM. Thoracic trauma in children: An indicator of increased mortality. J Pediatr Surg 1990;25(9):961–965; discussion 5–6

30. DiRusso SM, Sullivan T, Risucci D, Nealon P, Slim M. Intubation of pediatric trauma patients in the field: Predictor of negative outcome despite risk stratification. J Trauma 2005;59(1):84–90; discussion -1

31. Beaver BL, Colombani PM, Buck JR, Dudgeon DL, Bohrer SL, Haller JA, Jr. Efficacy of emergency room thoracotomy in pediatric trauma. J Pediatr Surg 1987;22(1):19–23

32. Sheikh AA, Culbertson CB. Emergency department thoracotomy in children: Rationale for selective application. J Trauma 1993;34(3):323–328
33. Lofland GK. Thoracic trauma in children. Philadelphia: WB Saunders Company; 2000
34. Green NE, Swiontkowski MF. Skeletal trauma in children, 3rd edn. Philadelphia: WB Saunders, 2003
35. Garcia VF, Gotschall CS, Eichelberger MR, Bowman LM. Rib fractures in children: A marker of severe trauma. J Trauma 1990;30(6):695–700
36. Grabb PA, Pang D. Magnetic resonance imaging in the evaluation of spinal cord injury without radiographic abnormality in children. Neurosurgery 1994;35(3):406–414; discussion 14
37. Pang D, Pollack IF. Spinal cord injury without radiographic abnormality in children – the SCIWORA syndrome. J Trauma 1989;29(5):654–664
38. Sartorelli KH, Rogers FB, Osler TM, Shackford SR, Cohen M, Vane DW. Financial aspects of providing trauma care at the extremes of life. J Trauma 1999;46(3):483–487
39. Allen GS, Cox CS, Jr. Pulmonary contusion in children: Diagnosis and management. South Med J 1998;91(12):1099–1106
40. Allen GS, Cox CS, Jr., Moore FA, Duke JH, Andrassy RJ. Pulmonary contusion: Are children different? J Am Coll Surg 1997;185(3):229–233
41. Fortenberry JD, Meier AH, Pettignano R, Heard M, Chambliss CR, Wulkan M. Extracorporeal life support for posttraumatic acute respiratory distress syndrome at a children's medical center. J Pediatr Surg 2003;38(8):1221–1226
42. Roux P, Fisher RM. Chest injuries in children: An analysis of 100 cases of blunt chest trauma from motor vehicle accidents. J Pediatr Surg 1992;27(5):551–555
43. Ball CG, Hameed SM, Evans D, Kortbeek JB, Kirkpatrick AW. Occult pneumothorax in the mechanically ventilated trauma patient. Can J Surg 2003;46(5):373–379
44. Enderson BL, Abdalla R, Frame SB, Casey MT, Gould H, Maull KI. Tube thoracostomy for occult pneumothorax: A prospective randomized study of its use. J Trauma 1993;35(5):726–729; discussion 9–30
45. Heniford BT, Carrillo EH, Spain DA, Sosa JL, Fulton RL, Richardson JD. The role of thoracoscopy in the management of retained thoracic collections after trauma. Ann Thorac Surg 1997;63(4):940–943
46. Tiao GM, Griffith PM, Szmuszkovicz JR, Mahour GH. Cardiac and great vessel injuries in children after blunt trauma: An institutional review. J Pediatr Surg 2000;35(11):1656–1660
47. Langer JC, Winthrop AL, Wesson DE, Spence L, Pearl RH, Hoffman MA, Loeff D, Price D, Wong A, Gilday D, Benson L, Filler RM. Diagnosis and incidence of cardiac injury in children with blunt thoracic trauma. J Pediatr Surg 1989;24(10):1091–1094
48. Dowd MD, Krug S. Pediatric blunt cardiac injury: Epidemiology, clinical features, and diagnosis. Pediatric Emergency Medicine Collaborative Research Committee: Working Group on Blunt Cardiac Injury. J Trauma 1996;40(1):61–67
49. Estes NA, III. Sudden death in young athletes. N Engl J Med 1995;333(6):380–381
50. Trachiotis GD, Sell JE, Pearson GD, Martin GR, Midgley FM. Traumatic thoracic aortic rupture in the pediatric patient. Ann Thorac Surg 1996;62(3):724–731; discussion 31–32
51. Harris GJ, Soper RT. Pediatric first rib fractures. J Trauma 1990;30(3):343–345
52. Dyer DS, Moore EE, Mestek MF, Dyer DS, Moore EE, Mestek MF, Bernstein SM, Iklé DN, Durham JD, Heinig MJ, Russ PD, Symonds DL, Kumpe DA, Roe EJ, Honigman B, McIntyre RC Jr, Eule J Jr. Can chest CT be used to exclude aortic injury? Radiology 1999;213(1):195–202
53. Spouge AR, Burrows PE, Armstrong D, Daneman A. Traumatic aortic rupture in the pediatric population. Role of plain film, CT and angiography in the diagnosis. Pediatr Radiol 1991;21(5):324–328
54. Bruckner BA, DiBardino DJ, Cumbie TC, Trinh C, Blackmon SH, Fisher RG, Mattox KL, Wall MJ, Michael E. Critical evaluation of chest computed tomography scans for blunt descending thoracic aortic injury. Ann Thorac Surg 2006;81(4):1339–1346
55. Karmy-Jones R, Hoffer E, Meissner M, Bloch RD. Management of traumatic rupture of the thoracic aorta in pediatric patients. Ann Thorac Surg 2003;75(5):1513–1517

56. Lowe LH, Bulas DI, Eichelberger MD, Martin GR. Traumatic aortic injuries in children: Radiologic evaluation. AJR 1998;170(1):39–42
57. Saad NE, Pegoli W, Alfieris G, Waldman DL, Davies MG. Endovascular repair of a traumatic aortic transection in a pediatric patient. J Vasc Interv Radiol 2007;18(3):443–446
58. Murala JS, Numa A, Grant P. Traumatic rupture of the aorta in children – stenting or surgical intervention? A word of caution. J Thorac Cardiovasc Surg 2006;132(3):731–732; author reply 2
59. Ramos CT, Koplewitz BZ, Babyn PS, Manson PS, Ein SH. What have we learned about traumatic diaphragmatic hernias in children? J Pediatr Surg 2000;35(4):601–604
60. Karnak I, Senocak ME, Tanyel FC, Buyukpamukcu N. Diaphragmatic injuries in childhood. Surg Today 2001;31(1):5–11
61. Sharma AK, Kothari SK, Gupta C, Menon P, Sharma A. Rupture of the right hemidiaphragm due to blunt trauma in children: A diagnostic dilemma. Pediatr Surg Int 2002;18(2–3):173–174
62. Brandt ML, Luks FI, Spigland NA, DiLorenzo M, Laberge JM, Ouimet A. Diaphragmatic injury in children. J Trauma 1992;32(3):298–301
63. Friese RS, Coln CE, Gentilello LM. Laparoscopy is sufficient to exclude occult diaphragm injury after penetrating abdominal trauma. J Trauma 2005;58(4):789–792
64. Nakayama DK. Abdominal and genitourinary trauma. In: O'Neill JA (ed.) Principles of pediatric surgery. 2nd edn. St Louis, MO: Mosby, 2003:159–176
65. Kristinsson G, Wall SP, Crain EF. The digital rectal examination in pediatric trauma: A pilot study. J Emerg Med 2007;32(1):59–62
66. Porter JM, Ursic CM. Digital rectal examination for trauma: Does every patient need one? Am Surg 2001;67(5):438–441
67. Esposito TJ, Ingraham A, Luchette FA, Sears BW, Santaniello JM, Davis KA, Poulakidas SJ, Gamelli RL. Reasons to omit digital rectal exam in trauma patients: No fingers, no rectum, no useful additional information. J Trauma 2005;59(6):1314–1319
68. Puranik SR, Hayes JS, Long J, Mata M. Liver enzymes as predictors of liver damage due to blunt abdominal trauma in children. South Med J 2002;95(2):203–206
69. Nadler EP, Gardner M, Schall LC, Lynch JM, Ford HR. Management of blunt pancreatic injury in children. J Trauma 1999;47(6):1098–1103
70. Isaacman DJ, Scarfone RJ, Kost SI, Gochman RF, Davis HW, Bernardo LM, Nakayama DK. Utility of routine laboratory testing for detecting intra-abdominal injury in the pediatric trauma patient. Pediatrics 1993;92(5):691–694
71. Holmes JF, Sokolove PE, Brant WE, Palchak MJ, Vance CW, Owings JT, Kuppermann N. Identification of children with intra-abdominal injuries after blunt trauma. Ann Emerg Med 2002;39(5):500–509
72. Patel JC, Tepas JJ, III. The efficacy of focused abdominal sonography for trauma (FAST) as a screening tool in the assessment of injured children. J Pediatr Surg 1999;34(1):44–47; discussion 52–54
73. Soudack M, Epelman M, Maor R, Hayari L, Shoshani G, Heyman-Reiss A, Michaelson M, Gaitini D. Experience with focused abdominal sonography for trauma (FAST) in 313 pediatric patients. J Clin Ultrasound 2004;32(2):53–61
74. Benya EC, Lim-Dunham JE, Landrum O, Statter M. Abdominal sonography in examination of children with blunt abdominal trauma. AJR 2000;174(6):1613–1616
75. Gaines BA, Ford HR. Abdominal and pelvic trauma in children. Crit Care Med 2002;30(11 Suppl):S416–S423
76. Feliz A, Shultz B, McKenna C, Gaines BA. Diagnostic and therapeutic laparoscopy in pediatric abdominal trauma. J Pediatr Surg 2006;41(1):72–77
77. Keller MS, Vane DW. Management of pediatric blunt splenic injury: Comparison of pediatric and adult trauma surgeons. J Pediatr Surg 1995;30(2):221–224; discussion 4–5
78. Peitzman AB, Ford HR, Harbrecht BG, Potoka DA, Townsend RN. Injury to the spleen. Curr Probl Surg 2001;38(12):932–1008

79. Hackam DJ, Potoka D, Meza M, Pollock A, Gardner M, Abrams P, Upperman J, Schall L, Ford H. Utility of radiographic hepatic injury grade in predicting outcome for children after blunt abdominal trauma. J Pediatr Surg 2002;37(3):386–389

80. Santucci RA, McAninch JW, Safir M, Mario LA, Service S, Segal MR. Validation of the American Association for the Surgery of Trauma organ injury severity scale for the kidney. J Trauma 2001;50(2):195–200

81. Gandhi RR, Keller MS, Schwab CW, Stafford PW. Pediatric splenic injury: Pathway to play? J Pediatr Surg 1999;34(1):55–58; discussion 8–9

82. Mooney DP. Multiple trauma: Liver and spleen injury. Curr Opin Pediatr 2002;14(4):482–485

83. Partrick DA, Bensard DD, Moore EE, Karrer FM. Nonoperative management of solid organ injuries in children results in decreased blood utilization. J Pediatr Surg 1999;34(11):1695–1699

84. Bond SJ, Eichelberger MR, Gotschall CS, Sivit CJ, Randolph JG. Nonoperative management of blunt hepatic and splenic injury in children. Ann Surg 1996;223(3):286–289

85. Stylianos S. Evidence-based guidelines for resource utilization in children with isolated spleen or liver injury. The APSA Trauma Committee. J Pediatr Surg 2000;35(2):164–167; discussion 7–9

86. Pearl RH, Wesson DE, Spence LJ, Filler RM, Ein SH. Shandling B, Superina RA. Splenic injury: A 5-year update with improved results and changing criteria for conservative management. J Pediatr Surg 1989;24(5):428–431

87. Bisharat N, Omari H, Lavi I, Raz R. Risk of infection and death among post-splenectomy patients. J Infect 2001;43(3):182–186

88. Shatz DV, Schinsky MF, Pais LB, Romero-Steiner S, Kirton OC, Carlone GM. Immune responses of splenectomized trauma patients to the 23-valent pneumococcal polysaccharide vaccine at 1 versus 7 versus 14 days after splenectomy. J Trauma 1998;44(5):760–765; discussion 5–6

89. Shatz DV, Romero-Steiner S, Elie CM, Holder PF, Carlone GM. Antibody responses in post-splenectomy trauma patients receiving the 23-valent pneumococcal polysaccharide vaccine at 14 versus 28 days postoperatively. J Trauma 2002;53(6):1037–1042

90. Melles DC, de Marie S. Prevention of infections in hyposplenic and asplenic patients: An update. Neth J Med 2004;62(2):45–52

91. Landgren O, Bjorkholm M, Konradsen HB, Söderqvist M, Nilsson B, Gustavsson A, Axdorph U, Kalin M, Grimfors G A. A prospective study on antibody response to repeated vaccinations with pneumococcal capsular polysaccharide in splenectomized individuals with special reference to Hodgkin's lymphoma. J Intern Med 2004;255(6):664–673

92. Lortan JE. Management of asplenic patients. Br J Haematol 1993;84(4):566–569

93. Uroz Tristan J, Poenaru D, Martinez Lagares F, Leclerc S, Sanchis Solera L. Selective splenic artery embolization or use of polyglycolic acid mesh in children with severe splenic trauma. Eur J Pediatr Surg 1995;5(5):310–312

94. Huscher CG, Mingoli A, Sgarzini G, Brachini G, Ponzano C, Paola MD, Modini C. Laparoscopic treatment of blunt splenic injuries: Initial experience with 11 patients. Surg Endosc 2006;20(9):1423–1426

95. Blaisdell WM. Liver resection. In: Madding GD, Kennedy PA (eds) Trauma to the liver: Philadelphia: WB Saunders Company, 1971:131–145

96. Landau A, van As AB, Numanoglu A, Millar AJ, Rode H. Liver injuries in children: The role of selective non-operative management. Injury 2006;37(1):66–71

97. Morris JA, Jr., Eddy VA, Rutherford EJ. The trauma celiotomy: The evolving concepts of damage control. Curr Probl Surg 1996;33(8):611–700

98. Giss SR, Dobrilovic N, Brown RL, Garcia VF. Complications of nonoperative management of pediatric blunt hepatic injury: Diagnosis, management, and outcomes. J Trauma 2006;61(2):334–339

99. Buckley JC, McAninch JW. The diagnosis, management, and outcomes of pediatric renal injuries. Urol Clin North Am 2006;33(1):33–40, vi

100. Snyder CM. Abdominal and genitourinary trauma. In: Ashcraft KW (ed) Pediatric surgery. Philadelphia: WB Saunders Company, 2000:204–216

101. Santucci RA, Wessells H, Bartsch G, Descotes J, Heyns CF, McAninch JW, Nash P, Schmidlin F. Evaluation and management of renal injuries: Consensus statement of the renal trauma subcommittee. BJU Int 2004;93(7):937–954

102. Moore EE, Shackford SR, Pachter HL, McAninch JW, Browner BD, Champion HR, Flint LM, Gennarelli TA, Malangoni MA, Ramenofsky ML, Trafton PG. Organ injury scaling: Spleen, liver, and kidney. J Trauma 1989;29(12):1664–1666

103. Canty TG, Sr., Canty TG, Jr., Brown C. Injuries of the gastrointestinal tract from blunt trauma in children: A 12-year experience at a designated pediatric trauma center. J Trauma 1999;46(2):234–240

104. Tso EL, Beaver BL, Haller JA, Jr. Abdominal injuries in restrained pediatric passengers. J Pediatr Surg 1993;28(7):915–919

105. Streck CJ, Lobe TE, Pietsch JB, Lovvorn HN, III. Laparoscopic repair of traumatic bowel injury in children. J Pediatr Surg 2006;41(11):1864–1869

106. Reid AB, Letts RM, Black GB. Pediatric chance fractures: Association with intra-abdominal injuries and seatbelt use. J Trauma 1990;30(4):384–391

107. Campbell DJ, Sprouse LR II, Smith LA, Kelley JE, Carr MG. Injuries in pediatric patients with seatbelt contusions. Am Surg 2003;69(12):1095–1099

108. Zaloshnja E, Miller TR, Hendrie D. Effectiveness of child safety seats vs safety belts for children aged 2 to 3 years. Arch Pediatr Adolesc Med 2007;161(1):65–68

109. Huntimer CM, Muret-Wagstaff S, Leland NL. Can falls on stairs result in small intestine perforations? Pediatrics 2000;106(2 Pt 1):301–305

110. Gaines BA, Shultz BS, Morrison K, Ford HR. Duodenal injuries in children: Beware of child abuse. J Pediatr Surg 2004;39(4):600–602

111. Stringer MD. Pancreatitis and pancreatic trauma. Semin Pediatr Surg 2005;14(4):239–246

112. Ladd AP, West KW, Rouse TM, Scherer LR III, Rescorla FJ, Engum SA, Grosfeld JL Surgical management of duodenal injuries in children. Surgery 2002;132(4):748–752; discussion 51–53

Chapter 20
Damage Control in Elderly Polytrauma Patients

Robert V. Cantu and Kenneth J. Koval

20.1 Decision-Making Factors

The elderly represent a unique group of trauma patients. How one defines the elderly is an important question. An active, healthy 65-year-old person may be physiologically more fit and better able to tolerate a high energy trauma than a 40-year-old person with multiple medical comorbidities and a sedentary lifestyle. On the other hand, a 75-year-old with a history of myocardial infarction, renal failure, and chronic obstructive pulmonary disease may not be able to tolerate even a slip-and-fall-type injury. Most studies of trauma in the elderly have used an age of at least 65 years in their definition.

Damage control surgery has been well established both in general surgery and in orthopedic literature. Little attention, however, has been focused on how damage control applies to the elderly patient. The principles of damage control are relatively simple. Once a person has sustained a trauma, the forces producing that injury cannot be changed, but the approach to treating that person is aimed at stabilizing the injuries while minimizing further physiologic insult. To perform damage control properly, one must understand both the benefit and the potential downside of any planned intervention. The concept of damage control typically applies to patients who have multiple injuries, the so- called "polytrauma" patients. These patients typically have an injury severity score (ISS) of at least 17.

20.2 Rationale

Mortality in trauma patients can be divided into three broad categories on the basis of timing. Immediate mortality is often due to overwhelming injury to the head or chest, or exsanguination from major arterial bleeding. Early mortality, defined as

R.V. Cantu (✉)
Department of Orthopedics, Dartmouth Hitchcock Medical Center, One Medical Center Drive, Lebanon, NH, 03756, USA
e-mail: Robert.V.Cantu@Hitchcock.org

H.-C. Pape et al. (eds.), *Damage Control Management in the Polytrauma Patient*,   357
DOI 10.1007/978-0-387-89508-6_20, © Springer Science+Business Media, LLC 2010

occurring within the first 24 h after injury, is most often due to inability to reverse ongoing hemorrhage. Late mortality, defined as occurring more than 24–48 h after injury, is typically caused by the development of Acute Respiratory Distress Syndrome (ARDS), Multiple System Organ Failure (MODS), or sepsis.

Major traumatic injury can lead to the Systemic Inflammatory Response Syndrome (SIRS), which is characterized by tachycardia, increased oxygen requirements, fever, and increased inflammatory markers such as inter-leukin 6 (IL-6) [1]. The duration of this inflammatory response is variable, but typically it is most apparent from 2 to 5 days post-injury. If the inflammatory response is severe enough, or if another insult during this period worsens the response, MODS and death can result. Following this inflammatory period, a time of relative decrease in immunonologic response has been described and given the name of Counter-Regulatory Anti-Inflammatory Response (CARS) [2]. During this anti-inflammatory state, the patient may be immunocompromised and at high risk of systemic sepsis and death.

20.3 Damage Control and the Elderly

Despite the increased emphasis by many experts on damage control orthopedics (DCO), little has been published regarding how the concept relates to the elderly. In general, elderly patients have less physiologic reserve and decreased ability to tolerate the ill effects of trauma. The limits of shock, acidosis, coagulopathy, hypoxia, inflammation, and hypothermia that the elderly can tolerate and still survive can be substantially lower than in younger adults. Although there are few studies looking at orthopedic damage control specifically in the elderly, it would make sense that the concepts would apply to them equally, perhaps even more, when compared to the younger trauma population.

20.3.1 Strategies and Recommendations

The initial approach to the elderly trauma patient is similar to that for any trauma victim. The ABCs of Advanced Trauma Life Support (ATLS®)[1] teaching should be followed. In the trauma bay, identified fractures should be splinted. Open fractures should be covered with saline soaked sterile gauze and splinted. Unstable pelvic fractures should be stabilized with a pelvic binder or an appropriately placed sheet. Femoral shaft fractures should be placed in traction if that has not beenalready done by EMS. Laboratory studies, including an arterial blood gas, can be helpful to identify patients who may be hypovolemic and consequently, acidotic.

---

[1]http://www.facs.org/trauma/atls/index.html.

Bosse has described three main factors that determine the clinical course of a polytrauma patient [3]. The first factor is the initial trauma or the "first hit." Nothing can be done to alter this factor for the elderly trauma patient other than prevention. The second factor is the patient's "biologic constitution" [3]. Here, the elderly demonstrate a wide range in their baseline health status. It is imperative to reverse the cascade of negative physiologic events as early as possible in the elderly. The third factor, closely tied to the second, is the timing and quality of any medical intervention. Surgical intervention can be thought of as an additional trauma or "second hit" to the patient. The goal of surgery is to maximize improvement of injuries while minimizing further insult due to blood loss, hypothermia, coagulopathy, etc.

For elderly patients, the ISS may underestimate the degree of injury. Pape and colleagues have reported that the most severely injured trauma patients or those "in extremis" are the ones that benefit most from the DCO approach [4–8]. An elderly patient may present with a lower ISS than a young adult and still be unstable or even in extremis, in the sense that minimal further insult or "second hit" can tip them past the point of recovery. At the same time, if ongoing injuries are not rapidly stabilized, the patient may deteriorate beyond the point at which they can survive. It is this tightrope that the orthopedic trauma surgeon must walk in treating the elderly patient with multiple fractures. In such cases, simple splinting or external fixation of upper extremity fractures and of lower extremity fractures may represent the best initial treatment.

Few studies have focused specifically on the impact of orthopedic injuries in elderly trauma patients [9–11]. One retrospective multicenter study did attempt to define the factors associated with increased morbidity and mortality in elderly patients who had sustained major trauma [9]. Of 326 patients with an average age of 72.2 years, there was an overall mortality rate of 18.1%. Of patients who required bony stabilization, 77% had this accomplished within 24 h of admission. The mortality rate for patients who underwent fracture stabilization within 24 h was 11%, and, for those who were fixed after more than 24 h, it was 18%; but this difference was not statistically significant [9]. The three complications with the highest mortality rates were ARDS (81%), myocardial infarction (62%), and sepsis (39%) (Table 20.1).

Limb salvage is an important topic in the elderly. For the elderly trauma patient with a mangled extremity, early amputation should be considered. Elderly patients may not be able to withstand the multiple surgeries required to salvage severe, open fractures, especially those with vascular insult (Fig. 20.1). If a severely injured limb

Table 20.1 Predictors of mortality in three studies of geriatric trauma

Tornetta et al. [9]	Horst et al. [23]	Zeitlow et al. [11]
ISS predictive ($P=0.008$)	ISS not predictive	Shock on admission predictive
GCS predictive ($P=0.007$)	Trauma score not predictive	GCS predictive
Transfusion requirement predictive ($P=0.01$)	Decreased hemoglobin predictive	Inotropic support predictive
Fluid requirement predictive ($P=0.06$)	Increased oxygen requirement predictive	Ventilatory support predictive

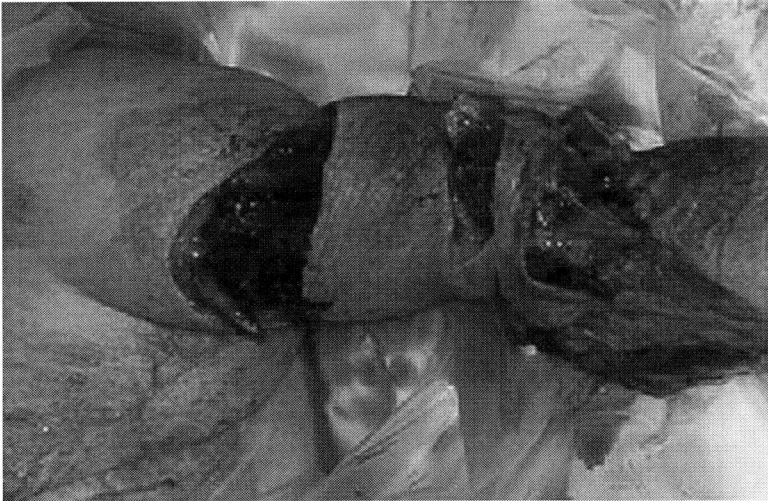

Fig. 20.1 Mangled upper extremity with vascular disruption and gross contamination from manure spreader in elderly polytrauma patient. Treatment was immediate amputation

becomes infected, the cascade of sepsis and MODS can proceed quickly. Although this is often a judgment call, early amputation in the elderly patient can be a life-saving procedure.

20.3.2   Timing of Converting External Fixator to IM Rod

For elderly patients who have undergone initial external fixation of fractures, the timing of conversion to definitive fixation must be considered. The main emphasis here is minimizing the "second hit" of the second operation. A large retrospective by Brundage and colleagues showed that patients who underwent intramedullary nailing of femur fractures during the 2–5-day window after injury had the highest mortality [12]. It is thought that many patients may have the greatest inflammatory response during this time, and therefore a second hit may tip them over the edge to ARDS or MODS. In the example of femoral shaft fractures, Pape and colleagues have shown that inflammatory markers such as IL-6 do increase substantially following reamed, intramedullary nailing [5]. To the authors' knowledge, no one has looked specifically at the elderly to see how their inflammatory response compares or to see if the 2–5-day window remains their most vulnerable time. It is safe to assume that if an elderly patient is within the first few days of a major trauma and is still requiring significant ventilatory support and close fluid management, this may not be the best time to return to the operating room for conversion of the fixator to an intramedullary nail. It may be that the elderly take longer to recover from the initial insult of the trauma and that delaying conversion of fixators to intramedullary nails or plates may best be performed more than 5 or even 7 days after injury. Further studies are needed to help answer this question.

20.4   Benefits and Risks

20.4.1   Pain Control

One impact of DCO in the elderly that should not be underemphasized is pain control. Pain control through provisional stabilization of fractures is an important factor, as minimization of narcotic use can improve respiratory function and mental status. Patients who have adequate pain control can be weaned from ventilators more easily, obtain a more upright posture, and have reduced delirium; these are all critical for survival in the elderly. Selective use of nerve blocks or catheters for continuous infusion, such as a femoral nerve block catheter following a femur fracture, can greatly aid in pain relief and minimize narcotic requirements.

20.4.2   Avoiding Infection

One concern when converting an external fixator to an intramedullary nail in the elderly is the potential for infection. The longer an external fixator has been in place, the higher the risk for infection, theoretically. Nowotarski and colleagues reported on a study of general trauma patients who had undergone initial external fixation of femur fractures followed by intramedullary nailing [13]. The average time to conversion was 7 days. There were 19 open fractures included in the study group. The overall infection rate was only 1.7%, suggesting that conversion of an external fixator to an intramedullary nail within the first 2 weeks is a relatively safe procedure with regard to infection [13]. This question has not been looked at specifically in elderly patients, but one can extrapolate from the previous data that it should be a safe procedure, at least when dealing with a femur fracture.

20.4.3   Controlling Hemorrhage

Management of unstable pelvic fractures in the elderly remains a challenging problem. Pelvic ring disruptions in general result in significant morbidity and mortality. Estimates of mortality for patients with pelvic fractures have ranged from 4.8 to 50% [14–16]. Early fracture stabilization is important to control bleeding from cancellous bone and promote clot formation for venous bleeding. Appropriate application of a pelvic binder or a well-placed sheet in the trauma bay is effective in provisionally stabilizing fractures and helping to control bleeding. Arterial bleeding, although less common than venous and cancellous bleeding, can be a major source of shock in patients with pelvic fractures. The retroperitoneum can hold up to 4 L of blood before the intravascular pressure is overcome by physiologic tamponade [17]. Often, however, the retroperitoneum is torn and disrupted, preventing any tamponade, and bleeding can progress to exsanguination. In such an instance, early angiography and arterial embolization can be a life-preserving measure. Angiography, while not without risk, is a minimally invasive procedure, and, when indicated, it is an important part of DCO. Its use has been shown to control bleeding, preventing the cascade of further coagulation disturbance, systemic inflammatory response, ARDS, multiple organ dysfunction syndrome, and death [18, 19]. If a patient has already been placed in a pelvic binder, it can simply be cut rather than removed, to maintain pelvic stability while allowing access to the femoral vessels for angiography.

For the elderly patient with an unstable pelvic fracture who is brought to the operating room for emergent laparotomy, it is important to maintain the stability of the pelvic fracture. If the patient is already in a pelvic binder, one option is to slide the binder inferiorly over the greater trochanteric region of the hips to allow the general surgeons to have access to the abdomen while still maintaining compression of the pelvic ring. Another option is to place a pelvic external fixator. The fixator can either be placed using 2–3 half-pins in each iliac wing or by placing one half-pin in each supra-acetabular region (Hannover frame) (Fig. 20.2a,b). Ideally, the frame should be placed quickly prior to laparotomy, as the process of opening the abdominal wall has been shown to further decrease stability of the pelvis and reduce intra-abdominal pressure that may be helping to tamponade bleeding in the retroperitoneum [17]. Here again, if a pelvic binder is in place, it can be cut, allowing access to the supra-acetabular region or iliac wing for placement of the external fixator half-pins.

The elderly polytrauma patient with a femoral shaft fracture represents a challenging scenario. Early stabilization of the femur fracture is important in order to limit bleeding, prevent or decrease fat embolism, control pain, and improve nursing care and patient mobility. The method of achieving this stabilization is a matter of controversy. Work by Pape and colleagues has suggested that as part of a damage control approach, patients who are either "unstable" or "in extremis" are best served with rapid external fixation of femur fractures followed later by definitive intramedullary nailing [4–8]. It is the next level down where, perhaps, more controversy exists. Patients with severe, potentially life-threatening injuries who have exhibited transient hemodynamic instability are the group for which it is not clear if initial application of an external fixator provides more benefit than intra-medullary nailing. The one prospective and randomized trial on patients with an ISS > 18 found that patients who underwent intramedullary nailing within 24 h had better results than those whose surgery was delayed [20]. This trial did not include a group with initial external fixation, however.

Recent study has shown that early stabilization of fractures is beneficial in preventing bacterial translocation [21]. Oztuna and colleagues used rat models, comparing one

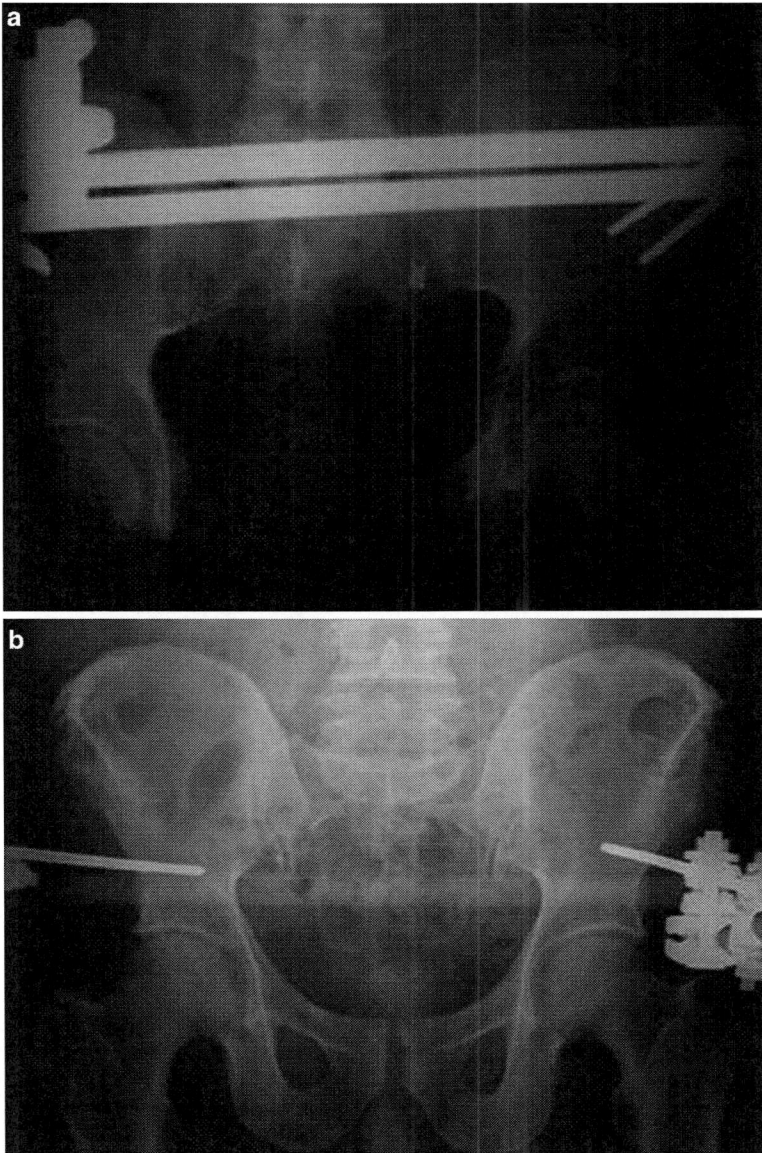

Fig. 20.2 (a) Comparison of iliac wing versus supra-acetabular pin (Hannover frame) (b) placement for pelvic external fixator

group with a "moderate head trauma" and tibia and femur fractures but no surgery to a second group with the same injuries that underwent fixation of the tibia and femur fractures [21]. They found that the "number of organs containing viable bacteria was significantly lower in the fixation group than in the trauma (alone) group" [21]. Assuming this finding has some correlation in humans, it may be particularly important in the elderly who are more prone to late sepsis and pneumonia.

20.5 Summary and Conclusion

The principles of DCO have evolved to treat the increasing numbers of severely injured patients in today's trauma centers. Trauma has increased in the United States to the point where a "paradigm shift" has been described with regard to medical advances in trauma care [22]. Throughout history, war time has led to major advances in fracture care, such as the advent of the Thomas splint in World War I or the Kuntschner rod in World War II. Currently, however, much of the care for American soldiers in Iraq "is being modeled after American urban trauma centers" [22].

Early stabilization of fractures, accomplished with as little insult to the patient as possible, is the hallmark of DCO. Although few studies have focused on the elderly trauma patient, it would make sense that the principles apply equally to them, as well. The elderly patient may not need to be "in extremis" or even "unstable" to benefit from the principles of damage control. Perhaps the concept of minimizing the "second hit" is even more important in the elderly than in the younger trauma patient. How the orthopedic traumatologist accomplishes fracture fixation is still a matter of debate. What seems clear, however, is that the sooner the fixation can be accomplished with the least amount of further insult, the better the outcomes will be.

References

1. Hildebrand F, Pape HC, van Griensven M, Meier S, Hasenkamp S, Krettek C, Stuhrmann M. Genetic predisposition for a compromised immune system after multiple trauma. Shock 2005;24(6):518–22.
2. Moore FA, Moore EE. Evolving concepts in the pathogenesis of post-injury multiple organ failure. Surg Clin North Am 1995;75:257–277.
3. Bosse M J. CAQ: Orthopaedic trauma "Damage Control". J Orthop Trauma 2007;21(1):1–4.
4. Pape H-C, Regel G, Dwenger A, Krumm K, Schweitzer G, Krettek K, Sturm JA, Tscherne H. Influences of different methods of intramedullary femoral nailing on lung function in patients with multiple trauma. J Trauma 1993;35:709–715.
5. Pape H-C, Grimme K, van Griensven M, Sott AH, Giannoudis P, Morley J, Roise O, Ellingsen E, Hildebrand F, Wiese B, Krettek C. Impact of intramedullary instrumentation versus damage control for femoral fractures on immunoinflammatory parameters: prospective randomized analysis by the EPOFF study group. J Trauma 2003;55(1):7–13.
6. Pape H-C, Schmidt RE, Rice J, van Griensven M, das Gupta R, Krettek C, Tscherne H. Biochemical changes following trauma and skeletal injury of the lower extremity: quantification of the operative burden. Crit Care Med 2000;28:3441–3448.
7. Pape HC, Giannoudis PV, Krettek C, Trentz O. Timing of fixation of major fractures in blunt polytrauma: role of conventional indicators in clinical decision making. J Orthop Trauma 2005;19(8):551–562.

8. Pape HC, Auf'm'Kolk M, Paffrath T, Regel G, Sturm JA, Tscheme H. Primary intramedullary femur fixation in multiple trauma patients with associated lung contusion: a cause of posttraumatic ARDS? J Trauma 1993;34:540–548.
9. Tornetta P, Mostafavi H, Riina J, Turen C, Reimer B, Levine R, Behrens F, Geller J, Ritter C, Homel P. Morbidity and mortality in elderly trauma patients. J Trauma 1999;46(4):702–706.
10. Lonner J, Koval K. Polytrauma in the elderly. Clin Orthop 1995;318:136–143.
11. Zeitlow S, Capizzi P, Bannon M. Multisystem geriatric trauma. J Trauma 1994;37:985–988.
12. Brundage SI, McGhan R, Jurkovich G, Mack CD, Maier RV. Timing of femur fracture fixation: effect on outcome in patients with thoracic and head injuries. J Trauma 2002;52(2):299–307.
13. Nowotarski PJ, CH Turen, RJ Brumback, Scarboro JM. Conversion of external fixation to intramedullary nailing for fractures of the shaft of the femur in multiply injured patients. J Bone Joint Surg (Am) 2000;82:781–788.
14. Eastridge BJ, Burgess AR. Pedestrian pelvic fractures: 5 year experience of a major urban trauma center. J Trauma 1997;42:695–700.
15. Flint L. Babikian G, Anders M, Rodriguez J, Steinberg S. Definitive control of mortality from severe pelvic fracture. Ann Surg 1990;211:703–707.
16. Rommens PM. Pelvic ring injuries: a challenge for the trauma surgeon. Acta Chir Belg 1996;96:78–84.
17. Grimm M, Vrahas M, Thomas K. Pressure-volume characteristics of the intact and disrupted pelvic retroperitoneum. J Trauma 1998;44:454–459.
18. Kadish L, Stein J, Kotler S. Angiographic diagnosis and treatment of bleeding due to pelvic trauma. J Trauma 1973;13:1083–1086.
19. Holting T, Buhr H, Richter G, Roeren T, Friedl W, Herfarth C. Diagnosis and treatment of retroperitoneal hematoma in multiple trauma patients. Arch Orthop Trauma Surg 1992;111:323–326.
20. Bone LB, Johnson KD, Weigelt J, Scheinberg R. Early versus delayed stabilization of femoral fractures: a prospective randomized study. J Bone Joint Surg Am 1989;71:336–340.
21. Oztuna V, Ersoz G, Ayan I, Eskandari MM, Colak M, Polat A. Early internal fracture fixation prevents bacterial translocation. Clin Orthop 2006;446:253–258.
22. Brooks J. "Damage control" surgery techniques used on soldiers. CMAJ 2006;175(7):727.
23. Horst H, Obeid F, Sorenson VJ, Bivins BA. Factors influencing survival of elderly trauma patients. Crit Care Med 1986;14:681–684.

Chapter 21
Mass Casualties: Military and Civilian

A Militarry Perspective

Alan D. Murdock and Donald H. Jenkins

21.1   Introduction

Mass casualty events are incidents incurring a large number of casualties and disrupting the normal deployment and operation of the emergency health care services, effectively overwhelming the system to the point that not all patients can receive immediate and complete care. The nature of the incident, its destructive force, and where it takes place determine the severity and diversity of injuries. Additionally, the number of victims will be a major factor in determining whether the mass casualty event overwhelms the local medical and public health services. Trauma centers are uniquely positioned to respond to mass casualty emergencies when compared to general hospitals, based on their resource availability, constant state of readiness, extra capacity, and strong connections with the local and regional emergency care community.

Military field medicine, due to the very nature of combat, is uniquely situated to deal with mass casualty scenarios, in part due to casualty surges during combat and in part due to the often austere circumstances found in deployed military medical treatment facilities and combat support hospitals [1]. Single battles during the civil war regularly produced thousands of casualties for each side in just a few hours. A more recent, infamous example was the bombing of the Marine barracks in Beirut in 1983, which killed or injured hundreds of Marines in an instant [2]. More recent experience includes Operation Phantom Fury in Fallujah, Iraq; during the first day of the assault, a single combat support hospital performed 70 major operations on combat injured casualties, half of whom were operated on first at a Forward Resuscitative Surgical System (FRS). More than 450 such operations were carried out over the next 10 days with a team of 12 surgeons in three operating rooms [3].

A.D. Murdock and D.H. Jenkins (✉)
Wilford Hall USAF Medical Center, Uniformed Services University, (Bethesda, Maryland), 59MDW/MCSG, 2200 Bergquist Drive, Suite 1, Lackland Air Force Base, TX, 78236, USA
e-mail: donald.jenkins@lackland.af.mil

H.-C. Pape et al. (eds.), *Damage Control Management in the Polytrauma Patient*,
DOI 10.1007/978-0-387-89508-6_21, © Springer Science+Business Media, LLC 2010

Although many of the characteristics of preparedness are in place in civilian trauma centers, many areas need improvement. In a recent survey sent to all designated or verified level I and level II trauma centers in the USA (33% or 175 trauma centers replied), only seven trauma centers scored 89% or better for mass casualty preparation, whereas the average overall preparedness score was 74% [4]. The lowest score was 31% on the self-reporting tool. There was disparity in the hospital's own rating of its preparedness and its data-derived overall preparedness score. Additionally, funding was directly related to the level of preparedness of the trauma centers, particularly those scoring in the upper 20%.

Another recent article outlines the position of The Eastern Association of the Surgery of Trauma (EAST) in defining the role of surgeons in the development of public health initiatives designed to deal effectively with acts of terrorism. All aspects of the surgeon's role in response to mass casualty incidents are considered — from prehospital response teams to the postevent debriefing. The role of the surgeon in response to Mass Casualty Incidents (MCIs) is substantial in response to threats and injury from natural, unintentional, and intentional disasters. The surgeon must take an active role in pre-event community preparation in training, planning, and executing the response to MCI. The marriage of initiatives among Departments of Public Health, the Department of Homeland Security, and existing trauma systems is necessary to provide for successful responses to terrorist acts [5].

Today's disasters, particularly those involving terrorism and weapons of mass destruction, may result in an austere environment in which the typically boundless resources, transportation, and access to immediate and definitive care for all will have severe constraints imposed upon them, affecting the adequacy of the immediate care for the population in need. This was never more evident than in the New Orleans area after Hurricane Katrina, where these limitations forced medical facilities to curtail services, triage resources, and patients, and attempt to provide continued lifesaving therapies. However, this type of disaster did not produce the type of injuries often seen in terrorism attacks, such as explosions, which result in more casualties and require extensive utilization of emergent trauma and surgical assets. It did, however, significantly test evacuation and hospital placement capabilities of regional disaster response and, in at least one significant instance, prove that trauma system planning for disaster was exceptionally successful [6].

Military field medical units and systems deal with mass casualties routinely in an austere environment through triage, graduated levels of care, and evacuation. Although no clear analogous civilian experience exists currently in the USA, these concepts of triage, initial stabilization, damage control surgery, and evacuation (if indicated) for definitive medical care are essential elements in the response to a mass casualty in the acute phase to achieve the primary objective of reducing mortality. *See* Table 21.1.

Table 21.1 Trauma Systems: Civilian vs Military: Comparative structure of trauma system components between civilian and military

	Civilian trauma system components	Military trauma system corollary
National level	American College of Surgeons, Committee on Trauma – Registry (National Trauma Data Bank: NTDB) – AAST (American Association for the Surgery of Trauma) EAST (Eastern Association for the Surgery of Trauma) – WEST (Western Trauma Association) – (Academic organizations influencing trauma care)	Department of Defense, Health Affairs, Joint Surgeon's Office/Joint Trauma System – Joint Theater Trauma Registry (JTTR) – Defense Medical Readiness Training Institute, Combat Trauma Surgery Committee and Committee on Tactical Combat Casualty Care
State level	State Trauma System – State Director (Texas: Governor's EMS and Trauma Advisory Committee Chair) – State registry – State Trauma System Plan	Combatant Command (COCOM, e.g., US CENTRAL COMMAND) – COCOM Surgeon – JTTR-derived COCOM data – Joint Theater Trauma System (JTTS); COCOM specific
Regional level	Regional Trauma Areas – Registry	Area of Responsibility (AOR, e.g., Operation Iraqi Freedom, Operation Enduring Freedom [Afghanistan]) – JTTR-derived AOR data
Local level	Lead Trauma Center – Trauma registry	JTTS Leadership at Combat Support Hospital (level III facility) – Local trauma database, begin capture JTTR data
Local/Regional Components	Regional Advisory Council (RAC) – RAC Chair – Rural/Urban Organizations – EMS (ground/air) – Hospital reps, all Levels – Performance Improvement, Communication, Rehabilitation, and Prevention committees	Medical Command (e.g., US Army MEDCOM, Air Force Central Command Surgeon, or Marine Expeditionary Force Surgeon) – JTTS director – Level II/III facilities – Level I/Medevac Battalion – Level II/III facilities – PI/Comm/Prev committees

21.2 Levels of Care

Military doctrine supports an integrated health services support system to triage, treat, and return injured combatants to duty in the most time-efficient manner. It begins with the injured combatant on the battlefield and ends in hospitals located within the continental USA. Care begins with buddy aid and field care following nationally accepted tactical combat casualty care standards [7], casualty evacuation, rapidly progresses to stabilizing surgery, and is followed by critical care transport out of the theater of operations.

There are five levels of care, which are different from the American College of Surgeons Committee on Trauma Levels of trauma centers. Different levels denote differences in capability, not the quality of care. Each level has the capability of the level forward of it and expands on that capability. Combatants with injury or illness effectively treated at any level should be returned to duty at that level; all others are prepared for safe transport to a higher level. These units are coordinated in a larger military trauma system across the theater of operations [8].

21.2.1 Level I

Level I care provides immediate first aid delivered at the scene, including immediate lifesaving measures, initial management of chemical casualties, primary disease prevention, combat stress control measures, and noncombat injury prevention. Care at Level I is administered by the injured combatant himself, "buddy aid," or via a combat lifesaver.

Battalion Aid Station (BAS) is often referred to as Level IB and is designed to provide triage, treatments akin to Advanced Trauma Life Support, and evacuation. Staffed by a physician or physician assistant, the primary goal of the BAS is stabilization and evacuation to the next level due to limited patient holding capability, usually up to 6 h. Patients treated may be returned to duty when appropriate. There is no surgical capability at this level of care.

21.2.2 Level II

Level II has increased medical capability and limited inpatient bed space, which includes basic primary care, optometry, psychiatry, dental, laboratory, surgical, and X-ray capabilities. Each service has a slightly different unit at this level and is 100% mobile. Forward surgical assets can be placed at this level (becoming a Level IIB in military parlance) to provide damage control surgery in an effort to reduce early mortality secondary to hemorrhage. Again, once stabilized, casualties are evacuated to the next level of care.

21.2.3   Level III

Level III care represents the highest level of medical care available within the combat theater, with the bulk of inpatient beds located here. Most deployable hospitals are modular, allowing the commander to tailor the medical response to the expected or actual demand by adding additional components as required. The mission of these hospitals is to provide resuscitation, initial and secondary surgery, and post-operative care including intensive care, and either to return the patient to duty or to stabilize for further evacuation. They are equipped with blood bank, laboratory, radiology (includes CT scanner), medical nutrition support, and physical therapy capability. Examples in the recent conflict include Combat Support Hospitals, Air Force Theater Hospitals, Navy Fleet Hospitals deployed across several countries in Operations Iraqi and Enduring Freedom.

21.2.4   Level IV

Level IV care involves definitive medical and surgical care outside the combat zone, yet within the communication zone of the theater of operations. The general hospital is usually a permanent or semipermanent facility. Capabilities include at least six operating rooms, oral surgery, and dental and optometry services; in addition, outpatient specialty and primary care services are also provided. Landstuhl Regional Medical Center, Germany, serves as the level IV in support of Operations Iraqi and Enduring Freedom. Patients requiring more intensive rehabilitation or special needs are evacuated to level V.

21.2.5   Level V

Level V represents continental US-based hospitals, including military medical centers, other federal hospitals such as Veteran Affairs, and civilian contracted hospitals. This represents the most definitive care possible and includes long-term convalescence and specialized rehabilitation.

21.3   Triage

The term triage applies to a wide spectrum of processes involved in the delivery of medical care. In broad terms, it is the process by which casualties are evaluated and classified, allowing appropriate distribution of medical care. This process is driven by the principle of accomplishing the greatest good for the greatest number of people. The discussion that follows outlines some of the basic tenants of triage and how these principles are applied to the unique situations that arise in the delivery of military medical care or care of civilians in an austere environment.

The process of triage is complex, requiring a working knowledge of multiple factors, including current casualty flow, expected casualty flow, current resources available, and the ability to replenish these resources in a timely fashion, all in the context of probability of survival of the casualty based on their injury patterns and physiologic state. When casualty numbers are low, this means that, with abundant resources, as in civilian trauma centers, the maximal effort can be expended on each patient because no other patients are put at risk during the resuscitation of casualties who might have a very small chance of survival; nothing is spared on any casualty in hopes of a good clinical outcome.

The decision process evolves as soon as a maximal effort cannot be applied to each additional patient. This results in casualties with catastrophic injuries, signifying limited chance of survival, being passed over until casualties with injuries that are life-threatening but correctable are addressed. This concept was known even when lifesaving surgical procedures were rare. In the mid-nineteenth century, John Wilson in "Outlines of Naval Surgery" said that lifesaving surgery could only be made available to those most in need if treatment was withheld from those whose injuries were likely to prove fatal and deferred for those whose injuries were slight [9]. These principles are universal and must be applied whenever the demand for medical care overwhelms the supply.

The unique aspects of military triage stem from the situations in which this medical care is delivered. Forward deployed medical teams and equipment must be mobile to adjust to changes in tactical conditions. This restriction means all medical care is delivered from limited resources. The potential for operating in a hostile environment introduces the concept of "reverse" triage. The primary role of medical support in these situations is to preserve the strength of the fighting force. Situations may arise in which standard medical triage decisions based on the greatest good is replaced by resource allocation redirected first to those casualties with injuries who could be treated and then returned to critical tactical duties.

21.3.1 Role of Forward Resuscitative Surgery in Triage Decision Making

The US military has incorporated forward resuscitative surgery (FRS) capabilities into doctrine and mission planning to provide limited yet lifesaving trauma surgical capability. The goal of these forward surgical teams (FSTs) is to provide "damage control" surgery in the select group of patients who would benefit on the battlefield. These teams, usually headed by a trauma surgeon, provide limited general and regional anesthesia, thoracoabdominal hemorrhage control and decontamination, emergent extremity stabilization, temporary limb revascularization, and limited intracranial procedures. Team members may include one or more general/trauma surgeons, anesthesia provider, operating room nurse or technician, medical corpsman, emergency medicine physician, orthopedic surgeon, and postoperative/critical care personnel. Each military branch has developed teams to meet specific requirements dictated by that service's mission.

The FST have been developed to be lightweight and rapidly deployable, allowing them to be quickly prepositioned or deployed. They are operational and can provide trauma resuscitative capability within 15 min of arrival at the deployed location. Operative limitations include consumable goods and the duration the surgical team can physically endure the challenges of operating in austere environments. They are deployed either as "stand-alone" medical resources or as an augmentation of existing medical facilities. The latter rapidly enhances operative capability and patient throughput during times of mass casualties and disaster scenarios. Access to rapid aeromedical evacuation to definitive care facilities is essential if the benefits of forward surgical intervention are to be maximized. FRS has been successfully employed in recent conflicts [10–14].

The challenge, from a triage perspective, is to identify the patients who will benefit from emergent stabilization and resuscitative surgical procedures. The patient who remains hemodynamically stable with no further continued blood loss and can tolerate transport to a definitive care facility should be rapidly transported. The patient with devastating intracranial and intrathoracic injuries who would not survive or would consume excess resources of these surgical teams may actually prevent the team from having a significant impact on other patients. The patient with thoracoabdominal hemorrhage or limb-threatening ischemia, unresponsive to conventional treatment measures (crystalloid infusion/fracture reduction or immobilization) is the ideal surgical candidate for these teams. These patients would not survive transport to definitive care facilities.

Knowledge of available resources is essential to the success of this treatment concept, in which selection and treatment of appropriate patients is driven by available medical intelligence. Scenarios in which a limited or fixed number of casualties are expected (such as a single vehicle accident with two patients and only one requiring operative intervention) would allow expanded use of equipment, consumable goods, and operative time, and differ from the situation of 20 casualties expected initially and the potential for continued arrival of injured patients. Such mass casualty cases require appropriate patient selection with limited use of consumable goods and minimized operative times. Most damage control operations require 1–2 h, and blood products may not be readily available except in the form of fresh whole blood, another critical factor in the care of the injured under such austere conditions [15].

Relatively few patients may actually benefit from forward surgical capability. However, these patients are treated to preserve life and limb and dramatically decrease "died of wounds" classification. During the Falklands Campaign, British military physicians reported 210 patients treated by four field surgical teams, and only three of these patients died. All three suffered serious multiple injuries [16]. This remarkably low mortality rate was related to the skill of the triage and resuscitation teams as they sorted the patients and prepared them for surgery, reverting to basic measures to adequately preserve life and limb function. Similarly, the Israeli's response to multiple mass casualty terrorist bombings involving 467 patients, 63 of whom were severely wound, cited a 2.6% mortality [17]. Again, this low mortality was attributed to well-developed protocols that place emphasis on stabilizing the airway, oxygenation, and hemodynamic stability. Examinations, techniques, devices, and drugs nonessential to a patient's survival or preservation of function are luxuries. CT scans are not performed on the majority of these casualties in the initial phase. The level of austerity is determined by the health care personnel, supplies, and equipment available [18]. The first victims treated are those with life-threatening injuries who can be readily stabilized without massive expenditure of limited resources. Unless the tactical situation dictates otherwise, the next priority is victims with injuries of significant morbidity. Early intervention appreciably decreases morbidity of these injuries.

21.3.2   The Triage Officer

Who should perform the triage function? Historically, the military advocated the use of the most experienced surgeon to perform this function [19]. Dental officers, obstetricians, and senior medical corpsmen have also been utilized in this capacity [16]. The residency-trained Emergency Medicine (EM) physician can be an ideal triage officer, extensively trained to initially evaluate, resuscitate, and manage trauma patients; this individual has the knowledge base and procedural competence to initially manage the combat casualty and make difficult triage decisions while the surgical team is engaged in the operating room [20, 21]. EM specialists frequently make triage decisions in civilian multiple casualty situations and are becoming the norm in military field medical systems as well [22, 23].

During Operation Desert Storm, EM physicians were utilized in the triage officer role. One military field trauma center had 461 coalition and enemy force personnel triaged as casualties. Only 7% of enemy forces and 2% of coalition casualties required retriage. Twelve of 302 (7%) enemy forces were retriaged from a delayed to minimal category representing "overtriage." Three (2%) of coalition forces were retriaged from delayed to immediate. Outcomes of these three patients were not reported [24].

With the EM physician in the triage role, the surgeons can concentrate on their duties and responsibilities in the operating theater. When operating, it is difficult for the surgeon to evaluate or treat a second patient [21]. The emergency physician, with appropriate communication techniques, can relay accurate diagnostic information to the surgeon for surgical or operative prioritization. Personnel performing triage must be competently trained in making such decisions, and there is no substitute for appropriate training and experience [9]. Psychological factors may affect this decision-making process. These factors may include a relationship with the patients or having personal ties with one or more of the patients. The concept of providing the greatest good for the greatest number of patients usually prevails, but this may be neither a comfortable nor an intuitively obvious decision [25]. The responsible physician must not allow emotion to influence triage decisions at the critical time of action.

21.3.3 Practical Considerations and Priorities of Treatment

In order to cope effectively and efficiently with large numbers of battle casualties that present almost simultaneously, the principles of triage must be universally accepted and routinely practiced throughout all echelons of collection, evacuation, and definitive treatment. The likely outcome of the individual casualty must be factored into the decision process prior to the commitment of limited medical resources. According to the NATO Emergency War Surgery Manual, casualties are sorted into four categories: immediate, delayed, minimal, and expectant [26]. Other sources cite three prioritization categories and assign each a color classification: immediate (red), urgent (yellow), and delayed (green) [27]. Other prioritization schemes call for different color assignments to categories wherein immediate becomes green and red becomes delayed [28].

Currently, US forces use a four categorization system: immediate (red), delayed (yellow), minimal (green), and expectant (black or blue) [29]. Obviously, the categorization and color assignments must be agreed to before the mass casualty strikes. This would necessarily be of utmost importance in coalition forces' mass casualty response, as the differing triage schemes and backgrounds of the triage and treatment teams would clearly add to the confusion of the scenario. Using colored casualty tags, colored pens, ribbons, clothespins, or "glow" sticks (particularly in nighttime) can facilitate the triage process and identification of patient category.

21.4 Triage in the Far Forward Environment

Initial mass casualty management at the FST triage point is critical to saving victims' lives, because once the number of patients is greater than the number of surgeons, care will be delayed. The entire FST should participate in the initial round of triage and resuscitation. Despite surgical specialty, all surgeons must address the injured combatants from a systematic and thorough evaluation perspective, not just "consult" from the perspective of their discipline; on mass casualty day, every doctor becomes a triage doctor first. The maximization of initial provider response and performance of initial lifesaving maneuvers (airway interventions, thoracic decompression, limb stabilization and immobilization, and obtaining intravenous access) save the most lives. Recognizing mental status as a sensitive indicator of tissue perfusion and identification of nonresponders and transient responders to initial resuscitative therapy will identify most patients requiring FRS. Surgical and transport prioritization can then be established [30].

One must take great care to evaluate the entire casualty scenario (as best as that can be accomplished in such situations) before committing vast resources to an individual casualty. A key factor and common pitfall to keep in mind is that the worst injured are the first evacuated. Utilizing tremendous resources on the first few futile casualties may not only unnecessarily deplete precious resources, but this may also cost the lives of potentially salvageable casualties who arrive in the next wave but whose operations are delayed.

Patients responding to initial crystalloid infusion and demonstrating no evidence of inadequate tissue perfusion will not routinely benefit from forward surgery. Obviously, emergent airway problems should be addressed immediately. These patients may not require any additional surgical management. Mechanical respiratory compromise, such as a tension pneumothorax, must be recognized immediately and treated without delay. Most thoracic trauma can be managed with the use of tube thoracostomy. Intra-abdominal hemorrhage, uncontrolled by noninvasive measures, requires laparotomy; the timing and prioritization of the operation depends on patient physiologic responsiveness to interventions. This requires reevaluation of such patients to assess for decline in physiologic status, emphasizing the dynamic nature of triage.

Casualties sustaining extremity injuries with vascular compromise are ideal candidates for FRS. The goal is to restore perfusion adequate for limb salvage while controlling hemorrhage; obviously, time is of the essence if the life and limb of the casualty are to be saved. Temporary vascular shunts and/or fasciotomies restore distal blood flow in many cases [31, 32]. Fracture stabilization with external fixation may also limit morbidity. Genitourinary and most facial injuries can be repaired at a definitive care facility. Spinal cord injury is relatively rare in penetrating trauma but is best cared for in a definitive facility. Head injuries in the combat casualty scenario are highly lethal. FSTs are limited to burr hole and cranial flap procedures, but these may be lifesaving.

Euthanasia is a difficult concept to consider for most health care providers. On the basis of beneficence of relieving the suffering of a dying person, it may be an ethically acceptable alternative in the rare situation in which a patient will die despite all possible attempts at saving his or her life [25]. Active euthanasia ("mercy killing") is the act of hastening or purposefully enhancing the dying process. Passive euthanasia is the act of allowing someone to die while alleviating suffering and pain with comfort measures. Passive euthanasia occurs during times of overwhelming casualties. It is affected by triaging these patients to expectant categories. Active euthanasia is documented at least once in modern military history. British soldiers of the 111th Indian Infantry Brigade in Burma euthanized their own companions during World War II [33].

21.4.1 Practical Utility of Forward Triage and Resuscitation

In the October 1973 War, Israeli forward field surgical hospitals operated on 3% of the casualties. The soldiers were in danger of losing their lives or viability of a limb without surgical intervention. A physician saw the wounded within 60 min of the time of injury. The indications for forward surgical procedures were

1. Massive hemorrhage in the abdomen, chest, or cranium
2. Progressive peritoneal irritation with reduction of vital signs
3. Extensive damage to a limb, requiring immediate amputation in order to save a life or longer stump
4. Arterial damage endangering a limb; and/or
5. Injuries endangering the upper respiratory tracts [34]

Naggan reported a 10–25% reduction in mortality from war injuries with medical officers at the front to perform triage and FRS using these criteria [20].

Retriage and surgical prioritization is a continuum of reassessment and treatment. Patients can deteriorate or improve based on the treatment they receive in triage and initial management phases. The goal of FRS is to maintain adequate tissue perfusion and prevent potential complications within its capability. Controversy remains regarding the use of crystalloid infusion in isolated thoracoabdominal trauma. Some proponents [35] argue establishment of intravenous access and limited or no fluid resuscitation until hemorrhage is surgically controlled; a single 250-cc infusion of 3% or 7.5% hypertonic saline is initially recommended in the combat casualty.

Colloid preparations appear to have size and weight advantages when compared to crystalloid preparations in the tactical field environment. Limited decontamination capability and nonsterile environments necessitate liberal use of antibiotics for combat casualties. Because of the limited resources, consumable goods may be utilized on more than one patient, with an increased risk of disease transmission. For example, if a casualty is to be given a 1-liter bolus of crystalloid but demonstrates adequate physiologic response after just 500 cc, the remaining fluid could be administered to another injured soldier with a greater physiologic need. Liberal use of analgesia and regional anesthesia is also encouraged. These patients may have prolonged time periods awaiting surgery and transport. Comfort measures are extremely important, even in austere environments.

Most recently, use of fresh whole blood, recombinant factor VIIa, and stored red cells to plasma transfusion ratios approximating 1:1 have all been demonstrated to be very beneficial in combat casualties presenting with massive injury and shock [36–40]. These advances have not been scrutinized in mass casualty situations, per se, but practical experience in the current conflict indicates they would be more successful than traditionally described resuscitation schemes [41].

21.4.2 Perioperative and IntraoperativeTriage

Triage is not isolated to initial evaluation. Critical decision points occur through the time of injury to stabilization at a definitive care facility. Identifying patients who require excess resources in order to salvage life or limb is difficult. During triage, physiologic and biochemical data available at the decision-making time may be limited. Available resources may be the single factor in the decision-making process. This is contrary to civilian practice, in which it is relatively rare to not have enough consumable goods to treat all victims. Because of the limitations in imaging capability, providers must rely on physical examination and changing hemodynamic parameters for triage decision making.

For the surgeon, casualties come in two broad categories: those who need immediate lifesaving or limb-saving surgery and those who do not. Prioritization then proceeds along urgency of the procedure and patient physiology. Few other disciplines can assess the surgical prioritization; however, the EM physician, intensivist, and anesthetist can assist greatly in the process. As outlined earlier, identifying nonsurvivable injuries or injuries with low likelihood of survival may not be accomplished until the patient has operative exposure and the specific injury is isolated. At this critical time, surgeons may find it difficult to cease the procedure after investing time and resources in this patient and to move to the next salvageable patient. Pressure from other personnel or command structure may demand "everything" be done for the patient. The surgeon must remain acutely aware of available resources, casualty flow, and evacuation intervals in order to make these decisions.

Another common pitfall belaying the surgeon is the inability to retriage the patient in midoperation to expectant. When the emergency and operative teams have expended significant time, energy, and resources on a given casualty, it becomes increasingly difficult to "let go" of that casualty. On-table triage decisions to expectant, in favor of casualties with more survivable injury awaiting surgery, should be considered after hemorrhage control has been established, when, despite aggressive resuscitative efforts, the patient has worsening physiology (acidosis, hypothermia, and coagulopathy).

Other anatomic considerations for such a decision can be taken from the civilian literature. Even in the civilian level I trauma center setting, there have been few survivors from combined aortocaval gunshots, retrohepatic caval injury, and traumatic arrest when the pathology is outside of the thorax [42–45]. Similarly, if a patient has dual sites of exsanguination, one of which is from the liver, the patient cannot be expected to survive in the FRS environment today [46]. Because of the relative shortage of consumable supplies in such situations, conservation limits can be determined prior to a mass casualty and communicated to the entire staff. Establishing such standards prior to the event will decrease the need for instantaneous decision making at the time of operative intervention. Available rapid evacuation may negate the need for salvage or resuscitative surgery.

21.4.3 Physiologic, Anatomic, and Historic Perspectives of Triage

Altered sensorium is a sensitive indicator of brain perfusion. In the initial phase of resuscitation, mental status changes may be subtle but provide a reliable means of determining oxygenation and perfusion of the brain. Tachycardia and systolic blood pressure do not correlate well with hypoperfusion. The young, otherwise healthy soldier may be able to compensate for volume loss until near death. A narrowing pulse pressure is a sensitive marker of hypovolemia. A resting tachypnea is an early sign of shock and related to a compensatory increase in tidal volume in an attempt to maintain minute ventilation [24].

Limited data are available to identify uniformly fatal traumatic injuries. Intuitive knowledge suggests that penetrating trans-hemispheric brain injury and aortic disruption are two anatomic injuries limiting the utility of operative intervention in a multiple casualty scenario of battlefield injuries. In the battlefield setting of salvage surgery with multiple casualties, it may be appropriate to stop further resuscitative efforts in patients with the following injuries: increasing intracranial pressure in spite of decompression and appropriate hemodynamic therapy; airway injuries with prolonged hypoxia; myocardial damage (other than single penetrating injuries easily repaired with staples or suture), and significant aortic injury. These patients may be revisited, if they survive until resources are available and the casualty flow has diminished. This exact scenario has occurred on several occasions in the current conflict (personal communication, Col. Steve Flaherty, Landstuhl, Germany). Ongoing resuscitative measures in these patients with limited chance of survival utilize a large portion of consumable goods, blood products, operative time, and postoperative critical care time.

Wound Data and Munitions Effectiveness Team (WDMET) database (Vietnam era) reflects fatal injuries by body region including head (38%), chest (24%), multiple (17%), and abdomen (9%). Nonfatal injury distribution was: superficial (47%); extremity (26%); abdomen (8%); and chest, face, and head, each with 4% [47]. Exsanguination was the most common cause of death for US ground forces in Vietnam. It accounted for approximately one-half of the combat mortality in the WDMET study. The most common sites of injury were heart, thoracic aorta, pulmonary artery, and intraparenchymal pulmonary vessels. However, in approximately 20% of casualties who exsanguinated on the battlefield, the site of bleeding was an artery in an extremity; femoral and brachial were the most common. Of the hospitalized casualties who died of shock, roughly equal numbers were categorized as dying of continued bleeding. The sites were most commonly the liver or pelvis, uncontrollable coagulopathy, and "irreversible shock" [47]. It is these patient populations, to which FRS is directed.

A trauma facility during the Persian Gulf War reported a low rate (2%) of chest injuries and a 45% rate of isolated extremity injuries. Approximately 29% had injuries limited to the head, neck, chest, or abdomen. Combination of multiple anatomic areas was seen in 26% of patients [24]. More recently in combat action in Afghanistan, chest injury was seen in 3.1% of casualties, isolated extremity injury in 30%, and multiple injuries in 49.7%. The introduction of improvised explosive devices by the enemy and the wear of newly developed body armor may account for a portion of this change in wound distribution [19].

In 1969, Cowley and colleagues attempted to identify biochemical markers in 300 shock patients while differentiating survivors and nonsurvivors. Measurements preceding death were identified. A statistical difference was found in the following areas: cardiac output, total peripheral resistance, serum glucose, osmolality, blood urea nitrogen (BUN), creatinine, lactic acid (demonstrated by metabolic acidosis, pH), pyruvic acid, transaminases, clotting time, and fibrinogen. Since this study, many authors have attempted to identify biochemical markers in order to predict increased morbidity, mortality, or survival [48].

Davis and colleagues found the base deficit calculation to be a useful indicator of volume deficit. The authors reviewed 2,615 trauma patients' charts. Inclusion criteria were the documentation of serial arterial blood gas determinations and a systolic blood pressure of <90 mmHg or an initial base deficit of <−3. One hundred ninety-four patients met these criteria, and 79 of these patients had a penetrating trauma mechanism. Base deficit was found to be a surrogate marker for lactic acid [49]. Serum lactate level was felt to be a reliable physiologic indicator of hypovolemia. While it was not statistically significant, a trend was noted, suggesting the greater the base deficit, the lower the probability of survival. More importantly, the authors noted patients with a worsening base deficit in spite of fluid resuscitation; 65% (32/49) had evidence of persistent hemorrhage [49]. This study did not correlate pH with base deficit.

Robertson and coworkers discussed severe acidosis (pH < 7.0) as a predictor of mortality. A trauma center registry of 3,996 patients was reviewed. Only 37 had an initial pH < 7.0 (incidence = 0.9%). This group of patients was differentiated into survivors and nonsurvivors. The severely acidotic group showed a higher mortality (70% vs 7.4%; $p < 0.0001$). This group also had a higher incidence of penetrating trauma (63% vs 40%; $p = 0.01$) and spent more time in the intensive care unit. Nonsurvivors were likely to present with a low systolic blood pressure, relative bradycardia, and depressed respiratory rate. Forty-nine percent of the severely acidotic patients survived initial resuscitation, with 30% of the entire group of acidotic patients surviving to discharge. The authors concluded that severe acidosis alone is not a sufficiently powerful predictor to withhold resuscitation. Resuscitation efforts did not consume excessive hospital resources even though ICU stays were longer. However, severe acidosis combined with coma (GCS < 8) and shock (SBP < 90 mmHg) was found to be uniformly fatal. Unfortunately, this study did not account for easily identifiable or correctable etiologies of acidosis, such as hypercarbia secondary to airway obstruction or ventilatory compromise. Additionally, 14% of patients in the severely acidemic group had evidence of sympathomimetic agents that can mimic acidosis [50].

The preceding conclusion may be appropriate in the civilian trauma center setting. When resources at the FRS unit are overwhelmed, it is reasonable to triage patients with a severe acidosis to an expectant category. In fact, data from a military level-I trauma center support this concept [51]. More than 2,100 patients were evaluated during a 42 month period; 3.2% were identified as having a pH < 7.0. Four patients were excluded because mechanisms of injury were inconsistent with combat trauma (hanging, smoke inhalation, and electrocution). Four patients were excluded because of relatively minor injuries with acidosis secondary to hypercarbia caused by inadequate airway control. Ethanol intoxication associated with minor injuries accounted for the exclusion of two patients. Of the remaining 33 patients with severe acidosis, only three survived. The survivors' injuries were: pulmonary artery stab wound with an ISS of 16 and probability of survival 0.93; a lower extremity near-amputation with an ISS of 20 and probability of survival of 0.99; and a gunshot wound to the duodenum and aorta with an ISS of 75 and a probability of survival of 0.17. Each of these patients presented to a trauma center with dedicated resources and personnel readily available. An excess of 30 units of blood products were utilized for each individual patient, with many hours of dedicated resuscitation resources, multiple surgeries, and extended intensive care unit hospitalizations, none of which are available in excess at the FRS unit.

Another recent review of more than 1,000 combat casualties identified that casualties arriving with a body temperature <34°C significantly correlated with mortality and the combination of low blood pressure, Glasgow Coma Scale score, and high Injury Severity Score on arrival also strongly correlated to mortality [52]. No prospective evaluation or use of such criteria in mass casualty scenarios has been undertaken. To categorize a soldier to the expectant category in these types of scenarios requires a resolve developed through experience in futile surgery using operating theaters and personnel while other more salvageable casualties wait, deteriorate, or die [53]. It is difficult to characterize a patient as unsalvageable when a pulse is palpable and respirations are spontaneous.

The experienced physician will realize and consider these difficult situations before facing them in the trauma resuscitation at the FRS unit. Triage saves lives. Unfortunately, rules, single physiologic markers, and critical pathways regarding triage are difficult to articulate and even more difficult to support with valid data. Anecdotal experiences are the most common form of education regarding triage principles. Effective triage requires knowledgeable personnel with the resolve to make difficult decisions based on limited data. Not everyone is capable of performing this skill. Education and practice in realistic environments with changing resources are the most effective means of learning these procedures.

21.5 Damage Control Surgery in Mass Casualty

The latest surgical innovation to translate from the civilian experience into the care of the traumatized patient in the military environment is damage control: the implication in this setting is the sum total of the maneuvers necessary to ensure patient survival above all else [54]. Damage control is defined as the initial control of hemorrhage and contamination followed by intraperitoneal packing and rapid closure, which allow for resuscitation to normal physiology in the intensive care unit and subsequent definitive re-exploration [55]. In the military environment, damage control takes a different twist, as the phases of damage control are undertaken by multiple surgical teams along the evacuation chain.

As currently described, damage control has three separate and distinct aspects. First, surgical control of hemorrhage and contamination is obtained quickly, definitive repairs are deferred, and the laparotomy is abruptly terminated. Temporary closure of the abdomen is performed after intra-abdominal packing (part I). The patient is then taken to the intensive care unit where core rewarming, correction of coagulopathy, and maximization of hemodynamic values take place (part II). When normal physiology has been restored, re-exploration is undertaken to complete the definitive surgical management of all intra-abdominal injuries (part III) [55, 56]. Packing of the abdomen for hemorrhage has undergone a rebirth since being soundly discouraged after military experience in World War II and the Vietnam War [57]. Since the recent review by Rotondo and Zonies [58], the total number of damage control patients described in the literature exceeds 1,000, and mortality is 50%.

Currently, damage control is encouraged in the mass casualty, far forward military environment, but it can take on a somewhat different connotation in these circumstances. Casualties with unfavorable physiology are treated as noted earlier. Tactical Abbreviated Surgical Control (TASC) is the application of damage control techniques in patients with favorable physiology in an attempt to shorten operative times and get more casualties into the operating room for lifesaving, abbreviated interventions [26]. These abbreviated, focused operative interventions can be used for peripheral vascular injuries, extensive bone and soft tissue injuries, and thoracoabdominal penetrations in patients expected to survive, instead of definitive surgery for every casualty. This has been demonstrated to conserve precious resources, such as time, operating table space, and blood. Obviously, this TASC philosophy relies on further definitive surgical care at the next echelon of care [59].

21.6 Summary and Conclusion

The management of mass casualty events in the military environment is challenging for even experienced military health care providers, is difficult to teach, and has not been well studied. Lessons learned in military conflict and civilian mass disasters need to be captured, codified, and made widely available. Physiologic parameters, anatomic injury patterns, and laboratory tests cannot be used alone as surrogates for experience in triage and mass casualty management. Identifying the risk for possible mass casualty in a local community should lead to development of management plans that include strategies for mitigation of the event, appropriate triage and treatment schemes, development of evacuation plans, notification of higher levels of disaster response for assistance, and education of all involved health care professionals in the disaster management plan.

References

1. Rhee P, Jenkins D, Holcomb J. Austere and battlefield surgery. In Feliciano D, Mattox K, Moore E eds: *Trauma*, Seventh Edition. Philadelphia: Lippincott Williams & Wilkins, 2007.
2. Frykberg ER, Tepas JJ, Alexander RH. The 1983 Beirut airport terrorist bombing: injury patterns and implications for disaster management. *Am Surg* 1989;54:134–141.
3. Stevens RA, Bohman HR, Baker BC, Chambers LW. The U.S. Navy's forward resuscitative surgery system during Operation Iraqi Freedom. *Mil Med* 2005;170:297–301.

4. National Foundation for Trauma Care. *The Study of the Impact of a Terrorist Attack on Individual Trauma Centers*. Las Cruces, New Mexico, 2006.
5. Ciraulo Dl, Barie PS, Briggs SM, Bjerke HS, Born CT, Capella J, Cancio L, Dennis A, DiGiacomo JC, Gross RI, Hammond JS, Holcomb JB, Jenkins D, Knuth TE, Letarte PB, Lynn M, O'Neill PA, Salomone JP, Shatz DV. An update on the surgeon's scope and depth of practice to all hazards emergencies. *J Trauma* 2006;60(6):1267–1274.
6. Epley E, Stewart R, Love P, Jenkins D, Siegworth GM, Baskin TW, Flaherty S, Cocke R. A regional medical operations center improves disaster response. *Am J Surg* 2006; 192(6):853–859.
7. NAEMT. *Prehospital Trauma Life Support, Military Issue*, Sixth Edition. St. Louis, MO: Mosby/JEMS, 2006.
8. Eastridge BJ, Jenkins DH, Flaherty S, Schiller H, Holcomb JB. Trauma system development in a theater of war: experiences from operation Iraqi Freedom and Operation Enduring Freedom. *J Trauma* 2006; 61(6):1366–1373.
9. Kennedy K, Aghababian RV, Gans L, Lewis CP. Triage: techniques and applications and decision making. *Ann Emerg Med* 1996; 282:136–144.
10. Bilski TR, Baker BC, Grove JR, Hinks RP, Harrison MJ, Sabra JP, Temerlin SM, Rhee P. Battlefield casualties treated at Camp Rhino, Afghanistan: lessons learned. *J Trauma* 2003;54:814–821.
11. Cho JM, Jotoi I, Alarcon AS, Morton TM, King BT, Hermann JM. Operation Iraqi Freedom: surgical experience of the 212th Mobile Army Surgical Hospital. *Mil Med* 2005;170:268–272.
12. Patel TH, Wenner KA, Price SA, Weber MA, Leveridge A, McAtee SJ. A U.S. Army Forward Surgical Team's experience in Operation Iraqi Freedom. *J Trauma* 2004;57:201–207.
13. Peoples GE, Jezior JR, Shriver CD. Caring for the wounded in Iraq: a photo essay. *N Engl J Med* 2004;351:2476–2480.
14. Place RJ, Rush RM Jr, Arrington ED. Forward surgical team (FST) workload in a special operations environment: the 250th FST in Operation ENDURING FREEDOM. *Curr Surg* 2003;60:418–422.
15. Kauvar DS, Holcomb JB, Norris GC, Hess JR. Fresh whole blood transfusion: A controversial military practice. *J Trauma* 2006;61(1):181–184.
16. Ryan JM. The Falklands War: triage. *Ann R Coll Surg Engl* 1984; 66:195–196.
17. Alfici, R, Ashkenazi I, Kessel B. Management of victims in a mass casualty incident caused by a terrorist bombing: treatment algorithms for stable, unstable, and in extremis victims. *Mil Med* 2006;171:1151–1162.
18. Noji EK. Military medicine. In Auerbach PS ed: *Wilderness Medicine: Management of Wilderness and Environmental Emergencies*, Third Edition. St. Louis, MO: Mosby, 1995.
19. Sorting of casualties. In Bowen TE and Bellamy RF eds: *Emergency War Surgery: Second United States Revision of the Emergency War Surgery NATO Handbook*. Washington, DC: United States Government Printing Office, 1988, pp. 181–192.
20. Naggan L. Medical planning for disaster in Israel. *Injury* 1976;7(4):279–285.
21. Walsh DP, Lammeright GR, Devoll J. The effectiveness of the advanced trauma life support system in a mass casualty situation by non-trauma experienced physicians: Granada, 1983. *J Emerg Med* 1989;7:175–180.
22. Llewellyn CH. Triage: in austere environments and echeloned medical systems. *World J Surg* 1992; 16:904–909.
23. Walsh DP, Mellon MM. The emergency medicine specialist in combat triage: a new and untapped resource. *Mil Med* 1990; 155:187.
24. Burkle FM, Orebaugh S, Barendese BR. Emergency medicine in the Persian Gulf War – Part I: preparations for triage and combat casualty care. *Ann Emerg Med* 1994;23:(4):742–747.
25. Iserson KV. Ethics of wilderness medicine. In Auerbach PS ed: *Management of Wilderness and Environmental Emergencies*, Third Edition. St. Louis, MO: Mosby, 1995.
26. Lounsbury DE, Bellamy RF eds. *Emergency War Surgery: Third United States Revision of the Emergency War Surgery NATO Handbook*. Washington, DC: Borden Institute, Walter Reed Army Medical Center, 2004.

27. Lumley JSP, Ryan JM, Baxter PJ, Kirby N. *Handbook of the Medical Care of Catastrophes.* London: The Royal Society of Medicine Press Limited, 1996, p. 94.
28. Personal communication. Alexander Partin, PhD, Chief of Disaster Response, Primorsky Krai, Vladivostok, Russia, 2001.
29. Operational Medicine CD. Washington, DC: Bureau of Medicine and Surgery, Department of the Navy, 2001.
30. Forward Resuscitative Surgery Report, January 1997. Prepared for the Joint Health Services Support Vision 2010.
31. Rasmussen T, Clouse W, Jenkins D, Peck M, Eliason JL, Smith DL. Echelons of care and the management of wartime vascular injury. *Perspect Vasc Surg Endovasc Ther* 2006;18(2):91–99.
32. Rasmussen TE, Clouse WD, Jenkins DH, Peck MA, Eliason JL, Smith DL. The use of temporary vasculars shunts as a damage control adjunct in the management of war time vascular injury. *J Trauma* 2006;61:8–15.
33. Swann SW. *Euthanasia on the Battlefield. Military Chaplain Revisits.* Spring 1991.
34. Rozin R. Triage of war casualties. *Harefuah* 1974;87:533.
35. Bickell WH, Wall MJ, Pepe PE, Martin RR, Ginger VF, Allen MK, Mattox KL. Immediate versus delayed fluid resuscitation for hypotensive patients with penetrating torso injuries. *N Engl J Med* 1994;331:1105–1109.
36. Borgman MA, Spinella PC, Perkins JG, Grathwohl KW, Repine T, Beekley AC, Sebesta J, Jenkins D, Wade CE, Holcomb JB. The ratio of blood products transfused affects mortality in patients receiving massive transfusions at a combat support hospital. *J Trauma* 2007;63(4):805–813.
37. Holcomb JB, Jenkins DH, Rhee P, Johannigman J, Mahoney P, Mehta S, Cox ED, Gehrke MJ, Beilman GJ, Schreiber M, Flaherty SF, Grathwohl KW, Spinella PC, Perkins JG, Beekley AC, McMullin NR, Park MS, Gonzalez EA, Wade CE, Dubick MA, Schwab CW, Moore FA, Champion HR, Hoyt DB, Hess JR. Damage control resuscitation: directly addressing the early coagulopathy of trauma. *J Trauma* 2007; 62(2):307–310.
38. Perkins JG, Schreiber MA, Wade CE, Holcomb JB. Early versus late recombinant factor VIIa in combat trauma patients requiring massive transfusion. *J Trauma* 2007;62(5): 1095–1101.
39. Gonzalez EA, Moore FA, Holcomb JB, Miller CC, Kozar RA, Todd SR, Cocanour CS, Balldin BC, McKinley BA. Fresh frozen plasma should be given earlier to patients requiring massive transfusion. *J Trauma* 2007;62(1):112–119.
40. Perkins J, Grathwohl K, Repine T, et al. Fresh whole blood use in combat casualties reduces mortality. J Trauma 2006;61(6):1570.
41. Jenkins D, Holcomb J. Resuscitation. In Irwin RS, Rippe JM eds: *Intensive Care Medicine*, Sixth Edition. Philadelphia: Lippincott Williams & Wilkins, 2006.
42. Feliciano D, Burch J, Spjut-Patrinely V, Mattox KL, Jordon FL Jr. Abdominal gunshot wounds. *Ann Surg* 1988;208:362–370.
43. Hirshberg A, Matto, KL. "Damage control" in trauma surgery. *Br J Surg* 1993;80:1501.
44. Rogers FB, Reese J, Shackford SR, Osler RM. The use of venovenous bypass and total vascular isolation of the liver in the surgical management of juxtahepatic venous injuries in blunt hepatic trauma. *J Trauma* 1997;43(3):530–533.
45. Coats TJ, Keogh S, Clark H, Neal M. Prehospital resuscitative thoracotomy for cardiac arrest after penetrating trauma: rationale and case series. *J Trauma* 2001;50(4):670–673.
46. May AK, Rotondo MF, Zonies DH, Reilly PM, Anderson HL, Schwab CW. Multifocal and multi-cavitary exsanguination: "The real double jeopardy." *Pan Am J Trauma* 1997 pp. 12–19.
47. Zajtchuck R, Grande CM. Combat trauma overview. In Zajtchuck R, Bellamy RF eds: *Textbook of Military Medicine: Part IV: Anesthesia and Perioperative Care of the Combat Casualty.* Falls Church, VA: Office of the Surgeon General (Department of the Army), 1996 pp. 33–39.
48. Cowley RA, Attar S, LaBrosse E. Some significant biochemical parameters found in 300 shock patients. *J Trauma* 1969;9(11):926–938.

49. Davis JW, Shackford SR, Mackersie RC, Hoyt DB. Base deficit as a guide to volume resuscitation. *J Trauma* 1988;28(10):1464–1467.
50. Robertson R, Eidt J, Bitzer L, Wallace B, Collins T, Pars-Miller C, Cone J, Saffle J, Asensio J, Hoyt D. Severe acidosis alone does not predict mortality in the trauma patient. *Am J Surg* 1995;170:691–695.
51. Jenkins D, Johannigman J, Kissinger D, et al. Arterial Blood Gas pH Facilitates Triage in Military Trauma Patients. Presented at Texas ACS, March 1995.
52. Eastridge BJ, Owsley J, Sebesta J, Beekley A, Wade C, Wildzunas R, Rhee P, Holcomb, J. Admission physiology criteria after injury on the battlefield predict medical resource utilization and patient mortality. *J Trauma* 2006;61(4):820–823.
53. Bowen TE and Bellamy RF eds. *Emergency War Surgery: Second United States Revision of the Emergency War Surgery NATO Handbook.* Washington, DC: United States Government Printing Office, 1988.
54. Pourmoghadam, KK, Fogler, RJ, Shaftan, GW. Ligation: an alternative for control of exsanguination in major vascular injuries. *J Trauma* 1997;43:126–130.
55. Rotondo M, Schwab CW, McGonigal M, Phillips III GR, Fruchterman TM, Kauder DR, Latenser BA, Angood PA. "Damage control": an approach for improved survival in exsanguinating penetrating abdominal injury. *J Trauma* 1993;35:375–383.
56. Morris J, Eddy V, Blinman T, Rutherford EJ, Sharp KW. The staged celiotomy for trauma: issues in unpacking and reconstruction. *Ann Surg* 1993;217:576–584.
57. Sharp K, Locicero R. Abdominal packing for surgically uncontrollable hemorrhage. *Ann Surg* 1992;215:467–475.
58. Rotondo MF, Zonies DH. The damage control sequence and underlying logic. *Surg Clin North Am* 1997;77:761–777.
59. Chambers LW, Rhee P, Baker BC, Perciballi J, Cubanc M, Compeggie M, Nace M, Bohman HR. Initial experience of US Marine Corps forward resuscitative surgical system during Operation Iraqi Freedom. *Arch Surg* 2005;140:26–32.

A Civilian Perspective

Yoram A. Weil and Rami Mosheiff

21.1 Decision-Making Factors: Overview and Applicability of Damage Control in Terrorist Attack Casualties

Civilian mass causality terror attacks have been steadily rising in recent years due to various geo-political reasons [1]. Despite the daunting threat of chemical and biological warfare, conventional terrorism is still the most common form of attack, resulting in high causality events [2]. This is augmented by the ease of obtaining high quality explosives and the relatively high degree of associated damage caused by them. Recent examples are the London attacks in 2005 [3] and the Madrid train attacks in 2004, [4] as well as the succession of suicide bombings during the Palestinian uprising in 2000–2005 [5, 6].

The typical pattern of the resultant injuries is distinct both in magnitude and severity when compared to the more "traditional" blunt trauma injuries [7, 8]. The extent of civilian terror attacks as well as the unpredictability of the events pose a significant challenge to health care facilities, exhausting the capacity of even large level-I trauma centers in certain instances [9–12]. Terror attack victims, in general, sustain a higher proportion of life-threatening injuries than those victims commonly seen in other trauma events [7, 10, 13].

Utilization of "damage-control" strategies is therefore crucial for the successful management of mass terror attack casualties. In that respect, damage control policy should dictate the tactics for triage, physical exam, imaging, and, eventually, treatment, including the general patient management and the specifics of damage control orthopedic surgery [14].

This chapter deals with implementation of damage control principles at the pre-hospital level, in management in the Emergency Department (ED) as the event further evolves, in triage, in management in other hospital departments and/or services, and, finally, in the surgical treatment of injuries, including orthopedic surgery.

Y.A. Weil (✉) and R. Mosheiff
Hadassah Hebrew University Hospital, Orthopaedic Trauma Service, POB 12000, Jerusalem, 91120, Israel
e-mail: yoramweil@gmail.com

21.2 Rationale

The mainstay of terror-related injury is blast. Blast injury is a multi-organ "disease" similar to blunt trauma, although specific site injuries tend to be more severe in nature, somewhat similar to high-energy multiple site penetrating trauma [8].

A few recent studies performed in Israel, comparing Terror-Related Injury (TRI) to "conventional" trauma, have demonstrated a distinctive pattern of injury, characterized by multi-system involvement, high morbidity and mortality, high requirement for acute surgery, and prolonged Intensive Care Unit (ICU) stay [15, 16]. The mortality pattern itself is different from the "classic" one observed in blunt trauma: Among other differences, it demonstrated a higher in-field and in-hospital immediate mortality [6].

The blast injury mechanism has been classified as the primary blast effect and the accompanying effects that follow it and increase the extent of injury [17, 18]. Although this classification has been mentioned in numerous instances, it is worth reviewing briefly due to its implications for the diagnosis and treatment of the resultant injuries.

The primary blast effect is related to the rapid pressure wave created during the detonation of an explosive [19]. The scene location and type of explosive used have a direct effect on the severity of injuries. Blast wave energy tends to decrease rapidly in space and dissipate [20]. When blast occurs in a closed or confined space such as in a bus or in a room, the blast waves reverberate from the walls instead of dissipating, [17, 20, 21] thus inflicting more damage on human victims. In a series of suicide bombings in Israel occurring in buses during the years 1995–1996, a threefold increase in primary blast injuries was observed when compared to open-space explosions, exemplifying this phenomenon [21].

When the pressure wave created by detonation encounters certain air-fluid interfaces, unique tissue damage may occur. The most common and perhaps the most life-threatening injury involves the lung. Surprisingly, before the 1980s, this type of injury was underreported, probably because of the rarity of confined space blast injuries [22]. Pressure differentials across the alveolar-capillary interface cause disruption, hemorrhage, pulmonary contusion, pneumothorax, hemothorax, pneumomediastinum, and subcutaneous emphysema [23].

The second most common type of primary blast injury affects the hollow viscera. The intestines, most usually the colon, are affected by the detonation wave. Mesenteric ischemia or infarct can cause delayed rupture of the large or the small intestine; these injuries are difficult to detect initially. Rupture, infarction, ischemia, and hemorrhage of solid organs such as the liver, spleen, and kidney are generally associated with very high blast forces or proximity of the patient to the blast center [24].

Tympanic membrane injury has been extensively discussed in the literature dealing with terror attacks. It is the most common non-lethal injury caused by relatively low-pressure blast waves. Traditionally, its presence was used to predict severe primary blast injuries (such as to the lung or bowel); however, this remains questionable and unreliable [25]. This will be further discussed in the triage section.

Limb injury due to terror attack is usually not caused by the primary blast effect. Blast usually affects air-fluid interfaces, and, therefore, limbs are probably less affected than the lungs or intestines. Hull and Cooper studied primary blast effects on the extremities that resulted in traumatic amputations in Northern Ireland [26]. Only nine of 52 victims with traumatic amputation survived, demonstrating the high level of energy needed to avulse a limb. In all 52 patients, the lower extremity amputation was at the level of the tibial tuberosity, and the limb was avulsed through the fracture site rather than through the joint. The coaxial forces produced the fracture, and dynamic forces (i.e., blast wind) caused the avulsion of the fractured limb. Practically, a limb injury caused solely by the primary blast effect is a rare entity.

The secondary blast effects comprise the core of the orthopedic injuries observed in the Middle Eastern experience [16, 27, 28]. Secondary blast effects are related to penetrating injuries caused by fragments ejected from the explosives or the foreign bodies impregnated within them. The extent of this effect depends on the subject's distance from the detonation center, the shape and size of the fragments, and the number of foreign bodies implanted in or created by the explosive. In contrast to most warfare injuries, the improvised explosives used by terrorists have multiple added fragments, including screws, bolts, nails, and other objects, which may increase the damage caused by penetrating injuries [29]. Open fractures, severe soft tissue injuries, and multi-organ penetrating injury are the more common injury patterns seen in the severely injured victim [29, 30].

Tertiary blast injury refers to the blunt trauma component of the explosion. Flying objects or falling can cause additional traumatic effects in addition to those discussed earlier. When structural collapse occurs, a high casualty and mortality event occurs [5]. The authors' experience in Israel did not demonstrate a significant proportion of additional blunt trauma, but reports from other parts of the world, such as the one originating from the Oklahoma City explosion, have indicated that this is the primary mechanism of the injury [31], usually with devastating results.

The quaternary blast effect is a recently added one and includes the thermal and chemical damage caused by fire and noxious substances occurring in the vicinity of the explosion. Confined-space explosions significantly increase these types of injuries [21].

Last but not least, the fact that more and more suicide bombers are involved in modern terrorism may increase the risk of biological contamination of the victims with tissues originating from the terrorists themselves, such as bone fragments [32]. The concerns of blood-borne infections such as Hepatitis B/C and HIV should be kept in mind when dealing with suicide bombers [33].

21.3   Strategies and Recommendations

21.3.1   Triage

Since the majority of terror attacks in civilian population occur in populated and crowded areas, the number of victims exceeds the treatment capacity allocated routinely at all levels. Therefore, the damage control strategy is the most appropriate one in this setting, and correct allocation of resources will ideally minimize undertriage, resulting in fewer missed fatal injuries and simultaneously avoiding overtriage, which can cause exhaustion of the system when minor injuries are being overtreated [34].

21.4   Pre-hospital Level

The recollection of an anesthesiology faculty member at the authors' institution when incidentally encountering a scene demonstrates some of the difficulties in the field level:

> I did not know what to do. Should I choose one survivor, giving him or her the best treatment I could, and abandon the others? My first aid kit seemed ridiculous among the multiple casualties[35]

Besides the frustration, there are some other considerations that need to be taken into account:

1. The existence of broken glass, sharp objects, and noxious materials may be dangerous for both the victims and the treating team at the scene
2. Many terrorists employ a "second wave" delayed bombing intended to kill and injure the rescue team as well as other people gathered at the scene, creating an unsecured zone
3. In an urban setting, the distance from the hospital is usually short and the number of available vehicles is usually sufficient for immediate evacuation of victims
4. Availability of a level I trauma center in most of the targets of terrorism attacks (major cities) rarely requires prolonged patient transport. Therefore, all efforts should concentrate on rapid evacuation of victims without any delay. Victims with amputated body parts who are not showing signs of movement and those who are pulseless with dilated pupils are considered dead. No further efforts should be spent on these victims, and attention should be directed to evacuating the remaining victims

Recommendations based on the authors' experience are to limit the number of interventions on the scene to:

1. Securing the airway
2. Tension pneumothorax relief
3. Major external bleeding control
4. Spine immobilization

All other measure can take place en route [8, 35].

In order to minimize chaos and maximize control, a well-accepted norm taken from the military experience is the following: The first team in the field takes responsibility at the scene after the arrival of additional teams and directs them in the emergency care and evacuation priorities in order to save time.

21.4.1 Evacuation

Unlike isolated events in which Emergency Medical Services (EMS) services should be instructed to evacuate patients to the nearest level I trauma center, this policy has not been implemented at all times when mass causalities occurred [36]. Therefore, due to the very rapid evacuation (average 5–10 min), the nearest hospitals and the nearest level I trauma should actually be converted from treating facilities into triage stations, receiving the bulk of patients and acting as referring centers for more critically ill patients [36]. In the damage control evacuation scenario, the triage is done only initially at the field due to the imminent danger of a "stay and play" policy [12]. Further triage takes place at the nearest hospital and en route by the EMS services in order to channel the patients to the correct treatment facilities.

21.4.2 Emergency Department Level

Unlike the events on September 11th 2001, and unlike the events in Oklahoma City, Madrid, and London, when analysis demonstrated that emergency departments were theoretically readily capable of handling the number of critically ill patients [37], the authors' experience proves that this was not the case in many of the attacks in Israel, and a scenario of an overcrowded and understaffed emergency rooms was possible. There are several explanations for these differences:

1. The distance from the hospitals as well as the training of the EMS services might add to the speed at which patients arrive in the OR. While in London the critically ill patients were received in the level I trauma center within 1–2 h [3], in Hadassah Hospital in Jerusalem, during one incident, 18 critically ill patients were evacuated within 6 min after the onset of the event [8], with a maximum arrival time of 43 min [11].

2. The mechanism of injury dictates different on-scene mortality and morbidity. When structural collapse occurs, as such as the World Trade Center event in 2001, the total number of critically ill (ISS > 15) patients admitted to the two nearest level I centers was 20 [38], while in an average suicide bombing explosion in Israel during 2000–2003, 26% of patients were critically ill [10], averaging about 4–8 per event. This is 90-fold less in magnitude. Thus, paradoxically, higher mortality due to a higher energy mechanism might lead to less load on the ED.

Despite this, the majority of patients in these causalities are "walking-wounded" and not critically injured [3, 11, 39]. Critically injured patients can be missed while attention is being given to the latter [40].

Logistics of ED management have a major impact on triage. The authors recommend evacuation of non-critical non-terror related patients temporarily to the hospital floors while the seriously ill patients can be treated in designated areas.

The trauma bays should then be dedicated only to resuscitative efforts on critically ill patients; the rest of the ED should be divided into admitting areas for the rest of the patients. Each area is designated with a Surgeon-in-Charge (SIC) of the other members of the treating team (surgical and orthopedic residents, nurses, medical students, etc.). The surgeon-in-charge directs in critical junctions as suggested by Almogy and colleagues [8] (Fig. 21.1):

- Triage at the initial admitting phase;
- Treatment cycles directed to the OR or admitting floors;
- Diagnostics constantly done until the general chaos is reduced.

Every hospital should explore and identify the logistics mechanism that provides the best available setting for disaster management for its capacity; this has been proven to be efficient when an actual disaster has occurred [15, 37, 39, 41]. Computer simulation has also been described in disaster management planning as an effective tool [41, 42]. As discussed earlier, correct triage will lead to the concentration of efforts on the critically ill patients who comprise 15–30% of the total number of victims in a typical suicide attack. Frykberg [43] had criticized overtriage as a source of misdiagnosing critically-ill patients. The authors' experience is that overtriage should be encouraged, provided that the personnel and space for doing so are allocated, therefore not interfering with the care of the more critically wounded patients [9].

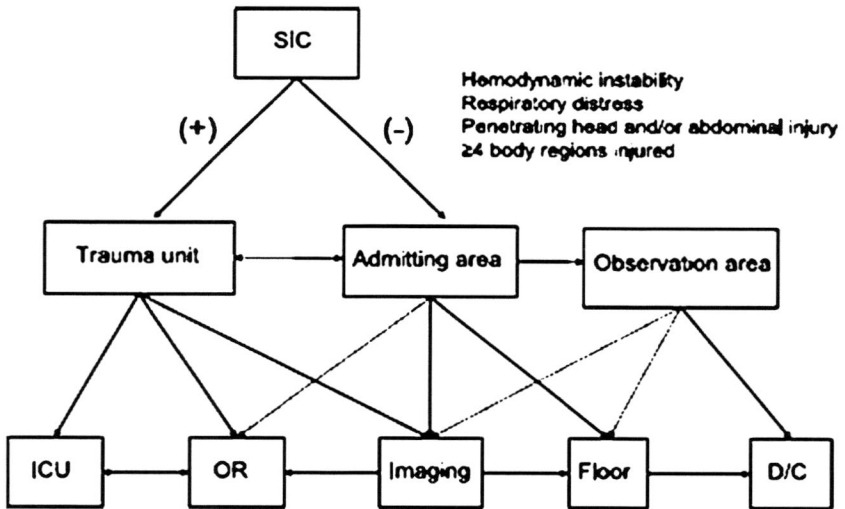

Fig. 21.1 Algorithm for the triage and initial management of victims of suicide bombing attacks. The presence of external signs of trauma is a considerable adjunct to triage. Flow of patients from the trauma room and admitting area is unidirectional. Slightly injured victims are transferred to an observation area and are examined once chaos subsides. *Solid lines:* primary pathways; *dotted lines:* secondary pathways; *D/C* discharge home; *OR* operating room; *SIC* surgeon-in-charge (Reproduced from [9]. With permission from Elsevier.)

A system in which the surgeon-in-charge of the event is gathering information in repeated rounds of triage and than delegating to the team the diagnostics and treatment until the next round allows for better control and allocation of resources. This is termed the "Accordion Method" [8] and was utilized successfully in numerous events in the authors' hospital (Fig. 21.2).

21.4.3   Diagnostics and Management

Some important and unique triage physical and diagnostic efforts have been taking place in recent years, giving a better perspective on the management of multiple casualty events. Since the number of patients may exceed the diagnostic capacity of the facility, the patients should be prioritized. The CT scanner is well known to be the "bottleneck" [41] in these scenarios, and many recommend restriction of its use solely to head injuries [3, 44].

In two recent studies originating from the authors' center, [24, 45] physical signs such as penetrating injury to the head and penetrating injury to four or more sites were highly predictive of blast lung injuries. It should be mentioned that since many of the victims in suicide bombings are facing away from the detonation, examination of the back is crucial [8].

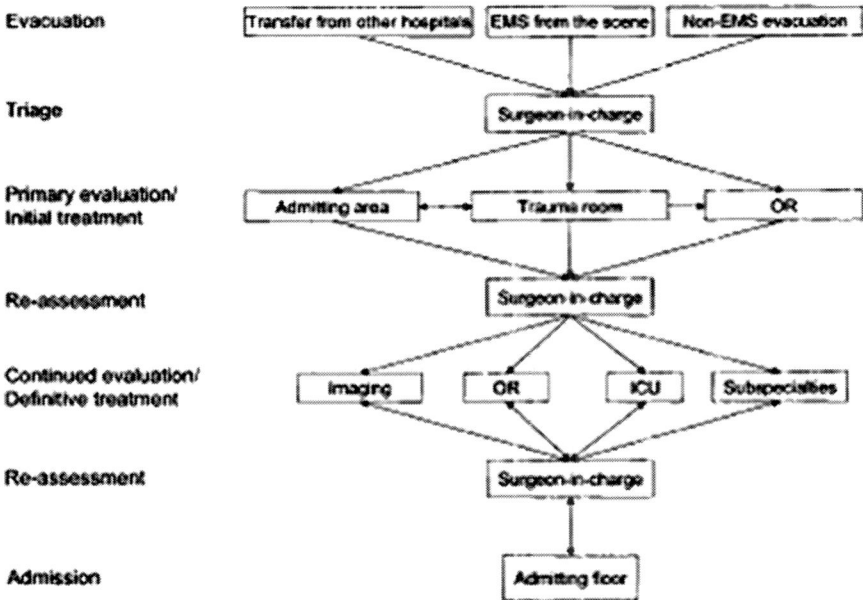

Fig. 21.2 The triage method in the authors' institution depicts the role of the surgeon-in-charge in mass casualty events, with converging and diverging decision points, similar to an accordion (Reproduced with permission of [8])

Penetrating torso injury as well as penetrating injury to four or more sites were highly predictive of intra-abdominal injury. For the London attack [3], CT was used only for the evaluation of head injuries, while laparotomies were performed only on the basis of ultrasound examination. Hypotension as a result of penetrating injury was also used as a guideline for laparotomy in an abbreviated damage-control strategy [8]. However, when the number of critically injured patients is small, normal diagnostic efforts can safely take place [46].

In a recent work [47] comparing gunshot wound injuries to blast injuries, the existence of a long bone fracture was indicative of a more severe ISS, morbidity, and mortality. Therefore, a long bone fracture may alert the surgeon that life-threatening injuries are imminent in this subgroup of patients.

Expedited flow of patients out of the trauma bay is an essential component of the care in a mass-casualty event [8, 24]. The patient flow should be directed in a "one-way" system, moving the patients after their diagnostics if needed either to the operating room or to the ICU, never back to the ED or the trauma unit [48]. Availability of multiple ORs simultaneously during such an event is a key factor, since up to 50% of admitted patients will need a form of a surgical intervention [7]. Whereas in a single event such as the Madrid and London bombings, having multiple ORs was feasible [3, 49], repetitive events may exhaust the system, as experienced in Israel [9].

Despite this, some events may result in a limited number of critically ill patients. In this case, a more systematic approach should be used, allowing a more liberal use of diagnostic studies and utilization of resources. These events have been termed "Limited Multi-Casualties Events." [46] Care should be taken, however, to recognize a true mass casualty event, and damage control strategies should be judiciously used to avoid unnecessary delays in triage and treatment.

Another bottleneck usually encountered in terror attacks is the Intensive Care Unit). Since blast-injured patients have significantly more critical injuries than the "traditional" blunt trauma victims [7], the authors' experience shows that ICU admittance is very predictable, ranging from four to eight patients per average event and usually comprising 50% of admissions [5], the very same proportion that was seen in the Madrid and World Trade Center data [49]. Provisional ICU beds such as those in the PACU (Post Anesthesia Care Unit) or other surgical care units should be available while evacuating the general or trauma ICU. In case ICU vacancy becomes an issue, the event workflow can be seriously affected [5]. Special ventilation considerations should be given to blast injured patients; Shamir and colleagues provide the current recommendations on this matter [5].

The suggested workflow demonstrating the Surgeon-in-Charge (SIC) and the different working areas is presented in Fig. 21.2.

21.4.4 Later Control

In the damage control strategy, secondary and tertiary surveys are of the utmost importance. As in the case of blunt trauma, the percentage of missed injuries can exceed 10–20% [50, 51], many of them (over 50%) being musculoskeletal injuries. The authors' experience confirms that secondary blast injuries are among the injuries most missed. The orthopedic trauma team (the authors' unpublished data) adopted the "morning after" rounds, in which records from the ED admitting area are used to allocate patients to all the hospitals. After a vigilant physical examination, all penetrating injuries were documented both literally and graphically using the burn-unit diagram to describe the distribution of skeletal injuries. More than once, fractures and foreign bodies requiring removal were found during that process. Most commonly, a general surgeon and a trauma nurse attended the "morning after" rounds in order to document and locate these injuries.

A thorough overview and control of the entire population of inpatients is crucial not only at the acute phase of the trauma but also during later stages in order to plan delayed reconstructive procedures, integration with other disciplines, and control over the OR and the ICU.

21.5 Damage Control Orthopedic Surgery in Terror Attacks

Although much has been written about the general concept of terror management in the general medical setting, very little has been written about managing orthopedic injuries in this scenario. In fact, most of the literature regarding blast injury has emerged from the military experience [14, 18]. Blast injuries to the extremities are highly unpredictable and diverse. This is due to the fact that the amount of foreign bodies impregnated in the explosive is erratic and to the variable distances of the victims from the detonation center. At a close proximity, the velocity of a fragment can be up to 1,800 m/s, but it decreases very rapidly because of lack of streamlining [14]. Therefore, both high and low energy injuries can be seen as well as isolated and multiple injuries (Fig. 21.3a, b).

Blast injury to the extremities is different from the more familiar one caused by a Gunshot Wound (GSW). The latter can be characterized by a fracture accompanied by a variable degree of soft tissue damage, depending on the energy and velocity of the bullet [52]. Gunshot wounds are usually successfully treated according to standard protocols, including modern treatments such as intramedullary nailing [53]. In a study conducted by the authors, both patient statistics as well as management of long bone fractures caused either by blast injury or GSW were examined. The blast injury group had significantly more multiple fracture involvement, higher ISS, and mortality, while the GSW had more severe localized tissue damage, such as high grade (IIIB and C) open fractures and compartment syndromes. The authors also compared the national trauma registry statistics in Israel of patients with terror-related orthopedic injuries ($n = 1,072$) and patients with blunt trauma injuries ($n = 17,307$) (Weil, unpublished data). Again, besides there being significantly more open fractures and amputations in terror victims than in blunt trauma patients, a higher ISS, mortality, and a higher requirement for surgery were found in terror victims.

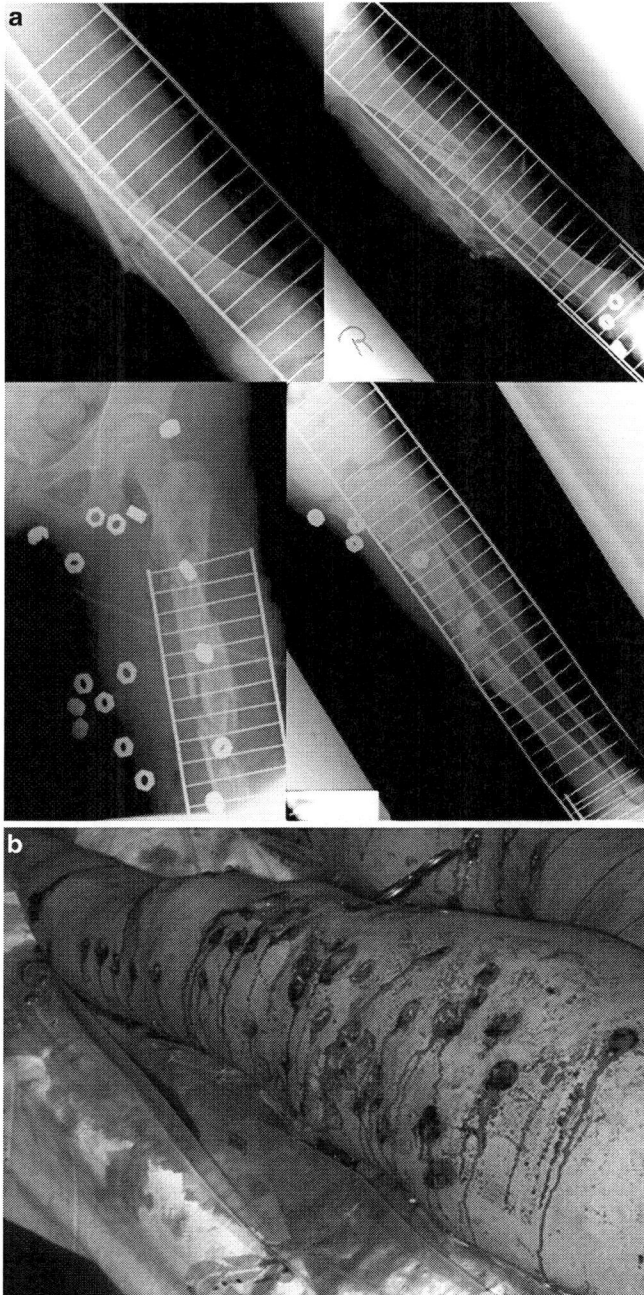

Fig. 21.3 Typical multiple fragment wounds to lower extremities with extensive skeletal (a) and soft-tissue damage (b)

The surgical principles advocated recently for damage control orthopedics are more than appropriate in treating a critically ill patient with a terror-related injury with a long bone fracture [54, 55]. The average ISS of patients with long bone injuries caused by blast is 20, with 75% associated injuries [47]. Besides the traditional markers, using the modified protocol of predicting blast lung injuries [24] can be helpful in determining the risk for a "second hit." Although the authors did not experience extensive morbidity attributed solely to an "early total care" approach that was widespread in the authors' institution, this may be masked by the severity of the accompanying injuries.

The following is a good illustrative case demonstrating the need for the adoption of the damage control orthopedics policy. After a suicide bombing in Jerusalem in 2001, a 14-year-old girl sustained multiple fragment wounds to her lower extremities with extensive soft-tissue damage (Fig. 21.3a, b). Her injuries included bilateral open fractures of the femora and tibiae, with bilateral obstruction of the posterior tibial artery. Following the injury, the patient was taken to the OR and had her fracture nailed in a 4-h procedure by multiple teams. Following that, she developed hypothermia and coagulopathy, the vascular injuries were not repaired, and she was transferred to the ICU. She continued to bleed profusely from multiple entry sites and received 57 units of red blood cells, 39 units of Fresh Frozen Plasma (FFP), 14 units of platelets, and 19 units of cryoprecipitate. Twenty-two hours after admission, she received 100 μg/kg of recombinant Factor VIIa with an immediate improvement of her INR from 2.11 to 0.64. The patient was complicated with Acute Respiratory Distress Symptom (ARDS), although initially her injuries were isolated to the lower extremities. The patient eventually recovered functionally, but the question of Early Total Care in extreme situations, despite the availability of OR and multiple surgical teams during these events, should be raised. Eventually, the patient healed, and she is ambulatory and functioning 4 years after her original injury (Fig. 21.4).

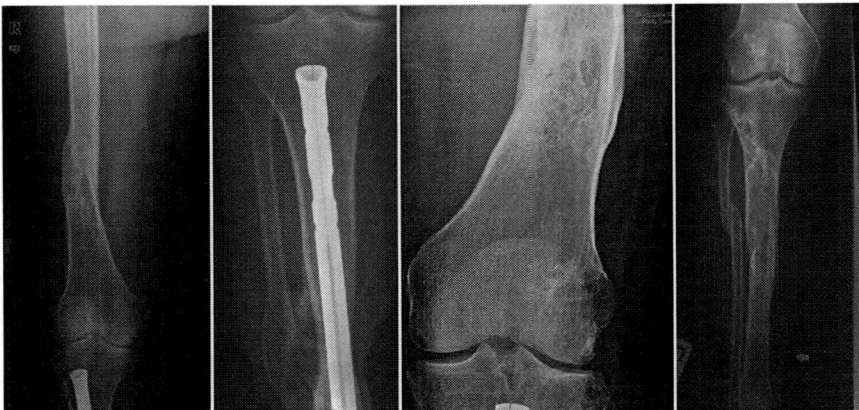

Fig. 21.4 Healed and remodeled left and right femora and tibiae at 4 years follow-up

Table 21.2 shows guidelines and recommendations for damage control orthopedics in blast injuries, based on the authors' experience and the current literature recommendations as to what are appropriate clinical guidelines for damage control orthopedics when long bone fractures are encountered with blast injuries

It should be stressed that the direct evidence for the use of this policy in a specific subset of patients is still lacking. It can be logically presumed that what may be the treatment of choice in blunt trauma may apply to these unique circumstances. The fact that the patients in question are generally more critically ill may even strengthen these assumptions. More data and evidence, including objective measures such as platelet counts, temperature, coagulation studies, and, finally, inflammatory profiles, are needed.

21.6   Benefits and Risks

As described earlier, some controversial issues exist when dealing with mass causality events. The authors' suggested protocols and experience are a bit different from those described elsewhere. Below is a discussion of these issues:

1. Pre-hospital care: Although increasing evidence supports the "scoop and run" [56] policy for general trauma care – in the face of a dangerous working zone that might be trapped with a timed second explosive or sharp objects – the minimum should be done at the scene. The risk associated with over-resuscitation is too high and outweighs the risk of under-resuscitation in the unsafe scene.
2. Evacuation to a trauma center or to the nearest hospital: Reality demonstrates that the nearest hospital might serve as an outpost triage hospital [11]. The question of the ideal evacuation pattern is still to be answered with the risks and benefits of each approach.
3. Implementing abbreviated diagnostic measures: Use of external signs for determining the severity of injury, relying heavily on US, and avoiding the unnecessary use of the CT scanner. In this setting, the risk is usually false positive surgery (so far in a minor amount of cases [8]), a risk that is far outweighed by the possibility of delaying treatment and creating bottlenecks.
4. Damage control orthopedic surgery: The risks of immediate intramedullary nailing of certain critically ill patients have been repeatedly demonstrated [57, 58].

Table 21.2 Guidelines and recommendations for damage control orthopedics in blast injuries

Damage Control Orthopedics
Penetrating injuries to >4 body areas with foreign bodies, penetrating head injuries
Multiple long bone injuries due to blast
ISS > 20
blast lung injury

There is no doubt that critically ill terror attack victims are usually "sicker" than their counterpart blunt trauma patients [7]. Given the open nature of these procedure mandates, repeat debridements should take place in any case. Thereafter, safe conversion to internal fixation can take place. Recently, it has been shown that performing this according to a reasonable timetable will add only a minimal risk of infection [59].

21.7   Summary and Conclusion

Unfortunately, terrorism is the war of the future for the human race. It achieves chaos and mass hysteria, and also occasionally overwhelms the medical care systems and other municipal public services. This battlefield is no longer remote [1]. Implementing damage control strategies is crucial in order to minimize mortality and morbidity of a significant proportion of critically injured victims of these events.

Damage control is not only a slogan: It is an approach to treating the victims at the immediate scene, using only airway-saving procedures, and then evacuating the patients to the nearest hospital as an outfield triage post. There, convergent and divergent control pathways are used as mandated by the most senior authority [60]. Control must be maintained at all times using the authors' suggested scheme. Limitation of resources such as imaging and the resuscitation bay at the trauma units requires dynamic and fast management of patients without delaying necessary emergency procedures. Implementing proper diagnostic studies and the judicious use of the CT scanner with priority to head injured patients are necessary.

Patients suffering from long bone fractures due to blast are more critically injured than their counterpart blunt trauma patients due to the high energy absorbed. Damage control orthopedic principles should be liberally used in this subset of the patient population. Following the acute event, re-rounding and locating all the patients using a tracking list and meticulous documentation minimizes the risk of missed injuries.

References

1. Stein M, Hirshberg A. Medical consequences of terrorism. The conventional weapon threat. *Surgical Clinics of North America* 1999;79(6):1537–52.
2. Lerner EB, O'Connor RE, Schwartz R, Brinsfield K, Ashkenazi I, Degutis LC, Dionne JP, Hines S, Hunter S, O'Reilly G, Sattin RW. Blast-related injuries from terrorism: an international perspective. *Prehospital Emergency Care* 2007;11(2):137–53.
3. Aylwin CJ, Konig TC, Brennan NW, Shirley P, Davies G, Walsh M, Brohi K. Reduction in critical mortality in urban mass casualty incidents: analysis of triage, surge, and resource use after the London bombings on July 7, 2005. *Lancet* 2006;368(9554):2219–25.

4. Gutierrez de Ceballos JP, Turegano Fuentes F, Perez Diaz D, Sanz Sanchez M, Martin Llorente C, Guerrero Sanz JE. Casualties treated at the closest hospital in the Madrid, March 11, terrorist bombings. *Critical Care Medicine* 2005;33(1 Suppl):S107–12.
5. Shamir MY, Rivkind A, Weissman C, Sprung CL, Weiss YG. Conventional terrorist bomb incidents and the intensive care unit. *Current Opinion in Critical Care* 2005;11(6):580–4.
6. Shapira SC, Adatto-Levi R, Avitzour M, Rivkind AI, Gertsenshtein I, Mintz Y. Mortality in terrorist attacks: a unique modal of temporal death distribution. *World Journal of Surgery* 2006;30(11):2071–7; discussion 8–9.
7. Kluger Y, Peleg K, Daniel-Aharonson L, Mayo A. The special injury pattern in terrorist bombings. *Journal of the American College of Surgeons* 2004;199(6):875–9.
8. Almogy G, Belzberg H, Mintz Y, Pikarsky AK, Zamir G, Rivkind AI. Suicide bombing attacks: update and modifications to the protocol. *Annals of Surgery* 2004;239(3):295–303.
9. Almogy G, Rivkind AI. Surgical lessons learned from suicide bombing attacks. *Journal of the American College of Surgeons* 2006;202(2):313–9.
10. Peleg K, Aharonson-Daniel L, Stein M, Michaelson M, Kluger Y, Simon D, Israeli Trauma Group (ITG), Noji EK. Gunshot and explosion injuries: characteristics, outcomes, and implications for care of terror-related injuries in Israel. *Annals of Surgery* 2004;239(3):311–8.
11. Einav S, Aharonson-Daniel L, Weissman C, Freund HR, Peleg K. In-hospital resource utilization during multiple casualty incidents. *Annals of Surgery* 2006;243(4):533–40.
12. Shamir MY, Weiss YG, Willner D, Mintz Y, Bloom AI, Weiss Y, Sprung CL, Weissman C. Multiple casualty terror events: the anesthesiologist's perspective. *Anesthesia and Analgesia* 2004;98(6):1746–52.
13. Peleg K, Aharonson-Daniel L, Michael M, Shapira SC. Patterns of injury in hospitalized terrorist victims. *The American Journal of Emergency Medicine* 2003;21(4):258–62.
14. Weil YA, Mosheiff R, Liebergall M. Blast and penetrating fragment injuries to the extremities. *The Journal of the American Academy of Orthopaedic Surgeons* 2006;14(10 Suppl):S136–9.
15. Kluger Y, Mayo A, Soffer D, Aladgem D, Halperin P. Functions and principles in the management of bombing mass casualty incidents: lessons learned at the Tel-Aviv Souraski Medical Center. *Eur J Emerg Med* 2004;11(6):329–34.
16. Peleg K, Aharonson-Daniel L. Blast injuries. *The New England Journal of Medicine* 2005;352(25):2651–3; author reply 3.
17. DePalma RG, Burris DG, Champion HR, Hodgson MJ. Blast injuries. *The New England Journal of Medicine* 2005;352(13):1335–42.
18. Covey DC. Blast and fragment injuries of the musculoskeletal system. *The Journal of Bone and Joint Surgery. American Volume* 2002;84A(7):1221–34.
19. Wightman JM, Gladish SL. Explosions and blast injuries. *Annals of Emergency Medicine* 2001;37(6):664–78.
20. Arnold JL, Halpern P, Tsai MC, Smithline H. Mass casualty terrorist bombings: a comparison of outcomes by bombing type. *Annals of Emergency Medicine* 2004;43(2):263–73.
21. Leibovici D, Gofrit ON, Stein M, Shapira SC, Noga Y, Heruti RJ, Shemer J. Blast injuries: bus versus open-air bombings – a comparative study of injuries in survivors of open-air versus confined-space explosions. *The Journal of Trauma* 1996;41(6):1030–5.
22. Katz E, Ofek B, Adler J, Abramowitz HB, Krausz MM. Primary blast injury after a bomb explosion in a civilian bus. *Annals of Surgery* 1989;209(4):484–8.
23. Mellor SG, Cooper GJ. Analysis of 828 servicemen killed or injured by explosion in Northern Ireland 1970–84: the Hostile Action Casualty System. *The British Journal of Surgery* 1989;76(10):1006–10.
24. Almogy G, Mintz Y, Zamir G, Bdolah-Abram T, Elazary R, Dotan L, Faruga M, Rivkind AI. Suicide bombing attacks: can external signs predict internal injuries? *Annals of Surgery* 2006;243(4):541–6.
25. Leibovici D, Gofrit ON, Shapira SC. Eardrum perforation in explosion survivors: is it a marker of pulmonary blast injury? *Annals of Emergency Medicine* 1999;34(2):168–72.
26. Hull JB, Cooper GJ. Pattern and mechanism of traumatic amputation by explosive blast. *The Journal of Trauma* 1996;40(3 Suppl):S198–205.

27. Barham M. Blast injuries. *The New England Journal of Medicine* 2005;352(25):2651–3; author reply 3.
28. Ashkenazi I, Olsha O, Alfici R. Blast injuries. T*he New England Journal of Medicine* 2005;352(25):2651–3; author reply 3.
29. Ad-El DD, Eldad A, Mintz Y, Berlatzky Y, Elami A, Rivkind AI, Almogy G, Tzur T. Suicide bombing injuries: the Jerusalem experience of exceptional tissue damage posing a new challenge for the reconstructive surgeon. *Plastic and Reconstructive Surgery* 2006;118(2):383–7; discussion 8–9.
30. Aharonson-Daniel L, Klein Y, Peleg K. Suicide bombers form a new injury profile. *Annals of Surgery* 2006;244(6):1018–23.
31. Teague DC. Mass casualties in the Oklahoma City bombing. *Clinical Orthopaedics and Related Research* 2004(422):77–81.
32. Leibner ED, Weil Y, Gross E, Liebergall M, Mosheiff R. A broken bone without a fracture: traumatic foreign bone implantation resulting from a mass casualty bombing. *The Journal of Trauma* 2005;58(2):388–90.
33. Wong JM, Marsh D, Abu-Sitta G, Lau S, Mann HA, Nawabi DH, Patel H.Biological foreign body implantation in victims of the London July 7th suicide bombings. *The Journal of Trauma* 2006;60(2):402–4.
34. Frykberg ER. Triage: principles and practice. *Scandinavian Journal of Surgery* 2005;94(4):272–8.
35. Shamir MY. Suicide bombing: professional eyewitness report. *Anesthesiology* 2004;100(4):1042–3.
36. Einav S, Feigenberg Z, Weissman C, Zaichik D, Caspi G, Kotler D, Freund HR.Evacuation priorities in mass casualty terror-related events: implications for contingency planning. *Annals of Surgery* 2004;239(3):304–10.
37. Rivara FP, Nathens AB, Jurkovich GJ, Maier RV. Do trauma centers have the capacity to respond to disasters? *The Journal of Trauma* 2006;61(4):949–53.
38. Cushman JG, Pachter HL, Beaton HL. Two New York City hospitals' surgical response to the September 11, 2001, terrorist attack in New York City. *The Journal of Trauma* 2003;54(1):147–54; discussion 54–5.
39. Alfici R, Ashkenazi I, Kessel B. Management of victims in a mass casualty incident caused by a terrorist bombing: treatment algorithms for stable, unstable, and in extremis victims. *Military Medicine* 2006;171(12):1155–62.
40. Frykberg ER. Medical management of disasters and mass casualties from terrorist bombings: how can we cope? *The Journal of Trauma* 2002;53(2):201–12.
41. Hirshberg A, Stein M, Walden R. Surgical resource utilization in urban terrorist bombing: a computer simulation. *The Journal of Trauma* 1999;47(3):545–50.
42. Hirshberg A, Scott BG, Granchi T, Wall MJ, Jr, Mattox KL, Stein M. How does casualty load affect trauma care in urban bombing incidents? A quantitative analysis. *The Journal of Trauma* 2005;58(4):686–93; discussion 94–5.
43. Frykberg ER. Terrorist bombings in Madrid. *Critical Care (London, England)* 2005;9(1):20–2.
44. Mayo A, Kluger Y. Terrorist bombing. *World Journal of Emergency Surgery* 2006;1:33.
45. Almogy G, Luria T, Richter E, Pizov R, Bdolah-Abram T, Mintz Y, Zamir G, Rivkind AI. Can external signs of trauma guide management? Lessons learned from suicide bombing attacks in Israel. *Archives of Surgery* 2005;140(4):390–3.
46. Almogy G. The approach to suicide bombing attacks: Changing concepts. In: R M, ed. Jerusalem; 2007.
47. Weil YA, Petrov K, Liebergall M, Mintz Y, Mosheiff R. Long bone fractures caused by penetrating injuries in terrorists attacks. *The Journal of Trauma* 2007;62(4):909–12.
48. Bar-Joseph G, Michaelson M, Halberthal M. Managing mass casualties. *Current Opinion in Anaesthesiology* 2003;16(2):193–9.
49. de Ceballos JP, Turegano-Fuentes F, Perez-Diaz D, Sanz-Sanchez M, Martin-Llorente C, Guerrero-Sanz JE. 11 March 2004: the terrorist bomb explosions in Madrid, Spain–an analy-

sis of the logistics, injuries sustained and clinical management of casualties treated at the closest hospital. *Critical Care (London, England)* 2005;9(1):104–11.
50. Buduhan G, McRitchie DI. Missed injuries in patients with multiple trauma. *The Journal of Trauma* 2000;49(4):600–5.
51. Brooks A, Holroyd B, Riley B. Missed injury in major trauma patients. *Injury* 2004;35(4):407–10.
52. Bartlett CS. Clinical update: gunshot wound ballistics. *Clinical Orthopaedics and Related Research* 2003(408):28–57.
53. Nowotarski P, Brumback RJ. Immediate interlocking nailing of fractures of the femur caused by low- to mid-velocity gunshots. *Journal of Orthopaedic Trauma* 1994;8(2):134–41.
54. Roberts CS, Pape HC, Jones AL, Malkani AL, Rodriguez JL, Giannoudis PV. Damage control orthopaedics: evolving concepts in the treatment of patients who have sustained orthopaedic trauma. *Instructional Course Lectures* 2005;54:447–62.
55. Giannoudis PV. Surgical priorities in damage control in polytrauma. *The Journal of Bone and Joint Surgery. British Volume* 2003;85(4):478–83.
56. Liberman M, Mulder D, Sampalis J. Advanced or basic life support for trauma: meta-analysis and critical review of the literature. *The Journal of Trauma* 2000;49(4):584–99.
57. Pape HC, Grimme K, Van Griensven M, Sott AH, Giannoudis P, Morley J, Roise O, Ellingsen E, Hildebrand F, Wiese B, Krettek C. Impact of intramedullary instrumentation versus damage control for femoral fractures on immunoinflammatory parameters: prospective randomized analysis by the EPOFF Study Group. *The Journal of Trauma* 2003;55(1):7–13.
58. Pape HC, Hildebrand F, Pertschy S, Zelle B, Garapati R, Grimme K, Krettek C. Changes in the management of femoral shaft fractures in polytrauma patients: from early total care to damage control orthopedic surgery. *The Journal of Trauma* 2002;53(3):452–61; discussion 61–2.
59. Harwood PJ, Giannoudis PV, Probst C, Krettek C, Pape HC. The risk of local infective complications after damage control procedures for femoral shaft fracture. *Journal of Orthopaedic Trauma* 2006;20(3):181–9.
60. Einav S, Spira RM, Hersch M, Reissman P, Schecter W. Surgeon and hospital leadership during terrorist-related multiple-casualty events: a coup d'etat. *Archives of Surgery* 2006;141(8):815–22.

Part IV
Complications and Outcomes

Chapter 22
Complications and Outcomes: Abdominal, General, and Extremity Complications

George C. Velmahos and Malek Tabbara

22.1 Introduction

The patient's outcome provides the final judgment on the surgeon's abilities and skills as well as on the effectiveness and safety of the health-care system. Some complications originate in errors or shortcuts, while some others are simply unavoidable. In this chapter, the authors focus on a few selected complications from the myriads that exist because of their importance and complexity. The authors aim to increase alertness on complications that would never arise if always suspected (e.g., muscle necrosis from extremity compartment syndrome) and improve outcomes by offering evidence-based solutions to the management of such mishaps.

22.2 Abdominal and General Complications

22.2.1 Abdominal Compartment Syndrome

Abdominal compartment syndrome (ACS) is defined as intraabdominal pressure greater than 20 mmHg in association with impairment in the pulmonary, renal, and cardiovascular functions [1–5]. ACS occurs in 2–25% of patients undergoing damage-control surgery (DCS) [6] and is seen typically in trauma patients with severe abdominal or pelvic injuries who required DCS. Nevertheless, cases of ACS with absence of any abdominal injury or abdominal operation have been described in trauma patients [3, 7]. This entity, also known as secondary ACS, is mainly related to the bowel edema that occurs due to the aggressive resuscitation (blood product and crystalloid) required for patients in shock [8, 9]. (See Chap. 4.)

G.C. Velmahos (✉)
Department of Surgery, Harvard Medical School, 165 Cambridge Street,
Suite 810, Boston, MA, 02115, USA
e-mail: gvelmahos@partners.org

H.-C. Pape et al. (eds.), *Damage Control Management in the Polytrauma Patient*,
DOI 10.1007/978-0-387-89508-6_22, © Springer Science+Business Media, LLC 2010

Although DCS is by itself a major cause of ACS, other predisposing factors have been identified: Complex and lengthy procedures, associated with blood loss and fluid administration; primary fascial closure when the abdomen is "tight"; need for extensive packing; large abdominal hematoma; significant bowel distention or edema; large-volume resuscitation; and multiple extra-abdominal injuries [7, 8, 10, 11]. Raeburn and colleagues found that post-DCS patients who had an early elevation in their peak airway pressure (PAP) were at higher risk for ACS. Patients who developed ACS were found to have a PAP of 44 ± 2 mmHg at the end of DCS as opposed to 33 ± 1 mmHg for those who did not develop ACS [4]. Similarly, McNelis and colleagues compared 22 patients who developed ACS with patients of equivalent age, diagnosis, and predictive outcome data and showed that the PAP on admission and net 24-h fluid balance were predictive of ACS. The authors developed an equation that can predict the probability of ACS. Using this equation they found that a patient with a PAP of 45 mmHg and a 12-L fluid balance would have a 41% probability of developing ACS. The likelihood of ACS increases to 100% with a PAP of 57 mmHg and 20-L fluid balance [12].

ACS can lead to visceral hypoperfusion and intestinal ischemia followed by bacterial translocation, cytokines, and production of free oxygen radicals. When left untreated, ACS may cause lethal multiple organ dysfunction. Decreased cardiac output, increased peripheral resistance, oliguria, anuria, increased PAP, decreased compliance, and hypoxia may all occur [5, 13, 14]. Therefore, careful monitoring and prompt recognition and management of increased intra-abdominal pressure are crucial to prevent the development of ACS [4, 15]. Even if treated promptly, patients who develop ACS after DCS have significantly increased risk for organ failure and a trend toward a longer hospital stay compared to non-ACS patients. This was described by Offner and colleagues, who recorded ACS in 33% (17 of 52) of their post-DCS patients and showed that ACS was associated with a higher incidence of adult respiratory distress syndrome and multiple organ failures (71 vs. 31% without ACS) [15].

The increased rate of complications in ACS patients is due to the direct compromise of organ function caused by abdominal hypertension, as well as by the greater severity of physiologic disturbance that led to ACS at the first place. It is important to identify the population at risk for ACS and monitor diligently for its development. The most widely applied method for abdominal pressure monitoring uses bladder pressure measurements through a three-way transurethral catheter [16–18]. These measurements should take place at least every 2–4 h in the postoperative period. With pressures above 20 mmHg, serious consideration should be given for decompressive laparotomy. Lower abdominal pressures can still be detrimental to organ function in the presence of hypotension, particularly if present for long periods of time. An abdominal perfusion pressure (defined as the difference between the mean arterial pressure and intraabdominal pressure) below 60 mmHg may cause tissue ischemia in important cellular beds, resulting in organ failure [19, 20].

The management of ACS aims to the immediate reduction of intraabdominal hypertension. This is achievable by abdominal decompression through a laparotomy. A review of publications identifying outcomes after abdominal decompression in patients with ACS showed that 84% of decompressed patients had an initial spontaneous improvement of their renal and respiratory functions. However, the mean survival rate for those patients was only 53% (17–75%), which possibly reflected the failure of sustainable benefit once ACS is established [21]. Patients with increasing intra-abdominal pressure and worsening organ failure should undergo decompressive laparotomy as soon as possible. The precise timing still relies on clinical judgment and is not set by widely acceptable guidelines [20]. Despite its life-saving potential, decompressive laparotomy is associated with many adverse events. The ischemia-reperfusion syndrome is almost unavoidable. Sudden metabolic disturbances due to the return of anaerobic byproducts from the abdominal and lower extremity circulation can lead to cardiac arrhythmias and asystolic arrest. The injection of mannitol and sodium bicarbonate before the procedure may be of benefit [11, 22]. Abdominal decompression may also cause bleeding, infection, and fluid loss from the large surface area of the open abdomen [11].

Although the treatment of ACS is important, there is usually some element of delay between recognition, decision-making, and final surgical decompression. Therefore, prevention becomes key. Avoiding primary fascial closure after DCS is advisable for many patients [3, 23–25]. Offner and colleagues showed that fascial closure following DCS was associated with an 11-fold increase in ACS compared with simple skin or Bogota bag closure of the abdomen [15]. Similarly, Ivatury and colleagues compared patients who underwent primary fascial closure with those who received prophylactic absorbable mesh closure and concluded that the latter group of patients had significantly lower incidence of abdominal hypertension, organ failure, and death [3].

22.2.2 Entero-Atmospheric Fistula

Exposed or entero-atmospheric fistula (EAF) is defined as an abnormal communication between gastrointestinal tract and skin. Its incidence ranges from 2 to 25% [6]. EAF is associated with substantial increase in morbidity and mortality [22, 26]. It has been established that the risk of fistula increases with prolonged exposure of open viscera to air, which causes dehydration and desiccation of the bowel. Frequent dressing changes required in such wounds contribute to the risk by causing abrasion and eventually perforation [27, 28]. Fabian and others reported cases of EAF in open abdomens occurring after erratic increase of the intra-intestinal pressure while coughing or performing a Valsalva mechanism [22]. The type of prosthetic mesh and the duration of its application have been associated with EAF formation [29, 30]. Schecter and colleagues noted that ongoing peritonitis from intestinal leaks causes inflammation of bowel, friability of its wall, and predisposition for EAF [28].

It is, therefore, desirable to protect the exposed bowel by closing the wound as soon as possible [22, 28]. A variety of techniques have been used. Simple skin grafting carries the disadvantage of a long period of bowel exposure until the wound granulates and is appropriate for a graft. It also results in complete loss of abdominal domain as the abdominal muscles are left to retract laterally with formation of a large hernia. Split-thickness skin grafting as the sole method of open abdominal wound coverage has been infrequently used in modern practice. Similarly, prosthetic meshes are being used with decreasing frequency because they are abrasive to the bowel surface and not resistant to infection, when placed in an abdominal environment that is by definition contaminated [31–33]. Jerningan and others suggested that by using an absorbable mesh instead of permanent one, effective temporary abdominal wall defect coverage can be achieved with a low fistula rate [29]. The component separation technique and biologic meshes are the most recent advancements for closure of these wounds and used extensively. The component separation technique has many iterations, but basically involves the release of the fascia laterally to allow the rectus muscle to approach at the midline and achieve primary fascial closure [31, 34, 35]. Biologic meshes are being harvested from human cadavers or animals. After proprietary processes, any cells are removed, and only the collagen structure remains. This is hypothesized to function as the matrix for the host's own cells to migrate and own fascia to regenerate [36–38]. Acellular dermal matrix from human cadaveric skin (Alloderm®, Lifecell, Branchburg, NJ) is the most widely used. Resistance to infection and lack of adhesions with the underlying bowel are valuable properties, but the long-term durability is questioned. Thinning and outstretching of these materials have led to hernia recurrence in the long-term, requiring reoperation [36, 39]. However, they remain a very useful alternative for the acute closure of the open abdomen. Often, a combination of component separation and biologic mesh is necessary. The vacuum-assisted closure technique [40, 41] has helped tremendously in the management and early closure of open abdomens. Studies describing the use of this technique in the management of open abdomen showed lower EAF rates (4.3–4.5%) compared with biosynthetic materials [42, 43].

Fistula closure is spontaneous in one-third of the cases with expectant management [44], whereas two-thirds will require surgical intervention. The management of EAF depends on its size and location. A small fistula on the lateral aspect of the wound is more likely to resolve spontaneously when the wound granulates and contracts over it [22]. However, EAF developing in the middle of an open abdomen is especially challenging to manage. Intubation of the fistula by a suction drain or Foley catheter in order to direct the flow and avoid spillage has often achieved the opposite result, i.e., enlarging the hole [45]. Subramrian and colleagues described the "floating stoma" that consists of covering the wound by a temporary silo (saline bag) and suturing the stoma directly to it, thus creating a physical barrier between the intestinal effluent and the peritoneal cavity [45]. Fabian and colleagues proposed skin grafting the entire wound around the fistula and applying a collection bag on the graft and around the fistula. They used this technique only for EAF originating in the distal small bowel. High-volume EAF occurring in the proximal small bowel was managed within the first 7 to 10 days by resection of the fistulous part, primary anastomosis, and placement of the anastomotic suture line deep between bowel loops. The authors found that patients have better outcomes with this early approach, rather than waiting several weeks to months and having their nutritional status and overall recovery continue to deteriorate while on total parenteral nutrition [22]. Recently, a number of studies described the successful use of the vacuum pack technique in controlling fistula effluent and eventual healing of the fistula. Goverman and colleagues described the "Fistula VAC" technique, which consisted of using a modified VAC®. (Vacuum Assisted Closure, VAC®, KCI Inc, San Antonio, TX) sponge, tailored to fit precisely on the wound, with a hole matching the enteric opening. A 75 mmHg continuous negative was applied through a polyurethane drape, and a 2 cm hole was cut in the drape directly over the enteric opening to allow the placement of an ostomy appliance adjacent to it. The authors used this technique on five patients and showed that by creating a barrier between the open abdominal wound bed and the enteric opening via confluent negative pressure, the system resulted in complete isolation of the fistula and 100% fecal diversion was achieved [46]. Studies by Erdmann and colleagues and Hyon and coworkers describing the use of the modified VAC® system in the management of high-output fistula showed complete fistula and wound closure after 56 and 50 days, respectively [47, 48].

22.2.3   Intra-Abdominal Abscess

Intra-abdominal abscess (IAA) after DCS was shown to increase mortality two-fold [49]. Its incidence ranges between 12 and 69% [2] and increases after multiple procedures or spillage from hollow visceral injuries (up to 82%) [50–52]. Swarpoo and colleagues showed significant difference in IAA rates when they compared patients who underwent multiple laparotomies with those who underwent only one (13.7 vs. 1.2 %) [53]. Increased rates of IAA are caused by the use of packing, especially if the laparotomy pads are not removed within 72 h [27, 50, 52]. IAA can lead to wound dehiscence and generalized sepsis and is associated with a mortality rate as high as 30 to 50% (in large disseminated IAA) [51].

Abdominal CT scan is the diagnostic standard of reference and has achieved 97.5% sensitivity in detecting intraabdominal foci of infection in trauma patients with suspected infection of unknown origin [54]. The management of IAA is dependent on its size, etiology, location, and patient physiology. Management options include percutaneous drainage, reoperation, and antibiotic therapy [55]. Small, localized, walled-off abscesses can be identified and are usually managed by CT-guided drainage [51]. Stylianos and colleagues used percutaneous drainage to treat 28 IAAs in 21 postoperative trauma patients [56]. There was only one complication (pneumothorax), and none of the patients required subsequent re-operation for an inadequately drained collection. Kim and colleagues assessed the effectiveness and safety of postoperative percutaneous drainage of IAA with limited accessibility by using a preexisting surgical drain as an access route. They showed an 86% success rate without need for additional percutaneous drainage or surgery in the 6 months of follow-up [57]. Percutaneous drainage of IAA with CT- or ultrasound-guided technique has become the method of choice in the management of postoperative abscesses, as it avoids re-operation and its associated morbidity.

Large, disseminated abscesses with subsequent peritonitis may require exploration and surgical control [51, 58]. The latter entity is also described as uncontrolled intra-abdominal infection that occurs from missed injuries or leaking intestinal repairs [51]. Diversion of the intestinal flow proximal to the leak remains the most suitable approach for these cases [51, 58]. In a collective review, Velmahos and colleagues noted that indications for relaparotomies for abdominal sepsis are still debated and recommended re-laparotomy at regular intervals (every 24–48 h) until complete eradication of sepsis in critically ill patients who cannot easily be assessed clinically and in which radiography was unable to give a diagnosis [59]. The recent advancement of percutaneous drainage has made the need for repeat laparotomies significantly less frequent than before.

Prompt and adequate initiation of empiric antimicrobial therapy concomitant with percutaneous drainage or surgery can help in decreasing the morbidity and mortality in critically ill patients with IAA [60, 61]. Ongoing clinical evidence of infection after 3–5 days of antibiotics should raise the concern of a new or recurrent infection or of inappropriate antibiotic selection [62]. Therapy of IAA by antibiotics alone was evaluated in the nontrauma population by Kumar and and colleagues. The authors concluded that patients with IAA diameter of more than 6.5 cm and a temperature more of than 101.2°F failed this conservative therapy and required percutaneous drainage [63]. Prophylactic use of antibiotics in trauma patients is well described in the literature. However, controversy regarding short vs. long course and single vs. multi-regimen therapy still exists. In a prospective study, long multi-regimen was compared to short single-regimen prophylaxis among critically injured patients; no difference in the multiple organ failure and sepsis was found [64]. In fact, multiple prophylactic antibiotics promoted drug resistance without any benefit. A similar study evaluating patients with penetrating abdominal trauma tested the same hypothesis and found no significant difference in intra-abdominal infections rates between patients treated with long versus a short course of antibiotic prophylaxis [65]. Several other studies also recommend prophylactic administration of a single broad-spectrum antibiotic only for 24 h after the operation [66–68].

22.2.4 Wound Complications

Wound complications such as infection, fascial dehiscence, and skin necrosis, are common in trauma patients undergoing DCS.

Wound infection (WI) occurs in 5–100% after DCS [6]. WI was shown to be associated with the emergent nature of this procedure, degree of contamination, need for blood transfusion, pro-inflammatory reaction, and resultant immunosupression state [69–73]. Other risk factors for WI include obesity, diabetes, hypertension, and steroid use [72]. WI has been associated with complex complications such as dehiscence, evisceration, and wound sinus formation [53, 74].

The wound can be managed by primary closure or delayed primary closure, or left open to heal by contraction and epithelialization. There is still controversy as to whether the skin wound should routinely be left open after DCS. In a prospective randomized trial, the WI rate was evaluated comparing primary skin wound closure vs. leaving the wound open to heal by secondary intention. WI developed in 65% of closed and 36% of open wounds. Primary wound closure, intraabdominal infection, and colectomy were found to be risk factors for development of WI [75]. Similar conclusions were shown by Cohn and colleagues who compared the 2 methods of closure (primary vs. delayed) in dirty abdominal wounds; they showed that delayed closure of these wounds 4 days after surgery yielded a decreased wound infection rate (21%) compared with primary closure (48%) without increasing the length of stay or cost [76].

Prevention of WI should take into consideration the patient's comorbidities and the other related factors. Maintenance of normoglycemia, normothermia, and adequate tissue oxygen tension are crucial in preventing post-operative infection [77–80]. The prophylactic use of antibiotics on arrival in the emergency department as part of resuscitation has been clearly demonstrated [81]. As mentioned earlier, delayed closure of the wound is considered to be a preventive measure when dealing with dirty abdominal wounds.

Treatment of WI often involves opening the wound, evacuation of pus, surgical debridement of any necrotic tissue, and digital exploration of the fascia to evaluate possible dehiscence [62]. Frequent dressing changes allow the tissues to granulate, and the wound heals by secondary intention over several weeks. Early closure of infected wounds that are seemingly improving is often associated with relapse of infection and wound dehiscence [75]. Infections related to complicated abdominal surgery, such as DCS, require broad-spectrum antibiotics [62].

Fascial dehiscence (FD) is defined as the separation of the abdominal musculoaponeurotic layers following surgery. The incidence of FD is much higher in post-DCS patients and has been reported to range between 9 and 25% [6]. This is due to extensive blood loss, tissue damage, and gross peritoneal contamination encountered in DCS [49]. Other anatomic and physiologic risk factors for FD are: Preexisting comorbidities, impaired wound healing, malnutrition, inappropriate technique in closing the wound, increased IAP, wound infection, and IAA [49, 82]. FD causes prolonged hospital stay and increased cost [82–84]. Various randomized studies have compared continuous vs. interrupted suture fascia closure. McNeil and Sugarman compared continuous, absorbable, coated, polyglycolic acid suture with interrupted, nonabsorbable, monofilament suture. The authors found no significant difference in the wound complication rate between the two closure methods, but recommended continuous absorbable suture closure for its economy of time [85]. Several other randomized trials showed no significant difference in incisional hernia or wound complication incidence between continuous and interrupted methods [85–88]. All studies favored the continuous closure method because it was found to be cost-effective, resulted in less foreign body suture material, and resulted in shorter operating time. Studies comparing the use of slowly absorbable vs. nonabsorbable suture material showed no significant difference in the incidence of wound dehiscence.

However, the incidence of prolonged wound pain and suture sinus increased when nonabsorbable material was used [89–91]. A recent meta-analysis of randomized controlled trials of abdominal fascial closures concluded that the best choice to reduce incisional hernia rates without increasing wound pain or the rate of dehiscence is a slowly absorbable continuous suture [92].

By direct pressure on the abdominal wall, ACS may cause ischemia to the fascia followed by necrosis and subsequent dehiscence [82, 83, 93]. Tillou and colleagues showed that 71% of the patients with FD had concurrent IAA [94]. In an earlier report looking at FD in both emergent and elective operations, 44% of patients with FD were found to have IAA [49]. Furthermore, trauma patients undergoing multiple laparotomies were reported to be at higher risk for FD [53]. They also noted that patients with multiple procedures were more prone to develop IAA, and they concluded that IAA could be considered the strongest predictor of FD in the setting of multiple procedures. Similarly, Velmahos and colleagues showed that IAA and WI are independent risk factors for FD [75].

The mainstay in prevention of FD is good technique. Closure of the abdomen under excessive tension causes ischemia of the fascial suture line. Delayed fascial closure after DCS, when the bowel edema has subsided, is preferable to a tight primary closure [26, 27]. The early application of the vacuum-assisted closure has increased the ability to close the fascia in 88% of the DCS patients with only 4.6% FD rate [95]. A similar study by Cothren and colleagues showed that 100% of DCS patients had successful fascial closure using a modified vacuum-assisted technique. However, the study did not report information on the FD rate encountered [96].

The treatment of FD in patients with multiple comorbidities and ongoing inflammation can be achieved only if the underlying problem (IAA, wound infection) causing the dehiscence is addressed in parallel with the establishment of a supportive environment for wound healing. Restoration of abdominal wall integrity by coverage and protection of exposed bowel and cutaneous closure of the wound are the paramount goals of the treatment [97, 98]. Abdominal wall closure can be achieved by secondary healing, surgical closure of all or some of the abdominal wall layer, placement of split-thickness graft, or the use of tissue flaps. When the fascia is involved, its closure can be achieved by delayed primary closure, component separation, prosthetic mesh placement, or a local tissue flap. Frequently, definitive reconstructions should not be performed in an immediate setting due to the wound condition or the general condition of the patient. In these cases, the closure of the wound is done in a delayed setting [97]. (Further details on wound closure will be discussed in Chap. 23.)

22.2.5 Multiple Organ Dysfunction Syndrome

Multiple organ dysfunction syndrome (MODS), also known as progressive systems failure, multiple organ failure, and multiple system organ failure, is characterized by progressive but potentially reversible physiologic dysfunction of two or more organ systems that arises after resuscitation from an acute life-threatening event. The incidence of MODS in high-risk trauma patients ranges from 14 to 43%. Patients with MODS have a poor prognosis, and the mortality rates in patients who develop more than two organ failures are in excess of 60% [6, 99–101].

Multiple factors have been incriminated in the development of MODS in trauma patients. Hietbrink and colleagues classified these as endogenous and exogenous factors. Endogenous factors comprise the genetic predisposition and physical condition, and determine the susceptibility of a trauma patient to MODS. Exogenous factors consist of: (1) The sustained injury (hypoxia, hypotension, organ and soft tissue injuries, fractures), which is considered as the "first hit" on the immune system; and (2) the subsequent burden of operations and resuscitation modalities (ischemia-reperfusion injury, compartment syndrome, operative interventions, infection), which is considered as a "second hit" that can exacerbate the inflammatory reaction [102]. The first hit consists of the release of pro-inflammatory mediators (cytokines, complement), which initiate the systemic inflammatory response syndrome (SIRS) and result in early MODS. This reaction can be worsened by additional insults (second hits). Later, post-injury, negative feedback systems down-regulate early SIRS to limit potential auto-destructive inflammation. This has been described as the compensatory anti-inflammatory response syndrome (CARS) and the mixed antagonist response syndrome (MARS), which can lead to delayed inhibition of the immune system and a late form of MODS [101, 103–105]. Tran and colleagues found that advancing age, preexisting chronic disease, malnutrition, coma on admission, number of blood transfusions, and the use of antacids and H2-blockers were primary predictors of poor outcome [106].

Sustained IAH and ACS can lead to simultaneous functional impairment of several vital systems: Respiratory, cardiovascular, cerebral, gastrointestinal, hepatic, and renal. Thus, patients who develop ACS are prone to develop MODS [11, 14, 107]. Furthermore, decreased mucosal blood flow and bacterial translocation resulting from ACS were shown to contribute to septic complications and MODS [13]. On the other hand, Balogh and colleagues showed that patients receiving supranormal resuscitation (oxygen delivery index ≥ 600 mL/min/m^2) had a higher MODS rate (22%) compared with patients who received normal resuscitation (9%) (oxygen delivery index ≥ 500 mL/min/m^2) [8]. The role of infection in MODS is still debated [101, 108]. Reports of blunt trauma patients demonstrated that MODS could occur in the absence of infection. Goris and colleagues reported that only 33% of trauma patients with MODS had bacterial sepsis [109]. Likewise, Waydhas and colleagues showed that infection and sepsis did not lead to an augmented release of mediators in patients with trauma; they concluded that the role of both entities remains unclear [104].

Prevention of MODS remains its best treatment. Adequate volume resuscitation, adequate nutrition, appropriate antibiotic coverage, and measures taken to prevent complications of DCS (ACS, IAA, EAF) are crucial to avoid the vicious circle that leads to MODS and results in death [110]. Earlier pulmonary and cardiovascular support beginning at the scene of the accident, and prevention and better treatment of head injury, respiratory failure, and sepsis are critical factors for preventing MODS and increasing survival [111].

22.3 Extremity Complications

22.3.1 *Extremity Compartment Syndrome*

Extremity compartment syndrome (ECS) is an acute emergency defined as an unremitting increase in the intracompartmental pressure that most commonly occurs following trauma to the extremities [112]. It is frequently associated with high-energy injuries and long-bone fractures, but may also be aggravated by a tight splint, cast, or dressing that compromises blood flows and causes pressures within a myofascial compartment to increase [113]. Patients at risk are young men who sustained injuries to the long bones [114]. Patients with bleeding disorders or on anticoagulant therapy are also shown to be at high risk for ECS [115]. On the other hand, ECS occurring in trauma patients in the absence of extremities injury has been described. Tremblay and colleagues described a series of 12,000 trauma patients over 5 years, of whom only 10 patients (0.08%) were found to have secondary ECS. ECS occurred in 10 upper extremities and 12 lower extremities. All 10 patients developed signs of SIRS and ARDS, and became noticeably edematous after aggressive fluid resuscitation. Mortality in patients with secondary ECS was 70% [116].

Increasing numbness, paresthesia, and pain out of proportion to examination (even in the presence of pulses) are the early clinical findings of ECS and should trigger immediate intervention to decrease the intra-compartmental pressure. Pallor, pulselessness, and paralysis occur in an advanced stage and imply a delay in diagnosis [117, 118]. If not identified and treated early, tissue necrosis, muscle death, and permanent nerve damage results, due to oxygen deprivation [119]. Studies have shown that physical exam has low sensitivity and positive predictive value in the diagnosis of ECS; however, its negative predictive value and specificity reach 98%. In addition, it was shown that the number of clinical findings correlate with the probability of ECS. When patients had 1 symptom or sign, the probability was 25%, but it reached 93% in the presence of 3 clinical findings [120]. However, by the time the patient develops 3 clinical findings, the diagnosis is usually delayed, and paralysis or even amputation may be unavoidable.

Missed ECS has devastating consequences and is considered a major liability risk for the treating surgeon, especially if there was failure to recognize and diagnose the injury. Since rapid treatment is the key to successful limb salvage, more reliable methods, such as compartmental pressure monitoring, should be used for a timely diagnosis and management of ECS. There are four techniques that have been utilized for tissue pressure measurements in compartment syndrome. These include the Whitesides infusion technique, the Stryker STIC® technique, the Wick catheter, and, finally, the Slit catheter technique. The Stryker® kit (Stryker, Kalamazoo, MI) is the most commonly used, although its reliability has come under question in clinical practice. The significance of measurement of compartment pressures becomes even greater in comatose, unresponsive, uncooperative, or sedated patients who are unable to respond to pain [121, 122]. Whitesides and Heckman showed that ischemic injury begins when tissue pressure is 10–20 mmHg below diastolic pressure and recommended that fasciotomy be performed when intra-compartmental pressures rise to 20 mmHg below diastolic pressure in any patient who has a worsening clinical condition, a documented rising tissue pressure, significant tissue injury, or a history of 6 h of total ischemia of an extremity [123]. In a prospective study, McQueen recommended decompression of the affected compartments when the difference between the diastolic and intracompartmental pressures is less than 30 mmHg [115].

Reduction of the fracture, immobilization, and placement of the injured extremity at the level of the heart are simple measures to be taken to prevent ECS. Complete fasciotomy of all the compartments involved is performed to normalize compartmental pressure and restore tissue perfusion [118]. Fasciotomy can be used as a prophylactic or therapeutic procedure. Therapeutic fasciotomy is usually performed when the intra-compartmental pressures rise and symptoms or signs of ECS are manifested. Fasciotomy is defined as prophylactic when there is anticipation but no presence of high intracompartmental pressures at the time of the fascial incision. The most commonly used criteria for a prophylactic fasciotomy are: A longer-than-6-h delay between injury and revascularization, a co-existing arterial and venous injury especially with ligation of the vein, and significant tissue damage surrounding a vascular injury [124].

The technique of fasciotomy involves an incision through the skin and fascia over the affected compartment. In the lower extremities, the four compartments of the lower leg are decompressed by two separate incisions (lateral and medial). The lateral and anterior compartments are decompressed through a lateral incision, and the superficial and deep posterior compartments are decompressed through a medial incision. Similarly, the thigh and the foot compartments are decompressed by two incision fasciotomy (lateral and medial). The gluteal compartment is usually decompressed by a semicircular incision, curving posteriorly around the acetabulum and often extending to the upper part of the postero-lateral thigh. For the distal upper extremity (forearm), volar or dorsal incisions (or both) are used. In the arm, lateral and medial straight incisions are used to decompress the anterior and posterior compartments, respectively. Five incisions (2 on dorsal, 1 on the thenar, 1 on the hypothenar, and 1 on the carpal tunnel) are used to decompress the hand compartments [124, 125]. Fasciotomy is not a benign procedure and can be associated with complications such as infection, bone necrosis, and malunion of an underlying fracture. Other complications include soft tissue necrosis, wound dehiscence after closure, skin graft-related problems (infection and partial or total graft necrosis), and the need for debridement of tissue after fasciotomy [124]. Velmahos and colleages showed that cases that received prophylactic fasciotomies were associated with trends towards a higher rate of fasciotomy site complications and nonclosure rates than therapeutic ones; they recommended caution against the liberal use of prophylactic fasciotomy [124].

22.3.2 Infection

After DCO surgery, infection occurs frequently and ranges from superficial pin-track infections (PTI) related to external fixation (EF) to deep infections after intramedullary nails (IMN). The latter is challenging and can lead to osteomyelitis and systemic infection [126]. Infection rates increase in open fractures mainly due to the fact that bacteria, debris, or necrotic tissue may often be deeply embedded within the tissue [119, 126].

EF is associated with a high risk of bacterial contamination and PTI [127]. These infections occur predominantly in pins located in the femur, upper tibia, and upper humerus [128]. Incidence rates of PTI in polytrauma patients range between 2.3 and 6.8% [126, 129, 130]. The contamination rate of the pin sites was shown to be substantially increased by the duration of EF. Harwood and colleagues showed that pin track contamination was more common when the external fixator was in place for more than 14 days before conversion to IMN (22.6 vs. 3.4% if conversion in less than 14 days). They concluded that conversion to definitive fixation should be carried out in a timely fashion (<14 days) as soon as the patient's overall physical condition and soft tissue healing allow [126]. The risk of PTI can be reduced if special pin care is taken. Davies and colleagues showed that avoiding thermal injury and local formation of hematoma during surgery and postoperative use of an alcoholic antiseptic and occlusive pressure dressings were associated with lower PTI rates [131]. In a prospective randomized trial comparing three different wound care regimens after EF for distal radial fractures, Egol and colleagues reported a high rate (19%) of local wound complications, including erythema, cellulitis, drainage, clinical or radiographic evidence of pin-loosening, the need for antibiotics, and the need for pin removal before fracture-healing due to infection around external fixation pin sites. However, these complications were minor and treated with oral antibiotics. They found that neither the use of hydrogen peroxide wound care or chlorhexidine-impregnated dressings helped to decrease these complications. On the basis of these results, the authors concluded that no additional wound care beyond the use of dry, sterile dressings for pin-track care after external fixation is needed [132].

Deep infection due to IMN is a complex and precarious complication. Its incidence ranges from 1.7 to 2.3% [129, 130]. Several studies looking at the safety of conversion from EF to IMN showed that prolonged EF and delayed conversion to IMN were associated with high risk of infection [85, 88, 89, 133–135]. Marshall and colleagues showed that PTI is not a contraindication to subsequent conversion to IMN, provided that underlying active osteomyelitis is not present [136]. In a recent report, Yokoyama and colleagues showed that early skin closure within 1 week can minimize deep infections when treating open tibial fractures with secondary IMN after EF [137]. Deep infection after IMN is usually managed with surgical treatment consisting of abscess drainage and soft tissue or bone debridement [126].

Prevention of infection at the site of the wound is a major concern, especially when dealing with an open fracture. Immediate application of sterile dressing can help protect these injuries from contamination and infections. Open fractures should be thoroughly debrided and irrigated under anesthesia [119]. Ostermann and colleagues showed that the timing of wound closure after treatment of an open fracture with antibiotic beads plays a significant role in preventing infection. In this study, patients who developed infection were closed after 18 days whereas those who did not develop infection were closed in the first 8 days [138].

22.4   Summary and Conclusion

The surgeons who take up the challenge of critically ill patients are destined to be unpleasantly confronted by serious complications. Following a catastrophic abdominal injury, abdominal hypertension is almost unavoidable. However, the ability to suspect it according to the type of degree of injuries, to monitor it by appropriate tools, to prevent it by choosing to leave the abdomen open, or to treat it early before it causes physiologic instability makes the difference between optimal and compromised outcomes. The list of interventions, tricks of the trade, and credible solutions for managing or preventing complications is endless. In this chapter, the authors focused on practical issues related to specific complications with the intent of offering guidelines to the clinician who is involved with these complex clinical problems.

References

1. Platell C, Hall J, Dobb G. Impaired renal function due to raised intraabdominal pressure. Intensive Care Med 1990;16:328–329
2. Morris JA, Eddy VA, Blinman TA, Rutherford EJ, Sharp KW. The staged celiotomy for trauma. Issues in unpacking and reconstruction. Ann Surg 1993;217:576–584; discussion 584–586
3. Ivatury RR, Diebel L, Porter JM, Simon RJ. Intra-abdominal hypertension and the abdominal compartment syndrome. Surg Clin North Am 1997;77:783–800
4. Raeburn CD, Moore EE, Biffl WL, Johnson JL, Meldrum DR, Offner PJ, Franciose RJ, Burch JM. The abdominal compartment syndrome is a morbid complication of postinjury damage control surgery. Am J Surg 2001;182:542–546
5. Burch JM, Moore EE, Moore FA, Franciose R. The abdominal compartment syndrome. Surg Clin North Am. 1996;76:833–842
6. Shapiro MB, Jenkins DH, Schwab CW, Rotondo MF. Damage control: Collective review. J Trauma 2000;49:969–978
7. Ertel W, Oberholzer A, Platz A, Stocker R, Trentz O. Incidence and clinical pattern of the abdominal compartment syndrome after "damage-control" laparotomy in 311 patients with severe abdominal and/or pelvic trauma. Crit Care Med 2000;28:1747–1753
8. Balogh Z, McKinley BA, Cocanour CS, Kozar RA, Valdivia A, Sailors M, Moore FA. Supranormal trauma resuscitation causes more cases of abdominal compartment syndrome. Arch Surg 2003;138:637–642; discussion 642–643
9. Kirkpatrick AW, Balogh Z, Ball CG, Ahmed N, Chun R, McBeth P, Kirby A, Zygun D. The secondary abdominal compartment syndrome: Iatrogenic or unavoidable? J Am Coll Surg 2006;202:668–679

10. McNelis J, Marini CP, Jurkiewicz A, Fields S, Caplin D, Stein D, Ritter G, Nathan I, Simms HH. Predictive factors associated with the development of abdominal compartment syndrome in the surgical intensive care unit. Arch Surg 2002;137:133–136

11. Moore AF, Hargest R, Martin M, Delicata RJ. Intra-abdominal hypertension and the abdominal compartment syndrome. Br J Surg 2004;91:1102–1110

12. McNelis J, Marini CP, Simms HH. Abdominal compartment syndrome: Clinical manifestations and predictive factors. Curr Opin Crit Care 2003;9:133–136

13. Diebel LN, Dulchavsky SA, Brown WJ. Splanchnic ischemia and bacterial translocation in the abdominal compartment syndrome. J Trauma 1997;43:852–855

14. Serpytis M, Ivaskevicius J. Intra-abdominal hypertension and multiple organ dysfunction syndrome. Medicina (Kaunas) 2005;41:903–909

15. Offner PJ, de Souza AL, Moore EE, Biffl WL, Franciose RJ, Johnson JL, Burch JM. Avoidance of abdominal compartment syndrome in damage-control laparotomy after trauma. Arch Surg 2001;136:676–681

16. Malbrain ML. Different techniques to measure intra-abdominal pressure (IAP): Time for a critical re-appraisal. Intensive Care Med 2004;30:357–371

17. Balogh Z, De Waele JJ, Malbrain ML. Continuous intra-abdominal pressure monitoring. Acta Clin Belg Suppl 2007;1:26–32

18. Balogh Z, Jones F, D'Amours S, Parr M, Sugrue M. Continuous intra-abdominal pressure measurement technique. Am J Surg 2004;188:679–684

19. Malbrain ML, Cheatham ML, Kirkpatrick A, Sugrue M, Parr M, De Waele J, Balogh Z, Leppäniemi A, Olvera C, Ivatury R, D'Amours S, Wendon J, Hillman K, Johansson K, Kolkman K, Wilmer A. Results from the international conference of experts on intra-abdominal hypertension and abdominal compartment syndrome. I. Definitions. Intensive Care Med 2006;32:1722–1732

20. Cheatham ML, Malbrain ML, Kirkpatrick A, Sugrue M, Parr M, De Waele J, Balogh Z, Leppäniemi A, Olvera C, Ivatury R, D'Amours S, Wendon J, Hillman K, Wilmer A. Results from the international conference of experts on intra-abdominal hypertension and abdominal compartment syndrome. II. Recommendations. Intensive Care Med 2007;33:951–962

21. Sugrue M, D'Amours S. Review of publications identifying outcomes after abdominal decompression in patients with ACS. J Trauma 2001;51:419

22. Fabian TC. Damage control in trauma: Laparotomy wound management acute to chronic. Surg Clin North Am 2007;87:73-93, vi

23. Sherck J, Seiver A, Shatney C, Oakes D, Cobb L. Covering the "open abdomen": A better technique. Am Surg 1998;64:854–857

24. Mayberry JC, Mullins RJ, Crass RA, Trunkey DD. Prevention of abdominal compartment syndrome by absorbable mesh prosthesis closure. Arch Surg 1997;132:957–961; discussion 961–962

25. Eddy V, Nunn C, Morris JA. Abdominal compartment syndrome. The Nashville experience. Surg Clin North Am 1997;77:801–812

26. Miller RS, Morris JA, Diaz JJ, Herring MB, May AK. Complications after 344 damage-control open celiotomies. J Trauma 2005;59:1365–1371; discussion 1371–1374

27. Martin RR, Byrne M. Postoperative care and complications of damage control surgery. Surg Clin North Am 1997;77:929–942

28. Schecter WP, Ivatury RR, Rotondo MF, Hirshberg A. Open abdomen after trauma and abdominal sepsis: A strategy for management. J Am Coll Surg 2006;203:390–396

29. Jernigan TW, Fabian TC, Croce MA, Moore N, Pritchard FE, Minard G, Bee TK. Staged management of giant abdominal wall defects: Acute and long-term results. Ann Surg 2003;238:349–355; discussion 355–357

30. Mayberry JC, Burgess EA, Goldman RK, Pearson TE, Brand D, Mullins RJ. Enterocutaneous fistula and ventral hernia after absorbable mesh prosthesis closure for trauma: The plain truth. J Trauma 2004;57:157–162; discussion 163

31. Joels CS, Vanderveer AS, Newcomb WL, Lincourt AE, Polhill JL, Jacobs DG, Sing RF. Abdominal wall reconstruction after temporary abdominal closure: A ten-year review. Surg Innov 2006;13:223–230

32. Aldridge AJ, Simson JN. Erosion and perforation of colon by synthetic mesh in a recurrent paracolostomy hernia. Hernia 2001;5:110–112
33. Voyles CR, Richardson JD, Bland KI, Tobin GR, Flint LM, Polk HC. Emergency abdominal wall reconstruction with polypropylene mesh: Short-term benefits versus long-term complications. Ann Surg 1981;194:219–223
34. Howdieshell TR, Proctor CD, Sternberg E, Cué JI, Mondy JS, Hawkins ML. Temporary abdominal closure followed by definitive abdominal wall reconstruction of the open abdomen. Am J Surg 2004;188:301–306
35. Shestak KC, Edington HJ, Johnson RR. The separation of anatomic components technique for the reconstruction of massive midline abdominal wall defects: Anatomy, surgical technique, applications, and limitations revisited. Plast Reconstr Surg 2000;105:731–738; quiz 739
36. Schuster R, Singh J, Safadi BY, Wren SM. The use of acellular dermal matrix for contaminated abdominal wall defects: Wound status predicts success. Am J Surg 2006;192:594–597
37. Patton JH, Berry S, Kralovich KA. Use of human acellular dermal matrix in complex and contaminated abdominal wall reconstructions. Am J Surg 2007;193:360–363; discussion 363
38. Kim H, Bruen K, Vargo D. Acellular dermal matrix in the management of high-risk abdominal wall defects. Am J Surg 2006;192:705–709
39. de Moya M, Dunham M, Inaba K, Bahouth H, Alam HB, Sultan B, Namias N. Long-term outcome of human acellular dermal matrix when used for large traumatic open abdomen. J Trauma 2008;65(2):349–353
40. Schein M, Saadia R, Jamieson JR, Decker GA. The "sandwich technique" in the management of the open abdomen. Br J Surg 1986;73:369–370
41. Brock WB, Barker DE, Burns RP. Temporary closure of open abdominal wounds: The vacuum pack. Am Surg 1995;61:30–35
42. Smith LA, Barker DE, Chase CW, Somberg LB, Brock WB, Burns RP. Vacuum pack technique of temporary abdominal closure: A four-year experience. Am Surg 1997;63:1102–1107; discussion 1107–1108
43. Barker DE, Kaufman HJ, Smith LA, Ciraulo DL, Richart CL, Burns RP. Vacuum pack technique of temporary abdominal closure: A 7-year experience with 112 patients. J Trauma 2000;48:201–206; discussion 206–207
44. Buechter KJ, Leonovicz D, Hastings PR, Fonts C. Enterocutaneous fistulas following laparotomy for trauma. Am Surg 1991;57:354–358
45. Subramaniam MH, Liscum KR, Hirshberg A. The floating stoma: A new technique for controlling exposed fistulae in abdominal trauma. J Trauma 2002;53:386–388
46. Goverman J, Yelon JA, Platz JJ, Singson RC, Turcinovic M. The "Fistula VAC," a technique for management of enterocutaneous fistulae arising within the open abdomen: Report of 5 cases. J Trauma 2006;60:428–431; discussion 431
47. Erdmann D, Drye C, Heller L, Wong MS, Levin SL. Abdominal wall defect and enterocutaneous fistula treatment with the Vacuum-Assisted Closure (V.A.C.) system. Plast Reconstr Surg 2001;108:2066–2068
48. Hyon SH, Martinez-Garbino JA, Benati ML, Lopez-Avellaneda ME, Brozzi NA, Argibay PF. Management of a high-output postoperative enterocutaneous fistula with a vacuum sealing method and continuous enteral nutrition. ASAIO J 2000;46:511–514
49. Graham DJ, Stevenson JT, McHenry CR. The association of intra-abdominal infection and abdominal wound dehiscence. Am Surg 1998;64:660–665
50. Abikhaled JA, Granchi TS, Wall MJ, Hirshberg A, Mattox KL. Prolonged abdominal packing for trauma is associated with increased morbidity and mortality. Am Surg 1997;63:1109–1112; discussion 1112–1113
51. Hirshberg A, Stein M, Adar R. Reoperation. Planned and unplanned. Surg Clin North Am 1997;77:897–907
52. Ivatury RR, Nallathambi M, Gunduz Y, Constable R, Rohman M, Stahl WM. Liver packing for uncontrolled hemorrhage: A reappraisal. J Trauma 1986;26:744–753
53. Swaroop M, Williams M, Greene WR, Sava J, Park K, Wang D. Multiple laparotomies are a predictor of fascial dehiscence in the setting of severe trauma. Am Surg 2005;71:402–405

54. Velmahos GC, Kamel E, Berne TV, Yassa N, Ramicone E, Song Z, Demetriades D. Abdominal computed tomography for the diagnosis of intra-abdominal sepsis in critically injured patients: Fishing in murky waters. Arch Surg 1999;134:831–836; discussion 836–838
55. Schöffel U, Häring R, Farthmann EH. Diagnosis and treatment strategy of intra-abdominal abscess. Zentralbl Chir 1993;118:303–308
56. Stylianos S, Martin EC, Starker PM, Laffey KJ, Bixon R, Forde KA. Percutaneous drainage of intra-abdominal abscesses following abdominal trauma. J Trauma 1989;29:584–588
57. Kim YJ, Han JK, Lee JM, Kim SH, Lee KH, Park SH, An SK, Lee JY, Choi BI, Percutaneous drainage of postoperative abdominal abscess with limited accessibility: Preexisting surgical drains as alternative access route. Radiology 2006;239:591–598
58. Sagraves SG, Toschlog EA, Rotondo MF. Damage control surgery – the intensivist's role. J Intensive Care Med 2006;21:5–16
59. Velmahos GC, Degiannis E, Souter I. Relaparotomies for abdominal sepsis – why, when, how? A collective review. S Afr J Surg 1998;36:52–56
60. Blot S, De Waele JJ. Critical issues in the clinical management of complicated intra-abdominal infections. Drugs 2005;65:1611–1620
61. Laterre PF, Colardyn F, Delmée M, De Waele J, Legrand JC, Van Eldere J, Vergison A, Vogelaers D. Antimicrobial therapy for intra-abdominal infections: Guidelines from the Infectious Disease Advisory Board (IDAB). Acta Chir Belg 2006;106:2–21
62. Schein M, Marshall J. Source control for surgical infections. World J Surg 2004;28:638–645
63. Kumar RR, Kim JT, Haukoos JS, Macias LH, Dixon MR, Stamos MJ, Konyalian VR. Factors affecting the successful management of intra-abdominal abscesses with antibiotics and the need for percutaneous drainage. Dis Colon Rectum 2006;49:183–189
64. Velmahos GC, Toutouzas KG, Sarkisyan G, Chan LS, Jindal A, Karaiskakis M, Katkhouda N, Berne TV, Demetriades D. Severe trauma is not an excuse for prolonged antibiotic prophylaxis. Arch Surg 2002;137:537–541; discussion 541–542
65. Cornwell EE III, Dougherty WR, Berne TV, Velmahos G, Murray JA, Chahwan S, Belzberg H, Falabella A, Morales IR, Asensio J, Demetriades D. Duration of antibiotic prophylaxis in high-risk patients with penetrating abdominal trauma: A prospective randomized trial. J Gastrointest Surg 1999;3:648–653
66. Fabian TC. Prevention of infections following penetrating abdominal trauma. Am J Surg 1993;165:14S–19S
67. Kirton OC, O'Neill PA, Kestner M, Tortella BJ. Perioperative antibiotic use in high-risk penetrating hollow viscus injury: A prospective randomized, double-blind, placebo-control trial of 24 hours versus 5 days. J Trauma 2000;49:822–832
68. Sarmiento JM, Aristizabal G, Rubiano J, Ferrada R. Prophylactic antibiotics in abdominal trauma. J Trauma 1994;37:803–806
69. Aprahamian C, Wittmann DH, Bergstein JM, Quebbeman EJ. Temporary abdominal closure (TAC) for planned relaparotomy (etappenlavage) in trauma. J Trauma 1990;30:719–723
70. Nichols RL, Smith JW, Klein DB, Trunkey DD, Cooper RH, Adinolfi MF, Mills J. Risk of infection after penetrating abdominal trauma. N Engl J Med 1984;311:1065–1070
71. Petersen K, Riddle MS, Danko JR, Blazes DL, Hayden R, Tasker SA, Dunne JR. Trauma-related infections in battlefield casualties from Iraq. Ann Surg 2007;245:803–811
72. Cheadle WG. Risk factors for surgical site infection. Surg Infect (Larchmt) 2006;7 Suppl 1:S7–S11
73. Sørensen LT, Hemmingsen U, Kallehave F, Wille-Jørgensen P, Kjærgaard J, Nørgaard Møller L, Jørgensen T. Risk factors for tissue and wound complications in gastrointestinal surgery. Ann Surg 2005;241:654–658
74. Bucknall TE. Factors influencing wound complications: A clinical and experimental study. Ann R Coll Surg Engl 1983;65:71–77
75. Velmahos GC, Vassiliu P, Demetriades D, Chan LS, Murray J, Salim A, Sava J, Katkhouda N, Berne TV. Wound management after colon injury: Open or closed? A prospective randomized trial. Am Surg 2002;68:795–801

76. Cohn SM, Giannotti G, Ong AW, Esteban Varela J, Shatz DV, McKenney MG, Sleeman D, Ginzburg E, Augenstein JS, Byers PM, Sands LR, Hellinger MD, Namias N. Prospective randomized trial of two wound management strategies for dirty abdominal wounds. Ann Surg 2001;233:409–413

77. Latham R, Lancaster AD, Covington JF, Pirolo JS, Thomas CS. The association of diabetes and glucose control with surgical-site infections among cardiothoracic surgery patients. Infect Control Hosp Epidemiol 2001;22:607–612

78. Hopf HW, Hunt TK, West JM, Blomquist P, Goodson WH III, Jensen JA, Jonsson K, Paty PB, Rabkin JM, Upton RA, von Smitten K, Whitney JD. Wound tissue oxygen tension predicts the risk of wound infection in surgical patients. Arch Surg 1997;132:997–1004; discussion 1005

79. Greif R, Akça O, Horn EP, Kurz A, Sessler DI. Supplemental perioperative oxygen to reduce the incidence of surgical-wound infection. Outcomes Research Group. N Engl J Med 2000;342:161–167

80. Kurz A, Sessler DI, Lenhardt R. Perioperative normothermia to reduce the incidence of surgical-wound infection and shorten hospitalization. Study of Wound Infection and Temperature Group. N Engl J Med 1996;334:1209–1215

81. Fullen WD, Hunt J, Altemeier WA. Prophylactic antibiotics in penetrating wounds of the abdomen. J Trauma 1972;12:282–289

82. Mäkelä JT, Kiviniemi H, Juvonen T, Laitinen S. Factors influencing wound dehiscence after midline laparotomy. Am J Surg 1995;170:387–390

83. Pavlidis TE, Galatianos IN, Papaziogas BT, Lazaridis CN, Atmatzidis KS, Makris JG, Papaziogas TB. Complete dehiscence of the abdominal wound and incriminating factors. Eur J Surg 2001;167:351–354; discussion 355

84. Rodríguez-Hermosa JI, Codina-Cazador A, Ruiz B, Roig J, Gironès J, Pujada M, Pont J, Aldeguer X, Acero D. Risk factors for acute abdominal wall dehiscence after laparotomy in adults. Cir Esp 2005;77:280–286

85. McNeil PM, Sugerman HJ. Continuous absorbable vs interrupted nonabsorbable fascial closure. A prospective, randomized comparison. Arch Surg 1986;121:821–823

86. Colombo M, Maggioni A, Parma G, Scalambrino S, Milani R. A randomized comparison of continuous versus interrupted mass closure of midline incisions in patients with gynecologic cancer. Obstet Gynecol 1997;89:684–689

87. Trimbos JB, Smit IB, Holm JP, Hermans J. A randomized clinical trial comparing two methods of fascia closure following midline laparotomy. Arch Surg 1992;127:1232–1234

88. Richards PC, Balch CM, Aldrete JS. Abdominal wound closure. A randomized prospective study of 571 patients comparing continuous vs. interrupted suture techniques. Ann Surg 1983;197:238–243

89. Gys T, Hubens A. A prospective comparative clinical study between monofilament absorbable and non-absorbable sutures for abdominal wall closure. Acta Chir Belg 1989;89:265–270

90. Larsen PN, Nielsen K, Schultz A, Mejdahl S, Larsen T, Moesgaard F. Closure of the abdominal fascia after clean and clean-contaminated laparotomy. Acta Chir Scand 1989;155:461–464

91. Wissing J, van Vroonhoven TJ, Schattenkerk ME, Veen HF, Ponsen RJ, Jeekel J. Fascia closure after midline laparotomy: Results of a randomized trial. Br J Surg 1987;74:738–741

92. van't Riet M, Steyerberg EW, Nellensteyn J, Bonjer HJ, Jeekel J. Meta-analysis of techniques for closure of midline abdominal incisions. Br J Surg 2002;89:1350–1356

93. Webster C, Neumayer L, Smout R, Horn S, Daley J, Henderson W, Khuri S, National Veterans Affairs Surgical Quality Improvement Program.Prognostic models of abdominal wound dehiscence after laparotomy. J Surg Res 2003;109:130-137

94. Tillou A, Weng J, Alkousakis T, Velmahos G. Fascial dehiscence after trauma laparotomy: A sign of intra-abdominal sepsis. Am Surg 2003;69:927–929

95. Miller PR, Meredith JW, Johnson JC, Chang MC. Prospective evaluation of vacuum-assisted fascial closure after open abdomen: Planned ventral hernia rate is substantially reduced. Ann Surg 2004;239:608–614; discussion 614–616

96. Cothren CC, Moore EE, Johnson JL, Moore JB, Burch JM. One hundred percent fascial approximation with sequential abdominal closure of the open abdomen. Am J Surg 2006;192:238–242

97. Heller L, Levin SL, Butler CE. Management of abdominal wound dehiscence using vacuum assisted closure in patients with compromised healing. Am J Surg 2006;191:165–172

98. McNeeley SG, Hendrix SL, Bennett SM, Singh A, Ransom S, Kmak DC, Morley GW. Synthetic graft placement in the treatment of fascial dehiscence with necrosis and infection. Am J Obstet Gynecol 1998;179:1430–1434; discussion 1434–1435

99. Durham RM, Moran JJ, Mazuski JE, Shapiro MJ, Baue AE, Flint LM. Multiple organ failure in trauma patients. J Trauma 2003;55:608–616

100. Montalvo JA, Acosta JA, Rodríguez P, Alejandro K, Sárraga A. Surgical complications and causes of death in trauma patients that require temporary abdominal closure. Am Surg 2005;71:219–224

101. Moore FA, Sauaia A, Moore EE, Haenel JB, Burch JM, Lezotte DC. Postinjury multiple organ failure: A bimodal phenomenon. J Trauma 1996;40:501–510; discussion 510–512

102. Hietbrink F, Koenderman L, Rijkers G, Leenen L. Trauma: The role of the innate immune system. World J Emerg Surg 2006;1:15

103. Keel M, Trentz O. Pathophysiology of polytrauma. Injury 2005;36:691–709

104. Waydhas C, Nast-Kolb D, Jochum M, Trupka A, Lenk S, Fritz H, Duswald KH, Schweiberer L. Inflammatory mediators, infection, sepsis, and multiple organ failure after severe trauma. Arch Surg 1992;127:460–467

105. Waydhas C, Nast-Kolb D, Trupka A, Zettl R, Kick M, Wiesholler J, Schweiberer L, Jochum M. Posttraumatic inflammatory response, secondary operations, and late multiple organ failure. J Trauma 1996;40:624–630; discussion 630–631

106. Tran DD, Cuesta MA, van Leeuwen PA, Nauta JJ, Wesdorp RI. Risk factors for multiple organ system failure and death in critically injured patients. Surgery 1993;114:21–30

107. Krivoruchko IA, Bo ko VV, Se dametov RR, Andreeshchev SA. Re-laparotomy and damage control during surgical treatment of postoperative intra-abdominal purulent-septic complications. Klin Khir 2004;8:5–8

108. Stillwell M, Caplan ES. The septic multiple-trauma patient. Infect Dis Clin North Am 1989;3:155–183

109. Goris RJ, te Boekhorst TP, Nuytinck JK, Gimbrère JS. Multiple-organ failure. Generalized autodestructive inflammation? Arch Surg 1985;120:1109–1115

110. Baue AE, Durham R, Faist E. Systemic inflammatory response syndrome (SIRS), multiple organ dysfunction syndrome (MODS), multiple organ failure (MOF): Are we winning the battle? Shock 1998;10:79–89

111. Faist E, Baue AE, Dittmer H, Heberer G. Multiple organ failure in polytrauma patients. J Trauma 1983;23:775–787

112. Middleton C. Compartment syndrome: The importance of early diagnosis. Nurs Times 2003;99:30–32

113. Mubarak SJ, Hargens AR. Compartment syndromes and Volkman's contracture. Monographs in clinical orthopedics 3. Philadelphia: WBSaunders, 1981:37–44, 66–68, 100–101

114. McQueen MM, Gaston P, Court-Brown CM. Acute compartment syndrome. Who is at risk? J Bone Joint Surg Br 2000;82:200–203

115. McQueen M. Acute compartment syndrome. Acta Chir Belg 1998;98:166–170

116. Tremblay LN, Feliciano DV, Rozycki GS. Secondary extremity compartment syndrome. J Trauma 2002;53:833–837

117. Gulli B, Templeman D. Compartment syndrome of the lower extremity. Orthop Clin North Am 1994;25:677–684

118. Olson SA, Rhorer AS. Orthopaedic trauma for the general orthopaedist: Avoiding problems and pitfalls in treatment. Clin Orthop Relat Res 2005;3:30–37

119. Bongiovanni MS, Bradley SL, Kelley DM. Orthopedic trauma: Critical care nursing issues. Crit Care Nurs Q 2005;28:60–71

120. Ulmer T. The clinical diagnosis of compartment syndrome of the lower leg: Are clinical findings predictive of the disorder? J Orthop Trauma 2002;16:572–577
121. Heckman MM, Whitesides TE, Grewe SR, Rooks MD. Compartment pressure in association with closed tibial fractures. The relationship between tissue pressure, compartment, and the distance from the site of the fracture. J Bone Joint Surg Am 1994;76:1285–1292
122. Heppenstall RB. An update in compartment syndrome investigation and treatment. UPOJ 1997;10:49–57
123. Whitesides TE, Heckman MM. Acute compartment syndrome: Update on diagnosis and treatment. J Am Acad Orthop Surg 1996;4:209–218
124. Velmahos GC, Theodorou D, Demetriades D, Chan L, Berne TV, Asensio J, Cornwell III EE, Belzberg H, Stewart BM. Complications and nonclosure rates of fasciotomy for trauma and related risk factors. World J Surg 1997;21:247–252; discussion 253
125. Velmahos GC, Toutouzas KG. Vascular trauma and compartment syndromes. Surg Clin North Am 2002;82:125–141, xxi
126. Harwood PJ, Giannoudis PV, Probst C, Krettek C, Pape HC. The risk of local infective complications after damage control procedures for femoral shaft fracture. J Orthop Trauma 2006;20:181–189
127. Roberts CS, Pape HC, Jones AL, Malkani AL, Rodriguez JL, Giannoudis PV. Damage control orthopaedics: Evolving concepts in the treatment of patients who have sustained orthopaedic trauma. Instr Course Lect 2005;54:447–462
128. Lerner A, Chezar A, Haddad M, Kaufman H, Rozen N, Stein H. Complications encountered while using thin-wire-hybrid-external fixation modular frames for fracture fixation. A retrospective clinical analysis and possible support for "Damage Control Orthopaedic Surgery." Injury 2005;36:590–598
129. Scalea TM, Boswell SA, Scott JD, Mitchell KA, Kramer ME, Pollak AN. External fixation as a bridge to intramedullary nailing for patients with multiple injuries and with femur fractures: Damage control orthopedics. J Trauma 2000;48:613–621; discussion 621–623
130. Nowotarski PJ, Turen CH, Brumback RJ, Scarboro JM. Conversion of external fixation to intramedullary nailing for fractures of the shaft of the femur in multiply injured patients. J Bone Joint Surg Am 2000;82:781–788
131. Davies R, Holt N, Nayagam S. The care of pin sites with external fixation. J Bone Joint Surg Br 2005;87:716–719
132. Egol KA, Paksima N, Puopolo S, Klugman J, Hiebert R, Koval KJ. Treatment of external fixation pins about the wrist: A prospective, randomized trial. J Bone Joint Surg Am 2006;88:349–354
133. Chen CE, Ko JY, Wang JW, Wang CJ. Infection after intramedullary nailing of the femur. J Trauma 2003;55:338–344
134. McGraw JM, Lim EV. Treatment of open tibial-shaft fractures. External fixation and secondary intramedullary nailing. J Bone Joint Surg Am 1988;70:900–911
135. Blachut PA, Meek RN, O'Brien PJ. External fixation and delayed intramedullary nailing of open fractures of the tibial shaft. A sequential protocol. J Bone Joint Surg Am 1990;72:729–735
136. Marshall PD, Saleh M, Douglas DL. Risk of deep infection with intramedullary nailing following the use of external fixators. J R Coll Surg Edinb 1991;36:268–271
137. Yokoyama K, Uchino M, Nakamura K, Ohtsuka H, Suzuki T, Boku T, Itoman M. Risk factors for deep infection in secondary intramedullary nailing after external fixation for open tibial fractures. Injury 2006;37:554–560
138. Ostermann PA, Henry SL, Seligson D. Timing of wound closure in severe compound fractures. Orthopedics 1994;17:397–399

Chapter 23
Critical Decision Points in Managing the Open Abdomen

Nathan T. Mowery and John A. Morris Jr

23.1 Post-operative Judgment in Damage Control Surgery

The outcome of the Damage Control Surgery (DCS) patient is equally dependent on decisions made at the initial operation and on a variety of post-operative decisions. Conceptually, DCS can be divided into three sequential phases:

1. Damage Control;
2. Restoration of Physiologic Reserve;
3. Reconstruction.

The goal of DCS is to have a patient who survives his injuries to ultimately undergo reconstruction and who subsequently returns to a productive lifestyle. Achieving this goal requires three critical judgments in three areas:

1. Success/adequacy of the damage control intervention;
2. Timing and location of subsequent operations;
3. Technique to be used when closing the patient.

The formulation of a plan to address these branch points will ultimately determine the mortality of the patient and can significantly impact the morbidity associated with the damage control technique. From the moment the surgeon decides to pursue damage control, a plan must be formulated that includes definitive repair and closure of the patient.

N.T. Mowery (✉)
Department of Surgery, Wake Forest University, Medical Center Boulevard,
Winston-Salem, NC, 27157, USA
e-mail: nmowery@wfubmc.edu

H.-C. Pape et al. (eds.), *Damage Control Management in the Polytrauma Patient*,
DOI 10.1007/978-0-387-89508-6_23, © Springer Science+Business Media, LLC 2010

23.2   Unplanned Reoperation

Whenthe goals of the first phase of DCS fail (control of hemorrhage and contamination), the surgeon must consider reexploration. This unplanned reexploration can be for clinical deterioration manifesting as either bleeding or secondary Abdominal Compartment Syndrome (ACS), and occurs in 15% of patients treated with damage control techniques [1]. The surgeon must show judgment in identification of the etiology for bleeding, as it may be a failure of surgical hemostasis or worsening medical bleeding from coagulopathy. Often, the distinction cannot be made easily without surgical exploration. In previous work, authors have shown that in patients requiring emergent reoperation, both surgical and medical bleeding are found at the time of exploration [1]. In addition, where and when this takes place can speed the process, leading to improved outcomes.

23.2.1   Continued Surgical Bleeding

Ongoing diffuse bleeding in this environment continues to be an ominous sign and a predictor of early trauma-related mortality [2, 3]. The markers of surgical bleeding are falling hematocrit, increasing drain output, and failure of the patient to achieve end points of resuscitation. Patients who underwent unplanned reoperation required more transfusion at the initial operation, in the Intensive Care Unit (ICU), and at the time of reoperation. This is despite the fact that acuity, measured by ISS, suggested similar injury patterns but diminished physiologic reserve [1].

23.2.2   Mechanical Bleeding vs. Medical Coagulopathy

The lethal triad of acidosis, hypothermia, and consumptive coagulopathy has been well established as a cause for ongoing bleeding in the trauma population and serves as the foundation for DCS [1, 4–14]. Determining the etiology of ongoing bleeding is challenging. The correction of hypothermia is the most urgent issue, as bleeding will continue despite fresh frozen plasma and platelets until the patient's temperature exceeds 35°C [15, 16]. Once hypothermia is corrected, unabated bleeding of greater than 2 units RBCs/hr suggests the need for reexploration, identification of surgical bleeding, and repacking [1]. Another useful landmark is the postoperative transfusion of greater than 10 units in a 24 h period, especially in the face of corrected thrombocytopenia or coagulopathy. Postoperative bleeding of greater than 10 units of packed red blood cells in 24 h or bleeding greater than 2 units an hour is an indication for reexploration.

23.2.3   How to Intervene

Once the decision has been made that the bleeding is due to ongoing surgical bleeding, the surgeon must decide upon the most appropriate intervention. Certain injury patterns may lend themselves to an interventional radiology approach. Studies have shown good outcomes in managing a variety of injuries with embolization including: Solid organ injuries [17, 18], pelvic injuries [19, 20], and even peripheral vascular injuries [21, 22]. These cases where bleeding is inaccessible or damage was caused by attempting to access them are often best treated with a combination of operative intervention (packing or ligation) combined with IR intervention. Velmahos and colleagues used this combined technique in penetrating abdominal trauma where surgical intervention had failed or where there was a late vascular complication after a successful operative intervention. They found that angiographic embolization after penetrating injuries to the abdomen is safe and effective for selected patients. It was a valuable tool for bleeding control when surgery had failed; it may be the treatment of choice for control of late vascular complications when reoperation is not desirable [23]. This staged approach to difficult bleeding has also been shown to be beneficial in controlling otherwise lethal injuries in hepatic injury [24].

Also, the geographic location of reexploration must be considered. In certain situations, such as vascular injuries and complex reconstructions, reexploration is best performed in the operating room. However, the majority of reexplorations can be performed at the bedside in the intensive care unit. This can only be done if Bedside Laparotomy (BL) protocols have been developed and practiced in advance [25]. Issues that require bedside reexploration include: High ventilatory requirements, hemodynamic instability that precludes transport or unstable intercranial hypertension. Bedside surgery has limitations: Inadequate lighting, a less sterile environment than the OR, absence of trained personnel, and limited surgical instruments. However, Diaz and colleagues were able to show that despite the high acuity of the population undergoing BSL, 50.7% of patients survived. Moreover, during bedside laparotomy, intra-abdominal abscess rate and fistula formation occurred at low rates [26]. In the end, defined criteria that preclude patient transport are lacking; the decision falls on clinical judgment to guide the surgeon, but he/she should feel confident that bedside laparotomy is a proven technique that is commonly practiced at a variety of trauma centers.

23.3   Planned Reexploration

The timing of reexploration and pack removal is important. It is important to view this as a decision that is independent of when to attempt definitive closure in these patients, which is a later intervention. Unpacking a patient before he/she is ready will lead to unnecessary bleeding and consumption of a limited resource in the form of blood loss. Late pack removal will result in unnecessary loss of abdominal domain and potentially increased infection and fistula formation. Traditionally, a time period, usually 24–48 h, was allowed to elapse before reexploration, with the thought that correction of physiology was not possible in less time [1]. Other authors have suggested definitive laboratory criteria, such as PT and PTT < 1.25 times normal, the platelet count > 100,000/mm³, and the fibrinogen level > 100 mg/ de [27]. However, more recent approaches suggest that the decision should allow for earliest possible time when normal physiology has been achieved and the patient has restored physiologic reserve [1, 3].

Control of contamination is another cornerstone of DCS. Each time the abdomen in unpacked, an attempt to irrigate to decrease bacterial counts should be made. This is often performed at the patient's bedside under full barrier precautions. The surgeon should use these windows into the abdomen to evaluate contamination, hemostasis, and degree of inflammation, all of which play key roles in determining progression to the next stage of the plan, which is reconstruction.

23.4   When to Consider Reconstruction

Damage control strategies often necessitate leaving the bowel in discontinuity. The decision to restore bowel continuity must balance the need for establishing enteral nutrition, with the risk of anastomotic failure. The surgeon must assess the patient's degree of bowel edema. Patients requiring more resuscitation will likely have persistent edema that would complicate an attempted anastomosis. It is imperative that the surgeon weigh the benefits of delaying an anastomosis to allow for decreasing edema with disadvantages of leaving the patient with an open abdomen. There was been an anecdotal belief that there is a window of 72 h to establish bowel continuity before morbidity increases. It is well documented that anastomoses performed in the face of shock and decompensation have a much higher rate of morbidity, including a higher leak rate and abscess formation [28, 29].

The decision to anastomose the patient is also predicated on the type of anastomosis being performed: Small bowel vs. colon. While a small bowel leak resulting in abdominal collections or fistula can be life threatening, it is often controllable. It is well accepted that small bowel anastomoses can be safely constructed at reoperation or when patient hemodynamics allow time for the procedure. The decision of when to address colonic injuries is more complex. The evolution for management of destructive colon injuries now favors anastomoses vs. colostomy [30–32]. While we use these data as evidence for primary anastomosis, it is important to note that these data examine colonic anastomoses exclusive of patients also undergoing DCS. The timing of the anastomosis can influence the associated morbidity in the event of a complication. Colonic leaks are associated with a higher mortality rate, often necessitating reoperation with diversion that now must be performed in the face of a hostile abdomen. Miller and colleagues reported that anastomotic leak rate, abscess rate, and colon-related death rate were similar among patients who had anastomosis performed at the time of initial surgery vs. in the reconstructive phase of a staged procedure. This leads the authors to suggest that delayed colonic anastomosis is safe, with a similar complication rate [33].

23.5   When to Close

After the threat of surgical bleeding has been eliminated and source control of infectious contamination has been obtained, the operating surgeon should begin to formulate a plan for expedited fascial closure of the abdomen. A marked increase in the risk of associated complications has been shown to rise if the abdomen is unable to be closed within 8 days. The percentage of complications significantly increased in patients closed after 8 days from the time of the initial celiotomy. Twenty-two of 185 patients (12%) who had their fascia closed in 8 days or less developed a complication, whereas 47 of 91 patients (52%) closed after 8 days developed a complication [34] (see Fig. 23.1).

A variety of factors impact achievement of this 8-day deadline and affect the long-term success of the closure. Damage control must be implemented early in the initial operation to optimize outcome [35]. Application of Damage Control (DC) techniques prior to physiologic exhaustion resulted in less hypothermia and decreased abscess and fistula formation. These patients were also subjectively noted to have less bowel edema and were able to undergo definitive abdominal wall closure during their hospital stay [36].

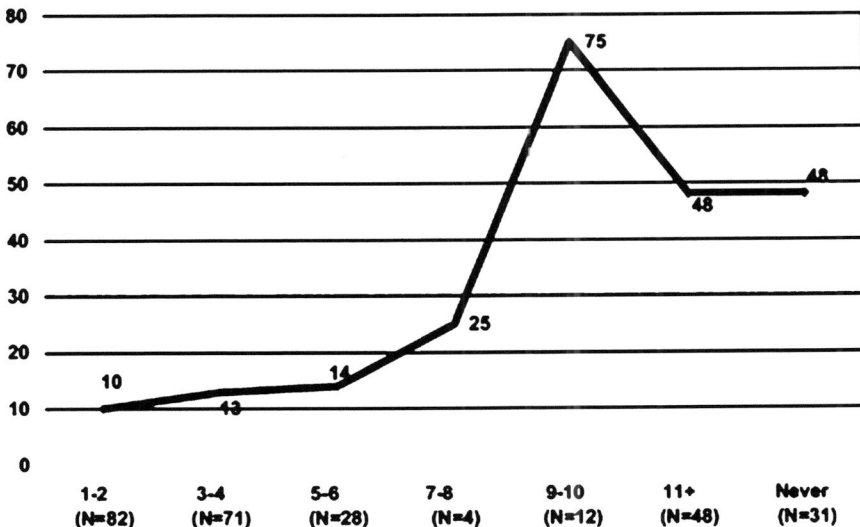

Fig. 23.1 The percentage of complications compared with the timing of fascial closure. (Reproduced with permission of Wolters Kluwer from [34]; discussion 1371–1374)

It is important to preserve the integrity of the fascia leading up to the time of closure. Over the evolution of DCS, a variety of techniques have been employed for temporary closure of the abdomen. Many of these techniques involved directly suturing or fastening material to the patient fascia. While these met the short-term needs of maintaining abdominal domain, repeated manipulation of the fascia led to decreased strength and increased morbidity.

In contrast, preservation of the abdominal domain by employing sutureless negative pressure dressing has been seen as a major advance in expediting the closure of these patients' abdomens. The maintenance of the abdominal domain has been reported, whether employing a makeshift negative pressure dressing or more elaborate pre-manufactured dressings. In a recent report by Stone and colleagues, delayed primary closure with vacuum assistance was achieved in 71.9% of trauma patients with open abdomens [37]. Miller and colleagues reported an abdominal closure rate in patients undergoing vacuum-assisted closure as 88%, with a mean time to closure being 9.5 days [38].

The need to supplement the patient's nutrition to prevent a catabolic state from developing in an already stressed patient is critical. The traditional means of providing calories, both enteral and paraenteral, have been proposed. Traditionally, patients with an open abdomen were fed by a parenteral route secondary to the fact that physicians assumed there would be decreased bowel motility and absorption with an open abdomen. Studies were able to show that enteral feedings with an open abdomen were safe and may lead to decreased bowel wall edema and early closure of the abdomen. Also paramount to the ability to close the patient is the overall fluid status of the patient. While the details of appropriate resuscitation of a trauma patient are outside the bounds of this chapter, carefully balancing the patient's fluid status can greatly affect the success rate of closure. Early resuscitation efforts based on invasive hemodynamic monitoring have been shown to result in the patient reaching earlier correction of the lethal triad, with improved mortality [39, 40]. This could result in less interstitial edema and in higher success rates of abdominal closure. The patient's overall degree of fluid resuscitation can have a profound effect on the success of abdominal closure. Maintaining a negative or total positive fluid balance of less than 20 L before the last attempted fascial closure improved successful closure rates, as seen in 19 of 22 patients (86.4%) [37].

In addition to limiting fluid resuscitation, authors have also suggested that active diuresis can increase the success of closure. There has been mention that the diuresis can be aided by the addition of albumin. This combination has been shown to be successful in removing fluid in other populations [41, 42]; it has not been validated in the open abdomen population.

While the patient's physiology often dictates the rate of transfusion, adopting a more restrictive transfusion strategy may lead to increased success in early abdominal closure. Transfusion of blood and blood products as well as excessive crystalloid resuscitation are known causative factors in the development of the abdominal compartment syndrome [43]. Despite no difference in injury severity between groups, the primary group required significantly less blood transfusions. This could be attributable to numerous factors including earlier initiation of damage control, fewer vascular injuries, or reduced intensive care unit length of stay with less phlebotomy. For whatever reason, this group had the lowest complication rate, most likely related to early primary fascial closure.

Another means to attempt to preserve abdominal domain has been the practice of maintaining chemical paralysis between subsequent trips to the operating theater with open abdomens. This practice stems from the belief that persistent contraction of the abdominal musculature in the nonparalyzed patient can lead to retraction of the fascia and abdominal musculature. There has not been good evidence to support the standard use of paralytics, and, often in this complex patient population, it may subject these patients to additional risks of hypercoagulability, positioning, and long-term polyneuropathy. In the end, the ability to close these patients falls on the shoulders of the surgeon. No amount of monitoring or strategy can substitute for an attentive surgeon who is constantly reassessing the patient and asking the question: Is the patient ready for definitive closure? While a variety of objective means can be applied, they only augment the physician in developing a plan for closure that both meets the patient's current needs and looks to avoid possible pitfalls that may develop in the patient's course and adapts when they develop.

23.6 Abdominal Wall Reconstruction

When reoperating on the patient, consider each time whether the patient can safely be closed. This is predicated on the determination of the degree of contamination and the amount of tension on the abdominal wall.

There are a variety of ways to determine if the amount of tension created will be excessive and lead to complications. The key is to make use of all information that is readily available in the operating room or at the bedside. While no technique has been validated by research, many employ a technique of using the change in the patient's Peak Airway Pressure (PAP) as a means of determining tension. Most anesthesia machines and bedside ventilators will report a constant PAP, and the authors have determined that if the change is greater than 20 cm H_2O with the temporary closure using towel clips, there is too much tension to proceed with closure.

At the time of closure, decisions must also be made regarding how to close the skin. The same tenants of general surgery that dictate closure apply in the damage control setting. Skin closure with a running suture, wide bites, and minimal tension on the stitch to avoid skin necrosis will protect the intestine from exposure to the atmosphere. Skin closure does not seem to increase the risk of infection. To the contrary, many wounds that cannot be closed at the initial laparotomy secondary to contamination may benefit from the multiple washouts and can be closed safely at the time of final closure.

23.7   Failure to Achieve Primary Closure

If the patient cannot be closed in the 7–10-day time frame, alternative means must be employed to reconstruct the abdominal wall and protect visceral contents. This may take many forms: Native tissue, biosynthetic meshed implants, and absorbable mesh. Most patients by this stage in their course have become "cocooned," so that evisceration is not a concern. Each of these closure methods has positives and negatives. Using the patient's native tissues, whether fascia or skin only, is preferred to any mesh, synthetic or biologic. There have been a variety of methods used, each with their pros and cons. Surgeons who frequently deal with this patient population should be experienced with multiple methods to allow them to tailor their approach to each patient's care [44]. Addressing closure occurs at the final operation of the patient's initial hospitalization. If definitive closure cannot be achieved at that time, the patient will require definitive reconstruction months later, generally 9–12 months postinjury.

23.8   Types of Definitive Abdominal Closures

23.8.1   Modified Component Separation

Component Separation (CS) uses a sliding myofascial flap to provide tension-free closure of large abdominal wounds without implantation of mesh [45]. This allows for a vascularized tissue to be brought together with little or no tension [46]. Fabian and colleagues used this method as part of a staged closure of complex open abdomens. They found that there was only a 11% hernia recurrence rate as compared to 33% in mesh reconstructions, and they recommended its use in moderate-sized defects [47].

23.8.2   Polypropylene Mesh (Marlex®, Prolene®)

Brandt and colleagues argued that polypropylene mesh placement is an effective alternative for abdominal closure after emergency laparotomy, even when intraabdominal sepsis is present. They reported a fistulas rate of 7.1% that they postulated could be effectively eliminated by the interposition of omentum between bowel and mesh. They reported no cases of infected mesh, but they did report an incidence of 15% of the mesh necessitating removal [48]. Other authors have argued that polypropylene mesh use in this setting has resulted in an unacceptably high complication rate, including fistula rates up to 50% [49, 50]. Also, long-term complications of infected mesh creating a catabolic drain are described, which can brew in a indolent manner for months [47]. While the short-term goal of abdominal closure is obtained, the long-term wound complications make the use of polypropylene mesh in this setting unacceptable when alternatives exist.

23.8.3 Polytetrafluoroethylene (Gore-Tex®)

Some authors have used Polytetrafluoroethylene (PTFE) mesh as a temporary patch to prevent evisceration and allow for the development of granulation tissue to serve as a bed for Split-Thickness Skin Graft (STSG) [47]. Its advantages are that it is relatively poorly incorporated, allowing for easier removal if the need arises. It has the same drawbacks of other permanent meshes in that infection often necessitates removal and there is a significant cost difference when compared to alternatives. Consequently, the authors no longer use permanent synthetic mesh in the damag-control process.

23.8.4 Polyglycolic Acid Mesh (Vicryl®)

A majority of patients in the literature who are unable to be primarily closed undergo abdominal closure with polyglycolic acid mesh with subsequent split thickness skin grafting before leaving the hospital [51]. Polyglactin mesh is tightly woven. Healthy granulation tissue occurs within 7–10 days of insertion. However, the mesh itself usually is not incorporated tightly, as is the case with polypropylene [47]. This technique of abdominal closure is associated with an increased risk for infection and fistula formation. Recent studies on abdominal closure in the open abdomen in trauma report an enterocutaneous fistula rate of 7–8%. These studies, however, were not limited to damage control patients [14, 37, 38, 52].

23.8.5 Biosynthetic Reconstruction

A variety of new biosynthetic meshes are available that have the advantage of being able to be placed in the contaminated wound without the fear of mesh contamination. These meshes are being employed more often with good initial results in patients who are unable to be closed [53, 54]. Scott and colleagues showed success with only minor superficial wound infections in employing the early application of human acellular dermal matrix (Alloderm®) to open abdomens when closure was not possible [55]. Some questions have arisen about the long-term durability of this type of mesh [56]. As long-term data continue to accumulate for the use of this biosynthetic mesh, its applications and its efficacy continue to be more accurately described.

23.9   Special Situations in Damage Control Surgery

23.9.1   Fistulas in the Open Abdomen

Despite attention to detail and vigilant surveillance, complications arise in staged surgery including fistula formation. This not only complicates nutritional plans in these patients, but it also can make the planning of abdominal closure even more complicated. The best plan for dealing with fistula formation is prevention. Techniques that can decrease the rate of formation include: Early closure, protecting the bowel, avoidance of permanent mesh, and placing any anastomosis deep within the abdomen, away from any skin/fascial closure or the atmosphere.

Early closure has been shown to decrease fistula formation [34]. Measures to protect the bowel include using bowel bag and decreased manipulation of the bowel on subsequent washouts. Also, the type of closure technique can have dramatic impact on fistula rate. Using absorbable mesh as discussed earlier in this chapter can reduce the fistula rate when compared to permanent mesh [57]. The act of burying your anastomosis may seem relatively simple, but it can have an effect on fistula formation and can ease the treatment should one develop [58].

The treatment of fistulas in the open abdomen follows the same tenants of surgery in other situations. The primary goal is to isolate the output and decrease the flow through the output. Isolation can be complicated by the fact that repeated washouts and dressing changes can disturb the body's attempt to wall off the collection. Also, the fact that these abdomens often progress to a "cocooned" appearance can make intervention problematic. Fortunately, the best plan is usually the simplest: Simple drainage. Attempting to resect or repair an enterocutaneous fistula in the hyper-inflammatory setting usually leads to worsening of the problem unless this takes place very early in the process [59]. In addition to isolation, most authors would advocate a trial of NPO (Nothing By Mouth) for the patient to allow decreased output via the fistula. This requires supplementation with paraenteral nutrition. Supplementation of key vitamins may also speed the wound healing.

23.9.2   Ostomy in the Open Abdomen

If the patient's physiologic reserve cannot be restored and bowel edema persists, an anastomosis is not safe and an ostomy needs to be performed. While ostomies can make dressing changes and care a challenge, they often are the safest option for the patient. When ostomies are performed in conjunction with a split thickness skin graft, the patient will need a tertiary operation, for reversal of an ostomy and repair of a planned hernia. The decision to combine such procedures vs. separating them will depend on the patient's condition and the choice of abdominal closure technique employed.

23.10 Long-term Outcome

Beyond initial hospitalization, damage control patients often require a significant follow-up. Sutton and colleagues followed damage control patients for 2 years to quantify and describe the outcomes associated with damage control laparotomy, with only two patients lost to follow-up. The most common reason for the readmission was the expected elective ventral hernia repair in patients who were unable to be primarily closed. Within 24 months of injury, only 50% of the patients had completed definitive organ repairs with abdominal wall closure. They concluded that delaying definitive abdominal wall reconstruction by at least 6 months allows for resolution of all inflammatory changes and gives the best chance for successful reconstruction without further complication [60]. It is critical to understand that the patient gets one optimal opportunity for definitive repair of the large abdominal hernia. This procedure must not be performed under suboptimal conditions with a higher risk of failure. This also allows for a multi-specialty approach to optimize and plan this often complex and lengthy reconstruction. Early involvement of plastic surgery can help with planning for reconstruction of these complex wounds. The options for reconstruction include primary fascial closure (not usually possible because of tension), advancement skin flaps, component separation techniques, or tensor fascia lata supplementation.

In addition to those already suspected reasons for admission, there is a risk of extra-abdominal infectious risks. Sutton showed that the majority of patients required readmission (31 out of 41), most often for infectious complications. Nearly half (47%) of the patients treated for infection were diagnosed with bacteremia or line sepsis, a complication of treatment with long-term antibiotics or parenteral nutrition. Reducing risk factors for line sepsis may represent the easiest means of reducing this morbidity. Because this therapy is instituted as a result of the high fistula rate, reducing the incidence of enterocutaneous fistulae has the potential for the greatest impact on morbidity reduction [60].

Mortality related to damage control laparotomy is generally restricted to the patient's initial hospitalization. In a 2-year follow-up, no deaths occurred following discharge [60]. Thus, the long-term survival after DCS appears to justify the initial high cost. In other words, patient survival is traded for the morbidity associated with a damage control approach. Unfortunately, no information currently exists that defines the probability of the patient returning to a productive lifestyle.

23.11 Summary and Conclusion

The management of the open abdomen does not stop once the initial life-saving effort ends. This marks the beginning of what will often become the most complex portion of the patient's care. The post-operative decisions will have a dramatic impact on the morbidity and mortality of the patient. While algorithms and advice can help guide the surgeon in making decisions, nothing can replace a vigilant surgeon reassessing the patient and adapting to changes in the patient's physiology and presentation. When an individually tailored approach is taken, this patient population can be safely navigated through the course with resultant improved outcomes. Although this surgical approach is associated with a significant complication and readmission rate, the patient's long-term survival is the benefit.

References

1. Morris JA, Jr., Eddy VA, Blinman TA, Rutherford EJ, Sharp KW. The staged celiotomy for trauma. Issues in unpacking and reconstruction. Ann Surg 1993; 217(5):576–584
2. Hoyt DB, Bulger EM, Knudson MM et al. Death in the operating room: An analysis of a multi-center experience. J Trauma 1994; 37(3):426–432
3. Rotondo MF, Schwab CW, McGonigal MD, Phillips GR III, Fruchterman TM, Kauder DR, Latenser BA, Angood PA. "Damage control": An approach for improved survival in exsanguinating penetrating abdominal injury. J Trauma 1993; 35(3):375–382
4. Abramson D, Scalea TM, Hitchcock R, Trooskin SZ, Henry SM, Greenspan J. Lactate clearance and survival following injury. J Trauma 1993; 35(4):584–588
5. Baker WF, Jr. Clinical aspects of disseminated intravascular coagulation: A clinician's point of view. Semin Thromb Hemost 1989; 15(1):1–57
6. Davis JW, Shackford SR, Mackersie RC, Hoyt DB. Base deficit as a guide to volume resuscitation. J Trauma 1988; 28(10):1464–1467
7. Harrigan C, Lucas CE, Ledgerwood AM. The effect of hemorrhagic shock on the clotting cascade in injured patients. J Trauma 1989; 29(10):1416–1421
8. Jurkovich GJ, Greiser WB, Luterman A, Curreri PW. Hypothermia in trauma victims: An ominous predictor of survival. J Trauma 1987; 27(9):1019–1024
9. Luna GK, Maier RV, Pavlin EG, Anardi D, Copass MK, Oreskovich MR. Incidence and effect of hypothermia in seriously injured patients. J Trauma 1987; 27(9):1014–1018
10. McClelland RN, Shires GT, Baxter CR, Coln CD, Carrico J. Balanced salt solution in the treatment of hemorrhagic shock. Studies in dogs. JAMA 1967; 199(11):830–834
11. Shapiro MB, Jenkins DH, Schwab CW, Rotondo MF. Damage control: Collective review. J Trauma 2000; 49(5):969–978
12. Sharp KW, Locicero RJ. Abdominal packing for surgically uncontrollable hemorrhage. Ann Surg 1992; 215(5):467–474
13. Valeri CR, Feingold H, Cassidy G, Ragno G, Khuri S, Altschule MD. Hypothermia-induced reversible platelet dysfunction. Ann Surg 1987; 205(2):175–181
14. Johnson JW, Gracias VH, Schwab CW, Reilly PM, Kauder DR, Dabrowski GP, Shapiro MB, Rotondo MF. Evolution in damage control for exsanguinating penetrating abdominal injury. J Trauma 2001; 51(2):261–269
15. Patt A, McCroskey BL, Moore EE. Hypothermia-induced coagulopathies in trauma. Surg Clin North Am 1988; 68(4):775–785
16. Gentilello LM, Cortes V, Moujaes S, Viamonte M, Malinin TL, Ho CH, Gomez GA. Continuous arteriovenous rewarming: Experimental results and thermodynamic model simulation of treatment for hypothermia. J Trauma 1990; 30(12):1436–1449
17. Demetriades D, Hadjizacharia P, Constantinou C, Brown C, Inaba K, Rhee P, Salim A. Selective nonoperative management of penetrating abdominal solid organ injuries. Ann Surg 2006; 244(4):620–628
18. Velmahos GC, Toutouzas KG, Radin R, Chan L, Demetriades D. Nonoperative treatment of blunt injury to solid abdominal organs: A prospective study. Arch Surg 2003; 138(8):844–851
19. Panetta T, Sclafani SJ, Goldstein AS, Phillips TF, Shaftan GW. Percutaneous transcatheter embolization for massive bleeding from pelvic fractures. J Trauma 1985; 25(11):1021–1029

20. Velmahos GC, Chahwan S, Hanks SE, Murray JA, Berne TV, Asensio J, Demetriades D. Angiographic embolization of bilateral internal iliac arteries to control life-threatening hemorrhage after blunt trauma to the pelvis. Am Surg 2000; 66(9):858–862

21. Panetta T, Sclafani SJ, Goldstein AS, Phillips TF. Percutaneous transcatheter embolization for arterial trauma. J Vasc Surg 1985; 2(1):54–64

22. Aksoy M, Taviloglu K, Yanar H, Poyanli A, Ertekin C, Rozanes I, Guloglu R, Kurtoglu M. Percutaneous transcatheter embolization in arterial injuries of the lower limbs. Acta Radiol 2005; 46(5):471–475

23. Velmahos GC, Demetriades D, Chahwan S, Gomez H, Hanks SE, Murray JA, Asensio JA, Berne TV. Angiographic embolization for arrest of bleeding after penetrating trauma to the abdomen. Am J Surg 1999; 178(5):367–373

24. Johnson JW, Gracias VH, Gupta R, Guillamondegui O, Reilly PM, Shapiro MB, Kauder DR, Schwab CW. Hepatic angiography in patients undergoing damage control laparotomy. J Trauma 2002; 52(6):1102–1106

25. Mayberry JC. Bedside open abdominal surgery. Utility and wound management. Crit Care Clin 2000; 16(1):151–172

26. Diaz JJ, Jr., Mauer A, May AK, Miller R, Guy JS, Morris JA, Jr. Bedside laparotomy for trauma: Are there risks? Surg Infect (Larchmt) 2004; 5(1):15–20

27. Moore EE, Burch JM, Franciose RJ, Offner PJ, Biffl WL. Staged physiologic restoration and damage control surgery. World J Surg 1998; 22(12):1184–1190

28. Demetriades D, Murray JA, Chan L, Ordonez C, Bowley D, Nagy KK, Cornwell EE, Velmahos GC, Munoz N, Hatzitheofilou C, Schwab CW, Rodriguez A, Cornejo C, Davis KA, Namias N, Wisner DH, Ivatury RR, Moore EE, Acosta JA, Maull KI, Thomason MH, Spain DA. Penetrating colon injuries requiring resection: Diversion or primary anastomosis? An AAST prospective multicenter study. J Trauma 2001; 50(5):765–775

29. Murray JA, Demetriades D, Colson M, Song Z, Velmahos GC, Cornwell III EE, Asensio JA, Belzberg H, Berne TV. Colonic resection in trauma: Colostomy versus anastomosis. J Trauma 1999; 46(2):250–254

30. Sasaki LS, Allaben RD, Golwala R, Mittal VK. Primary repair of colon injuries: A prospective randomized study. J Trauma 1995; 39(5):895–901

31. Sasaki LS, Mittal V, Allaben RD. Primary repair of colon injuries: A retrospective analysis. Am Surg 1994; 60(7):522–527

32. Gonzalez RP, Merlotti GJ, Holevar MR. Colostomy in penetrating colon injury: Is it necessary? J Trauma 1996; 41(2):271–275

33. Miller PR, Chang MC, Hoth JJ, Holmes JH, Meredith JW. Colonic resection in the setting of damage control laparotomy: Is delayed anastomosis safe? Am Surg 2007; 73(6):606–609

34. Miller RS, Morris JA, Jr., Diaz JJ, Jr., Herring MB, May AK. Complications after 344 damage-control open celiotomies. J Trauma 2005; 59(6):1365–1371

35. Asensio JA, McDuffie L, Petrone P, Roldan G, Forno W, Gambaro E, Salim A, Demetriades D, Murray J, Velmahos G, Shoemaker W, Berne TV, Ramicone E, Chan L, Biffl WL. Reliable variables in the exsanguinated patient which indicate damage control and predict outcome. Am J Surg 2001; 182(6):743–751

36. Asensio JA, Petrone P, Roldan G, Kuncir E, Ramicone E, Chan L. Has evolution in awareness of guidelines for institution of damage control improved outcome in the management of the posttraumatic open abdomen? Arch Surg 2004; 139(2):209–214

37. Stone PA, Hass SM, Flaherty SK, Deluca JA, Lucente FC, Kusminsky RE. Vacuum-assisted fascial closure for patients with abdominal trauma. J Trauma 2004; 57(5):1082–1086

38. Miller PR, Meredith JW, Johnson JC, Chang MC. Prospective evaluation of vacuum-assisted fascial closure after open abdomen: Planned ventral hernia rate is substantially reduced. Ann Surg 2004; 239(5):608–614

39. Bishop MH, Shoemaker WC, Appel PL, Meade P, Ordog GJ, Wasserberger J, Wo C-J, Rimle DA, Kram HB, Umali R, Kennedy F, Shuleshko J, Stephen CM, Shori SK, Thadepalli HD. Prospective, randomized trial of survivor values of cardiac index, oxygen delivery, and oxygen consumption as resuscitation endpoints in severe trauma. J Trauma 1995; 38(5):780–787

40. Scalea TM, Simon HM, Duncan AO, Atweh NA, Sclafani SA, Phillips TF, Shaftan GW. Geriatric blunt multiple trauma: Improved survival with early invasive monitoring. J Trauma 1990; 30(2):129–134

41. Martin GS, Moss M, Wheeler AP, Mealer M, Morris JA, Bernard GR. A randomized, controlled trial of furosemide with or without albumin in hypoproteinemic patients with acute lung injury. Crit Care Med 2005; 33(8):1681–1687

42. Martin GS, Mangialardi RJ, Wheeler AP, Dupont WD, Morris JA, Bernard GR. Albumin and furosemide therapy in hypoproteinemic patients with acute lung injury. Crit Care Med 2002; 30(10):2175–2182

43. Balogh Z, McKinley BA, Cocanour CS, Kozar RA, Valdivia A, Sailors RM, Moore FA. Supranormal trauma resuscitation causes more cases of abdominal compartment syndrome. Arch Surg 2003; 138(6):637–642

44. Vogel TR, Diaz JJ, Miller RS, May AK, Guillamondegui OD, Guy JS, Morris JA. The open abdomen in trauma: Do infectious complications affect primary abdominal closure? Surg Infect (Larchmt) 2006; 7(5):433–441

45. Ramirez OM, Ruas E, Dellon AL. "Components separation" method for closure of abdominal-wall defects: An anatomic and clinical study. Plast Reconstr Surg 1990; 86(3):519–526

46. Vargo D. Component separation in the management of the difficult abdominal wall. Am J Surg 2004; 188(6):633–637

47. Fabian TC, Croce MA, Pritchard FE, Minard G, Hickerson WL, Howell RL, Schurr MJ, Kudsk KA. Planned ventral hernia. Staged management for acute abdominal wall defects. Ann Surg 1994; 219(6):643–650

48. Brandt CP, McHenry CR, Jacobs DG, Piotrowski JJ, Priebe PP. Polypropylene mesh closure after emergency laparotomy: Morbidity and outcome. Surgery 1995; 118(4):736–740

49. Fansler RF, Taheri P, Cullinane C, Sabates B, Flint LM. Polypropylene mesh closure of the complicated abdominal wound. Am J Surg 1995; 170(1):15–18

50. Voyles CR, Richardson JD, Bland KI, Tobin GR, Flint LM, Polk HC, Jr. Emergency abdominal wall reconstruction with polypropylene mesh: Short-term benefits versus long-term complications. Ann Surg 1981; 194(2):219–223

51. Dayton MT, Buchele BA, Shirazi SS, Hunt LB. Use of an absorbable mesh to repair contaminated abdominal-wall defects. Arch Surg 1986; 121(8):954–960

52. Mayberry JC, Burgess EA, Goldman RK, Pearson TE, Brand D, Mullins RJ. Enterocutaneous fistula and ventral hernia after absorbable mesh prosthesis closure for trauma: The plain truth. J Trauma 2004; 57(1):157–162

53. Patton JH, Jr., Berry S, Kralovich KA. Use of human acellular dermal matrix in complex and contaminated abdominal wall reconstructions. Am J Surg 2007; 193(3):360–363

54. Kim H, Bruen K, Vargo D. Acellular dermal matrix in the management of high-risk abdominal wall defects. Am J Surg 2006; 192(6):705–709

55. Scott BG, Welsh FJ, Pham HQ, Carrick MM, Liscum KR, Granchi TS, Wall MJ, Mattox KL, Hirshberg A. Early aggressive closure of the open abdomen. J Trauma 2006; 60(1):17–22

56. Gupta A, Zahriya K, Mullens PL, Salmassi S, Keshishian A. Ventral herniorrhaphy: Experience with two different biosynthetic mesh materials, Surgisis and Alloderm. Hernia 2006; 10(5):419–425

57. Jernigan TW, Fabian TC, Croce MA, Moore N, Pritchard FE, Minard G, Bee TK. Staged management of giant abdominal wall defects: Acute and long-term results. Ann Surg 2003; 238(3):349–355

58. Fabian TC. Damage control in trauma: Laparotomy wound management acute to chronic. Surg Clin North Am 2007; 87(1):73–93, vi

59. Fabian TC. Damage control in trauma: Laparotomy wound management acute to chronic. Surg Clin North Am 2007; 87(1):73–93, vi

60. Sutton E, Bochicchio GV, Bochicchio K, Rodriguez ED, Henry S, Joshi M, Scalea TM. Long term impact of damage control surgery: A preliminary prospective study. J Trauma 2006; 61(4):831–834

Chapter 24
Functional Long-Term Outcomes in Polytrauma Patients with Orthopedic Injuries

Boris A. Zelle, Andrew Marcantonio, and Ivan S. Tarkin

24.1 Outcome Research in Polytrauma Patients

Outcome research is the process of data collection, analysis, and interpretation of the efficiency and effectiveness of patient treatment [1]. The purpose of outcome research is to improve the quality of patient care, and clinical outcome research should be an integral component of orthopedic research. For several reasons, thorough outcome evaluations in polytrauma patients provide important data for physicians, physical and occupational therapists, as well as for insurance and hospital administrations:

- A detailed analysis of the long-term results following polytrauma provides important information for the development or improvement of treatment guidelines and the allocation of resources.
- A broad knowledge of long-term outcomes following polytrauma will help the trauma surgeons and therapists to better manage and advise their patients regarding discharge planning, rehabilitation plans, or career planning, and the patients may benefit from a more thorough consultation.
- With increased health-care costs, the length of rehabilitation, the length of physical disability, and employment status following polytrauma are of economical interest.

Thorough outcome evaluations in polytrauma patients require the use of appropriate outcome measures. In general, outcome measures in polytrauma patients can be divided into the following groups:

- Process outcomes;
- Early clinical outcomes including morbidity and mortality;
- Functional long-term outcomes and patient satisfaction.

B.A. Zelle (✉)
Department of Orthopedic Surgery, University of Pittsburgh School of Medicine,
Kaufmann Building, 3471 Fifth Avenue, Suite 1011, Pittsburgh, PA, 15213, USA
e-mail: zelleba@upmc.edu

H.-C. Pape et al. (eds.), *Damage Control Management in the Polytrauma Patient*,
DOI 10.1007/978-0-387-89508-6_24, © Springer Science+Business Media, LLC 2010

Process outcomes represent the utilization of resources and include measures such as the duration of care, length of hospital stay, number of outpatient visits, and number and type of interventions provided to the patient. These data are of major socioeconomical interest. The evaluation of process outcomes provides important information on clinician and organizational performance. The sources of process outcomes data may include scheduling and billing databases and patient records.

Early clinical outcomes in polytrauma patients, such as morbidity and mortality, are usually the primary focus when attempting to demonstrate the effectiveness of immediate surgical interventions. The number one goal in polytrauma care is to prevent death and morbidity, and, therefore, these variables must be monitored carefully. With regard to Damage Control Orthopaedics (DCO) and the timing of surgery in polytrauma patients, the evaluation of mortality and morbidity rates are crucial, since the main goal of DCO is to improve survival rates in polytrauma patients.

Functional long-term outcomes and patient satisfaction represent other important outcome measures. Over the last decades, improved preclinical and clinical emergency care has decreased the mortality and complication rates of polytrauma patients [2, 3]. Given the increased survival rates, the long-term functional outcome and patient satisfaction have gained importance in polytrauma care. Today, long-term evaluation of Quality of Life (QOL), employment status, or residual complaints represents important data for evaluating the quality of polytrauma care.

While process outcomes and costs represent important aspects of polytrauma care, the main research focus has been the clinical outcomes in these patients. This chapter will focus on early clinical outcomes and long-term functional outcomes in polytrauma patients and the impact of DCO.

24.2   Functional Outcome Measures

Assessing the functional outcomes in polytrauma patients with multiple musculoskeletal injuries remains challenging. Polytrauma patients often face multiple problems during their rehabilitation process, which may include not only physical impairment, but also social, emotional, and economical issues. For that reason, evaluation of functional long-term outcomes in polytrauma patients must consider various aspects including activity and participation, patient satisfaction and QOL, and impairment of body function.

24.2.1   Activity and Participation

Activity and participation limitations in patients with multiple musculoskeletal injuries may include various aspects, such as the inability to participate in sports and hobbies, inability to perform activity of daily living, or the inability to return to work.

Activity and participation can be measured by the use of standardized self-reports of activity limitations and participation restrictions. In orthopedic patients, the Tegner Activity Score [4] is a widely used activity scale that allows grading and comparison of the pre-injury and the post-injury activity status.

24.2.2 Patient Satisfaction and QOL

Patient satisfaction and QOL measures are designed to measure the injured's perception of his or her physical, emotional, and social function following injury. Many QOL scoring systems have been developed and used in orthopedics. In general, they can be divided into general outcome measures and specific outcome measures. While general measures are designed to document the QOL in a wide range of individuals with the same or a different condition, specific measures are designed to document the status of specific injuries or specific body regions. Well-designed studies of functional outcomes in orthopedic patients should include both general and specific measures of QOL.

Multiple general measures for the evaluation of QOL have been designed and used in the evaluation of outcomes in polytrauma patients. These outcome measures are designed to be applicable across different injuries and interventions, and across demographic and cultural subgroups. The use of many of these instruments has been limited by the lack of validation psychometric testing. Validated scoring systems that are commonly used in trauma outcome research include the Short-Form 36-Item Health Survey (SF-36) [5], the Sickness Impact Profile (SIP) [6], the POLO chart [7], and the Short Musculoskeletal Function Assessment questionnaire (SMFA) [8]. Since general measures of health-related quality of life measure a broad range of health functions, such as emotional or social function, the content of the questionnaires often appears less relevant to patients and clinicians. Moreover, an important limitation that is associated with the use of general outcome measures is that they tend to be less sensitive to detect subtle differences of orthopedic conditions than in specific outcome measures [9]. Thus, using only a general health status outcome measure would make it more difficult to detect minor differences between patients with orthopedic conditions.

Numerous specific outcome measures have been used in the evaluation of outcomes in orthopedic patients, and multiple scoring systems have been suggested. Specific outcome measures have been developed for specific diseases (e.g., osteoarthritis), specific patient populations (e.g., elderly patients), specific functions (e.g., level of physical activity), specific impairments (e.g., pain), and specific body regions [9]. The use of specific outcome measures in polytrauma patients becomes important when the functional outcomes of specific subgroups are evaluated, such as patients with lower extremity injuries etc. Specific outcome measures are usually sensitive to small differences and are easy to administer and interpret [10].

24.2.3   Impairment of Body Function

Impairment of body function in polytrauma patients may include specific clinical evaluations of injured body regions. The impairment of body function in polytrauma patients may play a role when subgroups of patients with specific injuries are assessed. The evaluation may include range of motion, muscle strength, joint laxity, or pain with weight bearing. These outcome measures are usually incompletely covered in most available outcome scoring systems. Measures of clinical outcome at the level of impairment of body function may include goniometry to measure the range of motion and isometric or isokinetic testing to measure muscle strength.

24.2.4   The Hannover Score for Polytrauma Outcome

These concerns illustrate that defining the appropriate outcome measures in polytrauma patients is complicated by the large variety of social, psychological, economical, and physical problems in this patient population as well as the large variety of injury patterns. Most general measures of QOL do not encompass these specific social, psychological, and economical states of the polytrauma population. Moreover, previously suggested scoring systems do not include a specific clinical evaluation of the injured body regions. For this reason, the Hannover Score for Polytrauma Outcome (HASPOC) was implemented [11]. The HASPOC is a validated scoring system that was specifically designed for the evaluation of the functional long-term outcome after polytrauma [11]. The HASPOC includes a patient-reported questionnaire with items on the QOL as well as the social, psychological, and economical rehabilitation status. In addition, the HASPOC requires a clinical examination by a physician of all injured body regions.

24.3   Early Clinical Outcomes in Polytrauma Patients

The term "polytrauma" is used for severely injured patients with two or more injuries of at least two body regions, with at least one injury or the sum total of all injuries being life-threatening [12]. This emphasizes that the number one goal in polytrauma care is to avoid death and morbidity. The mortality and complication rates in polytrauma patients have been investigated in several studies [3, 13–18]. Independent from trauma system and management protocols, most reported mortality rates of polytrauma patients vary between 20 and 40%. Over the last decades, improvements in prehospital care, intensive care medicine, and surgical techniques have decreased the mortality and complication rates of polytrauma patients [2, 3, 17]. The optimal timing of long bone fixation in polytrauma patients and the impact of orthopedic interventions on the mortality and complication rates have been the topics of several recent and ongoing investigations, and a brief synopsis will be provided in this chapter.

In the early half of the twentieth century, polytrauma patients were considered to be too ill to undergo prolonged surgical procedures, and operations were avoided as it was felt that the patients would not be able to tolerate major surgery [18]. At the same time, surgical techniques available for fracture fixation were few and not in widespread use. An important contributory factor was the fear of generating fat embolism, hypotension/hypoperfusion, additional hemorrhage, and surgical stress [19]. However, the subsequent prolonged periods of bed rest were complicated by pneumonia, thromboembolic complications, and decubital ulcers.

In the 1970s, reproducible fracture fixation techniques developed and improved intensive care medicine facilitated the medical management of patients with significant physiologic compromise. A number of reports suggested improved outcomes in polytrauma patients undergoing immediate fracture fixation [20–24]. This episode is often referred to as the "era of early total care." In a retrospective review, Johnson and colleagues suggested that a delay of more than 24 h in the stabilization of a femur fracture was associated with a fivefold increase in the incidence of adult respiratory distress syndrome [23]. In a prospective randomized study of early vs. delayed stabilization of femur fractures, Bone and colleagues concluded that early stabilization in polytrauma patients reduced the incidence of pulmonary failure while no effect on mortality rates was observed [20]. In a multicenter study, Bone and colleagues compared the outcomes of 676 polytrauma patients undergoing immediate fixation of their long bone fracture with a "similar" group of 906 patients from the American College of Surgeons database [21]. These authors reported decreased mortality in the patients who had early total care of all their injuries.

In the early 1990s, several authors noted that early total care was associated with a high rate of complications in a certain subset of patients, and reports from the early 1990s suggested temporary external fixation and delayed definitive fracture fixation in polytrauma patients with long bone injuries and associated cardiopulmonary compromise [25–27]. The concepts of damage control surgery that had been widely used by general surgeons [28] were subsequently translated into the orthopedic field, and the term Damage Control Orthopaedics (DCO) was coined [29, 30]. Pape and colleagues [26] conducted a retrospective study of a series of 106 polytrauma patients with an injury severity score (ISS) [31] >18 and femoral shaft fractures treated by reamed intramedullary nailing. They found that, in patients with severe chest trauma, there was a significantly higher incidence of posttraumatic adult respiratory distress syndrome (33 vs. 7.7%) and mortality (21 versus 4%) when early intramedullary femoral nailing was done. These authors stated that the pulmonary function after polytrauma was significantly influenced by (1) the severity of the injury (e.g., shock); (2) the presence of a chest trauma; (3) intramedullary reaming of the femur. Subsequently, Pape and colleagues [17] conducted a retrospective cohort study in polytrauma patients with an ISS > 18 and an associated femoral shaft fracture. The authors divided their patients into the early total care period (1981–1989), an intermediate period (1990–1992), and a DCO group (1993–2000). They found that the incidence of systemic complications decreased significantly from the early total care period to the DCO period. Within the DCO group, there was also a higher incidence of adult respiratory distress syndrome when immediate intramedullary nailing was used as compared to temporary external fixation. Of note, the authors did not observe any increased local complications related to temporary external fixation, such as pin track infections, delayed unions, or nonunions. This is in accordance with the investigations from other authors who did not observe any major increase in local complications when temporary external fixation was used as a bridge to definitive intramedullary fixation [29, 30, 32].

24.4   Functional Long-Term Outcomes in Polytrauma Patients

The functional long-term outcome following polytrauma has been reported in multiple previous studies, and several aspects of recovery have been investigated [33–39]. The impact of DCO on the functional long-term outcome following polytrauma has gained little attention in the literature. It must be emphasized that the primary goal of optimizing the timing of surgery is to decrease the mortality and complication rates of polytrauma patients. With regard to long-term functional outcome, no major difference can be expected between patients managed according to DCO protocols and patients managed with early total care. However, increased survival rates of polytrauma patients have sparked the interest in the long-term functional outcome, and several recent investigations have focused on this issue. It has been suggested that various variables, such as female gender, older age, high ISS, injuries to the lower extremities, head injuries, lower educational level, and workers' compensation status are associated with unfavorable outcomes [33–39]. However, an evaluation of the long-term outcome following polytrauma should be based on an adequate sample size, an adequate follow-up period, and appropriate outcome measures, including patient-reported outcome scales as well as physical examinations. Given these difficulties, long-term functional recovery following polytrauma remains the topic of ongoing investigations. The Lower Extremity Assessment Project (LEAP study) [40–45] and the Hannover Rehab Study [46–49] are two large sophisticated outcome studies that have recently been conducted. The study design and the main conclusions of these studies will be discussed in this chapter.

24.4.1   The Lower Extremity Assessment Project

The LEAP study was a multicenter study investigating the functional outcomes in patients with severe lower extremity trauma at 2-year and 7-year follow-ups [40–45]. Six hundred one patients from eight level I trauma centers admitted for the treatment of high-energy trauma below the distal femur were included in the study. This included patients with open fractures, dysvascular limbs, major soft-tissue injuries, and severe foot and ankle injuries. The principal outcome measure was the Sickness Impact Profile, a multidimensional measure of self-reported health status [6]. Functional outcomes were compared between patients undergoing reconstruction vs. amputation.

Although few differences between the two groups were found, the overall functional outcomes were equivalent for patients undergoing amputation versus reconstruction [40, 42, 43]. Overall, functional outcomes were poor in both groups. Approximately one half of all patients had physical subscores on the Sickness Impact Profile ≥ 10, indicative of significant disability; only 34% of patients achieved scores typical of a member of the general population of similar age and sex; only 58% of the patients employed pre-injury were working at seven years post-injury; of those patients who returned to work, 20–25% were limited in their ability to perform the demands of their pre-injury status. Interestingly, the outcomes at the 7-year follow-up had not significantly improved compared to the 2-year data.

An important finding from the LEAP study was that the patient's social, economical, and emotional status had a stronger impact on the functional outcomes than the actual treatment of amputation versus reconstruction. The LEAP study identified several demographic variables that were significantly associated with poor functional outcomes. These included older age, female gender, non-white race, low educational level, low income, smoker, poor self-reported pre-injury health status, and involvement with the legal system for obtaining disability [40, 42, 43]. Moreover, LEAP study revealed that, besides these demographic variables, psychological disorders were a significant predictor of a poor functional long-term outcome [40, 42, 43]. At 2 years follow-up, 42% of the patients in the LEAP study screened positive for a likely psychological disorder; almost 20% of the patients reported severe phobic anxiety and/or depression [44]. A multivariate analysis demonstrated that emotional variables, such as anxiety, pain distress, and depression, had a significant impact on the long-term functional outcome, as measured by the Sickness Impact Profile, and return to work [40, 42, 43]. It was found that self-efficacy was one of the strongest predictors of the Sickness Impact Profile and return to work. Self-efficacy refers to the confidence in being able to perform specific tasks or activities. It can be assumed that persons with low self-efficacy are not actively participating in the social reintegration and physical rehabilitation process since failure is expected.

These results from the LEAP study suggest that, in severely injured patients, more attention to the social and psychological aspects of recovery may be needed. The authors hypothesize that further improvements in functional outcome may be achieved by interventions that directly address the patients' psychosocial needs and assist them in managing the multifactorial consequences of their injury [43].

24.4.2 The Hannover Rehab Study

The functional outcome following polytrauma has been widely investigated in the literature, and several well-designed studies have contributed to our understanding of the functional recovery in polytrauma patients [33–39]. However, most of these aforementioned studies focused on the outcomes following the first 2 years after the injury.

Given the multiple social, psychological, and physical problems in this patient population, further changes of the functional status over several years can be anticipated. Moreover, most previous studies mainly focused on patient-reported outcomes. As discussed earlier, the physical examination of the body function is an important outcome measure in orthopedic patients. Given these limitations of previous reports from the literature, the Hannover Rehab Study [46–49] was initiated at the Department of Trauma Surgery at Hannover Medical School, with the goal of evaluating the functional outcomes with a minimum follow-up of 10 years and including a physical examination of all injured body regions by a physician. A major challenge of this investigation was the recruitment of patients several years after the injury. For that reason, the method of patient recruitment will be illustrated in this chapter as well.

24.4.2.1 Study Population

The patients were identified using the database of the authors' institution. The inclusion criteria were as follows:

- Multiple blunt injures between 1973 and 1990;
- Treatment at the author's level one trauma center;
- Three to sixty years of age at time of injury;
- Minimum follow-up of at least 10 years;
- Discharged alive.

A total of 1,131 patients matched the inclusion criteria and were contacted by mail (Fig. 24.1). Patients, who did not respond to the first letter received a subsequent second and, if necessary, a third letter. Patients who did not respond to the third

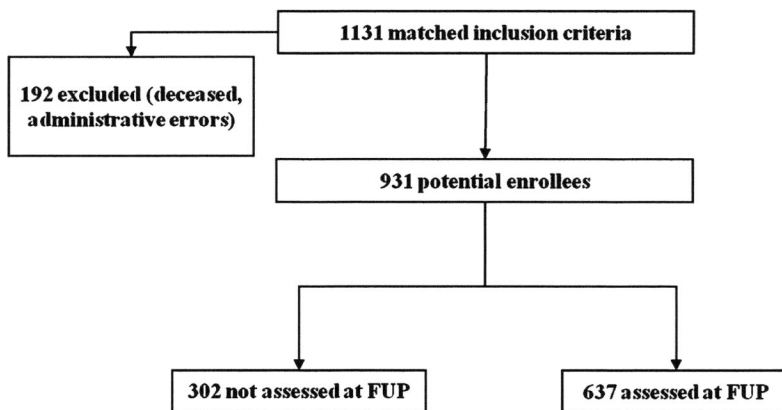

Fig. 24.1 Patients recruited for the Hannover Rehab Study. FUP: Follow-Up

letter were contacted by phone to schedule a follow-up exam. If the letters were undeliverable and the patients did not respond to several consecutive phone calls, the local government office for registration of residents was contacted. This government office can provide the new address within the community, date of death, or the new community for patients who had moved to another community. If the patient had moved to another community, the next responsible local government office for registration of residents was contacted to find the new address. No further attempt of recruitment was made for patients who were not registered at the local government office for registration of residents and for patients who had moved to more than three different communities since their injuries. As many as 89 patients could not be located for administrative reasons, and 103 patients had died after discharge; thus 192 patients were excluded from this study. Therefore, 939 patients matched the inclusion criteria, were alive at follow-up, could be successfully located, and thus presented the potential enrollees for this study. As many as 637 patients (68% of the potential enrollees) accepted the invitation and returned to our trauma center for the follow-up exam. Three hundred and two patients (32% of the potential enrollees) could not be evaluated. The reasons included administrative/logistic problems, medical problems, or no interest in study participation. The demographic data of these non-assessed patients were collected and compared to the demographic data of the assessed patients.

24.4.2.2   Outcome Measures

The primary outcome measurement was the Hannover Score for Polytrauma Outcome (HASPOC). The HASPOC is a validated scoring system that is specifically designed for the evaluation of polytrauma patients [11]. It is based on the evaluation of a patient-reported questionnaire with items on the QOL as well as the social, psychological, and economical rehabilitation status (HASPOC-Subjective). In addition, the HASPOC requires a clinical examination by a physician of all injured body regions. The questions of the SF-12 have been included in the patient questionnaire of the HASPOC. The SF-12 is based on the evaluation of a Physical Component Summary score and a Mental Component Summary score [50]. A transformed scale score of 0 to 100 can be calculated for these two health concepts. The SF-12 has been validated in trauma patients [51] and has been used in trauma outcome studies [52].

24.4.2.3   Functional Long-Term Outcomes

Between September 2000 and May 2002, 637 polytrauma patients (480 male and 157 female) were examined by a physician at the Department of Trauma Surgery at Hannover Medical School. The average follow-up was 17.5 years (range, 10–28 years); the average age at the time of injury was 26.4 years (range, 3–60 years); the average ISS was 20.7 (range, 4–54).

Table 24.1 Social and economic aspects at follow-up as part of the Hannover Rehab Study

Limited in recreational activities	65.4%
Less friends than before injury	44.6%
Less income than before injury	26.6%
Significant financial losses due to injury	36.9%
Switched to lighter job after injury	80.1%
Retired due to physical disability	26.9%

The evaluation of social and economic outcomes demonstrated the significant impact of the injury on social and economical status (Table 24.1). At follow-up, approximately two thirds of the study population felt limited in their recreational activities, and approximately one fourth of the patients were retired due to physical disability. More than 80% of the patients switched to a lighter job after the injury. The injured body regions that were most often responsible for physical disability included head injuries (40%) and injuries to the lower extremities (34%).

Further evaluation of the patients with lower extremity injuries showed that, in particular, injuries below the knee joint seemed to limit functional recovery [48]. Patients with lower extremity fractures below the knee joint showed significantly lower outcome scores than patients with lower extremity fractures above the knee joint as measured by the HASPOC, the SF-12, the Tegner Activity Score, the modified Karlstrom-Olerud Score [53], the Lysholm Score [54], and the ability to work. It was assumed that various factors, such as delayed treatment of foot injuries, the thin soft tissue envelope below the knee joint, unfavorable blood supply, and complex fracture patterns of many foot and ankle injuries, contributed to the unfavorable outcomes in patients with fractures below the knee joint.

Further analysis of the outcomes demonstrated the significant impact of demographic and social variables on the long-term functional outcome. The impact of the workers' compensation status on the functional outcome was evaluated in a multivariate analysis, with adjustments for age, sex, injury severity, and injury pattern [49]. This multivariate analysis demonstrated that, independent from potentially confounding demographic variables, workers' compensation patients achieved significantly worse outcomes than the remaining patient population as measured by the HASPOC, the SF-12, and the physical disability status.

24.5 Summary and Conclusion

Over the last decades, improvements in pre-hospital care, intensive care medicine, and surgical techniques have decreased the mortality and complication rates of polytrauma patients. With improved survival rates of polytrauma patients, the long-term functional outcomes have gained importance. Thorough evaluations of the long-term functional outcome require an appropriate follow-up period and adequate outcome measures.

Outcome measures should include general patient-reported measures of the QOL as well as specific outcome measures of the injured body regions. The impairment of body function represents an important outcome measure in orthopedic patients. Recently published large outcome studies have emphasized the important impact of psychosocial variables on the long-term functional outcome following polytrauma.

References

1. Dobrzykowski EA. The methodology of outcomes measurement. J Rehabil Outcomes 1997; 1:8–17
2. Kinzl L, Gebhard F, Arand M. Polytrauma and economics. Unfallchirurgie 1996; 22:179–185
3. Regel G, Lobenhoffer P, Grotz M, Pape HC, Lehmann U, Tscherne H. Treatment results of patients with multiple trauma: An analysis of 3406 cases treated between 1972 and 1991 at a German Level I Trauma Center. J Trauma 1995; 38:70–78
4. Tegner Y, Lysholm J, Odensten M, Gillquist J. Evaluation of cruciate ligament injuries: A review. Acta Orthop Scand 1988; 59:336–341
5. Ware JE Jr. Sherbourne CD. The MOS 36-item short-form health survey (SF-36). I. Conceptual framework and item selection. Med Care 1992; 30:473–483
6. Bergner M, Bobbitt RA, Carter WB, Gilson BS. The Sickness Impact Profile: Development and final revision of a health status measure. Med Care 1981; 19:787–805
7. Pirente N, Bouillon B, Schafer B, Raum M, Helling HJ, Berger E, Neugebauer E. Systematic development of a scale for determination of health-related quality of life in multiple trauma patients. The Polytrauma Outcome (POLO) Chart. Unfallchirurg 2002; 105:413–422
8. Swiontkowski MF, Engelberg R, Martin DP, Agel J. Short musculoskeletal function assessment questionnaire: Validity, reliability, and responsiveness. J Bone Joint Surg Am 1999; 81:1245–1260
9. Guyatt GH, Feeny DH, Patrick DL. Measuring health-related quality of life. Ann Int Med 1993; 118:622–629
10. McSweeny AJ, Creer TL: Health related quality-of-life assessment in medical care. Dis Month 1995; 41:6–71
11. Zelle B, Stalp M, Weihs C, Müller F, Reiter FO, Krettek Ch, Pape HC. Arbeitsgemeinschaft "Polytrauma" der Deutschen Gesellschaft für Unfallchirurgie. Validation of the Hannover Score for Polytrauma Outcome (HASPOC) in a sample of 170 polytrauma patients and a comparison with the SF-12. Chirurg 2003; 74:361–369
12. Tscherne H, Oestern HJ, Sturm JA. Stress tolerance of patients with multiple injuries and its significance for operative care. Langenbeck Arch Chir 1984; 364:71–77
13. Frink M, Probst C, Hildebrand F, Richter M, Hausmanninger C, Wiese B, Krettek C, Pape H-C, AG Polytrauma der DGU. The influence of transportation mode on mortality in polytraumatized patients: An analysis based on the German Trauma Registry. Unfallchirurg 2007; 110:334–340
14. Gomberg BF, Gruen GS, Smith WR, Spott M. Outcomes in acute orthopaedic trauma: A review of 130,506 patients by age. Injury 1999; 30:431–437
15. Hildebrand F, Giannoudis PV, Griensven M, Zelle B, Ulmer B, Krettek C, Bellamy MC, Pape HC. Management of polytraumatized patients with associated blunt chest trauma: A comparison of two European countries. Injury 2005; 36:293–302
16. Matthes G, Seifert J, Bogatzki S, Steinhage K, Ekkernkamp A, Stengel D. Age and survival likelihood of polytrauma patients. Local tailoring of the DGU prognosis model. Unfallchirurg 2005; 108:288–292
17. Pape HC, Hildebrand F, Pertschy S, Zelle B, Garapati R, Grimme K, Krettek C, Reed RL 2nd. Changes in the management of femoral shaft fractures in polytrauma patients: From early total care to damage control orthopedic surgery. J Trauma 2002; 53:452–462

18. Pape HC, Giannoudis PV, Krettek C. The timing of fracture treatment in polytrauma patients: Relevance of damage control orthopedic surgery. Am J Surg 2002; 183:622–629
19. Renne J, Wuthier R, House E, Cancro JC, Hoaglund FT. Fat macroglobulemia caused by fractures or total hip replacement. J Bone Joint Surg Am 1978; 60-A:613–618
20. Bone LB, Johnson KD, Weigelt J, Scheinberg R. Early versus delayed stabilisation of femoral fractures: A prospective randomized study. J Bone Joint Surg Am 1989; 71-A:336–340
21. Bone LB, McNamara K, Shine B, Border J. Mortality in multiple trauma patients with fractures. J Trauma 1994; 37:262–264
22. Goris RJ, Gimbrere JS, van Niekerk JL, Schoots FJ, Booy LH. Early osteosynthesis and prophylactic mechanical ventilation in the multitrauma patient. J Trauma 1982; 22:895–903
23. Johnson KD, Cadambi A, Seibert GB. Incidence of adult respiratory distress syndrome in patients with multiple musculoskeletal injuries: Effect of early operative stabilization of fractures. J Trauma 1985; 25:375–384
24. Riska EB, von Bonsdorff H, Hakkinen S, Jaroma H, Kiviluoto O, Paavilainen T. Primary operative fixation of long bone fractures in patients with multiple injuries. J Trauma 1977; 17:111–121
25. Ecke H, Faupel L, Quoika P. Considerations on the time of surgery of femoral fractures. Unfallchirurgie 1985; 11:89–93
26. Pape HC, Auf'm'Kolk M, Paffrath T, Regel G, Sturm J, Tscheme H. Primary intramedullary femur fixation in multiple trauma patients with associated lung contusion – a cause of posttraumatic ARDS? J Trauma 1993; 34:540–548
27. Reynolds MA, Richardson JD, Spain DA, Seligson D, Wilson MA, Miller FB. Is the timing of fracture fixation important for the patient with multiple trauma? Ann Surg 1995; 222:470–481
28. Rotondo MF, Schwab CW, McGonigal MD, Phillips GR, Fruchterman TM, Kauder DR, Latenser BA, Angood PA. "Damage control": An approach for improved survival in exsanguinating penetrating abdominal injuries. J Trauma 1993; 35:375–382
29. Nowotarski PJ, Turen CH, Brumback RJ, Scarboro JR.Conversion of external fixation to intramedullary nailing for fractures of the shaft of the femur in multiply injured patients. J Bone Joint Surg Am 2000; 82-A:781–788
30. Scalea TM, Boswell SA, Scott JD, Mitchell KA, Kramer ME, Pollak AN. External fixation as a bridge to intramedullary nailing for patients with multiple injuries and with femur fractures: Damage control orthopedics. J Trauma 2000; 48:613–623
31. Baker SP, O'Neill B. The injury severity scores: An update. J Trauma 1976; 16:882–885
32. Bhandari M, Zlowodzki M, Tornetta P, Schmidt A, Templeman DC. Intramedullary nailing following external fixation in femoral and tibial shaft fractures. J Orthop Trauma 2005; 19:140–144
33. Anke AG, Stanghelle JK, Finset A, Roaldsen KS, Pillgram-Larsen J, Fugl-Meyer AR. Long-term prevalence of impairments and disabilities after multiple trauma. J Trauma 1997; 42:54–61
34. Brenneman FD, Redelmeier DA, Boulanger BR, McLellan BA, Culhane JP. Long-term outcomes in blunt trauma: Who goes back to work? J Trauma 1997; 42:778–781
35. Holbrook TL, Anderson JP, Sieber WJ, Browner D, Hoyt DB. Outcome after major trauma: 12-month and 18-month follow-up results from the Trauma Recovery Project. J Trauma 1999; 46:765–771
36. Lehmann U, Gobiet W, Regel, G, al Dhaher S, Krah B, Steinbeck K, Tscherne H. Functional. Neuropsychological and social outcome of polytrauma patients with severe craniocerebral trauma. Unfallchirurg 1997; 100:552–560
37. Rhodes M, Aronson J, Moerkirk G, Petrash E. Quality of life after the trauma center. J Trauma 1988; 28:931–938
38. Seekamp A, Regel G, Tscherne H. Rehabilitation and reintegration of multiply injured patients: An outcome study with special reference to multiple lower limb fractures. Injury 1996; 27:133–138
39. Seekamp A, Regel G, Bauch S, Takace J, Tscherne H. Long-term results of therapy of polytrauma patients with special reference to serial fractures of the lower extremity. Unfallchirurg 1994;97:57–63

40. Bosse MJ, MacKenzie EJ, Kellam J, Burgess AR, Webb LX, Swiontkowski MF, Sanders RW, Jones AL, McAndrew MP, Patterson BM, McCarthy ML, Travison TG, Castillo RC. An analysis of outcomes of reconstruction or amputation of leg-threatening injuries. N Engl J Med 2002; 347:1924–1931

41. MacKenzie EJ, Bosse MJ, Castillo RC, Smith DG, Webb LX, Kellam JF, Burgess AR, Swiontkowski MF, Sanders RW, Jones AL, McAndrew MP, Patterson BM, Travison TG, McCarthy ML. Functional outcomes following lower extremity amputation for trauma. J Bone Joint Surg Am 2004; 86-A:1636–1645

42. MacKenzie EJ, Bosse MJ, Pollak AN, Pollak AN, Webb LX, Swiontkowski MF, Kellam JF, Smith DG, Sanders RW, Jones AL, Starr AJ, McAndrew MP, Patterson BM, Burgess AR, Castillo RC. Long-term persistance of disability following severe lower limb trauma: Results of a seven year follow-up. J Bone Joint Surg Am 2005; 87-A:1801–1809

43. MacKenzie EJ, Bosse MJ. Factors influencing outcome following limb-threatening lower limb trauma: Lessons learned from the lower extremity assessment project (LEAP). J Am Acad Orthop Surg 2006; 14(10 Suppl):S205–S210

44. McCarthy M, MacKenzie EJ, Edwin D. Psychological distress associated with severe lower limb injury. J Bone Joint Surg Am 2003; 85:1689–1697

45. Smith JJ, Agel J, Swiontkowski MF, Castillo R, MacKenzie E, Kellam JF, The LEAP Study Group. Functional outcome of bilateral limb threatening lower extremity: Injuries at two years post injury. J Orthop Trauma 2005; 19:249–253

46. Pape HC, Zelle B, Lohse R, Hildebrand F, Krettek C, Panzica M, Duhme N, Sittaro N. Evaluation and outcome of patients after polytrauma: Can patients be recruited for long-term follow-up? Injury 2006; 37:1197–1203

47. Sittaro NA, Lohse R, Panzica M, Probst C, Pape H-C, Krettek C. Hannover-polytrauma-longterm-study HPLS. Versicherungsmedizin 2007; 59:20–25

48. Zelle BA, Brown SR, Panzica M, Lohse R, Sittaro N, Krettek C, Pape H-C. The impact of injuries below the knee joint on the long-term functional outcome following polytrauma. Injury 2005; 36:169–177

49. Zelle BA, Panzica M, Vogt MT, Sittaro N, Krettek C, Pape H-C. Influence of workers' compensation eligibility upon functional recovery 10 to 28 years after polytrauma. Am J Surg 2005; 190:30–36

50. Ware JE, Kosinski M, Keller SD. A 12-item short-form-health survey: Construction of scales and preliminary tests of reliability and validity. Med Care 1996; 34:220–233

51. Alter HJ, Braun R, Zazzali JL. Health status disparities among public and private emergency department patients. Acad Emerg Med 1999; 6:736–743

52. Andresen EM, Fouts BS, Romeis JC, Brownson C. Performance of health-related quality-of-life instruments in a spinal cord injured population. Arch Phys Med Rehabil 1999; 80:877–884

53. Schandelmaier P, Krettek C, Rudolf J, Tscherne H. Outcome of tibial shaft fractures with severe soft tissue injury treated by unreamed nailing versus external fixation. J Trauma 1995; 39:707–711

54. Lysholm J, Gillquist J. Evaluation of knee ligament surgery results with special emphasis on use of a scoring scale. Am J Sports Med 1982; 10:150–154

Index